The Ethics and Regulation of Research with Human Subjects

Carl H. Coleman
Professor of Law and Director of the Health Law and Policy Program,
Seton Hall Law School

Jerry A. Menikoff
Associate Professor of Law, Ethics, and Medicine and Director
of the Institute for Bioethics, Law, and Public Policy, University
of Kansas School of Medicine, and Associate Professor of Law,
University of Kansas School of Law

Jesse A. Goldner
John D. Valentine Professor of Law, Saint Louis University School
of Law, Professor of Law in Psychiatry and Professor of Pediatrics,
Saint Louis University School of Medicine, and Professor of Health Care
Administration, Saint Louis University School of Public Health

Nancy Neveloff Dubler
Director of the Division of Bioethics, Department of Epidemiology
and Population Health, Montefiore Medical Center, and Professor
of Epidemiology and Population Health at the Albert Einstein
College of Medicine

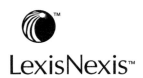

LexisNexis™

Library of Congress Cataloging-in-Publication Data

The ethics and regulation of research with human subjects / Carl H. Coleman ... [et al.].
    p. cm.
Includes index.
ISBN 1-58360-798-6 (softbound)
1. Human experimentation in medicine — Law and legislation — United States.
    2. Human experimentation in medicine — Moral and ethical aspects — United States.
    I. Coleman, Carl H..
KF3827.M38E86 2005
344.7304'196 — dc22   2005013163

This publication is designed to provide accurate and authoritative information in regard to the subject matter covered. It is sold with the understanding that the publisher is not engaged in rendering legal, accounting, or other professional services. If legal advice or other expert assistance is required, the services of a competent professional should be sought.

Editorial Offices
744 Broad Street, Newark, NJ 07102 (973) 820-2000
201 Mission St., San Francisco, CA 94105-1831 (415) 908-3200
701 East Water Street, Charlottesville, VA 22902-7587 (804) 972-7600
www.lexis.com

(Pub.03620)

ACKNOWLEDGMENTS

Numerous individuals provided help with the research, drafting, and production of this book. For valuable research assistance, we would like to thank Leslie Bailey, Victoria Brancoveanu, Moira Brennan, Anne Cooper, Margot Eves, August Heckman, Michael Long, Graham Pechenik, Anna Pomakala, Michael Welch, and Lauren Zell. For comments on draft chapters and other advice, we thank Gaia Bernstein, Maria Frankowska, Dan Hulsebosch, Sandra Johnson, Mary Faith Marshall, and Harry Ostrer, as well as participants in a faculty workshop at Saint Louis University School of Law. Finally, we wish to thank our deans and department chairs for the support they provided us: Barbara Atkinson, Christopher Crenner, Patrick Hobbs, Jeffrey E. Lewis, and Steven R. Smith.

The New York Community Trust and the United Hospital Fund provided partial support for Nancy Dubler's work on this book, as part of a grant to develop an independent certificate program for non-affiliated "community" members of institutional review boards.

PREFACE

In the last decade, the ethics and regulation of biomedical research has moved from a sleepy backwater to center stage. As concerns mount about the inability of existing regulatory structures to protect the rights and welfare of human subjects, those involved in designing, conducting, and overseeing research have come under increasing scrutiny. In this environment, lawyers, administrators, and other professionals who may never have thought much about research are finding it necessary to become conversant with the relevant ethical and regulatory issues.

The genesis of this book was our desire to develop a set of teaching materials that could be used in an academic course on human subject research in a broad range of professional school settings. In developing these materials, we were mindful that our readers would include tomorrow's advisers, managers, and regulators of researchers and research institutions. If students are to be effective in these roles, they must not only understand the history of human subject protection and the relevant ethical and regulatory issues; they must begin to think critically about the existing regulatory system and to consider the desirability of policy reform.

We have, therefore, adopted as a model for this book a variation of the traditional law school "casebook," which has been used successfully by generations of law students. These books are designed to foster critical thinking about the subject matter involved at least as much as to familiarize students with a given body of law and regulations. That does not mean that we have designed this book primarily with law students in mind; on the contrary, we have gone to great lengths to make the material accessible to non-law students, including those at schools of medicine, nursing, public health, and health administration. All of us have taught in one or more of those settings, and we have found that the law school casebook format works remarkably well there. Nonetheless, recognizing that the book will be used by students in a variety of disciplines, we have modified the traditional casebook approach to make it equally accessible to those who have had no legal training whatsoever. As a result, some basic legal concepts that may seem obvious to law students or lawyers are accompanied by brief explanations. In like fashion, understanding that some readers will have little or no clinical background, we have provided similar basic explanations, where appropriate, of clinical concepts. Outside of degree-granting programs, we envision that the book will be useful in training programs for professionals whose work requires an appreciation of the ethical and regulatory issues surrounding human subject research, such as members and professional staff of institutional review boards.

The book is largely comprised of primary source documents, including governmental regulations, guidance statements, and court decisions, and excerpts from the voluminous commentary produced by scholars, advisory commissions, and others. These materials are accompanied by extensive notes and questions, which expand on some of the issues raised in the primary readings and ask the reader to think about the gaps, ambiguities, and conflicts those readings raise. In true law school style, many of the questions have no indisputably correct answer. Instead, they are offered to stimulate discussion, provoke independent thinking, or simply lead to quiet moments of thoughtful puzzlement by students as they review the readings outside of class.

We wanted to keep the book to a manageable size. As a consequence, we made a number of not-painless decisions in terms of coverage. One of those relates to research conducted outside the United States, which has rapidly been growing in importance. We resisted the temptation to explore international research in any significant way, although we occasionally raise international comparisons when doing so seemed highly relevant to a discussion of a domestic issue. Similarly, we decided to focus solely on biomedical research, as opposed to research in the social sciences. Although most of this book's content should be equally applicable to both types of research, to the extent that there are special issues that arise in social science research, those issues are not discussed at any significant length here. Finally, because this is a book about the use of human subjects in research, it provides little coverage of research integrity issues that are not unique to research involving human subjects, such as falsification of data or authorship practices.

Organization of the Book

This book is divided into three parts. Part I provides a general overview of the history of research with human subjects, the existing regulatory framework, and the major entities involved in overseeing research. Part II examines the key ethical and regulatory issues that arise in every research protocol. Part III looks at special situations that raise issues beyond the general considerations addressed in Part II. Finally, the Appendices contain a variety of primary source materials discussed throughout the book, including portions of the federal regulations known as the Common Rule.

Stylistic Conventions

Most of the excerpts that appear in this book have been edited. Citations or footnotes appearing in the original text have in most cases been deleted without any notation. (Excerpted pieces commonly omit text that appeared in the original before or after the excerpted portion, and no notations have been used to indicate such deletions.) Where text has been deleted within the excerpted piece, however, ellipses have been inserted. Recognizing that students will sometimes wish to read the unedited original source, we have tried to provide web citations for many of the excerpts. All URLs provided in this book were functional as of the close of 2004. Even if you encounter a URL that is no longer functional, you can often still find the original web page by going to the Internet Archive at http://www.archive.org. Although we have not provided web citations for statutes or judicial opinions, the full text of those sources often can be found at FindLaw (http://www.findlaw.com/casecode) or at Cornell University Law School's Legal Information Institute (http://www.law.cornell.edu).

The journal whose full name is *IRB: Ethics & Human Research* (previously known as *IRB: A Review of Human Subjects Research*) is cited throughout this book, for simplicity purposes, with the shortened name *IRB*.

For Readers Without a Legal Background: A Brief Description of the U.S. Legal System

The basic structure of the American legal system is established by the United States Constitution. It creates a *federal* system, a term that refers to a system of government in which a group of smaller political units join together and agree to give up some of their power to a centralized government. In the case of the United States, the smaller units are each of the separate states, and the centralized government is the national (sometimes called federal) government. On the one hand, the Constitution spells out the details of how power is shared between the national government and the states. Under the Constitution's "supremacy clause," federal laws will generally override any conflicting laws enacted by the states. On the other hand, the Constitution does not say much about how each of the state's own internal governments will operate: for that very reason, each state has its own constitution.

In most instances, law is created from one of three sources: legislatures, administrative agencies, and courts. (Contracts — legally binding agreements created by private parties — represent an additional source of law, although one that is binding only on parties who voluntarily agree to accept a contract's terms.) The legislature for the national government is, of course, the United States Congress, which is comprised of the Senate and the House of Representatives. It has the authority to enact statutes, which in most cases need to be signed by the President before they become effective. Each state's constitution determines the structure of that state's legislature, which has the power to enact state statutes.

Statutes, whether on the federal or state level, often will only provide a broad outline of what the law is supposed to be. The fleshing out of the details of the law, together with performing the day-to-day implementation of what a particular statute requires, is often left to administrative agencies. One of the most important functions of administrative agencies is to issue regulations and to interpret those regulations. As will be explained in this book, a great deal of the law relating to protecting research subjects is found in regulations issued and interpreted by two federal administrative agencies, the Office for Human Research Protections (OHRP) and the Food and Drug Administration (FDA), both of which are part of the Department of Health and Human Services (DHHS).

Controversies often arise over the interpretation of state or federal laws, and in those instances the courts often are asked to resolve the dispute. There are separate court systems at the federal and state levels. In the federal court system, the initial trial of a case usually takes place in what are called "district courts." Any party who is not satisfied with the decision of a federal district court can appeal the decision to one of the circuit courts of appeals. Decisions of the court of appeals can be reviewed by the United States Supreme Court, but in contrast to the court of appeals, which is usually required to take appeals from the federal district courts, the U.S. Supreme Court has a great deal of discretion in deciding which cases it wishes to review. The U.S. Supreme Court has the final word in interpreting federal law, and in resolving conflicts between federal laws and state laws. Each state has its own system of trial and appellate courts, including one highest court similar to the U.S. Supreme Court, which has the authority to make a final determination of how that state's laws should be interpreted.

Courts also establish and enforce legal principles that do not derive from statutes or regulations. These principles, known as the "common law," can be traced back to old English judicial decisions, although they have been revised substantially over the centuries. Common-law principles are particularly important in resolving disputes over personal injuries (a body of law known as "torts") and contracts. Each state develops its own body of common-law principles. While there is a great deal of similarity in the common law of the various states, some important state-by-state variations exist.

ABOUT THE AUTHORS

Carl H. Coleman is Professor of Law and Director of the Health Law and Policy Program at Seton Hall Law School. Before joining the Seton Hall faculty, he served as Executive Director of the New York State Task Force on Life and the Law, a nationally recognized interdisciplinary commission with a mandate to develop policy recommendations on issues raised by medical advances. He received a J.D., magna cum laude, from Harvard University, where he also received an A.M. in East Asian Studies. He holds a B.S.F.S., cum laude, from Georgetown University's School of Foreign Service. He has written and lectured extensively on legal and regulatory issues related to human subject research, assisted reproductive technologies, genetic testing and screening, and medical decision making at the end of life. He has served on the Institutional Review Boards at Seton Hall University and the University of Medicine and Dentistry of New Jersey, and has also served as co-chair of the Committee on Ethical Issues in the Provision of Health Care of the New York State Bar Association.

Jerry A. Menikoff is Associate Professor of Law, Ethics, and Medicine and Director of the Institute for Bioethics, Law, and Public Policy, University of Kansas School of Medicine, where he serves as chairperson of the Human Subjects Committee, and Associate Professor of Law, University of Kansas School of Law. He received A.B., J.D. (both magna cum laude) and M.P.P. degrees from Harvard University, and an M.D. from Washington University. He has been a fellow at the University of Chicago's McLean Center for Clinical Medical Ethics, and at Harvard's Center for Ethics and the Professions. He is the author of *Law and Bioethics: An Introduction* (Georgetown University Press), now in its second printing, which was chosen in 2002 by the Association of American University Presses as one of "The Best of the Best from the University Presses: Books You Should Know About." He is also the author of a book about human subject research forthcoming from Oxford University Press, is a member of the Advisory Board for the *Medical Research Law & Policy Report* (BNA), and has served as a special expert for the Office for Human Research Protections.

Jesse A. Goldner is the John D. Valentine Professor of Law at Saint Louis University, where he also holds joint appointments as Professor of Law in Psychiatry and Professor of Pediatrics at the University's School of Medicine, and Professor of Health Care Administration in the University's School of Public Health. He has taught at Saint Louis University since 1973. He was a founder of and served for many years as

Director of the School of Law's Center for Health Law Studies. In addition, for 17 years he was a member of the University's Institutional Review Board, including six years as its chair. Since 2002, he has been a member and is now chair of the Council on Accreditation of the Association for the Accreditation of Human Research Protection Programs and has chaired site visits for the organization. Since 1976, he has served on the Ethics Committee of Cardinal Glennon Children's Hospital in St. Louis. Professor Goldner serves as co-editor-in-chief of the *Journal of Health Law*, published by the American Health Lawyers Association. In 2004, he received the Jay Healy Distinguished Health Law Teacher of the Year award from the American Society of Law, Medicine & Ethics. He received his A.B. (in political science) and M.A. (in psychology) from Columbia University and his J.D. from Harvard Law School.

Nancy Neveloff Dubler is the Director of the Division of Bioethics, Department of Epidemiology and Population Health, Montefiore Medical Center, and Professor of Epidemiology and Population Health at the Albert Einstein College of Medicine. She received her B.A. from Barnard College and her LL.B. from Harvard Law School. She directs the Bioethics Consultation Service at Montefiore Medical Center (founded in 1978), which provides analysis of difficult clinical cases presenting ethical issues in the health care setting. She lectures extensively and is the author of numerous articles and books on termination of care, home care and long-term care, geriatrics, prison and jail health care, and AIDS. She is Co-Director of the Certificate Program in Bioethics and the Medical Humanities, conducted jointly by Montefiore Medical Center/Albert Einstein College of Medicine and Cardozo Law School of Yeshiva University. She was a liaison from the Health Sciences Policy Board of the Institute of Medicine (IOM) to the IOM panel *Responsible Research: A Systems Approach to Protecting Research Participants*. She was the co-chair, with Mark Barnes, of the subcommittee on prison research of the Secretary's Advisory Committee on Human Research Protections (an advisory committee to the federal Office for Human Research Protections), and is an expert advisor to a new IOM committee on prison research. She was also Principal Investigator on a grant funded by the United Hospital Fund of New York City and the New York Community Trust to create a certificate program for non-affiliated and independent members of institutional review boards. She has been a member of the Montefiore Medical Center Institutional Review Board since 1976 and a vice-president of that Board since 1999. Her most recent books are: *Bioethics Mediation: A Guide to Shaping Shared Solutions* (with Carol

Liebman) (2004); *Ethics for Health Care Organizations: Theory, Case Studies, and Tools* (with Jeffrey Blustein and Linda Farber Post) (2002); and *Ethics On Call: Taking Charge of Life-and Death Choices in Today's Health Care System* (with David Nimmons) (1993). She consults often with federal agencies, national working groups, and bioethics centers.

COPYRIGHT ACKNOWLEDGMENTS

Excerpted material appearing in this book is reprinted by
permission, as listed below.

TABLE OF CONTENTS

Acknowledgements iii

Preface v

About the Authors xi

Copyright Acknowledgements xv

PART I:
BACKGROUND AND REGULATORY CONTEXT

Chapter 1 HISTORICAL ANTECEDENTS   3
§ 1.01 Early Examples of Human Experimentation   4
  [A] Ancient Activity   4
  [B] Approaches through the Mid-Twentieth Century   6
    [1] European Medical Education and Practice   6
    [2] Statistics and Research   7
    [3] The Revolution in American Medical Education   8
    [4] Early Experiments on Venereal Disease   9
    [5] Rabies and Yellow Fever   12
§ 1.02 American Judicial Reaction to Experimentation   14
§ 1.03 Nazi Germany and the Nuremberg Code   16
  [A] Introduction   16
  [B] The Indictment   17
  [C] Opening Argument   19
  [D] The Trial   22
    [1] Testimonial Evidence (Excerpts)   22
    [2] Documentary Evidence (Excerpts)   24
  [E] Defendants' Final Statements   25
  [F] Excerpts from the Judgment of the Tribunal, including
      the Nuremberg Code   26
§ 1.04 Medical Research in the United States from 1900 to
       the Early 1970s   31
  [A] Pre- and Post- World War I Research Activities   31
  [B] Funding of U.S. Research through World War II   32
  [C] The Developing Public Role In Research   34
  [D] The Need to Conduct Appropriate Research:
      Thalidomide and DES   35
  [E] The Beecher Article (1966)   37
  [F] Jewish Chronic Disease Hospital (1963) and
      Willowbrook (1956-1971)   39
  [G] Tuskegee (1932-1972)   41
  [H] Radiation Experiments (1944-1974)   44

[I] Behavioral and Social Science Research:
The Milgram Experiments 48

**Chapter 2 THE CHANGING FACE OF RESEARCH:
NEW REGULATIONS, NEW PLAYERS,
NEW PLACES, NEW AGENDAS** 51
§ 2.01 Governmental Oversight of Research 51
[A] Federal Oversight: 1960s to 1990s 51
[B] New Directions in Federal Regulation: 1996-2003 57
§ 2.02 Biomedical Advances, New Funding, New Places,
New Players 61
[A] Research Successes of the 1980s and 1990s 61
[B] How Much Do We Spend on Research? 63
[C] The Changing Role of Academic Health Centers
in Research 65
[1] Bayh-Dole 67
[2] Current Clinical Research Funding Streams 69
[D] Federal Sources of Research Funding 73
[1] National Institutes of Health 73
[2] Other DHHS Departments 74
[3] Other Federal Agencies 75
[E] Private Industry Funding of Research 76
[1] Pharmaceutical Companies 76
[2] Biotech Companies 76
§ 2.03 The Movement of Research from Academic Health
Centers To Private Physicians' Offices and the Rise
of Contract Research Organizations 77
§ 2.04 Developing New Research Agendas 86
[A] Setting NIH Priorities 87
[B] The Role of Advocacy 95
[1] Legislative Advocacy 96
[2] Advocacy Regarding the Manner in Which Research
Is Conducted 100

**Chapter 3 THE FEDERAL AND STATE
REGULATORY STRUCTURE** 105
§ 3.01 Overview of the Legal Structure 105
§ 3.02 Department of Health and Human
Service Regulations 106
[A] The Common Rule 106
[1] Scope of Coverage 107
[2] Definition of Research 107

[a] What Is a Research Protocol?   108
[b] Research versus Clinical Innovation   109
[c] Research versus Quality Improvement   115
[d] Research versus Public Health Initiatives   119
[3] Definition of Human Subject   121
[4] Exempt Studies   123
[B] Additional DHHS Regulations Governing
Vulnerable Populations   125
[C] The DHHS Office for Human Research Protections   136
§ 3.03 Food and Drug Administration Regulations   142
[A] Human Subject Protections   143
[B] The Drug Approval Process   144
[C] The Device Approval Process   157
[D] FDA Office for Good Clinical Practice   160
§ 3.04 Research Not Covered by Federal Regulations   161
§ 3.05 State Laws   163

Chapter 4 INSTITUTIONAL REVIEW BOARDS   169
§ 4.01 Purpose and Duties   169
§ 4.02 Composition   175
§ 4.03 Process of IRB Review   179
[A] Full Review   179
[B] Expedited Review   195
§ 4.04 Proprietary and Independent IRBs   197
§ 4.05 Accreditation   202

Chapter 5 CONFLICTS OF INTEREST   207
§ 5.01 Investigator Conflicts   207
§ 5.02 Institutional Conflicts   232
§ 5.03 IRB Conflicts   237
§ 5.04 Disclosing Conflicts of Interest to Subjects   239

PART II:
REVIEWING RESEARCH PROPOSALS: GENERAL CONSIDERATIONS

Chapter 6 RISK-BENEFIT ASSESSMENT   245
§ 6.01 The Role of Risk-Benefit Assessment in
Research Oversight   245
§ 6.02 Identifying Risks   247
[A] The Concept of Risk   247
[B] Risks to Research Subjects   250
[1] Introduction: A Typology of Research Risks   250

[2] Distinguishing the Risks of Research from the
    Risks of Interventions That Would Otherwise
    Be Performed 254
[3] The Concept of Clinical Equipoise 256
[4] Clinical Equipoise and the Use of Placebo Controls .. 262
[5] Washouts and Challenge Studies 271
[C] Risks to Others 279
[D] "Minimal Risk" Research under the
    Federal Regulations 280
§ 6.03 Identifying Benefits 282
[A] Potential Benefits to Research Subjects 282
[B] The Production of Knowledge as a Benefit
    of Research 286
§ 6.04 Balancing Risks and Benefits 289
§ 6.05 Minimizing Risks 295

Chapter 7 INFORMED CONSENT 297
§ 7.01 From Consent to Medical Care to Consent
    to Research 298
[A] Informed Consent to Medical Care 298
    [1] Case Law 298
    [2] Medical Practice Guidelines 303
[B] Informed Consent to Innovative Treatment 304
[C] Informed Consent to Research 307
§ 7.02 Federal Regulations Governing Informed Consent
    to Research 312
[A] General Requirements 312
[B] Waivers and Alterations of the Usual Requirements 313
    [1] General Waivers 313
    [2] Waivers in Emergency Research 318
§ 7.03 Implementing the Federal Regulations 327
[A] The Consent Form 327
[B] Informed Consent as a Process 344
[C] An Informed Consent Script 351
§ 7.04 Deficiencies in the Informed Consent Process 355
[A] The Therapeutic Misconception 355
[B] Failure to Convey Information 363
[C] Cultural and Gender-Based Barriers to
    Informed Consent 366

Chapter 8 RECRUITING AND PAYING SUBJECTS 371
§ 8.01 Recruiting Subjects 371
   [A] Overview of the Issues 371
   [B] Agency and Institutional Guidance 378
      [1] FDA 378
      [2] OHRP 381
   [C] Institutional Policies 384
   [D] Recruiting Normal Healthy Subjects 386
   [E] Soliciting Students or Employees of Researchers 391
§ 8.02 Paying Subjects 395
   [A] Agency Guidance 395
      [1] FDA 395
      [2] OHRP 397
   [B] Determining an Appropriate Level of Payment 402
   [C] Structuring Payments 405

**Chapter 9 RESEARCH AND JUSTICE: PROMOTING
             THE INCLUSION OF WOMEN AND
             RACIAL MINORITIES** 409
§ 9.01 The Concept of Justice in Research with
      Human Subjects 409
§ 9.02 Justice and Women 415
   [A] Federal Policy Before 1993 415
   [B] Revisions in Government Policies 426
      [1] FDA 426
      [2] NIH 430
      [3] Further FDA Revisions 432
§ 9.03 Justice and Racial Minorities 433

Chapter 10 CONFIDENTIALITY 443
§ 10.01 Overview of Medical Confidentiality 443
   [A] Confidentiality as an Ethical Principle 443
   [B] Legal Sources of Medical Confidentiality 446
      [1] State Laws 446
      [2] Federal Law 447
§ 10.02 Confidentiality Issues in Research 448
   [A] Maintaining the Confidentiality of Research Data 448
      [1] General Issues 448
      [2] Certificates of Confidentiality 452
   [B] Overseeing the Use and Disclosure of
      Medical Records 456
      [1] Human Subject Protection Regulations 456
      [2] HIPAA Regulations 459

Chapter 11 MONITORING OF ONGOING RESEARCH ... 465

§ 11.01 Continuing Review 465

§ 11.02 Adverse Event Reporting 470

§ 11.03 Data and Safety Monitoring Boards 475

Chapter 12 COMPENSATION FOR
RESEARCH INJURIES 487

§ 12.01 Ethical Considerations 487

§ 12.02 The Regulatory Framework 495

§ 12.03 Tort Liability 495

[A] The Emerging Role of Tort Litigation in Human
Subject Research 496

[B] Defining Researchers' Duties to Subjects 502

[C] Additional Issues in Informed Consent Cases 510

§ 12.04 No-Fault Compensation 519

[A] Voluntary No-Fault Compensation Schemes 520

[B] Proposals for Comprehensive No-Fault
Compensation Systems 522

PART III:
REVIEWING RESEARCH PROPOSALS: SPECIAL SITUATIONS

Chapter 13 CHILDREN 527

§ 13.01 Research with Children: Past and Present 527

§ 13.02 The Regulatory Framework 533

[A] Decision-Making Authority of Parents
and Children 533

[1] Parental Authority: Permission and Refusal 533

[2] Soliciting a Minor's Assent 538

[3] Allocating Decision-Making Authority in Research
with Adolescents 541

[B] Categories of Permissible Risk 544

[1] General Principles 544

[2] Applying the Standards: The Fenfluramine Studies ... 551

[C] DHHS Review of Research Not
Otherwise Approvable 554

[1] Cystic Fibrosis in Neonates 555

[2] Smallpox Vaccination in Young Children 562

§ 13.03 Pediatric Research in the Courts:
The *Kennedy Krieger* Case 567

Chapter 14 ADULTS WHO LACK DECISION-MAKING CAPACITY 585

§ 14.01 The Appropriateness of Conducting Research with Adults Who Lack Decision-Making Capacity 586

§ 14.02 Determining Whether Subjects Lack Decision-Making Capacity 591

[A] Defining Decision-Making Capacity 591

[B] Assessing Decision-Making Capacity 598

§ 14.03 Informed Consent 601

[A] Surrogate Decision Making 601

[B] Research Living Wills 609

[C] Subject Assent and Refusal 612

§ 14.04 Limitations on Permissible Risks 613

§ 14.05 Constitutional Considerations 621

Chapter 15 PRISONERS 629

§ 15.01 General Considerations 629

[A] The U.S. Prison Population 629

[B] History of Medical Research in Prisons 635

§ 15.02 Federal Regulation of Prison Research 642

[A] Overview of Subpart C 642

[B] OHRP Questions to NHRPAC on the Interpretation of Subpart C 645

§ 15.03 The Shift From Protection to Access 647

§ 15.04 Research with Incarcerated Children 650

Chapter 16 FETUSES AND EMBRYOS 655

§ 16.01 Fetal Research 655

[A] Research on Fetuses in Utero 655

[B] Research on Tissue from Aborted Fetuses 657

[1] Federal Law 657

[2] State Law 658

§ 16.02 Embryo and Embryonic Stem Cell Research 661

[A] Perspectives on Embryo and Embryonic Stem Cell Research 662

[B] Federal Law and Policy 672

[1] General Federal Policy on Embryo Research 672

[2] Application of Federal Embryo Research Policies to Research on Embryonic Stem Cells 676

[C] State Law and Policy 681

[D] Consent to Embryo and Embryonic Stem Cell Research 683

§ 16.03 Cloning 686

[A] What Is Cloning? 686
[B] Perspectives on Cloning 688
[C] Federal Law 693
[D] State Law 695

Chapter 17 GENETICS RESEARCH 697
§ 17.01 Research Designed to Learn About the Genome 697
    [A] What the Genome Can Tell Us: The Power and
        Perils of Genetic Information 698
    [B] Sources of Biological Materials for Genetics Research ... 701
    [C] Necessity of IRB Review of Genetic Testing Research ... 703
        [1] Definition of "Human Subject" 703
        [2] Exempt Research 706
    [D] Risk Assessment 707
        [1] Risks to Subjects 707
        [2] Risks to Others 709
        [3] Risk Assessment and Eligibility for
            Expedited Review 714
    [E] Informed Consent 715
        [1] Research Involving the Collection of New Tissue
            Samples ("Prospective Studies") 715
        [2] Research Using Existing Tissue Samples
            ("Retrospective Studies") 717
    [F] Confidentiality Issues 720
    [G] Informing Subjects of Study Results 723
    [H] Sharing the Profits from Research 729
§ 17.02 Gene Transfer Research 741

Appendix A: 45 C.F.R Part 46 .... A-1
Appendix B: Expedited Review Criteria B-1
Appendix C: Comparison of FDA and DHHS Regulations C-1
Appendix D: The Nuremberg Code D-1
Appendix E: The Declaration of Helsinki E-1
Appendix F: The Belmont Report F-1
Author Index AI-1
Index I-1
Table of Cases TC-1

PART I
BACKGROUND AND REGULATORY CONTEXT

Chapter 1

HISTORICAL ANTECEDENTS

The history of biomedical research must be examined through the lens of the history of medicine itself. When physicians had little more than intuition and anecdotal experience on which to rely, they were, quite understandably, perceived as being not very different from sorcerers. With the advent of the scientific method and the use of sophisticated clinical trial methodologies, that image has been transformed. To understand this history, the compound question that must be asked is, "How have physicians viewed themselves, and what have been the implications of such a self-image for patients and research subjects?"

For many generations, the principal ethic of medicine focused on the Hippocratic Oath, which sets forth an array of ethical norms and functions as the pledge of the medical profession to uphold ethical standards of care. Many medial school students still take some form of the Oath at graduation ceremonies. The Hippocratics, an organized group of third- and fourth-century B.C. physicians and followers of the philosopher Hippocrates, probably are best known for formulating that Oath. Many wrongly believe that the famous dictum, "First, do no harm" appears in the Oath. Actually, it is thought to have been derived from another of Hippocrates' writings, *Epidemics, Bk. 1, Sect. XI*. There are many versions of the Oath; one, for example, contains the following language:

> I will use my power to help the sick to the best of my ability and judgment; I will abstain from harming or wrongdoing any man by it. I will not give a fatal draught [drugs] to anyone if I am asked, nor will I suggest any such thing.

Oath of Hippocrates, in HIPPOCRATIC WRITINGS (translated by J. Chadwick and W.N. Mann, 1950), available at http://www.med.umich.edu/irbmed/ethics/Hippocratic/Hippocratic.html.

Yet the Nazi doctors viewed themselves quite differently: as tools of the state. And, while it might be comfortable to think that it was only they and a few other rare, twisted minds that engaged in unethical activities, Henry Beecher's article, discussed below at page 37, demonstrates that such has not been the case at all. As a physician, Beecher might well have paraphrased the philosopher-cartoon character Pogo, "I have met the enemy and it is us." The natural drives to explore new knowledge and to achieve fame, at practically any cost, may, on occasion, simply be part of the human condition. Moreover, the "at any cost" feature of this phenomenon has often had a disparate impact on particular socioeconomic classes, genders, and races.

In addition to exploring these issues, this chapter highlights the role of law and public policy in the oversight of research with human subjects. Consider, for example, the extent to which judicial decisions, such as the Nuremberg Code, have played a role in shaping current attitudes. That certainly continues today. While congressional inquiries and legislation also have played a role, it is policies and practices engendered by federal administrative agencies or presidential commissions, part of or appointed by the executive branch of government, that have had the greatest influence.

§ 1.01 EARLY EXAMPLES OF HUMAN EXPERIMENTATION

[A] Ancient Activity

The Hippocratics contributed much more than the Oath to Western medicine. Theorizing that illness had natural, not supernatural, causes, they were the first to view "humors," or liquids, as the key agents of health and disease. They reached this conclusion from regular observations of sick patients — fevers produced sweats, liver disease yielded jaundice, respiratory illness could result in phlegm, and the quality and color of urine and feces were all indicative of illness or wellness. These humors were seen as part of the healing process and thus were promoted. The physician's role was that of observer and advisor. The Hippocratics' theory that successful diagnosis and treatment depended on observation and understanding of the individual patient remains a guiding principle of medicine today.

The Hippocratics performed little human experimentation as we currently understand it. However, as William Bynum notes, the word "experimental" comes from the same Latin root as "experience," and these physicians very much valued experience:

> Any encounter between a doctor and a patient can be *experiential* and thus experimental, if only in a passive sense. The Hippocratics, who were interested in the rhythms and natural histories of disease, and in carefully observing sick people, were increasing their own experience. Further, any therapeutic innovation, even if the doctor believed it to be in the patient's best interest, was an experiment.

William Bynum, *Reflections on the History of Human Experimentation, in* THE USE OF HUMAN BEINGS IN RESEARCH 32 (Stuart F. Spicker et al. eds., 1988). Bynum proceeds to explain that the Hippocratics occasionally treated those who could not pay, but they drew a distinction between their obligations to paying and charity patients. "[T]heir motives were *philanthropia* (love of man) and *philotechnia* (love of the art [of healing]). The latter also embraced the desire to extend knowledge and easily encompassed experimentation with new procedures and drugs." Thus, he concludes, early on, the socially and economically disadvantaged were subjects of human experimentation. In Greek times,

Bynum relates, some physicians engaged in a limited number of human vivisectional experiments in order to better understand the "position, color, shape, size, arrangement, hardness, softness, smoothness, relation, processes and depressions" of body parts. The subjects were condemned prisoners who, through criminal conduct, had forfeited their rights. *Id.* at 32-33.

Similarly, Christianity in the Middle Ages reflected a continuing dichotomy between medicine provided to the rich and poor. Moral theologians of that era devoted much effort to defining moral responsibilities, both generally and of those in certain walks of life, such as physicians and surgeons. They particularly condemned experimentation on the poor. *See* Darrel W. Amundsen, *Casuistry and Professional Obligations: The Regulation of Physicians by the Court of Conscience in the Late Middle Ages, Part I*, in Series 5, vol. 3, TRANSACTIONS AND STUDIES OF THE COLLEGE OF PHYSICIANS OF PHILADELPHIA 22, 34-35 (1981). Bynum notes that the development of hospitals during this period enabled doctors to observe far more than was previously available: "the receipt of Christian charity often carried with it reciprocal obligations; those who received it were expected to be suitably docile, cooperative and grateful, thereby demonstrating their worthiness." Bynum, *supra* at 34.

The Middle Ages also witnessed the beginning of testing of new drugs. Initially, physicians themselves were the subjects. This practice, however, carried with it a risk that the physician could harm his own body during the experiment, thereby diminishing his effectiveness as a health care provider within the community. Accordingly, physicians began to use animal models, despite their obvious limitations, before progressing on to human subjects. Thus, Bynum recounts Bernard de Gordon's suggestion of "a hierarchy of drug testing; from birds, to brute animals, to 'those in the hospital,' to the 'lesser brethren,' and then on to others 'in order, because if it [the drug] should be poisonous it would kill.' " Bynum, *supra*, at 34.

The use of the socially disadvantaged as experimental subjects continued in this period. David Rothman reports that:

> Lady Mary Wortley Montagu, wife of the British ambassador to Turkey, . . . learned about Turkish successes in inoculating patients with small amounts of the smallpox material to provide immunity. Eager to convince English physicians to adopt the procedure, she persuaded King George I to run a trial by pardoning any condemned inmate at the Newgate Prison who agreed to the inoculation. In August 1721, six volunteers were inoculated; they developed local lesions but no serious illness, and all were released.

DAVID J. ROTHMAN, STRANGERS AT THE BEDSIDE: A HISTORY OF HOW LAW AND BIOETHICS TRANSFORMED MEDICAL DECISION MAKING 21 (1991). Rothman observes that, "[a]s science went, the trial was hardly satisfactory and the ethics were no better — the choices between death or enrollment in the experiment was not a freely made one." *Id.* at 22.

The search for a cure for smallpox continued through the eighteenth century. The most famous of the smallpox experiments was conducted by Dr. Edward Jenner. In 1796, a dairymaid consulted Jenner about a case of cowpox she had received from her diseased cow. He had previously noted that farmhands who contract the pox from swine or cows appeared to be immune to the more dangerous smallpox. Jenner then performed an experiment on a boy in which he rubbed one of the pox from the dairymaid's hand into the boy's scratched skin, in essence inoculating the boy with cowpox, in order to confirm that cowpox could travel from human to human, not just cow to human. Next, Jenner "challenged the boy with smallpox material." When the boy did not show any symptoms, Jenner concluded that the boy was immune because of his prior cowpox exposure. *Id.* at 20.

NOTES AND QUESTIONS

1. The history of human subject research has been marked by a constant tension between the search for knowledge and the protection of subjects' rights and welfare. This tension stems from the underlying conflict of medical research: the fact that developing knowledge often requires exposing some people to risks for the benefit of others. As you proceed through this book, consider how our society's approach to this conflict has changed over the years. What sorts of issues seem to have been resolved and which ones remain current?

2. Immanuel Kant's "categorical imperative" states, "So act as to treat humanity, whether in thine own person or in that of any other, in every case as an end withal, never as a means only." IMMANUEL KANT, FUNDAMENTAL PRINCIPLES OF THE METAPHYSIC OF MORALS 57 (1838) (Thomas K. Abbott trans., Liberal Arts Press 1949). Did the experiments described above violate this maxim? Is it fair to say that *whenever* a person participates as a subject in research, that individual is being treated as a means to an end? In that case, must a Kantian necessarily be opposed to medical research?

3. The practice of physician self-experimentation did not end with the Middle Ages. For an interesting account of its use during more modern times, see LAWRENCE K. ALTMAN, WHO GOES FIRST? THE STORY OF SELF-EXPERIMENTATION IN MEDICINE (1998).

[B] Approaches through the Mid-Twentieth Century

[1] European Medical Education and Practice

Sociologist Paul Starr observes that Europe in the nineteenth century saw significant changes in the medical profession. Reformers of medical education and practice in France "called for an end to metaphysical abstractions and an emphasis on clinical observation." In large hospitals, physicians came to be influenced by the work of surgeons, who emphasized localized rather than systemic pathology. The period between 1800 and 1830 witnessed a departure from "vague 'systems' of classical medicine" and the development of contemporary clinical approaches. By merging clinical observation with pathological anatomy, physicians proceeded to correlate patients' signs and symptoms with the internal lesions they observed at autopsy. In 1816, the use of crude stethoscopes began and auscultation (listening to sounds in the chest, abdomen etc. to determine the condition of the heart, lungs, or other organs) allowed physicians to "penetrate behind the externally visible to 'see' into the living." As a consequence, while "doctors previously observed patients[,] now they examined them." Moreover, and most critically, Parisian physicians "began to evaluate the effectiveness of therapeutic techniques statistically."

The effects of these new approaches to studying and curing diseases were profound. As Starr comments, "The nature of the debate . . . changed. Empirical evidence rather than dogmatic assertions of personal or traditional authority became the grounds for assessing truth. The early empirical investigations showed that accepted techniques had no therapeutic value, yet there were no effective alternatives available to replace them." The emphasis on localized pathology directed attention to specific organs, and this, in turn, "aroused interest in medical instrumentation and provided foci for the development of medical specialties. . . . [One consequence was the development of] modern clinical medicine." PAUL STARR, THE SOCIAL TRANSFORMATION OF AMERICAN MEDICINE 54-55 (1982).

[2] Statistics and Research

Nathan Hershey and Robert Miller discuss the effects of the recognition of the significance of statistics in medical research:

> Statistics, the theoretical basis for most elements of research design, did not begin developing until the late eighteenth century. Pierre Simon La Place, a French mathematician, suggested the application of statistics to experimentation in 1814, proposing the use of two groups of subjects, one treated and the other serving as a control. Over fifty years earlier, the Irish philosopher George Berkeley had suggested a similar design in an effort to prove the curative powers of his favorite remedy, tarwater. A few great men of science conducted controlled studies in the eighteenth century, most notably James Lind's study of the effects of citrus fruits on scurvy in the 1750s and the English physician Edward Jenner's study of inoculation with cowpox as a preventive for smallpox in the 1790s. There may have been some other earlier controlled studies. However, controlled studies were not widely pursued until the twentieth century. One of the first uses of randomization in the assigning of subjects to the control group was in nutritionist Horace Fletcher's study of the effect of dietary factors on beriberi in 1907.

NATHAN HERSHEY & ROBERT MILLER, HUMAN EXPERIMENTATION AND THE LAW 4 (1976).

The "chi-square" test[1] was developed in 1900 by Karl Pearson, and the "student's t-test," to be used in research involving a small number of subjects, emerged in 1908. The publication in 1935 of British scientist Ronald A. Fisher's book on study design and statistical analysis proved to be a milestone, as was a series of articles on medical statistics written by Sir Austin Bradford Hill, which appeared in *The Lancet* in 1937. But the initial double-blind controlled study, under which both subjects and investigators are unaware of who is in the control group, did not take place until the 1940s. *Id.* For a history of the use of statistics to test various scientific and commercial hypotheses, see DAVID SALSBURG, THE LADY TASTING TEA: HOW STATISTICS REVOLUTIONIZED SCIENCE IN THE TWENTIETH CENTURY (2001).

[3] The Revolution in American Medical Education

These early efforts of applying statistics to science were accompanied by a far more significant revolution in medical education. This, too, ultimately had an enormous effect on research with human subjects. Starr observes, for example, that before 1869, Harvard Medical School had only a faint relationship to Harvard University. It functioned similarly to the other proprietary medical colleges of the day, which Kenneth Ludmerer, an outstanding medical historian, later describes as having focused largely on inculcating medical facts through memorization. But in 1869, Charles Eliot became president of Harvard, and within a short time the school became far more integrated with the greater university. Soon thereafter, medical education changed significantly. The academic year was extended from four months to nine. By 1893, practically all medical schools had increased the time required to obtain a degree from two to three years. Perhaps most importantly, laboratory work was added to or replaced didactic lectures on physiology, chemistry and pathological anatomy. The effect, Ludmerer notes, was an emphasis on self-education and learning-by-doing that would produce critical thinkers and problem solvers. STARR, *supra*, at 114-115; KENNETH M. LUDMERER, TIME TO HEAL: AMERICAN MEDICAL EDUCATION FROM THE TURN OF THE CENTURY TO THE ERA OF MANAGED CARE 6 (1999).

Another milestone was the opening of the medical school at Johns Hopkins University in 1893. In addition to requiring four years of training, Starr observes, Hopkins "embodied a conception of medical education as a field of graduate study, rooted in basic science and hospital medicine that was eventu-

---

[1] Chi square is a test of statistical significance that can establish the degree of confidence in accepting or rejecting a hypothesis – whether or not two different samples (e.g., of people) are different enough in some characteristic or aspect of their behavior that we can generalize from the samples that the populations from which the samples are drawn are also different in the behavior or characteristic.

ally to govern all institutions in the country. Scientific research and clinical instruction now moved to center stage." The faculty no longer was comprised of local practitioners, but rather "were accomplished men of research." Students were required to spend two years studying basic laboratory sciences and then two years on hospital wards. "A hospital was built in connection with the school, and the two were conducted as a joint enterprise. . . . Here were the glimmerings of the great university-dominated medical centers of the next century."

In addition, the two most significant figures at the school — William Welch, who earlier had been an important pathology researcher, and William Osler, an outstanding clinician — were both committed to research. The implications of all of this were important.

> The significance of Johns Hopkins Medical School lay in the new relationships it established. It joined science and research ever more firmly to clinical hospital practice. While apprentices had learned the craft of medicine in their preceptor's offices and the patient's home, now doctors in training would see medical practice almost entirely on the wards of teaching hospitals. . . . [Hopkins] sent its graduates to medical institutions all over the country and abroad, where, as professors and scientists, they took a major part in shaping the character of medical education and research in the twentieth century.

STARR, *supra*, at 115-16. In a similar vein, Ludmerer concludes that the "presence of bedside clinical investigation led to more careful study of patients, which benefited not only the immediate patient, but also other patients, should something new be discovered." LUDMERER, *supra*, at 19.

[4] Early Experiments on Venereal Disease

Not all physicians were enamored with the effects of early attempts at conducting research with human subjects, particularly when such efforts were not accompanied by the subjects' consent. In 1901, a Russian doctor, Vikenty Veressayev, wrote a book describing the daily life of a Russian physician in the late nineteenth century. In it, he devotes a chapter to "Experiments on Living Men and Women."

THE MEMOIRS OF A PHYSICIAN
VIKENTY VERESSAYEV
(translated from Russian by Simeon Linden) 332-348 (1916)

I will now occupy myself with a question to which but one answer is possible, and that a perfectly straight one. It deals with gross and entirely conscious disregard for that consideration which is due to the human being. . . . I shall restrict myself to the venereal diseases. . . . [V]enereal complaints are the exclusive lot of man, and not a single one of them can be transmitted to lower animals. Owing to this, many questions which, in other branches of medicine, find their answer in experiments on animals, can, in venerology, only be decided through human inoculation, and venerologists have not hesitated to take the plunge: crime stains every step by their science. . . .

The first to inoculate man with gonococcus was Dr. Max Bockhart. . . .

Bockhart [it was reported in 1883] inoculated a patient suffering creeping paralysis in its last stages with a pure culture of gonococcus: a few months previously the patient had lost his sense of feeling and his death was awaited very shortly.

The inoculation proved successful, but the discharge was very insignificant. To increase it, the patient was given a half litre of beer. "The success was brilliant," writes Bockhart; "the discharge became very copious. . . . Ten days after inoculation the patient died of a paralytic fit. Autopsy showed acute gonorrhoeic inflammation of the urethra and bladder with incipient kidney mortification, and a large number of abscesses in the left kidney; numerous gonococci were found in the pus taken from these abscesses." . . .

The first undoubtedly pure culture of gonococcus was obtained by Ernst Bumm [reported in 1887]. To prove that it was the specific agent, Bumm, by means of a platinum wire introduced the culture into a woman's urethra, which had been found perfectly healthy after repeated examinations. Typical urethritis developed which required six weeks for its cure. . . . Bumm inoculated his gonococcus upon another woman in the same manner, obtaining an identical result. . . . Here we must note that more than twenty years previously, Noeggerath proved how serious and painful were the effects—especially in the case of women, following so-called "innocent" gonorrhoea. . . . Bumm himself declares in the preface to his work, that "gonorrhoeic infection is one of the most important causes of painful and serious affections of the sexual organs"; which knowledge did not, however deter him from subjecting two of this patients to such a risk. . . .

[In an effort to establish that secondary syphilis was contagious, William Wallace, an Irish physician, gave a series of lectures describing experiments that] are remarkable for the classical shamelessness with which their author tells us of his criminal experiments in inoculating healthy people with syphilis. . . .

[H]e gives a detailed account of his inoculations performed upon five healthy individuals from 19 to 35 years of age. All developed characteristic syphilis. . . .

First experiment: Durst, a boy of 12, registration number 1396, suffered for a number of years from sores on the head. Otherwise quite healthy, never had rash or scrofula. As his disease required his detention in hospital for several months, and as he had not suffered from syphilis in the past, I found him to be very suitable for inoculation, which was performed on August 6th. The skin of the right thigh was incised and the pus taken from a syphilitic patient introduced into the fresh and slightly bleeding wounds. I rubbed the matter into the abrasions with a spatula, then I rubbed the scarified surface with lint soaked in the same matter, and having covered it with the same lint, applied a bandage. About the beginning of October the child developed a typical syphilitic rash. . . .

[After describing still another series of gruesome experiments conducted between 1851 and 1858 by Professor H. von Hubbenet, also designed to investigate the contagiousness of secondary syphilis, Veressayev quotes Hubbenet as noting that the publication of his observations:]

> will perhaps restrain others, even with such a skeptical nature of my own, from making further experiments, often leading to the complete wrecking of the lives of the persons subjected to them. It would add considerably to my peace of mind in respect to the victims' fate, if these experiments were to spread the conviction that the secondary stage is contagious. If they lead to the establishing of such an important truth, the sufferings of a few individuals were not too high a price to be paid by mankind for the attainment of such a truly beneficial and practical result.

NOTES AND QUESTIONS

1. Assuming that the series of studies did prove that secondary stage syphilis was contagious, did the end justify the means? What if the subjects had consented to the research? Would that solve the ethical problems?

2. Many, though by no means all, of the experiments described above were conducted on individuals who were very close to death. Does that fact alter your assessment of the ethical acceptability of the studies? *See* Lila Guterman, *Crossing the Line? Medical Research on Brain-Dead People Raises Ethical Questions,* CHRONICLE HIGHER EDUC., August 1, 2003 (discussing dilemmas involving experiments on the soon-to-be dead and the newly dead); *see also* Chapter 3, at page 122.

3. Jay Katz, a psychiatrist and psychoanalyst on the faculty of Yale Law School, has been one of the most influential modern scholars to address the issue of human subject protection. His landmark volume, EXPERIMENTATION WITH HUMAN BEINGS (1972), played a key role in awakening the American legal, academic, and bioethics communities to concerns about the way in which research had been and continued to be conducted. In a section of his book titled "The Authority of the Investigator as Guardian of Science, Subject and Society," Katz presents a series of research studies from different disciplines, including those described above by Veressayev. He concludes that "[w]henever subjects are too helpless or ignorant to resist participation, the investigator is in a position to pursue his scientific interests constrained only by his personal and professional conscience and values." JAY KATZ, EXPERIMENTATION WITH HUMAN BEINGS 281-83 (1972). If you wanted to protect those who were "too helpless or igno-

rant," how would you identify these potential subjects and what would you do to protect them?

[5] Rabies and Yellow Fever

Louis Pasteur was the French chemist credited with conceiving the "germ theory of disease" and developing the first rabies and anthrax vaccines. In speculating about how his prior animal research to find a treatment for rabies might proceed further, he wrestled with the predicament that research with human subjects poses:

> But even when I shall have multiplied examples of teerophylaxis of rabies in dogs, I think my hand will tremble when I go on to Mankind. It is here that the high and powerful initiative of the head of a State might intervene for the good of humanity. If I were King, and Emperor, or even the President of a Republic, this is how I should exercise my right of pardoning criminals condemned to death. I should invite the counsel of a condemned man, on the eve of the day fixed for his execution, to choose between certain death and an experiment which would consist in several preventative inoculations of rabic virus, in order to make the subject's constitution refractory to rabies. If he survived this experiment — and I am convinced that he would — his life would be saved and his punishment commuted to a lifelong surveillance, as a guarantee towards that society which had condemned him. All condemned men would accept these conditions, death being their only terror.

RENE VALLERY-RADOT, THE LIFE OF PASTEUR 304-05 (1923).

While European investigators conducted many of the studies that have been discussed so far, Americans were by no means immune from using human beings for research purposes. One of the most famous experiments was the yellow fever work of the American army surgeon, Walter Reed, at the beginning of the twentieth century.

STRANGERS AT THE BEDSIDE
DAVID J. ROTHMAN
25-27 (1991)

Reed's goal was to identify the source of transmission of yellow fever, which was taking a terrible toll among North and South Americans. When he began his experiments, mosquitoes had been identified as crucial to the transmission, but their precise role was still unclear. . . . In time-honored tradition, members of the research team first subjected themselves to the mosquito bites; but it soon became apparent that larger numbers of volunteers were needed, and the team adopted a pull-them-off-the-road approach. No sooner was the decision made to use volunteers than a soldier happened by. "You still fooling with mosquitoes?" he asked one the doctors. "Yes," the doctor replied. "Will you take a bite?" "Sure, I ain't scared of 'em," responded the man. And with this feeble effort to inform a subject about the nature of the experiment, "the first indubitable case of yellow fever . . . to be produced experimentally" occurred. . . .

After two of the team's members died of yellow fever from purposeful bites, the rest, who had not yet contracted the disease, including Reed himself, decided "not to tempt fate by trying any more [infections] upon ourselves. . . . We felt we had been called upon to accomplish such work as did not justify our taking risks which then seemed really unnecessary." Instead, Reed asked American servicemen to volunteer, which some did. He also recruited Spanish workers, drawing up a contract with them: "The undersigned understands perfectly well that in the case of the development of yellow fever in him, that he endangers his life to a certain extent but it being entirely impossible for him to avoid the infection during his stay on this island he prefers to take the chance of contracting it intentionally in the belief that he will receive . . . the greatest care and most skillful medical service." Volunteers received $100 in gold, and those who actually contracted yellow fever received a bonus of an additional $100, which, in the event of their death, went to their heirs.

Reed's contract was traditional in its effort to justify the research by citing benefits for the subjects — better to be sick under Reed's care than left to one's own devices. But the contract was also innovative, in that intimacy gave way to a formal arrangement that provided an enticement to undertake a hazardous assignment, and the explanation in subtle ways distorted the risks and benefits of the experiment. Yellow fever endangered life only "to a certain extent"; the likelihood that the disease might prove fatal was unmentioned. So, too, the probability of contracting yellow fever outside the experiment was presented as an absolute certainty, an exaggeration to promote subject recruitment.

NOTES AND QUESTIONS

1. What do you make of Pasteur's suggestion of using criminals condemned to death as subjects in high-risk studies? As discussed in Chapter 15, federal regulations now place significant limits on research with prisoners.

2. What types of limits, if any, should society place on the conduct of research such as that conducted by Reed? What is your reaction to Reed's "informed consent" document? How might the document have been improved? Would improving the document have made the research ethically acceptable?

§ 1.02 AMERICAN JUDICIAL REACTION TO EXPERIMENTATION

An Overview of Legal Controls on Human Experimentation and the Regulatory Implications of Taking Professor Katz Seriously
Jesse A. Goldner
38 SAINT LOUIS U. L.J. 63, 71-72 (1993)

The earliest American court cases discussing experimentation did not deal with research in the way we have come to think about it today, namely as a systematic investigation designed to develop or contribute to generalizable knowledge. For the most part, these cases arose before the days of sophisticated research protocols. Rather, experimentation, or innovative treatment, was then seen by the courts merely as deviations from accepted or standard medical practice during the course of therapeutic interventions, and courts long struggled with the issue of what constraints should be placed on such new therapies.

Prior to the Second World War, very few reported appellate opinions in malpractice cases dealt with such experimentation. The almost uniform attitude of those decisions was that such deviations were presumed to be reckless or careless. At best, there would be absolute liability for the consequences of experimentation, and, at worst, it would be viewed as prima facie improper.

In an 1871 case, *Carpenter v. Blake*, a patient sued a physician to recover damages for malpractice in the setting and treatment of a dislocated limb. The argument was made that a surgeon had the right to exercise his own judgment regarding treatment methods, because methods adopted by other physicians might not necessarily apply in each case. Despite the claim that if such action was "not allowed . . . all progress in the practice of surgery . . . must cease," the court concluded that such a "danger is more apparent than real" and that "some standard . . . must be adopted; otherwise . . . the reckless experimentalist would take the place of the educated, experienced practitioner." The court proceeded to state that:

> [w]hen the case is one as to which a system of treatment has been followed for a long time, there should be no departure from it, unless the surgeon who does it is prepared to take the risk of establishing, by his success, the propriety and safety of his experiment.

The rule protects the community against reckless experiments, while it admits the adoption of new remedies and modes of treatment only when their benefits have been demonstrated, or when, from the necessity of the case, the surgeon or physician must be left to the exercise of his own skill and experience. . . .

A 1935 Michigan appellate opinion in *Fortner v. Koch* reviewed a malpractice award in a case in which syphilis was misdiagnosed as bone cancer because the physician failed to perform a standard Wassermann test. In the course of reversing the judgment on other grounds, the court stated, "we recognize the fact that, if the general practice of medicine and surgery is to progress, there must be a certain amount of experimentation carried on." In so noting, this may have been the first case to suggest that experiments could be seen in a positive light and possibly as legitimate. Nonetheless, the court proceeded to note that "such experiments . . . must not vary too radically from the accepted method of procedure." Interestingly enough, in addition to raising the issue of variance from accepted methods of procedure, the court in *Fortner* also stated that "any such experiments must be done with the knowledge and consent of the patient or those responsible for him."

In practically all of these innovative therapy cases the courts seemed to understand that the physician was seeking to alleviate the suffering of his patient; but, nonetheless, the physician was held to a standard whereby he would be strictly liable for any deviation from standard or accepted practice, even if done for the purpose of developing improved therapy for the patient. If a new therapy failed, the courts were likely to rule that the therapy did, in fact, represent an extreme departure such that even if the patient had knowledge of the experimental nature of the procedure, he was not capable of authorizing it. The line of cases then did not rule out the possibility that some experimentation was necessary in order to develop innovative therapies, but in order for these therapies to be acceptable, they had to be introduced when standard therapies were deficient, and then, in an incremental and not a drastic manner.

NOTES AND QUESTIONS

1. How would you characterize the American judicial approach toward medical experimentation on humans between 1871 and 1935? Why do you think courts approached the concept of human experimentation as a combination of medical malpractice and strict liability (i.e., liability regardless of fault)? Might the courts have been better off viewing these cases simply as a form of the intentional tort of battery, which applies when an individual intentionally engages in harmful or offensive conduct with another person?

2. During this period, how could a physician or surgeon legally treat a patient with innovative or experimental therapies? Did the approach described above adequately protect patients from the dangers of experimentation? What specific limitations on new medical techniques did the courts establish to ensure that patients, even those with knowledge of an experimental procedure, were protected from unlawful practices? Did the courts place the physicians in a "Catch-22" situation, under which they could not "experiment" in uncharted areas lest

there be a poor outcome, but poor outcomes were likely to result without such experimentation?

3. Under current law, "innovative treatment" is no longer held to a standard of strict liability. Rather, with the development of the doctrine of informed consent, liability for experimentation depends on the patient's knowledge of the risks, benefits, and alternatives, as well as the reasonableness of the procedure, given the circumstances involved. The reasonableness of the procedure, in turn, depends on the patient's prognosis, the likelihood of success with the experimental procedure, and the probability and severity of the risks involved. Juries and judges are required to assess those risks and benefits against the traditional standard of care used in malpractice cases. If the physician can prove that it was reasonable to deviate from accepted practice, there is no malpractice, even if there are bad outcomes. *See* Goldner, *supra*, at 87-88.

§ 1.03 NAZI GERMANY AND THE NUREMBERG CODE

[A] Introduction

At the conclusion of World War II, a variety of plans were developed for bringing war criminals to justice. Ultimately, the U.S. War Department proposed treating the Nazi regime as a criminal conspiracy directed to committing war crimes involving a variety of atrocities and a war of aggression. A series of criminal statutes relating to wars of aggression and crimes against humanity was drafted to punish acts that Justice Robert Jackson, the chief prosecutor, described as having been "regarded as criminal since the time of Cain and [that had been] so written in every civilized code." REPORT OF ROBERT H. JACKSON TO THE PRESIDENT, June 7, 1945, available at http://www.ibiblio.org/pha/war.term/trib_07.html. Ultimately, more than one hundred defendants were tried before a variety of courts between 1945 and 1949 in the city of Nuremberg.

On December 9, 1946, an American military tribunal opened criminal proceedings against 23 leading German physicians and administrators for their willing participation in war crimes and crimes against humanity.

According to the charges, German physicians conducted pseudoscientific medical experiments on thousands of concentration camp prisoners without their consent. Most of these victims, who were Jews, Poles, Russians, and Roma (Gypsies) died or were permanently disabled as a result of the "experiments." As with criminal cases that would be brought in the United States, prosecutors initiated charges by bringing an indictment. Subsequently, the case proceeded in the manner of a typical common law criminal trial, with opening statements, testimony through live witnesses subject to direct and cross-examination, documentary evidence, and closing statements and briefs. After almost 140 days of proceedings, including the testimony of 85 witnesses and the submission of almost 1,500 documents, the American judges pronounced their verdict on August 20, 1947. Sixteen of the doctors were found guilty. Seven were sentenced to death. They were executed on June 2, 1948. A portion of the Nuremberg Military Tribunal's decision in this series of cases has come to be known as the Nuremberg Code. In addition to the importance of the document ultimately produced, the Doctors Trial was significant because it proved to be a milestone in the judicialization of human subject protection violations. *See* Introduction to the United States Holocaust Memorial Museum's Online Exhibit Commemorating the Fiftieth Anniversary of the Doctors Trial, available at http://www.ushmm.org/research/doctors/index.html.

[B] The Indictment

1 TRIALS OF WAR CRIMINALS BEFORE THE NUERNBERG MILITARY TRIBUNALS UNDER CONTROL COUNCIL LAW NO. 10, 8-17
(U.S. Gov't Printing Office 1946-1949)

The United States of America, by the undersigned Telford Taylor, Chief of Counsel for War Crimes, duly appointed to represent said Government in the prosecution of war criminals, charges that the defendants herein participated in a common design or conspiracy to commit and did commit war crimes and crimes against humanity, as defined in Control Council Law No. 10, duly enacted by the Allied Control Council on 20 December 1945. These crimes included murders, brutalities, cruelties, tortures, atrocities, and other inhumane acts, as set forth in counts one, two, and three of this indictment. . . .

COUNT ONE — THE COMMON DESIGN OR CONSPIRACY

Between September 1939 and April 1945 all of the defendants herein, acting pursuant to a common design, unlawfully, willfully, and knowingly did conspire and agree together and with each other and with diverse other persons, to commit war crimes and crimes against humanity, as defined in Control Council Law No. 10, Article II. . . .

COUNT TWO — WAR CRIMES

Between September 1939 and April 1945 all of the defendants herein unlawfully, willfully, and knowingly committed war crimes, as defined by Article II of Control Council Law No. 10, in that they were principals in, accessories to, ordered, abetted, took a consenting part in, and were connected with plans and enterprises involving medical experiments without the subjects' consent, upon civilians and members of the armed forces of nations then at war with the German Reich and who were in the custody of the German Reich in exercise of belligerent control, in the course of which experiments the defendants committed murders, brutalities, cruelties, tortures, atrocities, and other inhuman acts. Such experiments included, but were not limited to, the following:

. . . *Malaria Experiments.* From about February 1942 to about April 1945 experiments were conducted at the Dachau concentration camp in order to investigate immunization for and treatment of malaria. Healthy concentration-camp inmates were infected by mosquitoes or by injections of extracts of the mucous glands of mosquitoes. After having contracted malaria the subjects were treated with various drugs to test their relative efficacy. Over 1,000 involuntary subjects were used in these experiments. Many of the victims died and others suffered severe pain and permanent disability. . . .

Sterilization Experiments. From about March 1941 to about January 1945 sterilization experiments were conducted at the Auschwitz and Ravensbrueck concentration camps, and other places. The purpose of these experiments was to develop a method of sterilization which would be suitable for sterilizing millions of people with a minimum of time and effort. These experiments were conducted by means of X-ray, surgery, and various drugs. Thousands of victims were sterilized and thereby suffered great mental and physical anguish. . . .

The said war crimes constitute violations of international conventions, particularly of Articles 4, 5, 6, 7, and 46 of the Hague Regulations, 1907, and Articles 2, 3, and 4 of the Prisoner-of-War Convention (Geneva, 1929), the laws and customs of war, the general principles of criminal law as derived from the criminal laws of all civilized nations, the internal penal laws of the countries in which such crimes were committed, and Article II of Control Council Law No. 10[.]

[Count Two included descriptions of a variety of other experiments involving humans: High-Altitude Experiments, Freezing Experiments, Lost (Mustard) Gas Experiments, Sulfanilamide Experiments, Bone, Muscle, and Nerve Regeneration and Bone Transplantation Experiments, Sea-water Experiments, Epidemic Jaundice Experiments, Spotted Fever (Fleckfieber) Experiments, Experiments with Poison, Incendiary Bomb Experiments.]

COUNT THREE — CRIMES AGAINST HUMANITY

Between September 1939 and April 1945 all of the defendants herein unlawfully, willfully, and knowingly committed crimes against humanity, as defined by Article II of Control Council Law No. 10, in that they were principals in, accessories to, ordered, abetted, took a consenting part in, and were connected with plans and enterprises involving medical experiments, without the subjects' consent, upon German civilians and nationals of other countries, in the course of which experiments the defendants committed murders, brutalities, cruelties, tortures, atrocities, and other inhuman acts.

The said crimes against humanity constitute violations of international conventions, including Article 46 of the Hague Regulations, 1907, the laws and customs of war, the general principles of criminal law as derived from the criminal laws of all civilized nations, the internal penal laws of the countries in which such crimes were committed, and of Article II of Control Council Law No. 10. . . .

Wherefore, this indictment is filed with the Secretary General of the Military Tribunals and the charges herein made against the above named defendants are hereby presented to MILITARY TRIBUNAL NO. I.

TELFORD TAYLOR
Brigadier General, USA
Chief of Counsel for War Crimes
Acting on Behalf of the United States of America

Nuernberg, 25 October 1946

[C] Opening Statement

1 TRIALS OF WAR CRIMINALS BEFORE THE NUERNBERG MILITARY TRIBUNALS UNDER CONTROL COUNCIL LAW NO. 10, 27-28, 37-38, 68-71
(U.S. Gov't Printing Office 1946-1949)

Opening Statement of the Prosecution by Brigadier General Telford Taylor, 9 December 1946

The defendants in this case are charged with murders, tortures, and other atrocities committed in the name of medical science. The victims of these crimes are numbered in the hundreds of thousands. A handful only are still alive; a few of the survivors will appear in this courtroom. But most of these miserable victims were slaughtered outright or died in the course of the tortures to which they were subjected. . . .

The defendants in the dock are charged with murder, but this is no mere murder trial. We cannot rest content when we have shown that crimes were committed and that certain persons committed them. To kill, to maim, and to torture is criminal under all modern systems of law. These defendants did not kill in hot blood, nor for personal enrichment. Some of them may be sadists who killed and tortured for sport, but they are not all perverts. They are not ignorant men. Most of them are trained physicians and some of them are distinguished scientists. Yet these defendants, all of whom were fully able to comprehend the nature of their acts, and most of whom were exceptionally qualified to form a moral and professional judgment in this respect, are responsible for wholesale murder and unspeakably cruel tortures.

It is our deep obligation to all peoples of the world to show why and how these things happened. It is incumbent upon us to set forth with conspicuous clarity the ideas and motives which moved these defendants to treat their fellow men as less than beasts. The perverse thoughts and distorted concepts which brought about these savageries are not dead. They cannot be killed by force of arms. They must not become a spreading cancer in the breast of humanity. They must be cut out and exposed for the reason so well stated by Mr. Justice Jackson in this courtroom a year ago — "The wrongs which we seek to condemn and punish have been so calculated, so malignant, and so devastating, that civilization cannot tolerate their being ignored because it cannot survive their being repeated." . . .

CRIMES COMMITTED IN THE GUISE OF SCIENTIFIC RESEARCH

[Here General Taylor details the various experiments charged as war crimes and as crimes against humanity. He notes that many were related to air raid and battlefield medical problems, or diseases which German armed forces encountered.]

But our proof will show that a quite different and even more sinister objective runs like a red thread through these hideous researches. We will show that in some instances the true object of these experiments was not how to rescue or to cure, but how to destroy and kill. The sterilization experiments were, it is clear, purely destructive in purpose. The prisoners at Buchenwald who were shot with poisoned bullets were not guinea pigs to test an antidote for the poison; their murderers really wanted to know how quickly the poison would kill. This destructive objective is not superficially as apparent in the other experiments, but we will show that it was often there. . . .

This policy of mass extermination could not have been so effectively carried out without the active participation of German medical scientists. . . .

SUMMARY

. . . Final judgment as to the relative degrees of guilt among those in the dock must await the presentation of the proof in detail. Nevertheless, before the introduction of evidence, it will be helpful to look again at the defendants and their part in the conspiracy. What manner of men are [the defendants] and what was their major role?

The 20 physicians in the dock range from leaders of German scientific medicine, with excellent international reputations, down to the dregs of the German medical profession. All of them have in common a callous lack of consideration and human regard for, and an unprincipled willingness to abuse their power over the poor, unfortunate, defenseless creatures who had been deprived of their rights by a ruthless and criminal government. All of them violated the Hippocratic commandments which they had solemnly sworn to uphold and abide by, including the fundamental principle never to do harm — "primum non nocere."

Outstanding men of science, distinguished for their scientific ability in Germany and abroad, are the defendants Rostock and Rose. Both exemplify, in their training and practice alike, the highest traditions of German medicine. Rostock headed the Department of Surgery at the University of Berlin and served as dean of its medical school. Rose studied under the famous surgeon, Enderlen, at Heidelberg and then became a distinguished specialist in the fields of public health and tropical diseases. Handloser and Schroeder are outstanding medical administrators. . . .

The part that each of these 20 physicians and their 3 lay accomplices played in the conspiracy and its execution corresponds closely to his professional interests and his place in the hierarchy of the Third Reich. . . . The motivating force for this conspiracy came from two principal sources. Himmler, as head of the SS, a most terrible machine of oppression with vast resources, could provide numberless victims for the experiments. By doing so, he enhanced the prestige of his organization and was able to give free rein to the Nazi racial theories of which he was a leading protagonist and to develop new techniques for the mass exterminations which were dear to his heart. The German military leaders, as the other main driving force, caught up the opportunity which Himmler presented them with and ruthlessly capitalized on Himmler's hideous overtures in an endeavor to strengthen their military machine.

And so the infernal drama was played just as it had been conceived in the minds of the authors. . . . Under Himmler's authority, the medical leaders of the SS — Grawitz, Genzken, Gebhardt, and others — set the wheels in motion. They arranged for the procurement of victims through other branches of the SS, and gave directions to their underlings in the SS medical service such as Hoven and Fischer. Himmler's administrative assistants, Sievers and Rudolf Brandt, passed on the Himmler orders, gave a push here and a shove there, and kept the machinery oiled. Blome and Brack assisted from the side of the civilian and party authorities. . . .

I intend to pass very briefly over matters of medical ethics, such as the conditions under which a physician may lawfully perform a medical experiment upon a person who has voluntarily subjected himself to it, or whether experiments may lawfully be performed upon criminals who have been condemned to death. This case does not present such problems. No refined questions confront us here.

None of the victims of the atrocities perpetrated by these defendants were volunteers, and this is true regardless of what these unfortunate people may have said or signed before their tortures began. Most of the victims had not been condemned to death, and those who had been were not criminals, unless it be a crime to be a Jew, or a Pole, or a gypsy, or a Russian prisoner of war.

Whatever book or treatise on medical ethics we may examine, and whatever expert on forensic medicine we may question, will say that it is a fundamental and inescapable obligation of every physician under any known system of law not to perform a dangerous experiment without the subject's consent. In the tyranny that was Nazi Germany, no one could give such a consent to the medical agents of the State; everyone lived in fear and acted under duress. I fervently hope that none of us here in the courtroom will have to suffer in silence while it is said on the part of these defendants that the wretched and helpless people whom they froze and drowned and burned and poisoned were volunteers. If such a shameless lie is spoken here, we need only remember the four girls who were taken from the Ravensbrueck concentration camp and made to lie naked with the frozen and all but dead Jews who survived Dr. Rascher's tank of ice water. One of these women, whose hair and eyes and figure were pleasing to Dr. Rascher, when asked by him why she had volunteered for such a task replied, "rather half a year in a brothel than half a year in a concentration camp."

[D] The Trial

The prosecution relied on a number of survivors of the Nazi experiments to testify about the atrocities alleged in the indictment. In addition, they also used numerous documents to prove the cases. Examples of each type of evidence follow.

[1] Testimonial Evidence (Excerpts)

Excerpts from the testimony of
FATHER LEO MIECHALOWSKI

The transcription of this document comes from U.S. National Archives & Records Administration, Record Group 238, M887, as reproduced at: http://www.ushmm.org/research/doctors/miechptx.htm

Q: Now, father, did there come a time when you were experimented on [in] the concentration camp at Dachau?

A: Yes. Malaria experiments and also on one occasion we were engaged in high altitude experiments. . . .

Q: Now, father, will you tell the Tribunal just what happened when you were experimented on with malaria? That is, when it happened and how you happened to be selected?

A: . . . I thought to myself that perhaps this was going to be some detail for easier work in the hospital. We were told that we should undress and after we had undressed ourselves our numbers were taken down and then we asked what was going on and they told us, smilingly, "this is for air detail." But we were not told what was going to be done with us. . . . I was given malaria in such a manner that there were little cages with infected mosquitoes and I had to put my hand on one of the little cages and a mosquito stung me and afterwards I was still in the hospital for five weeks. However, for the time being no symptoms of the disease showed themselves. Somewhat later, I don't exactly recall, two or three weeks, I had my first malaria attack. Such attacks recurred frequently and several medicines were given to us for against malaria. I was given such medicine as neo-salvasan. I was given two injections of quinine. On one occasion I was given atabrine and the worst was that one time when I had an attack, I was given so-called perifer. I was given nine injections of that kind, one every hour and that every second day through the seventh injection. All of a sudden my heart felt like it was going to be torn out. I became insane. I completely lost my language — my ability to speak. This lasted until evening. In the evening a nurse arrived and wanted to give me the eighth injection. I was then unable [sic] to speak and I told the nurse about all of the complications I had had and that I did not want to receive the injection. The nurse had already poured out the injection and said that he would report this to Dr. Schilling. After approximately ten minutes another nurse arrived and said that he would have to give me the injection after all. Then I said the same thing again, that I was not going to have the injection. However, he told me that he had to carry out that order. Then I replied that no matter what order he had, I would not be willing to commit suicide. Then he went away and returned once again after ten minutes. He told me, "I know you know what can happen if you don't accept the injection." Then I said in spite of everything, "I refuse to receive another injection . . . I said, "Hauptsturmfuehrer, I refuse to be given that injection." The physician turned around after I had said that and looked at me and said, "I am responsible for your life, not you." . . . [T]he nurses complied with his order and it was then they gave me this injection. It was the same one to whom I had previously told that I did not want to have another injection. . . .

Q: Father, do I understand you to say that you were injected with malaria in the middle of 1942?

A: It was approximately in the middle of 1942 when I was infected with malaria.

Q: And you were not asked your consent to the malaria experiment?

A: No. I was not asked for my consent.

Q: And you did not volunteer for this experiment?

A: No. I was taken in the manner which I have just described. . . .

Q: And do you know the approximate total number of inmates experimented on with malaria in Dachau?

A: Towards the end I heard that approximately one thousand two hundred prisoners were subjected to these experiments.

Q: Do you know whether or not any of those inmates died as a result of the malaria experiments?

A: Several have died, but if this was the direct result of malaria, I do not know. I know of one case when the patient died after having been given Perifere injections. Then I still know another priest who died, but afterwards — and prior to his death he was sent to another room.. . .

Q: How many recurrences of malaria fever did you have, Father?

A: I cannot give you the exact number any more. However, those attacks recurred frequently, I think about five times, and then I still had treatment in bed for some time, and then there were several more, and altogether I had ten attacks, one every day. Then I reached a temperature of 41.6. [nearly 107 degrees Farenheit] . . .

Q: Well, will you tell the tribunal about this other experiment?

A: [Fr. Miechalowski then proceeded to describe another experiment that occurred later in 1942 where he was kept in ice water for at least ninety minutes. The temperature was lowered over time and his body temperature dropped to 30 degrees centigrade (84 degrees Farenheit). After begging to be taken out, a physician gave him a few drops of liquid, he became unconscious, and sometime later awakened with a warming lamp over him. This resulted in ongoing cardiology problems and limitations in his ability to walk. Due to the experiments and starvation his weight dropped from 220 pounds to 125 pounds.]

[2] Documentary Evidence (Excerpts)

1 TRIALS OF WAR CRIMINALS BEFORE THE NUERNBERG MILITARY TRIBUNALS UNDER CONTROL COUNCIL LAW NO. 10, 228
(U.S. Gov't Printing Office 1946-1949)

Report by Prof. Dr. Holzloehner, Dr. Rascher, and Dr. Finke, regarding cooling experiments, 10 October 1942

If the experimental subject was placed in the water under narcosis [a state of deep stupor or unconsciousness], one observed a certain arousing effect. The subject began to groan and made some defensive movements. In a few cases a state of excitation developed. This was especially severe in the cooling of head and neck. But never was a complete cessation of the narcosis observed. The defensive movements ceased after about 5 minutes. There followed a progressive rigor, which developed especially strongly in the arm musculature; the arms were strongly flexed and pressed to the body. The rigor increased with the continuation of the cooling, now and then interrupted by tonic-clonic twitchings. With still more marked sinking of the body temperature it suddenly ceased. These cases ended fatally, without any successful results from resuscitation efforts.

[E] Defendants' Final Statements

2 TRIALS OF WAR CRIMINALS BEFORE THE NUERNBERG MILITARY TRIBUNALS UNDER CONTROL COUNCIL LAW NO. 10, 160-63
(U.S. Gov't Printing Office 1946-1949)

[Among the verbal and written closing statements submitted to the Tribunal by the various defendants was the following of Defendant Gerhard Rose.]

A subject of the personal charges against myself is my attitude toward experiments on human beings ordered by the state and carried out by other German scientists in the field of typhus and malaria. Works of that nature have nothing to do with politics or with ideology, but serve the good of humanity, and the same problems and necessities can be seen independently of any political ideology everywhere, where the same dangers of epidemics have to be combated. . . .

The fact is undoubted that human experiments, which were exactly the same as those, the participation in which I am unjustly charged with, have been carried out in other countries, above all, in the United States which has indicted me. That has led the prosecution to place the center of gravity of its charges upon the outside conditions of the persons put at my disposal for experiments by the German authorities. In that connection the question of whether they were voluntary was put into the foreground. I shall not discuss the question as to what extent the doctor who is charged with the experiments is responsible for these external, formal questions, at least a doctor who was so far removed from the experiments themselves as I was. But in connection with the principal question of subjects being volunteers, I have to make a few statements. A trial of this kind presents probably the most unsuitable atmosphere to discuss questions of medical ethics. But since these questions have been raised here, they have to be answered. Everyone who, as a scientist, has an insight into the history of dangerous medical experiments knows with certainty the following fact. Aside from the self-experiments of doctors, which represent a very small minority of such experiments, the extent to which subjects are volunteers is often deceptive. At the very best they amount to self-deceit on the part of the physician who conducts the experiment, but very frequently to a deliberate misleading of the public. In the majority of such cases, if we ethically examine facts, we find an exploitation of the ignorance, the frivolity, the economic distress, or other emergency on the part of the experimental subjects. I may only refer to the example which was presented to the Tribunal by Dr. Ivy when he presented to the forms for the American malaria experiments.

You yourselves, gentlemen of the Tribunal, are in a position to examine whether, on the basis of the information contained in these forms, individuals of the average education of an inmate of a prison can form a sufficiently clear opinion of the risks of an experiment made with pernicious malaria. These facts will be confirmed by any sincere and decent scientists in a personal conversation, though he would not like to make such a statement in public. . . .

The state, however, or any human community which, in the interest of the well-being of the entire community, did not want to forego the experiments on human beings, only bases itself on ethical principles as long as it openly assumes the full responsibility which arises therefrom, and imposes sacrifices on enemies of society to atone for their crimes and does not choose the method of apparent voluntary submission, which it imposes the risk of the experiment on the experimental subjects, who are not in a position to foresee the possible consequences.

[F] Excerpts from the Judgment of the Tribunal, including The Nuremberg Code

2 TRIALS OF WAR CRIMINALS BEFORE THE NUERNBERG MILITARY TRIBUNALS UNDER CONTROL COUNCIL LAW NO. 10, 181-83
(U.S. Gov't Printing Office 1946-1949)

THE PROOF AS TO WAR CRIMES AND CRIMES AGAINST HUMANITY

Judged by any standard of proof the record clearly shows the commission of war crimes and crimes against humanity substantially as alleged in counts two and three of the indictment. Beginning with the outbreak of World War II criminal medical experiments on non-German nationals, both prisoners of war and civilians, including Jews and "asocial" persons, were carried out on a large scale in Germany and the occupied countries. These experiments were not the isolated and casual acts of individual doctors and scientists working solely on their own responsibility, but were the product of coordinated policy-making and planning at high governmental, military, and Nazi Party levels, conducted as an integral part of the total war effort. They were ordered, sanctioned, permitted, or approved by persons in positions of authority who under all principles of law were under the duty to know about these things and to take steps to terminate or prevent them.

PERMISSIBLE MEDICAL EXPERIMENTS

The great weight of the evidence before us is to the effect that certain types of medical experiments on human beings, when kept within reasonably well-defined bounds, conform to the ethics of the medical profession generally. The protagonists of the practice of human experimentation justify their views on the basis that such experiments yield results for the good of society that are unprocurable by other methods or means of study. All agree, however, that certain basic principles must be observed in order to satisfy moral, ethical and legal concepts: [The following items, numbered 1-10, comprise what commonly is referred to as the Nuremberg Code:]

1. The voluntary consent of the human subject is absolutely essential.

   This means that the person involved should have legal capacity to give consent; should be so situated as to be able to exercise free power of choice, without the intervention of any element of force, fraud, deceit, duress, over-reaching, or other ulterior form of constraint or coercion; and should have sufficient knowledge and comprehension of the elements of the subject matter involved as to enable him to make an understanding and enlightened decision. This latter element requires that before the acceptance of an affirmative decision by the experimental subject there should be made known to him the nature, duration, and purpose of the experiment; the method and means by which it is to be conducted; all inconveniences and hazards reasonably to be expected; and the effects upon his health or person which may possibly come from his participation in the experiment.

   The duty and responsibility for ascertaining the quality of the consent rests upon each individual who initiates, directs or engages in the experiment. It is a personal duty and responsibility which may not be delegated to another with impunity.

2. The experiment should be such as to yield fruitful results for the good of society, unprocurable by other methods or means of study, and not random and unnecessary in nature.

3. The experiment should be so designed and based on the results of animal experimentation and a knowledge of the natural history of the disease or other problem under study that the anticipated results will justify the performance of the experiment.

4. The experiment should be so conducted as to avoid all unnecessary physical and mental suffering and injury.

5. No experiment should be conducted where there is an a priori reason to believe that death or disabling injury will occur; except, perhaps, in those experiments where the experimental physicians also serve as subjects.

6. The degree of risk to be taken should never exceed that determined by the humanitarian importance of the problem to be solved by the experiment.

7. Proper preparations should be made and adequate facilities provided to protect the experimental subject against even remote possibilities of injury, disability, or death.

8. The experiment should be conducted only by scientifically qualified persons. The highest degree of skill and care should be required

through all stages of the experiment of those who conduct or engage in the experiment.

9. During the course of the experiment the human subject should be at liberty to bring the experiment to an end if he has reached the physical or mental state where continuation of the experiment seems to him to be impossible.

10. During the course of the experiment the scientist in charge must be prepared to terminate the experiment at any stage, if he has probable cause to believe, in the exercise of the good faith, superior skill and careful judgment required of him that a continuation of the experiment is likely to result in injury, disability, or death to the experimental subject.

Of the ten principles which have been enumerated our judicial concern, of course, is with those requirements which are purely legal in nature — or which at least are so clearly related to matters legal that they assist us in determining criminal culpability and punishment. To go beyond that point would lead us into a field that would be beyond our sphere of competence. However, the point need not be labored. We find from the evidence that in the medical experiments which have been proved, these ten principles were much more frequently honored in their breach than in their observance. Many of the concentration camp inmates who were the victims of these atrocities were citizens of countries other than the German Reich. They were non-German nationals, including Jews and "asocial persons," both prisoners of war and civilians, who had been imprisoned and forced to submit to these tortures and barbarities without so much as a semblance of trial. In every single instance appearing in the record, subjects were used who did not consent to the experiments; indeed, as to some of the experiments, it is not even contended by the defendants that the subjects occupied the status of volunteers. In no case was the experimental subject at liberty of his own free choice to withdraw from any experiment. In many cases experiments were performed by unqualified persons; were conducted at random for no adequate scientific reason, and under revolting physical conditions. All of the experiments were conducted with unnecessary suffering and injury and but very little, if any, precautions were taken to protect or safeguard the human subjects from the possibilities of injury, disability, or death. In every one of the experiments the subjects experienced extreme pain or torture, and in most of them they suffered permanent injury, mutilation, or death, either as a direct result of the experiments or because of lack of adequate follow-up care.

Obviously all of these experiments involving brutalities, tortures, disabling injury, and death were performed in complete disregard of international conventions, the laws and customs of war, the general principles of criminal law as derived from the criminal laws of all civilized nations, and Control Council Law No. 10. Manifestly human experiments under such conditions are contrary to "the principles of the law of nations as they result from the usages established among civilized peoples, from the laws of humanity, and from the dictates of public conscience."

Whether any of the defendants in the dock are guilty of these atrocities is, of course, another question.

NOTES AND QUESTIONS

1. There is a factual basis to the argument set forth by Defendant Rose concerning malaria experiments conducted in the United States. Jonathan Moreno describes in detail a number of experiments involving human subjects that were conducted under governmental auspices prior to and during World War II. The malaria experiment, which was conducted in the early 1940s, involved the use of Atabrine, an antimalarial drug. At the time, malaria was a threat to the Americans' ability to succeed in the war against Japan. The studies were conducted on inmates of various prisons, as well as patients in civilian hospitals and conscientious objectors relieved of military service. Moreno notes that all the prison subjects signed contracts, which were akin to consent forms. The technical language downplayed the risks. Some 800 prisoners were enrolled. Motives for participation were mixed. Some subjects had relatives or friends in the armed services and wanted to help the soldiers; others hoped their sentences would be reduced; some did it to earn the $100 payment provided to subjects; others did it for patriotic motives.

In addition to the malaria experiments, Moreno describes other experiments during this era. One study on dysentery was carried out on adolescents and mentally retarded residents at the Ohio Soldiers and Sailors Orphanage. A hospitalized patient dying of lymphosarcoma was injected with nitrogen mustard, which was known to be poisonous to cells. Two hundred "volunteers" at a federal penitentiary were given gonorrhea in an effort to find a cure for the disease. A sailor was offered a three-day pass in exchange for participating in a test of navy clothing, where he was locked in a gas chamber filled with mustard gas, which causes sneezing, vomiting, blistering of the skin and temporary blindness. When he became nauseous and asked to be released, the request was denied. He finally passed out. In fact, during World War II, more than 60,000 servicemen were used in chemical research, 4,000 with mustard gas or its equivalent. Included were patch tests of the outer surfaces of the body for burn prevention and treatment, tests of the protective abilities of different types of clothing, and tests contaminating areas of land. Many of these studies were conducted at universities, and a number of subjects died or were badly burned as a result. Many later suffered various health problems that they did not link to the mustard gas studies until after many years. *See* JONATHAN D. MORENO, UNDUE RISK: SECRET STATE EXPERIMENTS ON HUMANS 21-40, 63-75 (2000).

2. What arguments might be made for using soldiers as subjects in experiments designed to better the war effort? When a person enrolls in the military, doesn't he or she agree to follow orders, whatever they may be? Don't the risks

of medical experiments often pale in comparison to those encountered in battles? In the First World War, sexually transmitted disease was almost as much of a problem in disabling soldiers as the cannons and guns they faced on the battlefield. Would it not make military sense to find a cure for this scourge, and wouldn't soldiers be the perfect subjects? Recall Reed's use of soldiers decades earlier. Should members of the military be required to become subjects in certain types of experiments? Or should military research be limited to "volunteer" subjects? Is the distinction between mandatory and voluntary meaningful in the military context?

3. The appropriateness of using soldiers as research subjects was recently debated within the context of the anthrax vaccine. In a case brought by six unnamed plaintiffs, presumably military service members, a federal district court judge ordered the Defense Department to stop its requirement that members of the armed forces be vaccinated against anthrax, even without their consent. Between 1999 and the court's decision, more than five hundred service members had refused the vaccine and faced disciplinary action, including discharge from the military and imprisonment. *See Judge Halts Forcing of Anthrax Shots*, N.Y. TIMES, Oct. 28, 2004, Sec. A, at 20; Doe v. Rumsfeld, 2004 U.S. Dist. LEXIS 21668 (2004).

4. What differences exist between the studies described above and those conducted by the Nazis? Do they have to do with the "endpoints" of the studies? (Endpoints are what is actually being measured, such as hard clinical events like strokes, or surrogate markers of health status like blood pressure.) The reasons the various subjects were "invited" to participate? Do you have concerns about the racial and political backgrounds of the various groups of subjects? In thinking about these questions, remember that, until relatively recently, the army was drafted, so that sons of the rich and famous served next to farm boys. Does that make a difference in your answer? Can you judge from the excerpts the extent to which the researchers had any regard for the subjects' well-being?

5. One significant difference between the "subjects" of the Nazi Doctors' experiments and that of subjects of other experiments is that, in the former situation, the subjects were all meant to be destroyed, either as a result of the experiments themselves or otherwise. In practically all other biomedical research, no such evil intent existed.

6. Jay Katz notes that much of the Western medical community dismissed the Nuremberg Code, particularly its uncompromising first principle, "viewing it as a code for barbarians and not for civilized physician-investigators." However, Katz argues that the Nuremberg Code, promulgated by the three U.S. judges who presided over the proceedings, was not needed to adjudicate the facts, but rather was intended to set forth principles that would apply to all human research in civilized societies. "The Nuremberg judges spoke not only to the past but to the present and future as well when it formulated its principle on voluntary consent. Being lawyers, the judges wanted to be precise about the quality of consent required when human beings are asked to make sacrifices

for the sake of others." According to Katz, the medical research community, today, still finds the stringency of the Code's first principle of voluntary consent "all too onerous." *See* Jay Katz, *The Nuremberg Code and the Nuremberg Trial: A Reappraisal*, 276 JAMA 1662 (1996). Is the first principle of the Nuremberg Code too burdensome for researchers? If you or a family member were considering whether to participate in a research study, would a less exacting standard be acceptable?

7. The Nuremberg Code did not specifically address research in the context of the patient-physician relationship. In 1964, the World Medical Association promulgated the Declaration of Helsinki, a series of recommendations to guide physicians in biomedical research involving human subjects, including patients participating in research related to their conditions. Its principal purpose was to assert the primacy of the interests of individual patients, declaring them to be paramount to those of society. Review the Declaration of Helsinki in Appendix E. In what ways could it be viewed as reducing some of the more stringent ethics requirements of the Nuremberg Code? Does that change in emphasis likely reflect the distance of the discussion from the reality of the concentration camps, or does it reflect some renewed faith in the ethical stature of physicians as a profession? Is the Declaration of Helsinki an improvement over the Nuremberg Code?

§ 1.04 MEDICAL RESEARCH IN THE UNITED STATES FROM 1900 TO THE EARLY 1970s

[A] Post-World War I Research Activities

By World War I, research had become a major activity at American medical schools, and by the 1920s the United States was the world leader in new medical discoveries. At Harvard Medical School, the amount spent on research had increased from $21,000 in 1910 to $2 million in 1947.

After World War I a number of factors led to the boom in biomedical research in the United States. The period between the wars saw major advances in the study of the causes and mechanisms of disease, such as the discovery of disease-producing organisms, including fungi, viruses, and parasites. New diseases became recognized and their courses made clearer. More significantly, major therapeutic advances took place. These ranged from advances in endocrinology, such as the discovery of insulin, to the rise of nutritional knowledge regarding the roles that vitamins play both in preventing and curing disease. During the 1920s and 1930s, the pharmaceutical industry came into its own.

Kenneth Ludmerer describes four characteristics of medical research in the United States during this period. The first is the significant boom in the research accomplishments of the preclinical sciences, such as biochemistry and physiology, which looked to medicine for questions to ask in conducting research, thus leading to a maturing of clinical scientists. Second, traditionally, clinical research had involved the passive study of patients, including descriptions of diseases and developments of tests and procedures. The primary sources of data were bedside observations of patients, retrospective review of hospital charts, and the use of the hospital's diagnostic labs, with an emphasis on maintaining thorough clinical records. After World War I, however, clinical research came to involve actively applying experimental methods to the study of diseases and therapeutics to explain the physiological mechanisms of disease. Clinical investigators took questions developed from observations of patients and searched for answers in their laboratories. The answers that they found often explained the pathophysiology of disease and led to direct applications of diagnostic procedures or therapeutic interventions to the patients. Third, a strong connection developed between the substance of the teaching in standard medical school courses and the research problems with which faculty were involved. Fourth was the demonstrable authority that medical research came to have despite the absence of biostatistics. This was a result of medicine's early success in curing acute diseases, such as meningitis, that previously had been untreatable. In turn, this led to a public infatuation with medicine.

Ludmerer observes that reinforcing this adulation of medical research was the researcher's clear contempt for commercialism and a lack of interest in personal financial reward.

> Medical scientists . . . sought non-monetary rewards: approval and recognition from their peers and . . . from society. The currency of academic medicine was not dollars but publications, appointments, titles, memberships and awards. . . . [In the view of medical schools] the objective of medical research was to promote the public welfare, not to enable individuals or institutions to profit financially from inventions or discoveries. Most medical schools would not hold patents or accept royalties from patents that arose from university work. . . .
>
> [The policy at most medical schools was similar to that expressed by the dean at Johns Hopkins who said that] "universities (and particularly medical schools) do not belong in business. . . . [A]ny commercialization of the institutions will in the long run do the institutions great harm. Universities being supported by philanthropy and by State grants should not sell themselves in any way." Neither the school nor individual faculty members owned patents, and the school refused royalties from patents growing out of medical school research. . . . In research, as well as in education, American medical schools acted as a public trust.

LUDMERER, *supra*, at 30-39.

[B] Funding of U.S. Research through World War II

Between 1900 and 1940, private sources provided most of the financing for medical research, largely through foundations and endowed research centers such as the Rockefeller Institute, which did much of the basic research. Universities themselves, often using foundation grants, endowment income, and "special" research funds, were key sponsors of medical research. After the 1920s, pharmaceutical companies began to play a role, particularly in the area of applied research. Initial support from the federal government was quite small.

The federal sponsorship of research had its earliest roots in the federally funded Hygienic Laboratory, which was established in 1887 to help in the control of epidemics. In 1891 this laboratory was moved to Washington and expanded to include laboratories in the study of chemistry, pharmacology, and zoology. By 1912, it was authorized to study chronic diseases as well. In 1930, it became known as the National Institute of Health, a part of the Public Health Service. Until the 1930s, practically all research supported by the federal government took place in government laboratories. In 1937, however, when Congress passed legislation to promote cancer research, it authorized the Public Health Service (PHS) to make grants to outside researchers. This legislation also set up the National Cancer Institute under the National Institute of Health.

World War II provided an enormous boost to biomedical research. Historically, disease was a more significant threat to soldiers than was the enemy. While the conditions that existed in World War I had improved, disease remained a major threat, and medical research became a priority. In 1941, President Roosevelt created an Office of Scientific Research and Development (OSRD) with two parallel committees, one on national defense and the other on medical research. The Committee on Medical Research (CMR) initiated an extensive research program to deal with the medical problems of the war, which ultimately came to cost approximately $15 million. These efforts led to improved therapeutics for malaria, the development of gamma globulin (to prevent and treat measles and other infectious diseases, including hepatitis) and an enormous increase in the ability to produce penicillin, previously a rare antibiotic. Much of the war research occurred in academic medicine. Before the end of the war, the President asked the OSRD to recommend plans for postwar government aid to science, including what could be done to aid "the war of science versus disease." The resulting report noted that basic research was "scientific capital" and that, while federal money should be used for research as well as scholarships, science had to be kept free from government influence as well as that of various pressure groups. In 1944, Congress authorized the PHS to make further grants for research in fields of medicine other than cancer research. By the end of World War II, the CMR's projects were transferred to the NIH. That transfer increased the NIH research budget from $180,000 in 1945 to $4 million in 1947. *See* STARR, *supra,* at 338-343.

As a result of World War II and its aftermath, two phenomena occurred that have had an enormous impact on medical research. First, "[t]he ties formed between the federal government and academic medical centers during World War II irrevocably altered the scale of medical research in the United States." LUDMERER, *supra,* at 139. Second, the development of biostatistics, which stemmed largely from post-World War II research into chronic diseases, would "help structure studies, eliminate investigator and participant bias, control for multiple interacting factors, and determine levels of statistical significance." *Id.* at 37.

The twenty-five-year period following the war saw massive infusions of federal support for education, mostly in the research area. The effect was an enormous change in emphasis in medical schools, away from developing physicians and toward medical research, with an increasing reliance on federal funding. The instruction of medical students came to play a much smaller role in academic medical centers, which instead favored the research enterprise and the education of house officers (physicians who had completed medical school and were obtaining further training as "residents"), clinical fellows, and graduate students.

The direction of medical research itself began to shift in the 1950s and 1960s away from the observational style of clinical investigation into a far more analytical or physiological approach. Efforts were now focused largely at the subcellular and molecular level in an effort to understand life processes in physical and chemical terms. This led to the emergence of the term *biomedical*. *See id.* at 142-148.

[C] The Developing Public Role in Research

Another phenomenon that began in the late 1940s was the development of a strong lay lobby for medical research. Wealthy individuals, by developing groups such as the American Cancer Society and the National Foundation for Infantile Paralysis (March of Dimes), encouraged the imposition of public pressure in these arenas. Paul Starr notes that "[p]ublic opinion polls confirmed the breadth of [the sentiment in favor of medical research] and politicians were not insensible to the possibilities. Opponents of national health insurance could display their deep concern for health by voting generous appropriations for medical research." STARR, *supra*, at 343. Soon there was a growing recognition that one method of fueling the demand for increased funding was to direct Congressional attention to individual diseases. This led to the creation of a number of institutes within the National Institute of Health, thereby changing the name of the research entity to the plural National Institutes of Health (NIH), as it is known today, and also caused a significant increase in funding for the NIH.

As an example of how the public viewed these developments, Starr discusses the success of the March of Dimes in raising money that ultimately led to an effective vaccine against polio. He writes:

> Probably no event in American history testifies more graphically to public acceptance of scientific methods than the voluntary participation of millions of American families in the 1954 trials of the Salk vaccine. The methodological conscience of epidemiologists had demanded that

these trials be double-blind. Neither doctors nor teachers, neither parents nor children, knew whether the children were receiving vaccine or placebo. And when on April 12, 1955, epidemiologists at the University of Michigan announced the results showing that the vaccine worked, pandemonium swept the country. "More than a scientific achievement, the vaccine was a folk victory," observes Richard Carter in his biography of Jonas Salk. "People observed moments of silence, rang bells, honked horns . . . smiled at strangers, forgave enemies."

The magic of science and money had worked. And if polio could be prevented, Americans had reason to think that cancer and heart disease and mental illness could be stopped too. Who knew how long human life might be extended. Medical research might offer passage to immortality. Between 1955 and 1960, unswerving congressional support pushed the NIH budget from $81 million to $400 million.

STARR, *supra*, at 342-47.

[D] The Need to Conduct Appropriate Research: Thalidomide and DES

A critical piece in the history of biomedical research in the United States actually began in Germany, where by 1957 a drug, Thalidomide, which was both a sleeping pill and a treatment for pregnant women suffering from morning sickness, was being sold over the counter. Its manufacturer claimed that it was non-addictive, caused no hangover, and was safe for pregnant women. By 1960 it was being sold throughout the world, and the Richardson-Merrell pharmaceutical company of Cincinnati applied to the FDA to sell it in the United States. The FDA assigned Frances Oldham Kelsey as the medical officer to conduct the review. She delayed granting approval, requesting more data because she was concerned that the chronic toxicity studies were not long enough and absorption and excretion data were inadequate.

At the end of 1960, the *British Medical Journal* reported seeing cases of peripheral neuritis, a painful tingling in the extremities, in patients on the drug for a long period of time. Kelsey requested still more data, suspicious that a drug that could damage nerves could also affect a developing fetus. Soon thereafter, European physicians began reporting that an increasing number of women were miscarrying, giving birth to infants who died shortly thereafter, or giving birth to severely deformed babies. By the end of 1961 it was established that half of the mothers with deformed children had taken Thalidomide in the first trimester of pregnancy. By March 1962, Richardson-Merrell withdrew its application for approval, but more than 10,000 children in forty-six countries had already been born with birth defects due to Thalidomide. In the United States, only seventeen children were born with Thalidomide-associated deformities, due to some doctors obtaining it on an "investigational" basis from Richardson-Merrell. The Thalidomide experience led to the passage, in late

1962, of the Kefauver-Harris Amendments to the earlier federal Food, Drug and Cosmetic Act of 1938, strengthening the FDA's control of drug experimentation on humans, requiring informed consent from patients, and mandating that drug companies report adverse reactions to the FDA. Kelsey became the head of the FDA's investigational drug branch, which was created to monitor clinical trials for compliance. *See* L. Bren, *Frances Oldham Kelsey: FDA Medical Reviewer Leaves Her Mark on History*, 35 FDA CONSUMER MAGAZINE (March-April 2001), available at http://www.fda.gov/fdac/features/2001/201_kelsey.html.

NOTES AND QUESTIONS

1. Thalidomide is used today to treat leprosy and a variety of cancers. It is dispensed only under very tight controls. Among other requirements, patients of childbearing potential must be sexually abstinent or use two forms of contraception. One form must be highly effective (hormonal methods, IUD, bilateral tubal ligation, vasectomy), and the other must be a barrier form of contraception. *See* Brad L Neiger, *The Re-emergence of Thalidomide: Results of a Scientific Conference*, 62 TERATOLOGY 432 (2000).

2. Diethylstilbestrol (DES) is a synthetic estrogen hormone that was prescribed to treat women for the prevention of spontaneous abortions and premature delivery. It was first produced in England in 1938, and it was approved by the FDA in 1947. By one estimate between five and ten million women in the United States and England received DES during pregnancy or were exposed to the drug in utero, and the doses prescribed differed by a factor of ten or more. Although a randomized clinical trial in the early 1950s showed it to be ineffective, it nonetheless continued to be prescribed. Should the government have removed the drug from the market at that point? Does the fact that a drug is ineffective mean that it should be banned? In 1971, evidence was reported demonstrating that the use of DES was strongly associated with the occurrence of vaginal clear cell adenocarcinoma in exposed female offspring. In November 1971, the FDA issued a drug bulletin warning against its use in pregnancy, and several studies since then have followed DES-exposed daughters for the occurrence of cancer, precursor lesions and reproductive effects. *See* NATIONAL CANCER INSTITUTE, DES RESEARCH UPDATE 1999: CURRENT KNOWLEDGE, FUTURE DIRECTIONS, July 19-20, 1999; E.E. Hatch et al., *Cancer Risk in Women Exposed to Diethylstilbestrol in Utero*, 1280 JAMA 630 (1998). Some DES-exposed daughters successfully sued the manufacturers of the drug. *See* Anna C. Mastroianni, *HIV, Women, and Access to Clinical Trials: Tort Liability and Lessons from DES*, 5 DUKE J. GENDER L. & POL'Y 167, 178 (1998).

3. What could have been done to prevent the harms to daughters of women who took DES during pregnancy, both before and after the drug was approved for marketing? For discussion of the FDA's current system of overseeing drugs, see Chapter 3, at page 144.

[E] The Beecher Article (1966)

In 1966, Henry Beecher, a Harvard physician and researcher, published a six-page article in the *New England Journal of Medicine* in which he described a series of experiments on human subjects conducted by American researchers. All of these experiments had been published in medical journals, suggesting that they were studies about which people in the medical world would have known. The experiments, he claimed, involved "unethical or questionably ethical procedures." Henry Beecher, *Ethics and Clinical Research*, 274 NEW ENG. J. MED. 1354 (1966). He argued that the subjects in many of the studies never received satisfactory explanations of the risks involved or even were told that they were participating in an experiment, and that "grave consequences" were suffered as a direct result of the experiments.

Beecher found that consent was mentioned in only two of the fifty articles he originally compiled, but he expressed skepticism about how realistic it would be to place much stock in such claims at all. Rather, he argued, any statements concerning consent would have no meaning "unless one knows how fully the patient was informed of all risks, and if these are not known, that fact should also be made clear. A far more dependable safeguard than consent is the presence of a truly *responsible* investigator."

Beecher observed that while patients would often be willing to undergo some inconvenience and discomfort, most would not agree to jeopardize their health or lives for the sake of science. Nonetheless, he argued, in many of the studies it was clear that investigators did risk the health or life of the subjects, and that some of the experimental procedures had established death rates.

The article proceeded to describe each of twenty-two experiments culled, to save space, from the larger group of fifty he originally reviewed. Among those noted were a study in which mentally retarded children were deliberately infected with hepatitis virus (later revealed to have taken place at Willowbrook State Hospital) and a study in which live cancer cells were injected into patients at the Jewish Chronic Disease Hospital in Brooklyn. Each of those studies is described in more detail below at page 39.

Beecher concluded that, when the types of risks involved in these studies were taken into account, "and a considerable number of patients are involved, it may be assumed that informed consent has not been obtained in all cases." Furthermore, criticizing those who claimed that obtaining informed consent from research subjects would "block progress," Beecher quoted Pope Pius XII's observation that "science is not the highest value to which all other orders of values . . . should be subordinated."

NOTES AND QUESTIONS

1. As David Rothman explains:

> At a time when the media were not yet scouring medical journals for stories, Beecher's charges captured an extraordinary amount of public attention. Accounts of the *NEJM* article appeared in the leading newspapers and weeklies, which was precisely what he intended. A circumspect whistle-blower, he had published his findings first in a medical journal without naming names; but at the same time, he had informed influential publications (including the *New York Times*, the *Wall Street Journal*, *Time*, and *Newsweek*) that his piece was forthcoming. The press reported the experiments in great detail, and reporters, readers, and public officials alike expressed dismay and incredulity as they pondered what had led respectable scientists to commit such acts.

ROTHMAN, *supra*, at 17.

2. If research on human subjects is performed in an illegal or unethical manner, as described in many of the illustrations provided throughout this chapter, is it appropriate to use the scientific data derived from that research in further research or medical treatment? Beecher argued that such data should not be published. He maintained that "[e]ven though suppression of such data (by not publishing it) would constitute a loss to medicine, in a specific localized sense, this loss, it seems, would be less important than the far reaching moral loss to medicine if the data thus obtained were to be published." Beecher illustrated his belief with a reference to the United States Supreme Court's decision in *Mapp v. Ohio*. In *Mapp*, the evidence introduced against the defendant by the prosecution was seized during an illegal search of the defendant's residence in violation of the Fourth Amendment. The Supreme Court held that evidence that is unconstitutionally obtained cannot be used in any judicial proceeding. Beecher drew a parallel between the exclusion of this type of criminal evidence and his belief that data obtained improperly in a scientific setting should be excluded no matter how important the information is to the ends of science. Is Beecher's analogy to unconstitutionally obtained evidence persuasive? Should the rules of evidence for criminal proceedings guide the scientific and medical community's use of unethically or illegally obtained research data? What if data are characterized as "improperly obtained" due to de minimis procedural errors by the institutional review board or the principal investigator? Should a study in which the consent forms were drafted improperly be treated differently from the Nazi experiments? For further discussion of the use of data from unethical research, see Marcia Angell, *Editorial Responsibility: Protecting Human Rights by Restricting Publication of Unethical Research*, in THE NAZI DOCTORS AND THE NUREMBERG CODE 276 (George J. Annas & Michael Grodin eds., 1992).

3. Because the "conscientious" physician was not much of a protection for human subjects in the past, does it strike you as odd that Beecher would have relied on the integrity of the investigator as the primary safeguard against

unethical research? And if ordinary patients would not risk their health for the sake of science, what might that say about the entire research enterprise?

[F] Jewish Chronic Disease Hospital (1963) and Willowbrook (1956-1971)

Two of the studies described in the Beecher article generated particular controversy. The first was a 1963 study, partially funded by the Public Health Service and the NIH, in which investigators, led by a physician at the Sloan-Kettering Cancer Research Institute, injected live cancer cells into twenty-two indigent, chronically ill, and debilitated elderly patients at the Brooklyn Jewish Chronic Disease Hospital (JCDH) in New York. The participants were not informed that live cancer cells were being used or that the experiment was designed to measure the patients' ability to reject foreign cells — a test unrelated to their normal therapeutic program. Two of the physicians involved were censured by the state licensing authority and placed on probation for a year. The license revocation proceedings revealed that the reason the investigators did not inform the subjects that the injected material contained live cancer cells was to avoid refusals of participation and emotional responses from the patients. The study was not presented to the research committee of JCDH, and several physicians who were directly responsible for patients involved in the study were never contacted for approval for the injections. Several resident physicians who were presented with information about the study objected to the participation of JCDH patients because they could foresee problems obtaining informed consent. *See* HERSHEY & MILLER, *supra*, at 6-7.

The second study, which took place between 1956 and 1971, was led by Dr. Saul Krugman, an infectious disease researcher at the Willowbrook State School, a New York State institution for "mentally defective persons." The purpose of the study was to better understand the natural history of hepatitis and the effects of gamma globulin in preventing or moderating its effects. The subjects, all of whom were children, were deliberately infected with the virus. In early studies they were fed extracts of stools from infected children, while later subjects received injections of more purified virus preparations. As a result, Krugman's research established the distinctive features of Hepatitis A and Hepatitis B.

The investigators defended their experiment by arguing that because hepatitis was prevalent in the institution, most of the children would have acquired the infection in any event, and there was no known antidote. They also claimed to have signed consent forms from parents of all of the subjects. The *Journal of the American Medical Association*, which published the results of the study, commended Krugman for his "'judicious use of human beings.'" In response to the study, Franz Inglefinger, later the editor of the *New England Journal of Medicine*, argued that the children benefited from being infected under carefully controlled research conditions and receiving expert attention.

David and Sheila Rothman, in their book THE WILLOWBROOK WARS (1984), report the following:

> Many parents of children accepted at Willowbrook but still awaiting actual admission — a wait that could last for several years — did receive the following letter from Dr. H.H. Berman, then Willowbrook's director:
>
> November 15, 1958
>
> Dear Mrs. _____:
>
> We are studying the possibility of preventing epidemics of hepatitis on a new principle. Virus is introduced and gamma globulin given later to some, so that either no attack or only a mild attack of hepatitis is expected to follow. This may give the children immunity against this disease for life. We should like to give your child this new form of prevention with the hope that it will afford protection.
>
> Permission form is enclosed for your consideration. If you wish to have your child given the benefit of this new preventive, will you so signify by signing the form.
>
> . . . To send such a letter over the signature of Willowbrook's director appeared coercive. These parents wanted to please the man who would be in charge of their child. Moreover, an especially raw form of coercion may have occasionally intruded. When overcrowding at Willowbrook forced a close in regular admissions, an escape hatch was left — admission via Krugman's unit. A parent wanting to institutionalize a retarded child had a choice: Sign the form or forgo the placement.

DAVID J. ROTHMAN & SHEILA M. ROTHMAN, THE WILLOWBROOK WARS 265-266 (1984).

NOTES AND QUESTIONS

1. In what ways might the words and phrases in what today would be called a "recruitment statement" be seen as deceptive and inappropriate? What words or phrases would be more suitable than "studying hepatitis," the "[v]irus is introduced," or "gamma globulin given later to some"? The letter states that "no attack" or a "mild attack" of the disease "is expected to follow." But it was known by then that, without gamma globulin, an attack was likely and in some cases severe. Was feeding a child a live virus, in fact, a "new form of prevention"? Was finding "a new form of prevention" the goal of the study?

2. In 1965, Willowbrook's awful conditions were reported to the press by Senator Robert F. Kennedy, after he made an unannounced visit to the institution. He described the wards as "less comfortable and cheerful than the cages in which we put animals in a zoo. . . . We cannot tolerate a new snake pit." David and Sheila Rothman further describe this "snake pit," detailing how the overcrowded hallways of Willowbrook were filled with beds jammed together and with unattended children, some of whom were naked, covered in their own feces, and lying on the floors. ROTHMAN & ROTHMAN, *supra*, 15-17, 23.

3. Would the study have been ethically acceptable if the researchers had provided more complete information to the parents? What do you make of the argument that it was acceptable to infect the children with hepatitis because they probably would have become infected anyway?

[G] Tuskegee (1932-1972)

REPORT OF THE TUSKEGEE SYPHILIS STUDY
LEGACY COMMITTEE
(1996)
http://www.med.virginia.edu/hs-library/historical/apology/report.html

In 1932, the United States Public Health Service (USPHS) initiated the Tuskegee Syphilis Study to document the natural history of syphilis. The subjects of the investigation were 399 poor black sharecroppers from Macon County, Alabama, with latent syphilis and 201 men without the disease who served as controls. The physicians conducting the Study deceived the men, telling them that they were being treated for "bad blood." However, they deliberately denied treatment to the men with syphilis and they went to extreme lengths to ensure that they would not receive therapy from any other sources. In exchange for their participation, the men received free meals, free medical examinations, and burial insurance.

On July 1972, a front-page headline in the *New York Times* read, "Syphilis Victims in U.S. Study Went Untreated for 40 years." The accompanying article publicly revealed the details of the Tuskegee Syphilis Study — "the longest nontherapeutic experiment on human beings in medical history." . . . [S]ince its disclosure, the Study has moved from a singular historical event to a powerful metaphor. It has come to symbolize racism in medicine, ethical misconduct in human research, paternalism by physicians, and government abuse of vulnerable people.

———————

The *New York Times* story caused a public uproar, which resulted in the Assistant Secretary for Health and Scientific Affairs appointing an Ad Hoc

Advisory Panel to review the study. The panel concluded that the study participants were not given adequate treatment for their disease. Moreover, it found that the subjects were not given the option of withdrawing from the study when penicillin, a very effective drug treatment for syphilis, became widely used in 1947. In November 1972, based upon the strong recommendation of the advisory panel, the Assistant Secretary for Health and Scientific Affairs ordered that the Tuskegee Study be halted. *See* CDC Timeline, *The Tuskegee Syphilis Study: A Hard Lesson Learned*, available at http://www.cdc.gov/nchstp/od/ tuskegee/ time.htm.

BAD BLOOD
JAMES H. JONES
2-5, 12-13, 16-17, 22-24, 29 (1993)

The Tuskegee Study had nothing to do with treatment. No new drugs were tested; neither was any effort made to establish the efficacy of old forms of treatment. It was a nontherapeutic experiment, aimed at compiling data on the effects of the spontaneous evolution of syphilis on black males. . . .

Since the effects of the disease are so serious, reporters in 1972 wondered why the men agreed to cooperate. The press quickly established that the health officials had offered them incentives to participate. The men received free physical examinations, free rides to and from the clinics, hot meals on examination days, free treatment for minor ailments, and a guarantee that burial stipends would be paid to their survivors. Though the latter sum was very modest (fifty dollars in 1932 with periodic increases to allow for inflation), it represented the only form of burial insurance that many of the men had. . . .

What the health officials had told the men in 1932 was . . . difficult to determine. . . . Dr. J.W. Williams, who . . . assisted in the experiment's clinical work, stated that neither the interns nor the subjects knew what the study involved. "The people who came in were not told what was being done," Dr. Williams said. "We told them we wanted to test them. . . . We didn't tell them we were looking for syphilis. I don't think they would have known what that was." . . .

The specter of Nazi Germany prompted some Americans to equate the Tuskegee Study with genocide. A civil rights leader in Atlanta, Georgia, charged that the study amounted to "nothing less than [an] official, premeditated policy of genocide." . . .

The *Los Angeles Times* echoed this view. In deftly chosen words, the editors qualified their accusation that PHS officials had persuaded hundreds of black men to become "human guinea pigs" by adding: "Well, perhaps not quite that [human guinea pigs] because the doctors obviously did not regard their subjects as completely human." A Pennsylvania editor stated that such an experiment "could only happen to blacks."

Other observers thought that social class was the real issue, that poor people, regardless of their race, were the ones in danger. Somehow people from the lower class always seemed to supply a disproportionate share of subjects for scientific research. . . . And the *Washington Post* made much the same point when it observed, "There is always a lofty goal in the research work of medicine but too often in the past it has been the bodies of the poor . . . on whom the unholy testing is done."

. . . Nineteenth century physicians had ample opportunities to inject racial prejudice into their daily practices. . . . Physicians did not dissent as a group from white society's pervasive belief in the physical and mental inferiority of blacks. . . .

Physicians knew that syphilis was contracted through sexual intercourse. . . . Since most sexual intercourse involved a willful, voluntary activity, physicians believed that the responsibility for any disease acquired during the act rested solely upon the individual. . . .

Few physicians managed to discuss the problem without revealing an inordinate fascination with black sexuality. . . . They perpetuated the ancient myth that blacks matured physically at early ages and were more sexually active throughout their lives than whites. . . . The formidable penis of the black man with its long prepuce offered greater opportunity for venereal infection. Moreover, personal restraints on self-indulgence did not exist, physicians insisted, because the smaller brain of the Negro had failed to develop a center for inhibiting sexual behavior. . . .

In this atmosphere it was not surprising that physicians depicted syphilis as the quintessential black disease. . . .

The gross exaggerations and virulent attitudes in the medical literature discussing syphilis in blacks declined after World War I as medical discussions became more quantified and physicians concentrated on clinical manifestations. Yet the image of blacks as "a notoriously syphilis-soaked race" did not fade.

NOTES AND QUESTIONS

1. In 1969, an earlier ad hoc committee had been appointed to review the Tuskegee Study in order to decide if it should continue. The group met for a single afternoon session. While it concluded that such a study should never be repeated, it neither suggested that it be terminated nor that the consent of the subjects be obtained. *See* HERSHEY & MILLER, *supra*, at 10.

2. In the summer of 1973, a class-action lawsuit filed by the National Association for the Advancement of Colored People (NAACP) ended in a settlement that gave more than $9 million to the study participants. As part of the settlement, the U.S. government promised to give free medical and burial services to

all living participants. The Tuskegee Health Benefit Program was established to provide those services. It also gave health services to wives, widows, and children who had been infected because of the study. The CDC was given responsibility for the program, where it remains today in the National Center for HIV, STD, and TB Prevention. On May 16, 1997, President Clinton issued an apology to participants in the Tuskegee Study on behalf of the United States government.

3. Some scholars have suggested that it would be appropriate to have the "Tuskegee Study" renamed the "U.S. Public Health Service Study." Why do you think they have proposed this change?

4. Many people believe that a major impact of the Tuskegee experiments is a "legacy of mistrust" within the African American community toward the medical profession and public health authorities. In the 1993 edition of *Bad Blood*, the author devotes the final chapter to discussing the belief among African Americans, first reported in the *New York Times* in 1992, that, "AIDS [Acquired Immune Deficiency Syndrome] and the health measures against it are part of a conspiracy to wipe out the black race." JAMES JONES, BAD BLOOD 220-21 (1993). Similarly, Peter Clark, a Jesuit priest, notes that the Tuskegee experiments "authenticated a historically based pattern of medical mistreatment that has been well-known to the African-American community through their folklore tradition. . . . As a result, participation by African-Americans in clinical AIDS trials has been disproportionately small in comparison to the number of African-Americans who have been infected with HIV." Peter A. Clark, *A Legacy of Mistrust: African-Americans, the Medical Profession, and AIDS,* 65 LINACRE QUARTERLY 66 (1998). For further discussion of these issues, see Chapter 9, at page 459.

[H] Radiation Experiments (1944-1974)

Between 1944 and 1974, the federal government funded a series of radiation experiments, including the injection of plutonium into unsuspecting hospital patients as well as the intentional release of radiation into the environment for research purposes. Some were conducted to advance biomedical science, while others related to national interests in defense or space exploration. Most of the human experiments involved radioactive tracers administered in amounts similar to those used in research today and were unlikely to have caused physical harm. However, in some nontherapeutic tracer studies involving children, the exposures were associated with an increased lifetime risk of developing thyroid cancer. Moreover, in several studies, patients died shortly after receiving external radiation or radioisotope doses in the therapeutic range that were associated with acute radiation effects.

During the 1940s and 1950s, physicians typically used patients as subjects in radiation experiments without the patients' awareness or consent. Scant attention was paid to concerns regarding fairness in selection of subjects. Moreover, information about the radiation experiments was kept secret because the government worried about embarrassment and potential legal liability, and was concerned that public misunderstanding would negatively affect government programs. In some cases subjects and their families had no available avenues of redress for possible wrongdoing because the government actively kept the truth from them. Even in situations in which maintaining the classified nature of records was legitimately required on national security grounds, the government often failed to create or maintain adequate records, keeping the public and those at risk from learning about the programs.

Between 1944 and 1974, the federal government conducted research involving several hundred intentional releases of radiation into the environment. In general, these experiments were not done to study the effects of radiation on humans. Rather they were designed to test the operation of weapons, the safety of equipment, or the dispersal of radiation into the environment and the pathways that the radiation would take. The releases took place in secret and remained so for decades. There was little or no independent review of whether the studies were needed, risks were minimized, or records kept.

As a result of exposure to radon and related products in underground uranium mines — well in excess of levels known to be hazardous — at least several hundred miners died of lung cancer and surviving miners remained at elevated risk levels. These men were the subject of government study as they mined uranium for use in weapons manufacturing, but the government failed to require the reduction of the hazard by ventilating the mines and adequately warning the miners of the danger to which they were exposed. *See* ADVISORY COMMITTEE ON HUMAN RADIATION EXPERIMENTS, EXECUTIVE SUMMARY, KEY FINDINGS (1995), available at http://tis.eh.doe.gov/ohre/roadmap/achre/summary.html.

NOTES AND QUESTIONS

1. The material presented above summarizes the findings of the Advisory Committee on Human Radiation Experiments, which was appointed by President Clinton in 1994. Its members were fourteen private citizens from around the country. It included one representative of the general public and thirteen experts in bioethics, radiation oncology and biology, nuclear medicine, epidemiology and biostatistics, public health, history of science and medicine, and law. With the assistance of staff, the Committee was asked to engage in fact-finding, to identify the appropriate ethical and scientific standards for evaluating these events, and to make recommendations to ensure that whatever wrongdoing may have occurred in the past would not be repeated. While it was anticipated that the Committee's recommendations would form the basis of legislative or regulatory changes, as of this writing no legislative or regulatory proposals addressing the Committee's concerns have been put forth.

Might this lack of attention to the conclusions of the report have been affected by the fact that the report was issued on the day that O.J. Simpson was acquitted of murder? Was an advisory committee the appropriate vehicle for reviewing the radiation experiments and developing public policy recommendations? Why do you think President Clinton entrusted these tasks to an advisory committee, rather than to an administrative agency with regulatory authority? Might other approaches have been preferable?

2. The Advisory Committee made a number of recommendations, including that the government should personally apologize and provide financial compensation to those subjects or their next of kin in situations in which

efforts were made by the government to keep information secret from these individuals or their families, or the public, for the purpose of avoiding embarrassment or potential legal liability, and where this secrecy had the effect of denying individuals the opportunity to pursue potential grievances[; or]

there was no prospect of direct medical benefit to the subjects, or interventions considered controversial at the time were presented as standard practice, and physical injury attributable to the experiment resulted.

ADVISORY COMMITTEE ON HUMAN RADIATION EXPERIMENTS, EXECUTIVE SUMMARY, *supra*.

At the 1995 White House ceremony in which President Clinton accepted the Committee's report, he apologized to the victims:

"While most of the tests were ethical by any standards, some were unethical, not only by today's standards, but by the standards of the time in which they were conducted. They failed both the test of our national values and the test of humanity. . . . So today," he said, "on behalf of another generation of American leaders and another generation of American citizens, the United States of America offers a sincere apology to those of our citizens who were subjected to these experiments, to their families, and their communities."

Statement Of Tara O'Toole, M.D., M.P.H., before the Committee On Governmental Affairs United States Senate, March 12, 1996, available at http://www.eh.doe.gov/docs/testimony/031296.html. In 1997, the government provided $6.5 million in financial compensation. *See* "Administration Responds to Human Radiation Experiment Advisory Committee," available at http://www.eh.doe.gov/docs/synergy/97spr/sec3.html.

3. The recommendations were made in the face of a number of significant judicial opinions rendered prior to the Advisory Committee's report, arising out of lawsuits filed in connection with the experiments involved. These included, among others:

a. **United States v. Stanley**. In *Stanley*, a serviceman filed a negligence action against the government under the Federal Tort Claims

Act, which authorizes certain negligence lawsuits against the government, and under 42 U.S.C. § 1983, a cause of action for the violation of constitutional rights by federal officials. He alleged that he had volunteered for what was ostensibly a chemical warfare testing program designed to test the effectiveness of protective clothing and equipment against chemical warfare, but in which he was secretly administered lysergic acid diethylamide (LSD) pursuant to an Army plan to test the effects of the drug on human subjects. He claimed that, as a result of the testing, he had suffered from hallucinations and periods of incoherence and memory loss, and would on occasion "awake from sleep at night and, without reason, violently beat his wife and children, later being unable to recall the entire incident." These severe personality changes led to his discharge and the dissolution of his marriage. Stanley did not become aware that he had been given LSD in the study until 1975, when the Army sent him a letter soliciting his cooperation in a study of the long-term effects of LSD on "volunteers who participated" in the 1958 tests.

The Supreme Court denied the claims under legal doctrines that bar governmental liability for injuries to servicemen resulting from activity "incident to service." The court noted that it had previously determined that a constitutional claim would not lie where there are "special factors counseling hesitation" or an "explicit congressional declaration" of another, exclusive remedy. It then pointed to a number of "special factors" that indicate that, as a matter of policy, such lawsuits should not be permitted. These included "the constitutional authorization for Congress rather than the judiciary to make rules governing the military, the unique disciplinary structure of the Military Establishment," Congress's establishment of "a comprehensive internal system of military justice," and the degree of disruption that allowing such a suit would have on the government's military chain-of-command rules. The Court stated that its position was not affected by the fact that the laws would not give servicemen an "adequate" federal remedy for their injuries. *See* United States v. Stanley, 483 U.S. 669, 671-86 (1987).

A dissenting opinion by Justice Brennan stated:

> [T]he Government of the United States treated thousands of its citizens as though they were laboratory animals, dosing them with this dangerous drug without their consent. . . . The Court holds that the Constitution provides [Stanley] with no remedy, solely because his injuries were inflicted while he performed his duties in the Nation's Armed Forces. If our Constitution required this result, the Court's decision, though legally necessary, would expose a tragic flaw in that document. But in reality, the Court disregards the commands of our Constitution,

and bows instead to the purported requirements of a different master, *military discipline,* declining to provide Stanley with a remedy because it finds "special factors counseling hesitation." This is abdication, not hesitation.

483 U.S. at 686 (Brennan, J., dissenting). The dissent pointed out the irony that, although the military had played a critical role in the Nazi Doctors' case, the LSD experiments were conducted in defiance of the Nuremberg Code's first principle, which requires the subject's voluntary consent. It also noted that a 1959 Army study recognized that legal liability could be avoided by covering up the LSD experiments. *See id.* at 688-89.

b. **Central Intelligence Agency v. Sims**. Similarly, in 1985, the Supreme Court held that the CIA was not required, under the Freedom of Information Act, to release the names of institutions and individuals who had performed research under an Agency-sponsored project to counter Soviet and Chinese advances in brainwashing and interrogation techniques. Over the years the program had included various medical and psychological experiments. The court held that the CIA director had broad authority to protect all sources of intelligence information from disclosure. *See* Central Intelligence Agency v. Sims, 471 U.S. 159 (1985).

c. **In re Cincinnati Radiation Litigation**. Not all lawsuits against the government for involuntarily enrolling citizens in military research have been unsuccessful. In 1995, a federal district court in Ohio refused to dismiss a case brought by the heirs and representatives of cancer patients who were given radiation as part of a study to see what would happen to combat troops who had been irradiated. The patients were primarily indigent, poorly-educated African Americans who had inoperable cancer but were not near death. They were told they were getting the radiation to treat their cancer. *See* In re Cincinnati Radiation Litigation, 874 F. Supp. 796 (S.D. Ohio 1995).

[I] Behavior and Social Science Research: The Milgram Experiments

Ethically questionable research has not been limited to the biomedical field. In the early 1960s, behavioral psychologist Stanley Milgram, then a Yale doctoral student, carried out a controversial laboratory experiment designed to examine obedience and disobedience to authority under a variety of conditions. The study involved ordering naïve subjects to administer increasingly severe punishments involving what appeared to be an electrical generator with graded switches ranging from "Slight Shock" to "Danger: Severe Shock." In reality, the victim was a confederate of the experimenter, and no shocks were actually delivered. Instead, the study was designed to determine the maximum shock the subjects were willing to administer before they refused to continue. Twenty-six subjects obeyed the experimental commands to administer the highest shock, while fourteen subjects broke off the experiment at some point after the "victim" protested. The experiment created extreme nervous tension in some subjects. Milgram describes that a "mature and initially poised businessman" began his participation in a confident manner. Nonetheless,

> [w]ithin 20 minutes he was reduced to a twitching, stuttering wreck, who was rapidly approaching a point of nervous collapse. He constantly pulled on his earlobe and twisted his hands. At one point he pushed his fist into his forehead and muttered: "Oh God, let's stop it." And yet he continued to respond to every word of the experimenter, and obeyed to the end.

Stanley Milgram, *Behavioral Study of Obedience*, 67 J. ABNORMAL & SOCIAL PSYCHOLOGY 371 (1963).

Critics of the study have argued that the experiments should not have taken place because they exposed subjects to a significant loss of dignity. By virtue of subjects' comprehending what they did and having to live with the realization that they were capable of such brutal behavior, it has been claimed, Milgram exceeded the appropriate limits of a study in terms of the intensity and duration of psychological distress. A related criticism is that the experiment "disregard[ed] the special quality of trust and obedience with which the subject appropriately regards the experimenter." Diana Baumrind, *Some Thoughts on Ethics of Research: After Reading Milgram's "Behavioral Study of Obedience,"* 19 AM. PSYCHOLOGIST 421 (1964).

NOTES AND QUESTIONS

1. A similar situation occurred in an experiment conducted in the summer of 1971 at Stanford University by Philip Zimbardo, a professor of psychology. He sought to study the psychology of imprisonment through simulation. The participants were randomly assigned to be guards or prisoners. The prisoners were told to wait at home or another agreed-upon location on a certain Sunday, and that they would be contacted. They were not told how the experiment would begin. They were then arrested by real police and taken into a prison created for the purpose of the study on the campus of Stanford University. They were all divided into two groups by a flip of a coin: one made up of prisoners and the other group made up of guards. After only the first two days, the "prisoners" had become fed up with having roll calls in the middle of the night and rebelled. They pushed their beds against their cell bars and refused to come out. The "guards" pulled the prisoners from their cells, stripped them naked, and proceeded to humiliate and abuse them for hours. The situation only worsened, and after only six days of the planned two-week study, Zimbardo ended the experiment. *See* Philip Zimbardo, *Stanford Prison Experiment,* available at http://www.prisonexp.org; Philip G. Zimbardo et al., *Reflections on the Stanford*

Prison Experiment: Genesis, Transformations, Consequences, in THOMAS BLASS (ed.), OBEDIENCE TO AUTHORITY: CURRENT PERSPECTIVES ON THE MILGRAM PARADIGM, available at www.prisonexp.org/pdf/blass.pdf.

2. Subsequently, Zimbardo had the following to say about his own research: "[I]t was unethical because people suffered and others were allowed to inflict pain and humiliation on their fellows over an extended period of time. . . . And, yes, we did not end the study soon enough. We should have terminated it as soon as the first prisoner suffered a severe stress disorder on day two." Philip G. Zimbardo et al., *supra*.

3. Zimbardo recently compared his experiment to the 2004 Abu Ghraib prison scandal in Iraq. He has explained that his experiment and the Iraqi prison situation were based on the same foundations and had similar results. In both situations, he argued, inexperienced guards were given little instruction, extraordinary power, and limited oversight, which resulted in prisoner abuse, although in Abu Ghraib that dynamic was heightened by the stress of war and death and the need for information from Iraqi prisoners. *See id.* at http://www.prisonexp.org/slide-33.htm; *see also* NATIONAL PUBLIC RADIO, PRISON PSYCHOLOGY AND THE STANFORD PRISON EXPERIMENT, available at http://www.npr.org/templates/story/story.php?storyId=1870756.

Chapter 2

THE CHANGING FACE OF RESEARCH: NEW REGULATIONS, NEW PLAYERS, NEW PLACES, NEW AGENDAS

Chapter 1 detailed a variety of research scandals in the United States that occurred before the last quarter of the twentieth century. In response to these scandals, Congress and the executive branch recognized the need for greater regulatory controls over research. There is now mandatory oversight of most research with human subjects, including a review of the consent documents that will be presented to subjects. It is likely that these reviews have improved the quality of the research being undertaken, reduced risks to subjects, and increased the flow of information to individuals considering whether to become subjects. Particularly over the last decade, however, new questions have been raised about the effectiveness of the existing oversight system. The chapters that follow will explore many of these concerns.

It is not only the regulatory environment that has changed, however. The entire nature of the research enterprise has undergone a significant transformation over the past several decades. There has been a marked revolution in how research is funded, who conducts it, and where it occurs. The very nature of the research agenda and how that agenda is set have been dramatically altered. This chapter will explore some of these changes and their implications for the future of research regulation.

§ 2.01 GOVERNMENTAL OVERSIGHT OF RESEARCH

[A] Federal Oversight: 1960s to 1990s

An Overview of Legal Controls on Human Experimentation and the Regulatory Implications of Taking Professor Katz Seriously
Jesse A. Goldner
38 Saint Louis U. L.J. 63, 93-100 (1993)

Prior to 1972, relatively little in the way of formal legal requirements for reviewing protocols or for obtaining the consent of subjects was imposed on researchers. Studies in the early 1960s indicated that some limited efforts at institutional peer review procedures had been made at a very few institutions. In 1962, Congress had passed legislation requiring that consent be obtained from patients involved in studies seeking Food and Drug Administration approval of new drugs, but it allowed for broad exceptions where obtaining consent was "not feasible" or not in the best interests of the subjects. Consequently, the requirement proved to be largely ineffective. . . .

Ultimately, early in 1966, the Surgeon General issued a directive stating that clinical research would be supported only if the judgment of the investigator would be subject to prior review by institutional associates concerning the issues of: (1) the rights and welfare of research subjects; (2) the appropriateness of the methods used to assure informed consent; and (3) the risks and medical benefits of the investigation.

Later revisions of this policy required institutions to assure the Public Health Service that investigations complied with local community laws, and gave "due consideration to pertinent ethical issues." The committees that were established, however, were typically comprised entirely of scientists and physicians, and there was little in the way of specific mandates to them beyond the language of the directive. By 1969, the guidelines did require that committee membership reflect "varying backgrounds . . . [and possess] competencies . . . in terms of institutional regulations, relevant law, standards of professional practice, and community acceptance." In May 1974 the Department of Health, Education and Welfare issued regulations mandating specific numerical requirements for committee membership and requiring that no committee or quorum could be comprised entirely of institution employees or members of a single professional group. . . .

The National Research Act and the Belmont Report

At the same time that some advances were being made within the Public Health Service, the disclosures of many of the experiments [described in Chapter 1] led to U.S. Senate hearings on the control of research with human subjects and ultimately to the passage of the National Research Act of 1974. That legislation established the National Commission for the Protection of Human Subjects of Biomedical and Behavioral Research, which was to conduct a comprehensive investigation and study to identify basic ethical principles that would underlie the conduct of human subjects research and to recommend guidelines that could apply to human subjects research supported by the then Department of Health, Education and Welfare.

What emerged from the charge to the National Commission to identify relevant ethical principles was the 1979 *Belmont Report* (the Report). This document of twenty pages briefly discussed the line to be drawn between the practice of biomedical and behavioral therapy and research and identified three philosophical principles or prescriptive judgments which were particularly relevant to research involving human subjects: respect for persons, beneficence and justice. . . .

The National Research Act of 1974 also required

> that each entity which applies for a grant or contract which involves the conduct of biomedical or behavioral research involving human subjects submit . . . assurances satisfactory to the Secretary of Health, Education and Welfare that it has established a board (to be known as an Institutional Review Board) to review biomedical and behavioral research involving human subjects conducted or sponsored by the institution in order to protect the rights of the human subjects of research.

. . .

Current Federal Regulations for the Protection of Human Subjects

IRB Jurisdiction and Federal Oversight   Institutional Review Board

While by the terms of the regulations, IRB review is only required for federally funded research protocols, for the most part, institutions such as universities, medical schools and research hospitals which have "negotiated" these assurances with the federal government, pledging conformity with the regulations have made them applicable to all research, irrespective of the source of funding. In addition, a separate set of requirements, issued by the Food and Drug Administration, but which very closely tracks these regulations, mandates IRB review of all investigational studies designed to support applications to the FDA for the marketing of drugs and medical devices. There is no "negotiated assurance" procedure, but the FDA conducts on-site inspections in which compliance with the regulations is evaluated. The result is that hundreds of IRBs review thousands of research protocols each year.

The regulations give institutions wide discretion in establishing the structure, procedures and membership of the IRB, in order to be eligible for receipt of federal research funds. Each institution engaged in research covered by the regulations must provide satisfactory "written assurance" that it is meeting each of the requirements mandated by the federal government for the protection of human subjects of biomedical and behavioral research. . . . Apart from this . . . [assurance process and its requirements for reporting violations], there is no other formal mechanism whereby the activities of IRBs are in any way monitored by the federal government.

In its 1978 report on IRBs, the National Commission explained:

> The ethical conduct of research requires a balancing of society's interest in protecting the rights of subjects and in developing knowledge that can benefit the subjects or society as a whole. . . .
>
> [I]nvestigators should not have sole responsibility for determining whether research involving human subjects fulfills ethical standards. Others who are independent of the research must share this responsibility, because investigators are always in positions of potential conflict

by virtue of their concern with the pursuit of knowledge as well as the welfare of the human subjects of their research. . . .

[T]he rights of subjects should be protected by local review committees operating pursuant to federal regulations and located in institutions where research involving human subjects is conducted. Compared to the possible alternatives of a regional or national review process, local committees have the advantage of greater familiarity with the actual conditions surrounding the conduct of research.

At first blush, this decentralization of authority may appear to be extraordinary, in that non-governmentally appointed bodies, appointed by organizations within the private sector, are given significant control. In fact, however, this is not at all unusual. In fact, since 1935, the United States Supreme Court has not invalidated a public regulation delegation to the private sector. Generally, delegation of public powers is sustainable with "adequate procedural safeguards, appropriate legislative supervision or reexamination, and the accustomed scope of judicial review."

THE BELMONT REPORT: ETHICAL PRINCIPLES AND GUIDELINES FOR THE PROTECTION OF HUMAN SUBJECTS OF RESEARCH NATIONAL COMMISSION FOR THE PROTECTION OF HUMAN SUBJECTS OF BIOMEDICAL AND BEHAVIORAL RESEARCH
(1979)

The full text of this document is reproduced in Appendix F. Please read it before proceeding.

NOTES AND QUESTIONS

1. How does the Belmont Report address the distinction between practice and research? Does it deem all departures from accepted practice to be research? At what point should such departures become part of a formal research protocol? For further discussion of this distinction, see Chapter 3, at page 109.

2. What does the notion of "respect for persons" mean?

3. What does the principle of beneficence entail? How does it apply to an individual protocol? To research in general?

4. Can research on vulnerable populations (e.g., children or prisoners) ever be consistent with the principles of respect for persons or beneficence when the subjects will not benefit from participating in the study? If not, should such research be permitted? These issues are explored further in Part III of this book. .

5. What does the Report mean by the "principle of justice"?

6. In the Report's discussion of informed consent, what standard is proposed for determining the minimum level of information to be provided to subjects? How does this standard differ, if at all, from the standard governing informed consent to ordinary medical treatment?

7. What does the Report say about how the relationship between the risks and potential benefits of research ought to be assessed?

8. In the years following the National Commission, the federal government has convened eight other bioethics commissions. Some were chartered or appointed by Congress, others created by a presidential executive order or appointed by the Secretary of the Department of Health and Human Services (DHHS) or its predecessor, the Department of Health, Education and Welfare. Each was intended to assist in the national debate on bioethical issues, including research with human subjects. The results of their efforts have not been nearly as influential as the Belmont Report. Among the more notable such operations were the following:

a. The President's Commission for the Study of Ethical Problems in Medicine and Biomedical and Behavioral Research ("President's Commission") (1980-1983), which continued some of the work of the National Commission in examining issues regarding federal regulation of research with human subjects and compensation for research injuries. The Commission issued 11 reports addressing, among other topics, "whistleblowing" in biomedical research, genetic screening and counseling, the definition of death, and access to health care.

b. The National Bioethics Advisory Commission ("NBAC") (1995-2001), created by a Presidential executive order, published six reports: CLONING HUMAN BEINGS (1997), RESEARCH INVOLVING PERSONS WITH MENTAL DISORDERS THAT MAY AFFECT DECISIONMAKING CAPACITY (1998), RESEARCH INVOLVING BIOLOGICAL MATERIALS: ETHICAL ISSUES AND POLICY GUIDANCE (1999), ETHICAL ISSUES IN HUMAN STEM CELL RESEARCH (1999), ETHICAL AND POLICY ISSUES IN INTERNATIONAL RESEARCH: CLINICAL TRIALS IN DEVELOPING COUNTRIES (2001), and ETHICAL AND POLICY ISSUES IN RESEARCH INVOLVING HUMAN PARTICIPANTS (2001). All of these reports are available at http://www.georgetown.edu/research/nrcbl/nbac/.

c. The federal Advisory Committee on Human Radiation Experiments (ACHRE) (described in Chapter 1), issued its report in 1995. In addition to addressing matters specific to radiation experiments, ACHRE identified other problems related to the conduct of research with human subjects through a variety of empirical studies. These included findings that patients with serious illnesses often have unrealistic expectations about the prospect of benefiting directly from participating in research, and that consent forms are often overly optimistic about the likely benefits to subjects, insufficiently clear about the impact of research on subjects' quality of life and personal finances, and generally incomprehensible to laypeople.

d. The National Human Research Protections Advisory Committee (NHRPAC) (2000-2002), established by the Secretary of DHHS, issued one report, on confidentiality and research data protections. In addition, before its charter expired, it created a series of workgroups in a number of other areas. The groups dealing with subjects who lack decision-making capacity and with children issued final reports, and the genetics workgroup issued a draft report. These reports are available at http://www.hhs.gov/ohrp/nhrpac/ nhrpac.htm.

e. In 2002, NHRPAC was replaced by the Secretary's Advisory Committee on Human Subject Protections (SACHRP), which remains in existence as this book goes to press. Details about its activities are available at http://www.hhs.gov/ohrp/sachrp.

f. NBAC was replaced by the President's Council on Bioethics (the "Council"), which, like its predecessor, was created by Executive Order, issued in November 2001. The Council's mission was broadly defined as providing advice "on bioethical issues that may emerge as a consequence of advances in biomedical science and technology." It was specifically authorized to study questions regarding the protection of human subjects in research. The Council has issued reports on a variety of topics, including cloning, regulation of new reproductive technologies, stem cell research, and the uses and limitations of biotechnology. It also remains in existence as this book goes to press. Information about its activities, including the full text of most of its reports, can be found at http://bioethics.gov.

9. A variety of commissions have also been created at the state level. In New York, for example, Governor Mario Cuomo created the New York State Task Force on Life and the Law in 1985 to recommend public policy on issues raised by medical advances. The Task Force's reports on assisted reproductive technologies and genetic testing are discussed in Chapter 16 and 17, respectively. The New York State Department of Health also has convened several workgroups to develop policy recommendations on specific aspects of research, including research with normal, healthy subjects and subjects who lack decision-making capacity. In Maryland, the state Attorney General created a commission to recommend legislation on research with decisionally impaired subjects.

10. When national and state-level commissions and committees have commented, and their suggestions have not been turned into legislation or regulations, how should IRBs interpret that lack of action? Do these reports have some moral authority even if they have no regulatory or legal authority? Or does the government's failure to incorporate a commission's recommendations into law or policy suggest that the recommendations are somehow deficient?

[B] New Directions in Federal Regulation: 1996-2003

By the end of 1996, federal authorities had cited only seven institutions for violating rules regarding the conduct of research with human subjects. All of these institutions were permitted to continue to do research under close government supervision. *See* Paulette V. Walker, *Government Oversight on Research on Humans Draws Fire*, CHRONICLE HIGHER EDUC., November 8, 1996, at A29.

In 1998, the Office of the Inspector General (OIG) of DHHS issued a report charging that IRBs faced overwhelming workloads and often provided perfunctory oversight of studies. The OIG extensively reviewed federal records, interviewed government officials and members of 75 IRBs, and visited six academic health centers engaged in clinical research. The report claimed that IRBs assessed too many research proposals, too quickly, and with too little expertise. It noted that, over a five-year period, IRB workloads had increased by an average of 42 percent, with some panels overseeing as many as 2,000 experiments a year. During this period, the size of the boards and their budgets had remained the same. The report also asserted that potential conflicts of interest and inadequate training hindered the IRBs' effectiveness. *See* OFFICE OF THE INSPECTOR GENERAL, DEPARTMENT OF HEALTH AND HUMAN SERVICES, INSTITUTIONAL REVIEW BOARDS: A TIME FOR REFORM (1998), available at http://oig.hhs.gov/oei/reports/oei-01-97-00193.pdf.

U.S. Officials Order Duke Medical Center to Suspend Research Involving Humans
Paulette Walker Campbell
CHRONICLE HIGHER EDUC., May 21, 1999, at A35

Citing lax safety and oversight procedures, a federal agency has suspended nearly all government-sponsored research involving humans at the Duke University Medical Center, one of the nation's top locations for clinical research. . . .

This is only the fourth time in 10 years that the research-protection office has suspended an institution's federal license to conduct human research. The action came after the office concluded that Duke's medical center had failed to correct more than 20 deficiencies in its system for protecting human research subjects.

Many of the infractions may be common at research universities around the country, according to recent studies.

The problems involved Duke's institutional review board. . . . In June, the Inspector General of the Department of Health and Human Services issued a report on review boards nationwide specifying instances of conflicts of interest and inadequate training — two of the deficiencies found at Duke. The federal General Accounting Office identified similar lapses in a 1997 report.

Among the problems cited by the research-protection office was a failure by Duke's review board to monitor studies once they had begun. Such monitoring is the primary means of insuring that human subjects are not unexpectedly harmed by the research, explain federal officials. The review board was also criticized for having failed to insure that studies involving children included the safeguards required by federal regulations.

The research-protection office also found that the review board had failed to comply fully with federal conflict-of-interest rules. The membership of the Duke medical center's review board included the director and the assistant director of the university's Office of Grants and Contracts, which is responsible for bringing in grants.

NOTES AND QUESTIONS

1. The Duke suspension was just one of many involving major research centers between 1998 and 2000. Prior to the Duke shutdown, in October 1998, the Office for Protection from Research Risks (OPRR), the predecessor agency to the present Office for Human Research Protections (OHRP), suspended research at Rush-Presbyterian-St. Luke's Medical Center in Chicago, the West Los Angeles Veterans Affairs Medical Center, and the University of Illinois-Chicago. After Duke, federal authorities suspended or restricted research at the University of Alabama-Birmingham, the University of Pennsylvania, and Virginia Commonwealth University. Thereafter, either OPRR or the Food and Drug Administration (FDA) halted or restricted research at a variety of other institutions, including St. Jude's Children's Research Hospital, University of Colorado Health Sciences Center, the University of Oklahoma College of Medicine in Tulsa, the University of Texas Medical Branch at Galveston, and the University of Miami. *See IRBs: Facing a Crackdown*, 7 CENTER WATCH (ARTICLE # 165) (April, 2000); P.J. Hilts, *Safety Concerns Halt Oklahoma Research*, N.Y. TIMES, July 11, 2000, at F12; J. Brainard, *Federal Regulators Call on 2 Universities to Suspend Studies Involving Prisoners*, CHRONICLE HIGHER EDUC., Sept. 15, 2000, at A26.

The suspensions and restrictions by OPRR and by the FDA were based on findings that the institutions were not following regulations designed to protect the safety and dignity of research subjects. While the specific reasons for the federal agencies' finding of non-compliance varied from one institution to another, some of the common concerns included the following:

   a. IRBs acting improperly by approving inadequate protocols or informed-consent documents

   b. Insufficient information regarding plans for subject recruitment and enrollment

   c. Questions about the equitable selection of subjects

d. Protocol deficiencies in protecting subject privacy and confidentiality

e. Lack of quorums at IRB meetings

f. The inappropriate granting of exemptions from IRB review

g. Omissions of required elements in informed-consent documents and failure to provide adequate detail regarding certain elements

h. Inappropriately complex consent documents

i. Inadequate IRB resources

j. Overburdened IRBs

2. Duke University made a number of changes in the ten months immediately following the four-day suspension of its authority to conduct research with human subjects. These changes included: (a) increasing the number of IRBs, from one to two, and making plans to add at least two more; (b) sponsoring a ninety-minute course on the regulation and history of medical research with human subjects and requiring that all 1,350 clinical investigators at the medical center take the course; (c) providing up to forty hours of training for each IRB member; (d) increasing the size of the support staff for its IRBs, from two full-time positions to 11; and (e) increasing the staff support budget from approximately $100,000 to about $1 million. *See* Jeffrey Brainerd, *Duke Tries to Rebuild Confidence in Its System for Protecting Research Subjects*, CHRONICLE HIGHER EDUC., March 17, 2000, at A32.

3. In April 2000, the OIG issued a follow-up to its 1998 report. The new study concluded that only "minimal progress" had been made by the National Institutes of Health (NIH; at the time, the home of OPRR) and the FDA in improving IRBs during the interim period, and that these agencies could do more to monitor and assist IRBs. It also criticized the failure to streamline federal regulatory provisions so as to decrease the workload on IRBs. The study applauded OPRR's decision to suspend research at various institutions and urged such enforcement actions to continue. It noted that the FDA had increased its on-site inspections of IRBs from 213 in the 1997 fiscal year to 336 in 1999. *See* OFFICE OF THE INSPECTOR GENERAL, DEPARTMENT OF HEALTH AND HUMAN SERVICES, PROTECTING HUMAN SUBJECTS: STATUS OF RECOMMENDATIONS (2000), available at oig.hhs.gov/oei/reports/oei-01-97-00197.pdf.

4. One of the more highly publicized actions taken by OPRR occurred in July 2001, when it halted all federally financed medical studies on human subjects at Johns Hopkins University's School of Medicine, shortly after the death of a healthy young woman in a research study at that institution. Among the major findings were the failure to individually present and discuss most new protocols and the failure to conduct continuing reviews of previously approved studies at convened IRB meetings. The Johns Hopkins suspension is discussed further in Chapter 4, at page 182.

5. Are fines an appropriate remedy for violations of human subject protection regulations? If not, in addition to the suspension of an institution's authority to conduct research, what other actions ought to be available to regulatory authorities? *sus pulic qnts*

6. Because OHRP's findings are posted on the agency's Web site, should OHRP assume that IRBs at other institutions have received notice of problem areas, and therefore impose harsher penalties if the same problems arise in subsequent investigations?

7. How do you think IRB members reacted to these enforcement efforts? What about researchers? University officials? Were the regulators' actions necessary wake-up calls to research institutions? Or were they just unreasonable grandstanding? Note that several of the suspensions included no allegations that human subjects had been injured by risky experiments or had not given informed consent. Might the primary effect of the suspensions have been to encourage IRBs to spend inordinate amounts of time attending to procedural requirements, thus diluting efforts at substantive review of research protocols? Do the enforcement actions, which necessitated a significant increase in resources devoted to IRB activities, essentially impose an "unfunded mandate" on these largely not-for-profit institutions?

8. It can be argued that part of the reason for the surge in government actions during this period was a combination of government reports, such as the 1998 OIG document discussed at the beginning of this section, and Congressional hearings and investigations suggesting that IRBs were doing too little. OPRR had been portrayed during these hearings as being "bureaucratically impotent," and questions had been raised about whether the OPRR's position within the NIH, which sponsored much research regulated by OPRR, might have created "the appearance and actuality of a conflict of interest." Rick Weiss, *Panel Urges Major Upgrade for Medical Research Safety Office*, WASHINGTON POST, June 4, 1999, at A16. In June 2000, the Secretary of DHHS, following the recommendation of a committee that she had appointed, ordered that OPRR be moved out of the NIH. The office was renamed the Office for Human Research Protections (OHRP) and placed in the Office of the Assistant Secretary of Health, where it would have more clout and no longer be subject to the conflicts that arise when an office at the bottom of an organization is regulating entities high above itself. Shortly thereafter, Gary Ellis, the director of OPRR when most of the suspensions occurred, was assigned to other duties within NIH. Some speculated that this action was the result of NIH and university officials' perceptions that his enforcement activities were overzealous, and was a sign that future enforcement would be less strict. *See* Jeffrey Brainard, *Will 'Fresh Face' Bring a New Approach to Federal Protection of Human Subjects?* CHRONICLE HIGHER EDUC., July 21, 2000, at A21. During the next two years, Dr. Greg Koski, Ellis's successor, was viewed as having a friendlier, more cooperative relationship with academic institutions. *See* Jeffrey Brainerd, *New Human-Subjects Chief Will Face Challenges and Controversies,* CHRONICLE HIGHER

EDUC., Nov. 22, 2002, at A25. During Koski's tenure, only one institution (Johns Hopkins, as noted above) was subject to an enforcement action suspending research, but it was a rather significant one.

§ 2.02 BIOMEDICAL ADVANCES, NEW FUNDING, NEW PLACES, NEW PLAYERS

[A] Research Successes of the 1980s and 1990s

PHARMACEUTICAL INDUSTRY PROFILE
PHARMACEUTICAL RESEARCH AND MANUFACTURERS OF AMERICA
7-8 (2001)
http://www.phrma.org/publications/publications/profile01/index.phtml

The following is a partial chronology of drug innovations of the 1980s through 1990s:

1981 — ACE inhibitors and calcium channel blockers are approved. . . .

1986 — First genetically engineered interferons are approved for the treatment of hairy cell leukemia. Later these drugs will be approved to treat such diverse conditions as genital warts, AIDS-related Kaposi's sarcoma, hepatitis C, hepatitis B, and other diseases.

1987 — Zidovudine, the first medicine approved to treat AIDS, is introduced.

1987 — First statin, a cholesterol-lowering drug, is approved.

1987 — Fluoxetine — the first selective serotonin reuptake inhibitor, is introduced and revolutionizes the treatment of depression. . . .

1994 — A breakthrough drug for breast, ovarian, and other cancers, made from the bark of the Pacific yew tree, is introduced.

1995 — Saquinavir becomes the first protease inhibitor to be approved by the FDA for the treatment of AIDS. Over the next three years, combination of drug therapy, including a protease inhibitor, will reduce AIDS deaths in the U.S. by 70 percent.

1995 — The first vaccine for chicken pox is approved by the FDA.

1995 — The first vaccine against hepatitis A is introduced. . . .

1997 — The first monoclonal antibody to treat cancer is approved, for non-Hodgkins lymphoma.

1998 — FDA approved Fomivirsen, the first of a class of drugs that fights disease by switching off the gene that triggers it. Known as an antisense drug, Fomivirsen is injected into AIDS patients with CMV retinitis, a virus that can cause blindness.

Pharmaceutical developments have led to a significant decrease in cancer death rates since 1991, and even more rapid declines since 1995. As of 2001, over 402 new cancer drugs were in development. ACE inhibitors, introduced in 1981, and clot-dissolving drugs, pioneered in the 1980s, had cut the risk of coronary death by more than 40 percent, and 122 new medicines for cardio-vascular diseases were being developed. *See id.* at 3, 4, 7, 8.

SELECTED RESEARCH ADVANCES OF NIH
http://history.nih.gov/history/advances.htm#2002

[The NIH Web site lists a variety of research advances supported by the agency from its inception to the present. In 2002 alone, more than fifty such instances are described, including the following:]

Mouse Genome Sequenced — The international Mouse Genome Sequencing Consortium, jointly funded by several NIH Institutes along with the Wellcome Trust, published a high-quality draft sequence of the mouse genome — the genetic blueprint of a mouse — together with a comparative analysis of the mouse and human genomes. This is the first time scientists have compared the human genome with another mammal's. Because the mouse carries a very similar set of genes, this information will allow scientists to learn more about human genes and the proteins they encode, leading to a better understanding of human disease and improved treatments and cures. The sequence is posted on the Internet, where it is freely available. . . .

Detecting Ovarian Cancer — By uniting proteomics and an artificial intelligence program, scientists from NIH and the Food and Drug Administration reported that patterns of proteins found in patients' blood serum may reflect the presence of ovarian cancer, even at early stages. The test can be completed in 30 minutes and uses blood obtained from a finger prick. The emerging concept that an entire pattern of proteins can contain important diagnostic information is potentially applicable to any type of disease. . . .

Improved Diet and Exercise Delays Type 2 Diabetes — A major clinical trial sponsored by NIH found that people at high risk for type 2 diabetes can delay and possibly prevent the disease by improving their diet and exercising. Diet and exercise leading to weight loss of 5 to 7 percent reduced diabetes incidence by 58 percent in people at high risk. The study found that the oral diabetes drug metformin (Glucophage) also reduces type 2 diabetes risk, although not as effectively as lifestyle changes. . . .

Key Gene Identified in Cleft Lip and Palate — Scientists supported by NIH discovered the gene that causes Van der Woude syndrome, which causes cleft lip and palate along with other birth defects. The gene, called IRF6, seems to play a key role in the normal formation of the lips, palate, skin, and genitalia. Further study of the gene should provide molecular clues into normal human development and might suggest strategies to prevent birth defects such as cleft lip and palate. . . .

First Vaccine Against Deadly Staph Bacteria — NIH scientists and the company Nabi have developed the first successful vaccine against Staphylococcus aureus, a major cause of infection and death among hospital patients. This bacterium causes illnesses ranging from minor skin infections to life threatening diseases such as severe pneumonia, meningitis, and infections of the heart and bloodstream. Recently, researchers have discovered strains of the bacteria that are resistant to the antibiotics used to treat them, making a preventive vaccine critical. . . .

Eye Drops Treat Lazy Eye — Scientists supported by NIH found that atropine eye drops given once a day to treat moderate amblyopia, or lazy eye, work as well as the standard treatment of patching one eye.

[B] How Much Do We Spend on Research?

Significant public support for biomedical research in the United States is a relatively recent phenomenon. In 1940, the largest sources of biomedical research funding in the United States were corporations and nonprofit organizations. They spent $25 million and $17 million, respectively (not adjusted for inflation). On the other hand, federal agencies' spending for biomedical research was primarily directed to the agencies' own laboratories and equaled only $3 million, or less than seven percent of the total. *See* INSTITUTE OF MEDICINE, SOURCES OF MEDICAL TECHNOLOGY: UNIVERSITIES AND INDUSTRY (1995).

Obtaining precise figures on patterns of overall spending for various types of health-related research is a challenge. Nonetheless, some approximations are possible. For example, it has been reported that the total spending for biomedical research in 2000 was approximately $88 to $95 billion. Federal spending was estimated at approximately $25 billion, private foundation support contributed approximately $8 to $10 billion, and private industry contributed as much as $55 to $60 billion. While the NIH budget has increased significantly in recent years, expenditures by private organizations have increased even more rapidly. *See* INSTITUTE OF MEDICINE, ACADEMIC HEALTH CENTERS LEADING CHANGE IN THE 21st CENTURY 94 (2004). The Pharmaceutical Research and Manufacturers of America (PhRMA), which represents the country's leading research-based pharmaceutical and biotechnology companies, claims that its members alone invested an estimated $33.2 billion in research in 2003. *See* PhRMA, WHO WE ARE, available at http://www.phrma.org/whoweare/.

NOTES AND QUESTIONS

1. Can the figures presented by the pharmaceutical industry be trusted? Marcia Angell, a former editor-in-chief of the *New England Journal of Medicine*, argues that the industry's claims regarding how much it spends on research and development are vastly inflated, and that those costs are far exceeded by the industry's profits. She suggests that companies include in their research and development many activities that should be viewed as marketing. *See* MARCIA ANGELL, THE TRUTH ABOUT DRUG COMPANIES: HOW THEY DECEIVE US AND WHAT TO DO ABOUT IT 12, 156-72 (2004). Should we be concerned about how much the pharmaceutical industry spends on research as compared to marketing?

2. Irrespective of the precise amounts being spent, do such large investments in biomedical research make sense when compared to expenditures for other societal needs, both within health care (such as screenings and other forms of preventive medicine) and in other areas (such as education, job training, housing, etc.)?

3. The pharmaceutical industry uses its claims about the high research and development costs of new drugs to justify the high prices that are charged for them, and to fight efforts to impose price controls on the industry. Angell argues that "[i]mplicit in this claim is a kind of blackmail: If you want drug companies to keep turning out life-saving drugs you will gratefully pay whatever they charge. Otherwise you may wake up one morning and find there are no more new drugs." *Id.* at 37-38.

4. Americans pay more for drugs than individuals in any other industrialized country. The industry admits this, but, particularly whenever the issue of possible price controls in various American markets, such as Medicare, arises, it claims that the disparity exists because other countries regulate prices, leaving Americans to pay a disproportionate percent of research and development costs. The industry further argues that Americans must bear a disproportionate share of those costs because nobody else will. *See* ANGELL, *supra*, at 38, 217-223. What do you think about the fact that Americans pay more for drugs than people in other countries? Does it matter that, unlike the situation fifty years ago, many of the most popular and costly drugs are now crucial to the health and well-being of persons with chronic and acute illnesses?

5. What connection, if any, do you see between the high prices of drugs and human subject protection?

[C] The Changing Role of Academic Health Centers in Research

In the 1970s, American health care institutions began to experience a variety of financial pressures. These pressures had significant implications for academic health centers (AHCs) (formerly known as academic medical centers), where, until recently, the majority of medical research was conducted. Multiple causes contributed to these difficulties. Kenneth Ludmerer describes many of these causes in his 1999 book, TIME TO HEAL: AMERICAN MEDICAL EDUCATION FROM THE TURN OF THE CENTURY TO THE ERA OF MANAGED CARE, from which the following discussion is drawn.

In the late 1960s, in part to pay for the Vietnam War, the high annual increases in the growth of appropriations for the NIH began to decline. The double-digit inflation rates of the late 1970s and federal budget deficits in the 1990s meant that the growth rate of NIH funding frequently fell in real dollars. In the early days of the NIH, after World War II, the theory was that all meritorious research projects should be funded, and fifty percent of them, in fact, did receive support. By the early 1990s, the funding rate declined to twelve percent, even though ninety percent of the projects were viewed as being worthy of funding. Two-thirds of applications for renewal were denied.

Historically, many of the AHC facilities have been located in inner cities. As wealthier inhabitants of these areas began to move to the suburbs, they sought more sophisticated specialty care from some of the larger community hospitals. The result was a decline in the rate of increase of clinical income in the academically-oriented institutions. In addition, while state legislative efforts to minimize unnecessary building of expensive health care facilities had some early salutary effects, these requirements soon began to vanish. Reimbursements for Medicare, and especially for Medicaid — a critical source of support for inner-city hospitals with large poor populations — regularly began to grow more slowly, if not actually decline, both through changes in allocation formulas and through overall budgetary limitations. Large employers within the community, frequently principal payors of health care expenditures through employment-based health insurance, began to organize and insist that providers, both individual practitioners and institutions, compete for their employees/patients by offering bulk rate discounts. The advent of managed care throughout the insurance industry had similar effects.

At the same time, the development of faculty practice plans (group medical practices whose members are comprised of medical school faculty who offer services to patients on a fee-for-service basis) meant that individual faculty members could earn large amounts of compensation from clinical care, rather than allowing those monies to be used to support teaching and research. In addition, some basic scientists and clinicians became wealthy through entrepreneurial activities involving biotechnology operations and the like, royalties from patents that proved to have commercial value, large consulting fees from companies, and awards of stock and stock options. This sea change in financial arrangements seemed to indicate that, for many in medicine, the altruistic approaches of the past had become little more than a memory. Results of the commercialization of biomedical research have included a marked increase in the potential for conflicts of interest and scientific misconduct, including plagiarism, misrepresentation of results and fabrication of data, and a skewing of the scientific issues that investigators choose to explore.

Beginning in the 1970s, as a result of the decline in traditional sources of research funding, academic health centers began to look for research support from non-governmental sources. One likely source was the pharmaceutical industry, which had both increased in size and begun to develop better relations with academia. Large private foundations were also tapped. Increasingly, clinical practice income was used to support research and education, but relatively speaking, clinical income, as noted, has been on the decline. The result was increased tension between teaching and research in the 1970s and 1980s. From the point of view of advancement within academic medicine, success at research was more easily quantifiable than success in teaching, although the quality and significance of what was published often was dubious. A 1990 study of papers published in 1981-1985 showed that eighty percent of them were never cited more than once.

Finally, contrary to the situation that had existed previously, the attitude of medical schools toward developing relationships with industry began to change. Universities began entering into contracts permitting companies to license the research that had occurred within the universities in exchange for substantial funding streams for research. The federal government, through the passage of the Patent and Trademark Amendments (Bayh-Dole) Act of 1980, further encouraged these relationships by allowing universities and other not-for-profit entities to retain ownership of inventions from federally supported research. This fostered the promotion of technology transfer, which is designed to develop commercially useful products from government-sponsored basic research. In 1986, legislation gave universities the ability to own startup companies based on their faculties' work.

See KENNETH LUDMERER, TIME TO HEAL: AMERICAN MEDICAL EDUCATION FROM THE TURN OF THE CENTURY TO THE ERA OF MANAGED CARE, 260-79, 283-87, 310, 340-44 (1999).

[1] The Bayh-Dole Act

35 U.S.C. § 200, PATENTS: PART II. PATENTABILITY OF INVENTIONS AND GRANT OF PATENTS CHAPTER 18, PATENT RIGHTS IN INVENTIONS MADE WITH FEDERAL ASSISTANCE
(Bayh-Dole Act)

It is the policy and objective of the Congress to use the patent system to promote the utilization of inventions arising from federally supported research and development; to encourage maximum participation of small business firms in federally supported research and development efforts; to promote collaboration between commercial concerns and nonprofit organizations, including universities; to ensure that inventions made by nonprofit organizations and small business firms are used in a manner to promote free competition and enterprise without unduly encumbering future research and discovery; to promote free competition and enterprise without unduly encumbering future research and discovery; to promote the commercialization and public availability of inventions made in the United States by United States industry and labor; to ensure that the Government obtains sufficient rights in federally supported inventions to meet the needs of the Government and protect the public against nonuse or unreasonable use of inventions; and to minimize the costs of administering policies in this area.

Dealing with Conflicts of Interest in Biomedical Research: IRB Oversight as the Next Best Solution to the Abolitionist Approach
Jesse A. Goldner
28 J. L. MED. & ETHICS 379, 384, 385 (2000)

[T]he passage of the Bayh-Dole Act in 1980 . . . "encourages academic institutions supported by federal grants to patent and license new products developed by their faculty members and to share royalties with the researchers." The National Institutes of Health (NIH) has a standard process for determining who can take title to an invention and file a patent application. After notifying the NIH of an invention, the awardee institution has two years to determine if it will do so, and if the researcher himself will share any profits. If the institution does not elect to take title, then the NIH can choose to do so, in which case the individual inventor is also guaranteed a portion of any royalties received. However, if the NIH does not take title, then the researcher-inventor may file for a patent.

The passage of the Bayh-Dole Act has also compounded institutional conflicts of interest. Under the Act, sponsoring universities are given intellectual property rights in the inventions created with federal funding. These rights are then freely transferable to private companies. The purpose of the Bayh-Dole Act was to establish uniform vesting of patent rights in inventions resulting from federally funded research as well as to encourage the commercialization of such inventions. The result, however, has been to give academic institutions and researchers intellectual property rights. Thus, the institution may potentially obtain valuable patent rights as a direct result of research conducted at the university. Furthermore, the passage of the Bayh-Dole Act has also strengthened the ties between academic institutions and for-profit industries because academic institutions need an avenue to facilitate the movement of new products, such as drugs or devices, from the institution to the marketplace. Such ongoing relationships, however, may prove to be problematic in the long run as universities may become increasingly tempted to lose their objectivity.

NOTES AND QUESTIONS

1. Apart from the concerns about institutional conflicts of interest, on balance was the Bayh-Dole Act, designed to hasten the translation of basic research that was supported by tax dollars into useful new products, wise public policy? Angell argues that, before the legislation, all taxpayer-financed discoveries were in the public domain and available to whatever companies wanted to use them. Now, by contrast, universities, where most NIH-sponsored research takes place, can patent and license their discoveries and charge royalties for those who use them, allowing drug companies, to whom the patents are typically licensed, to cash in on the public investment. "While Bayh-Dole was clearly a bonanza for big pharma and the biotech industry, whether it is a net benefit to the public is arguable." ANGELL, *supra*, at 7-8.

2. To what extent should the cost of drugs that came to fruition largely with federal funding reflect the significant public investment in their development? Angell notes that many of the most significant drug discoveries now produced commercially, such as AZT (used to treat HIV/AIDS), Taxol (the best selling cancer drug), Epogen (to treat anemia in patients with kidney failure), and Procrit (to treat other forms of anemia), were developed with NIH funding. *See* ANGELL, *supra*, at 24-27, 57-62. Many such drugs have provided some of the largest profits to drug companies. The Bayh-Dole Act requires that work licensed to pharmaceutical companies be made "available to the public on reasonable terms." The significance of this phrase is not entirely clear but, as Angell points out, it could be interpreted to mean that the drugs should be priced reasonably. She claims that this and other public interest protections written into the legislation have been largely ignored, and that often the pricing of drugs that emerge from research supported by federal funds is exorbitant. *See id.* at 58-71.

3. In a recent article in the *New England Journal of Medicine*, Hamilton Moses and colleagues report that "[t]he relationships between academic insti-

tutions and private companies are strengthening. The decision of several large pharmaceutical companies, and many biotechnology companies, to build major new laboratories near U.S., European, and Asian universities is just one example of the growing commercial value of academic innovation in biomedicine and the talent that produces it." They note that academia and industry have similar needs. Each requires access to specialized talent at a variety of levels, from senior investigators through postdoctoral fellows. The growing scale of research also fosters collaboration between industry and the academy. There is increased dependence on sophisticated techniques and complex equipment, both of which have high initial and maintenance costs. Frequently, universities are unable to foot the bill, and thus they seek industry support or collaboration. At the same time, the increasing emphasis on genetics research requires access to well-characterized clinical populations and biological material from both "normal" and affected persons. It also requires sophisticated knowledge of bioinformatics and computational biology. Such resources, which are normally unavailable to industry, can readily be provided by academic health centers. *See* Hamilton Moses III et al., *Collaborating with Industry — Choices for the Academic Medical Center*, 347 NEW ENG. J. MED. 1371, 1371-72 (2002).

[2] Current Clinical Research Funding Streams

Curing Conflicts of Interest in Clinical Research: Impossible Dreams and Harsh Realities
Patricia C. Kuszler
8 WIDENER L. SYMP. J. 115, 115-23 (2001)

Although lack of funding is frequently decried as a barrier to research, little empirical evidence supports this hypothesis. Clinical research is simultaneously financed by several contemporaneous, intertwined funding streams. It is not unusual for federal grant dollars, private industry support, third-party payments, and direct patient payment to all be in play in a given clinical research project. . . .

1. Federal Funding

. . . On the individual front, research scientists and clinicians develop and test new drugs, devices, and procedures in research funded by federal grants. Typically, this is in the form of salary support, usually phrased as a percentage of total work effort. This compensation is funneled through the institutional employer — usually the university or the academic medical center. In the case of research clinicians, this salary support will apply to their income as employees of the university or academic medical center. It is likely only one of the several income streams enjoyed by the researcher.

The academic medical center will benefit financially from clinical research through compensation by the government grantor for the costs it incurs for the trial. These generally are skimmed off the top of the grant award as so-called "indirect costs" of the institution. It is not unusual for academic medical center and university indirect costs to consume half of the grant award. In addition, the academic medical center will benefit from federal grant awards by being able to recapture salary of researchers who are supported by the grant. Most academic researchers, although dependent on "soft money," do have the safety net of a guaranteed salary from the university or medical center. Thus, when a grantee receives a percentage of salary support from the grant, the institution will also indirectly benefit by being freed from this percentage of the salary expense.

2. Private Sponsor Funding

Although the federal government has been the primary source of funding for clinical research in the past, it has been superseded by private industry in the last decade. There is a pronounced trend toward a greater percentage of research being funded by the private sector. One study has shown that 28% of life sciences faculty received private sponsor funding. In 1986, the private sector funded 42% of health care research and development. By 1995, the private sector's allocation of research dollars had risen to 52%. . . .

Research clinicians receive compensation from the sponsor for their work on the clinical trial. This may be in the form of salary support, honoraria, or even in some cases, per-head payment for recruitment of human subjects. The researcher may also serve as the spokesperson for the new innovation. In return for this activity, the researcher may receive additional compensation for presenting the new technology or treatment at academic and industry meetings and conferences. . . .

3. Third-Party Payers Funding Clinical Research

In the case of clinical research, the cost may be further defrayed by seeking payment from a third party payer. Both the physician researcher and the academic medical center will typically seek additional reimbursement from third-party payers.

While we once saw health care payers as insurers, the health insurer payer of yesteryear has been supplanted by the self-insuring employer using a managed care organization to administer the employee health benefit plan. The other big payers, of course, are the federal and, to a lesser degree, state governments who finance the Medicare and Medicaid programs.

Health plans, whether public or private, seek to avoid paying for unproven or speculative treatments. At the time Medicare was enacted in 1965, one of the standards borrowed from the private health insurance market was the requirement that care must be medically necessary and reasonable in order to be covered and reimbursed by Medicare. Therapies and technologies that are "investigational" or "experimental" are not eligible for coverage. Although this coverage policy is frequently articulated by Medicare, Medicaid, and private third-party payers, there is considerable uncertainty as to how concretely this exclusion is administered and maintained, even in the setting of regular treatment.

Despite a few targeted national coverage policies excluding coverage for certain procedures, Medicare has been surprisingly forthcoming with support for costs of clinical research. In 1996, when an audit revealed that most of the audited hospitals had billed Medicare for care rendered in connection with implantable medical devices, the Health Care Financing Administration (HCFA) [now the Centers for Medicare and Medicaid Services (CMS)] chose to enter into an agreement with the Food and Drug Administration (FDA) and cover a large percentage of investigational devices. Indeed, the investigational devices that fall into this covered category include 96% of the devices in ongoing clinical trials.

In June, 2000, then-President Clinton issued an executive memorandum directing the Secretary of Health and Human Services to "explicitly authorize [Medicare] payment for routine patient care costs . . . and costs due to medical complications associated with participation in clinical trials." Pursuant to that memorandum, HCFA issued a national coverage decision in September 2000, authorizing coverage of the routine costs of qualifying clinical trials, including costs of diagnosis and treatment resulting from complications arising from participation in the trial. Routine costs include all items and services normally covered by Medicare and provided to subjects in either the experimental or control arm of the trial. The coverage does not extend to the investigational item or service itself, items or services related to data collection and analysis that are not integral to the clinical management of the patient, and anything customarily furnished by research sponsors free of charge to subjects.

With respect to private payers, whether an employer-provided health plan or an individually purchased plan, there is a long tradition of excluding "experimental" or "investigational" services and items. These exclusions, typically found in the policy contract, have been the subject of frequent and vigorous litigation. On balance, these exclusions have proven feeble in courts of law. They have also resulted in public relations disasters when used to deny care to a pitiable beneficiary. In recent years, payers, particularly the private payers — typically employee health plans administered by managed care organizations — have opted to cover the cost of these unproven therapies rather than engage in costly court and media battles.

In fact, in recent years, there has been willingness on the part of third-party payers to assume the costs of clinical research, especially the routine services associated with such research. For example, the American Association of Health Plans encourages its health plans to reimburse the routine costs of care associated with National Institutes of Health (NIH) sponsored trials. Several large private health plans cover costs of patient care in cancer research trials conducted under the National Cancer Institute (NCI).

Even absent the payers' increasing willingness to fund the routine patient costs of clinical research, the fact is that isolating costs associated with research from costs not associated with research is administratively difficult and costly. Because of this difficulty, both Medicare and private payers have actually been paying for a large proportion of research-related costs long before they affirmed their willingness to do so.

Indeed, according to a recent study published by the Institute of Medicine (IOM), coverage and reimbursement of medical services — especially routine services — associated with clinical trials is common. The IOM sought to verify this "widespread understanding" with a study commissioned by the Lewin Group, a health policy consulting firm. In the Lewin Group study, clinical trial investigators reported routine patient claims generated in clinical trials are routinely submitted and paid by plans. This finding was sustained across a variety of research areas. In fact, oncologists indicated claims would be routinely submitted for nearly all the routine services used in the course of the clinical trial. Similarly, cardiologists reported they commonly bill insurers for routine patient costs in clinical trials, although not necessarily for protocol-specific procedure costs. It appears a lack of clarity about what constitutes standard therapy versus research makes it difficult for both provider and payer to discern what is covered and reimbursable.

4. Patient "Out-of-Pocket" Payment

In some instances, the patient/subject will pay out-of-pocket for care and services received in the course of clinical research. This generally occurs in protocols in which a new experimental procedure is being offered. New procedures are typically not funded by federal agencies and there is frequently no new drug or device involved that might be under sponsorship by private industry. Alternatively, the new drug or device may be provided in concert with an experimental procedure that is not covered by third-party payers or part of the federal grant or industry sponsorship.

Perhaps the most timely example of this would be the use of autologous bone marrow or stem cell transplant for breast cancer. This procedure has been the subject of countless suits brought by patients seeking health plan coverage. Although highly touted as "cutting edge" therapy by the research and oncology community, it remained of unproven value by scientific standards for many years. Health plans, including Medicare, balked at covering the procedure, and patients desiring the procedure frequently had to cover the cost themselves, a cost typically well in excess of $100,000. Ironically, this cutting edge, much sought after therapy, has recently been discredited and shown to be no better, and perhaps worse, than conventional breast cancer treatments.

NOTES AND QUESTIONS

1. How billing for research actually works is not as precise as one might expect.

> A typical medical center, even an academic teaching facility, will lack the resources to adequately differentiate between costs applicable to research procedures versus other procedures. In most cases, third-party payers will be billed for all costs and will have the burden of reviewing claims to determine which services performed were routine and not research protocol-related, and thus eligible for coverage.

Patricia C. Kuszler, *Financing Clinical Research and Experimental Therapies: Payment Due, but From Whom?* 3 DePaul J. Health Care L. 441, 465 (2000).

2. Myriad sources currently provide external support for research conducted at AHCs. In addition to federal and industry sponsorship, investigators may obtain funding from an array of private foundations and endowments, such as the National Kidney Foundation, the March of Dimes, the Robert Wood Johnson Foundation, the American Cancer Society, and the American Diabetes Association. Some of these organizations focus on specific diseases, while others are far broader in purpose. Research funding also may come from the universities' own resources.

3. While the extent to which AHCs are able to cross-subsidize research with clinical revenues and other internal resources has declined, it remains a significant factor, particularly in supporting new investigators who have yet to develop research track records adequate to attract substantial government or industry money. Such research appears to play an important role in the development of basic ideas that, when better developed, may attract external funding. A recent survey of medical school faculty indicated that 43 percent received some institutional funding from university sources for the direct costs of research. This includes monies the university receives from clinical income and faculty practice plans, unexpended grant funds, and discretionary funds. *See* J.S. Weissman, et al., *Market Forces and Unsponsored Research in Academic Health Centers*, 281 JAMA 1093 (1999). The same study came to two other significant conclusions: (a) the greater the competition in the clinical market in which the AHC is located, the less the availability of institutional support for faculty research, and (b) it was not unusual for research to be conducted by working extra, uncompensated hours. *See id.* at 1096-97.

[D] Federal Sources of Research Funding

[1] National Institutes of Health

Within the Department of Health and Human Services, the Public Health Service (PHS) includes seven agencies, a number of which provide support for research with human subjects. Within the PHS, a principal source of research support is the NIH, which operates through twenty-seven separate components, mainly Institutes and Centers. In FY 2003, $27 billion was appropriated for the NIH's efforts. The goal of the NIH's research "is to acquire new knowledge, to help prevent, detect, diagnose, and treat disease and disability, from the rarest genetic disorder to the common cold." Nearly eighty-four percent of its research funds are used to make grants and contracts supporting research and training throughout the United States and abroad. Approximately ten percent of the NIH budget goes to its own Intramural Research Programs, involving more than 2,000 projects conducted in its own laboratories, while the remaining eight percent supports overhead. Overall, NIH estimates that it sponsors about 7,000 clinical research studies at any one time, including both clinical trials and more basic studies. *See* INSTITUTE OF MEDICINE, EXTENDING MEDICARE REIMBURSEMENT IN CLINICAL TRIALS 23 (2000).

The NIH's intramural research program involves studies in research laboratories on the NIH campus in Bethesda, Maryland, and at other locations. Within the NIH campus, the Warren Grant Magnuson Clinical Center, a research hospital, admits more than 7,000 inpatients annually and works with another 72,000 outpatients who are study subjects.

The NIH uses three methods to fund outside organizations: grants, cooperative agreements, and contracts. With the former two, individual scientists describe ideas for research in a written application for a research grant. With contracts, the Institute involved establishes the plans, protocols, and requirements. Any of these may involve the study of basic biological processes as well as new diagnostic or treatment modalities.

In total, about 43,400 research and training applications are reviewed annually through the NIH peer review system. According to the most recent update, NIH supports 46,700 grants in universities, medical schools, and other research and research training institutions both nationally and internationally. *See* NATIONAL INSTITUTES OF HEALTH: ABOUT NIH, available at http://www.nih.gov/about.

[2] Other DHHS Departments

The Centers for Disease Control and Prevention (CDC), which, like the NIH, operates through a variety of organizational components, spends about ten percent of its budget on health research. The National Institute for Occupational Safety and Health (NIOSH) is the primary research arm of CDC. NIOSH conducts research on the full scope of occupational disease and injury, ranging from lung disease in miners to carpal tunnel syndrome in computer users. An average of 9,000 U.S. workers sustain disabling injuries on the job each day, sixteen workers die from an injury sustained at work, and 137 workers die from work-related diseases. The economic burden of this continuing toll is high. Data from a NIOSH-funded study reveal $171 billion annually in direct and indirect costs of occupational injuries and illnesses ($145 billion for injuries and

$26 billion for diseases). These costs compare to $33 billion for AIDS, $67.3 billion for Alzheimer's disease, $164.3 billion for circulatory diseases, and $170.7 billion for cancer. *See* ABOUT NIOSH RESEARCH AND SERVICES, available at http://www.cdc.gov/niosh/about.html. In addition, through its National Center for HIV, STD, and TB Prevention (NCHSTP) and its National Center for Infectious Diseases (NCID), the CDC has become significantly involved in conducting research aimed at preventing and controlling the spread of HIV, as well as in dealing with bioterrorism and related threats.

[3] Other Federal Agencies

A variety of other federal agencies also provide significant biomedical and behavioral research funding. These include, for example, the Agency for Healthcare Research and Quality (AHRQ), which largely funds work designed to improve outcomes, quality, access to, cost and use of health care services and to enhance patient safety. About seventy-five percent of AHRQ's nearly $300 million budget supports researchers at universities, in clinical sites such as hospitals and physicians' offices, and in research institutions.

The Department of Defense manages a variety of medical research programs, including the Congressional Special Interest Medical Programs (CSI). The CSI programs include research in military infectious diseases, combat casualty care, military operational medicine research, and medical chemical and biological defense. *See* UNITED STATES ARMY MEDICAL RESEARCH AND MATERIEL COMMAND, available at https://mrmc-www.army.mil. In addition, the Department of Defense administers the Congressionally Directed Medical Research Programs (CDMRP). The story of how CDMRP came to fund research on the screening and diagnosis of breast cancer among military women and dependents is described at page 96 below. The CDMRP also manages other research programs in defense women's health, osteoporosis, neurofibromatosis, prostate and ovarian cancer, tuberous sclerosis, chronic myelogenous leukemia, as well as a variety of other specified areas. The total budget for these efforts exceeded $345 million for FY 2002. *See* DEPARTMENT OF DEFENSE: CONGRESSIONALLY DIRECTED MEDICAL RESEARCH PROGRAMS, available at http://cdmrp.army.mil.

The Department of Veterans Affairs, through its Office of Research and Development, has four Services that conduct health research. Its Medical Research Service (MRS), for example, focuses on diseases of significance to the veterans' population, such as diabetes, heart disease, cancer, neurological disorders, and serious mental illnesses.

[E] Private Industry Funding of Research

[1] Pharmaceutical Companies

As of 2001, the pharmaceutical industry had more than 1,000 medicines in development — either in human clinical trials or at the FDA awaiting approval. These included more than 400 for cancer; more than 200 to meet the special needs of children; more than 100 each for heart disease and stroke, AIDS, and mental illness; twenty-six for Alzheimer's disease; twenty-five for diabetes; nineteen for arthritis; sixteen for Parkinson's disease; and fourteen for osteoporosis. *See* PHARMACEUTICAL RESEARCH AND MANUFACTURERS OF AMERICA, ANNUAL REPORT 2001-2002 (2001), available at http://www.phrma.org/publications/publications/annualreport/2002/phrma_annreport2001.pdf.

As noted earlier, U.S. pharmaceutical companies claim to have spent $32 billion in research and development in 2002. They further contend that this was an increase of 7.7 percent over 2001 and four times that of 1990. This figure exceeds the total NIH FY 2002 budget of $24 billion. The companies claim that the average cost to develop a new drug has increased from $138 million in 1975 to $802 million in 2002. Only one out of every 5,000 screened compounds is approved, and only three out of ten marketed drugs produce revenues that match or exceed average research and development costs. In 2002, the FDA approved twenty-six new medicines with an average of 17.8 months of review time each. Typically, it takes ten to fifteen years to develop a drug from laboratory to FDA approval. *See* PHARMACEUTICAL RESEARCH AND MANUFACTURERS OF AMERICA, INDUSTRY PROFILE 2003, available at http://www.phrma.org/publications/publications/profile02/2003%20CHAPTER%201.pdf.

Once again, Marcia Angell takes issue with PhRMA's assertions of an $802 million cost per new drug. She observes not only that significant parts of a mass-marketing budget often are included in these costs, but also that the industry receives generous tax credits and deductions for research and development. Ultimately, she concurs with the results of an analysis performed by the consumer advocacy group, Public Citizen, which concluded that the real cost per drug is well under $100 million after taxes. *See* ANGELL, *supra* at 37-46.

[2] Biotech Companies

Biotechnology is the use of organisms and their smallest parts, cells and molecules, to solve problems or make products. For example, erythropoietin, a protein essential in red blood cell formation, has been isolated from human urine and is used to treat anemia. Anemia is a disease itself, and it can be a side effect of the treatment of various other diseases, such as cancer. The FDA has approved more than 155 biotechnology drugs and vaccines. Seventy percent of the biotech medicines on the market were approved between 1997 and 2003. There are more than 370 biotech drug products and vaccines currently in clinical trials targeting more than 200 diseases, including various cancers, Alzheimer's disease, heart disease, diabetes, multiple sclerosis, AIDS, and arthritis. *See* BIOTECHNOLOGY INDUSTRY ORGANIZATION, BIOTECHNOLOGY INDUSTRY FACTS, available at http://www.bio.org/speeches/pubs/er/statistics.asp.

Biotech products are used in a variety of diagnostic tools, including rapid testing for various infectious diseases. They also allow for detection of diseases at earlier times in the disease processes. Other uses of biotechnology-based tests include screening of donated blood for pathogens that cause AIDS and hepatitis. On the therapeutic side, biotech products are used to treat many diseases, including anemia, cystic fibrosis, growth deficiency, rheumatoid arthritis, hemophilia, hepatitis, genital warts, transplant rejection, and leukemia and other cancers. They are also used for treatment of burns, as adhesives in surgery, to reduce organ transplant rejection, to replace injured skin and cartilage, and to manufacture vaccines against diseases such as hepatitis B and meningitis. *See* BIOTECHNOLOGY INDUSTRY ORGANIZATION, HEALTH CARE APPLICATIONS, available at http://www.bio.org/speeches/pubs/er/healthcare.asp.

§ 2.03 THE MOVEMENT OF RESEARCH FROM ACADEMIC HEALTH CENTERS TO PRIVATE PHYSICIANS' OFFICES AND THE RISE OF CONTRACT RESEARCH ORGANIZATIONS

Even today, AHCs still "perform nearly thirty percent of all the health care research and development in the United States and more than fifty percent of research supported by the National Institutes of Health." Moreover, they serve as the principal training grounds for preparing clinicians

> to participate in and partake in the results of biomedical research and clinical innovation, . . . train the next generation of clinical and clinically oriented biomedical researchers, . . . provide their clinicians with the protected time necessary to conduct clinical research and to experiment with new forms of clinical care, . . . [and] test and implement nascent clinical practices when they are still relatively unproven.

THE COMMONWEALTH FUND TASK FORCE ON ACADEMIC HEALTH CENTERS, ENVISIONING THE FUTURE OF ACADEMIC HEALTH CENTERS 3, 31 (February 2003), available at http://www.cmwf.org/usr_doc/ahc_envisioningfuture_600.pdf.

Yet, while it is true that AHCs have increasingly joined with private industry for support in conducting research, more recently there also has been a major shift in research from AHCs to private hospitals and physicians in private practice. As noted above, at the end of World War II, the vast majority of research was supported with federal dollars, and the vast majority of that work was conducted at AHCs. That has changed significantly. An oft-cited article in the *New England Journal of Medicine*, written in 2000, reviewed why this shift has occurred as well as some of its implications. It noted that, previously, the pharmaceutical industry required the cooperation of academic physicians to perform drug trials for three reasons: the companies did not possess the expertise to devise studies themselves, hospitals affiliated with AHCs could provide subjects, and industry wanted the cachet of academic publications to promote their products. This is no longer the case. Pharmaceutical and device companies have hired competent research physicians to develop and analyze clinical studies, while physicians in private practice have become interested in participating in trials and recruiting their patients to be subjects. Moreover, the bureaucracy endemic to AHCs, which typically requires approval of research contracts by offices of sponsored research as well as by seemingly slow IRBs, often discourages industry from utilizing AHCs. In addition, physicians in AHCs must both teach and be involved in patient care, and such added responsibilities may delay further the completion of studies. The article notes that, on average, drug companies lose $1.3 million each day that there is a delay in obtaining FDA approval. As a result, the pharmaceutical industry is increasingly relying on for-profit contract research organizations (CROs) to assist in conducting research. CROs provide basic and applied research and technical services, including clinical trial monitoring and data management to industry, the government, and other private and public groups. In 1991, eighty percent of the dollars spent by the drug industry for clinical trials were directed to AHCs, while by 1998 that figure had dropped to forty percent. *See* Thomas Bodenheimer, *Uneasy Alliance — Clinical Investigators and the Pharmaceutical Industry*, 342 NEW ENG. J. MED. 1539 (2000).

Another impetus for the movement away from AHCs is the fact that much of the pharmaceutical industry's business is now focused on the prevention and treatment of chronic conditions, rather than acute infections. Meeting FDA requirements for the latter types of medication rarely requires large populations and lengthy studies but, for the former category, clinical trials must include many subjects over a long period, necessitating the use of numerous study sites instead of a single AHC and further encouraging the movement away from AHCs. *See id.*

Finally, in addition to the cost pressures that were brought to bear by reductions in Medicaid and Medicare reimbursement noted in Kuszler's article excerpted above, the emergence of managed care also has limited researchers' access to patients because managed care organizations often direct patients to lower-cost, non-academic institutions rather than to the higher-cost services found in AHCs. *See* THE COMMONWEALTH FUND TASK FORCE ON ACADEMIC HEALTH CENTERS, FROM BENCH TO BEDSIDE: PRESERVING THE RESEARCH MISSION OF ACADEMIC HEALTH CENTERS 11 (1999), available at http://www.cmwf.org/programs/taskforc/AHC_cwf_bench.PDF; E.G. Campbell et al., *Status of Clinical Research in Academic Health Centers: Views from the Research Leadership*, 286 JAMA 800 (2001).

NOTES AND QUESTIONS

1. What risks are there in the movement away from AHCs as the site of most research studies?

    a. Greater concerns about the integrity of the data?

    b. Questions regarding the competence and training of investigators?

    c. Possible biasing of inclusion and exclusion criteria or methods of drug delivery?

    d. Inappropriate selection of study endpoints?

    e. Concerns about controls over publication of results, particularly when the potential outcomes of studies might result in a decline in the sale of the drug?

2. As AHCs become more interested in the profits of research and more stressed by the financial constraints of managed care, might the concerns identified in the previous note apply with equal force to research conducted in universities? Might they become lax in protecting human subjects if too much regulation and protection interferes with data collection and profit? If this is a concern, how should the regulatory structure deal with it? Does the location of research really tell us much these days about the likelihood that human subject protections will be taken seriously?

3. For discussions of these issues, see, e.g., L.A. Bero and D. Rennie, *Influences on the Quality of Published Drug Studies*, 12 INT. J. OF TECHNOLOGY ASSESSMENT IN HEALTH CARE 209 (1996); L. Henderson, *The Ups and Downs of SMO Usage*; 6 CENTERWATCH 5 (May, 1999); J.R. Vogel, *Maximizing the Benefits of SMOs,* 8 APPLIED CLINICAL TRIALS 56 (1999); Thomas Bodenheimer, *supra*; P.A. Rochon et al., *A Study of Manufacturer-Supported Trials of Nonsteroidal Anti-Inflammatory Drugs in the Treatment of Arthritis*, 154 ARCH. INTERN. MED. 157 (1994).

The Industrialization of Clinical Research
Richard A. Rettig
19 HEALTH AFFAIRS 129, 134-35, 137-38 (2000)

Traditionally, drug firms have both sponsored and managed clinical trials. Indeed, trial management remains an internal function for some firms, and most use a mix of internal and outsourced clinical trial management. In the traditional mode, drug firms have been responsible for trial design and for recruiting investigators and patients, all organized to support an NDA [New Drug Application] submission to the FDA.

In the past decade, an increasing amount of clinical trial work has been contracted out. . . . [I]t is safe to say that at least $5 billion and perhaps as much as $8 billion of R&D is currently going to contract research organizations (CROs). . . . [One] source estimates outsourced R&D growth at 15-20 percent annually and increasing CRO penetration of total drug development research from 15 percent to 22.1 percent between 1995 and 2000, for year-to-year growth slightly over 20 percent.

A number of factors are driving the outsourcing of clinical trials. First, government and private-sector cost containment and marketplace globalization pressures on drug prices have generated an intensive search for efficiencies in the drug development cycle, which has not shortened, even though FDA review times are shorter. Industry has concluded that some bottlenecks can be managed more effectively by external than by internal resources. Second, pipeline management may pose a problem when the number of new compounds approaching market approval is large. Firms may find contract research an attractive way to escape the limits of existing organizational capacity. Third, industry consolidation may also be a CRO stimulus, as merged companies seek to manage costs by reducing jobs, centralizing R&D, and outsourcing to reduce fixed costs. It may be easier for a merged company to outsource clinical trials than to integrate two R&D units.

Fourth, biotechnology firms, with great scientific competence, often lack the internal resources and experience (capital, equipment, and staff) to conduct preclinical and clinical research. A number have chosen to outsource rather than to create these capabilities de novo. Fifth, as the market for new drugs has become increasingly global, the concurrent harmonization of U.S., European, and Japanese drug evaluation procedures has created the opportunity for drug firms to seek regulatory approval in various national markets simultaneously rather than sequentially. Coupled with an increase in multinational trials, international CROs often are better able than a drug firm's central regulatory affairs unit is to provide expertise about the regulatory requirements of a specific country and can help to tailor clinical trials accordingly. Finally, as clinical trials have become more complex in response to chronic disorders and life-threatening conditions, CROs with particular therapeutic expertise become attractive to drug firms with promising research but limited experience in a given therapeutic area. . . .

CROs' services can be grouped under drug development, related resources, and marketing. Drug development services include preclinical services (pharmacology, drug metabolism and pharmaco-kinetics, and toxicology and pathology); pharmaceutical sciences (formulations development and manufacturing, analytical chemistry, and quality control); and drug packaging, labeling, and distribution (both to support trials and to market-approved drugs). Quality control concentrates on compliance with international Good Laboratory Practice (GLP), Good Clinical Practice (GCP), and Good Manufacturing Practice (GMP) regulations, and International Standards Organization (ISO) 9000 quality system standards.

Clinical trial management services for all phases include project management, study and protocol design, case report form development, clinical database design, data entry and verification, data management, statistical analysis and reporting, investigator and site selection, healthy volunteer and special population recruitment, investigator meetings, clinical monitoring, centralized clinical trial laboratory, bioanalytical and clinical chemistry laboratory services, pharmacokinetics and pharmacodynamics, expert report writing, and regulatory applications.

Regulatory services deal with complying with FDA requirements in this country and those of relevant non-U.S. authorities. These requirements include drug safety surveillance; regulatory support of clinical trials; preparation of regulatory documents; interaction with regulatory authorities; submission strategies; training for GLP, GCP, and GMP; and determination of national and international regulatory requirements, including data evaluation requirements.

Related resources include studies of outcomes research, pharmacoeconomics, quality-of-life analysis, and patient satisfaction studies. . . .

Investigators and sites. The conduct of clinical trials requires investigators and patients, which has led to the creation of another market segment: site management organizations (SMOs). One commentator defined SMOs as "centrally managed groups of multiple investigative sites that work on behalf of biopharmaceutical companies or contract research organizations and focus on the front-end aspects of clinical studies." These include marketing investigative sites (to sponsors or CROs), negotiating contracts, obtaining IRB approval and handling regulatory documents, enlisting clinical investigators, training investigators and coordinators, recruiting and enrolling patients, and improving and standardizing sites and practices.

The Private Practicing Physician-Investigator: Ethical Implications of Clinical Research in the Office Setting
Jason E. Klein & Alan R. Fleischman
32 HASTINGS CENTER REP., July-Aug. 2002, at 22, 22-24

A new model for performing clinical investigations has emerged in the United States. No longer are academic medical centers the sole or even primary site for cutting-edge clinical research. Instead, over the past decade, the pharmaceutical industry has turned to commercially oriented networks of physicians practicing in private offices. In 1991, 80 percent of pharmaceutical industry money for clinical research went to investigators in academic medical centers. In 1998, that figure dropped by half, to only 40 percent.

As a result, thousands of private physicians have become physician-investigators, and their patients have become patient-subjects. In 1997, according to some estimates, the number of private physicians engaged in clinical research reached 11,662, triple what it had been in 1990.

The phenomenon has sparked much controversy because of the potential conflict between the physicians' two roles. The physician is a clinician, obligated to serve the well-being and interests of the patient. But the physician is now also an investigator, whose aim is to contribute to the development of generalizable knowledge. The conflict can be exacerbated if the pharmaceutical company is paying the physician directly to recruit and retain research subjects.

Changing the Locus of Research

. . . Today, pharmaceutical companies effectively bypass the academic medical centers. They employ their own research design experts and find subjects in the offices of private practicing community-based physicians, often organized in commercially oriented networks such as contract-research organizations (CROs) and site-management organizations (SMOs).

The major driving force for this change is the desire to contain the very high cost of developing new drugs. Contemporary clinical trials require large numbers of subjects, far more than drug studies performed only a decade ago. Because of new federal regulations that require better gender and ethnic representation, a trial must meet rigorous statistical criteria both to establish that the drug works and to assure that it is safe. And when conducting trials of medications for common disorders, pharmaceutical companies now often seek "medication naive" subjects. These demands necessitate large numbers of subjects, and engaging independent private practice-based physicians as clinical investigators provides a way of recruiting them rapidly and efficiently. . . .

Very little is known about what motivates privately practicing physicians to participate in clinical research studies. We can speculate that many of the reasons are rather innocuous and even laudable. For some physicians, serving as an investigator allows them to fulfill personal academic goals. For others it may provide a break from the day-to-day routine of patient care. Still others might choose to participate because it allows them to keep abreast of the most current treatments and offer them to their patients.

Some other possible motivations are more dubious. Consider the practice of providing physicians direct financial incentives to bring patients into the study. Typically, physicians receive a flat fee, which can vary widely depending on the complexity of the study, for each patient they enroll. Additionally, some pharmaceutical companies are reportedly offering bonuses to physician-investigators, nurses, and other members of the study teams to "speed up subject recruitment to meet industry-imposed study completion deadlines" and to retain subjects until the study is completed.

Such incentives may have grown more attractive as changes in health care financing and delivery have reduced physicians' personal income. But sometimes the incentives more than make up for the decline in income. Some physician practices are alleged to net profits as high as one million dollars a year from research trials. Patient recruitment into clinical trials has become so lucrative that entire professional conferences now address it. Among the topics at one conference: "Learning the benefit of social marketing," "Examining creative and media strategies for a successful recruitment campaign," and "Converting 'interested' subjects to 'enrolled' subjects." This business-like, profit-oriented approach to clinical trials stands in contrast to the claim of many physician-investigators that financial compensation is only "for services rendered for the filling out of reports and handling of other administrative details required for reporting purposes."

Incentives to physicians for patient recruitment and retention are not new. In academic medical centers, physician-investigators have for years accrued substantial secondary gain, for either themselves or their departments, by conducting clinical trials. Income from clinical trials can help support research nurses, fellows, laboratory technicians, and coordinators to enhance the academic work of the investigator. Unlike the private practice setting, however, direct personal financial gain has rarely been possible in academia. We ought not trivialize the potential for conflicts of interest in clinical research in the teaching setting, but the isolation of the private office setting, its lack of oversight and accountability, and the potential for direct financial benefit make the conflict there more worrisome. . . .

The Research Enterprise

Conducting clinical trials in the private office setting also has troubling implications for the research enterprise itself. Financial incentives can and do influence supposedly unbiased investigators, and therefore can influence the quality of research findings. A number of studies offer empirical evidence that industry funding of clinical research may bias the researchers' conclusions. No great leap of the imagination is required to worry that financial gain may influence physician-investigators' individual patient recruitment practices and data collection.

Again, this worry is not exclusively about private practicing physicians, but it is especially pertinent in this context. Because the research is taking place in a closed office environment, there may be greater potential for private practicing physician-investigators to alter or fabricate data in order to have their patients meet eligibility requirements. An extreme example was chronicled in a 1999 *New York Times* story about a physician who made a significant amount of money by inventing fictitious patients, using falsified X-rays, and even submitting a nurse's urine in place of the actual research subjects' because it met the requirements of a particular study. Although this story is surely the exception rather than the rule, it does demonstrate the potential worst-case abuses of a system that is extremely difficult to monitor.

Remaining Faithful to the Promises Given: Maintaining Standards in Changing Times
Nancy Neveloff Dubler
32 SETON HALL L. REV. 563, 564-66 (2002)

Review and Monitoring of Research in Diverse Settings

The extension of research protocols into the previously untapped resource of the physician's office is one of the prime features of the intellectual and logistical topography of the modern research enterprise. This development satisfies a number of goals for those planning and conducting large clinical trials. First, it provides a setting for pharmaceutical companies, which assures a supply of patients suited to particular protocols. Second, patients like to go to the small, private offices of their physicians because they are personal and non-intimidating. Third, in a well-run office, appointments are thoughtfully scheduled and often occur on time. Access is easy, parking is available, and more homogeneous populations may be served.

In contrast, the academic medical center has become the colossus of modern medicine: vast entryways lead to miles of corridors, and befuddling arrays of color-coded signs attempt to direct patients to the right destination. Who would want to participate in research in such an intimidating setting? Even clinical centers designed to attract possible research participants still retain some of these features of an academic medical center.

Conducting research in the private doctor's office generally distances the company from the review of an academic medical center's institutional review board (IRB) and places the review under the aegis of a private IRB. The extensive delays that accompany review by the academic medical center cannot plague private review; private review, however, lacks the in-depth scrutiny that adequate review by independent scholars should provide. I have recently heard presentations by the heads of two independent IRBs. Each has panels that meet frequently and each provides review and approval, in general, within one week. Each has experts available to review the science of the protocol and assess whether the "[r]isks to subjects are reasonable in relation to anticipated benefits, if any, to subjects, and the importance of the knowledge that may reasonably be expected to result."

There are two ways in which to approach this intellectual calculus, often referred to by the shorthand of the "risk/benefit ratio." It may be parsed from the basis of technically adequate expertise, or it may be approached from broad-based scholarship and, in some cases, from wisdom. Judgments about the importance of knowledge are distinctly difficult to make about new areas of research. Is the pursuit of another "me too" drug for the treatment of the symptoms of chronic illness an acceptable goal that justifies exposing subjects to risk? If adequate drugs already exist, will this one, if successfully tested and marketed, add anything to generalized knowledge? What if this drug will be far cheaper and will increase access to therapy? IRBs are directly precluded from considering whether the long-range public policy impact of their decision may be the raising or lowering of costs of medicine. In addition, the FDA regulations require the company to demonstrate that the drug is safe and effective, not that it is better. How should an IRB balance all of these factors? I would argue that this must be approached with the wisdom that comes as the result of years of research and thoughtful efforts at design and at patient care — that is, from experience.

Thus, in the "best of all possible worlds," as Candide might sing, the IRB would evaluate the protocol against the most elegant design and suggest changes that might bring results more quickly or produce results more definitively, thus limiting the exposure of subjects to risk. This type of review is less critical for two kinds of proposals: those developed by large drug companies, which have teams of designers assigned to create and refine the design of research; and those submitted to the National Institutes of Health ("NIH"), which undergo peer review by qualified study sections. But in-depth design review is absolutely essential for protocols initiated by academic investigators that have not endured these sorts of review. This is the case with protocols that will not be submitted for drug company or NIH funding because they require small amounts of money, or because they are submitted to private foundations with little expert capacity. Whether the commercial IRBs can muster this sort of deep expertise has not yet been demonstrated, though recent events prove that academic IRBs often fall far short of the mark. Ideally, review should be by a cohort of qualified researchers whose comments in a congregate setting encourage deep analysis. . . .

Finally, the diffusion of research to locations outside of the academic medical center scatters responsibility so that authority is not challenged. Historically, when most medical research was funded by the NIH, protocols were conceived of by groups of academics. These academics submitted the design for peer review, reviewed the data as they accumulated, and assessed the aggregate data before formulating the written product and submitting it to another layer of intense scrutiny by peers before publication. When research is diffused, the scrutiny by the company proposing the research is focused on accumulation of data quickly as a support for the FDA approval process — a good thing if the goal is to limit unnecessary risk to participants. All other aspects of the process, however, are also under the exclusive control of the company — including review of the data, analysis of the data, drafting the article, and reaching the conclusions. The company has one goal required by its fiduciary obligations to shareholders: maximizing profit. This goal is not compatible with dispassionate review of the data, reference to other like compounds and studies, and evenhanded conclusions. This process is further complicated by the fact that the names of well-recognized academics are frequently attached to the publication even when they have hardly participated in any stage of the process.

NOTES AND QUESTIONS

1. While CROs work extensively with physicians in private practice, often they also play a significant role in research at AHCs. Many of the private dollars financing clinical research are filtered to AHCs by CROs. CROs contract with several AHCs and handle the administrative aspects of the trial. They pay the AHCs and researchers for conducting the trial, cover the costs of recruiting, monitoring, and caring for the subjects, and supply the drug or device that is being researched. They also ensure that the research has been approved by the IRB and other necessary committees. *See* Kuszler, *Financing Clinical Research*, *supra*, at 465.

2. Chapter 7 examines the problem of the "therapeutic misconception," a term used to describe subjects' tendency to assume that research is no different from ordinary medical treatment, and that researchers are primarily devoted to promoting the subjects' individual needs. *See* Chapter 7, at page 355. Is it more likely that patients seen in a physician's office would be influenced by the therapeutic misconception than patients in AHCs? For example, might they be more likely to believe that the doctor will tailor the research interventions based on the patient's individual reactions — for example, by changing the dose of the study medications if they do not appear to be working?

3. In light of the issues raised in the Klein and Fleischman excerpt, what procedural protections ought to be put into place, either through voluntary accreditation requirements or regulatory mandates, to decrease the likely impact of the ethical problems posed by research in private practice settings? Required training of all clinical investigators? If so, what would the curriculum entail? What would be a reasonable minimal number of contact hours for such training? How should financial incentives be limited so as to minimize their influence on physician access? Would it be appropriate to cap per subject reimbursement so as to compensate for fixed costs and a reasonable, but limited, profit to the investigator? Should there be limits on or prohibition of bonuses for rapid recruitment and active retention of subjects? Should there be required independent consent or procedure monitors? Who should decide when such monitoring is warranted? What rules should be in place for disclosure to subjects of the dual role of the physician as a clinician and as an investigator? Ought there to be some direct communication with the patient-subject to alert him or her to the unseen dangers of research in a setting that was previously allocated to treatment alone? Should only certain sorts of risks be permitted in the office setting? What level of risk is appropriate and why? For additional discussion of conflicts of interest, see Chapter 5.

§ 2.04 DEVELOPING NEW RESEARCH AGENDAS

What factors determine what types of research are conducted in the United States? The private sector, particularly pharmaceutical and device companies, is likely to identify research priorities based largely on the goal of increasing profits. As a consequence, companies may invest heavily in the development of drugs or devices quite similar to those already available for a given condition, but for which a substantial market appears to exist for something with one or two fewer, perhaps even relatively minor, side effects. They are likely to eschew the development of agents designed to alleviate or cure rare conditions, or conditions largely affecting individuals in developing countries, as devastating as those conditions might be. While profit is not necessarily the only factor determining the research agenda in the private sector, few would deny that the factors that go into setting priorities for public spending on biomedical research are far more complex. They are governed at one level by the Presidential budget and Congressional appropriations. At the next level, the various federal agencies themselves have much to say about how, in terms of general research categories, appropriated funds will be used. Then within those categories there is a further selection made from among the various proposals that are submitted. Finally, this entire process can be greatly affected, both at the macro and micro levels, by various interest groups and advocates.

[A] Setting NIH Priorities

SETTING RESEARCH PRIORITIES
AT THE NATIONAL INSTITUTES OF HEALTH
NATIONAL INSTITUTES OF HEALTH
www.nih.gov/about/researchpriorities.htm

[T]he National Institutes of Health (NIH) must make choices about where and how it spends its money . . . Managing the NIH's budget requires many decisions.

There are 27 Institutes and Centers (called Institutes for convenience) within the NIH. By law, each must be funded. Each also has a statutory mission, which may be the investigation of a disease or a class of diseases (for example, the National Cancer Institute), inquiries into particular aspects of human life and health (for example, the National Institute on Aging and the National Center on Minority Health and Health Disparities), research on specific organs (for example, the National Heart, Lung, and Blood Institute), and broadly defined areas of research and technology (e.g., the National Institute of General Medical Sciences and National Institute for Biomedical Imaging and Bioengineering). Their existence and funding mandates set rough limits on both current and future budgets and thus set the framework for priorities in spending.

The appropriations process, from the President's request through final passage of the bill by the Congress, obligates each Institute to determine how to allocate its own funds among many different activities of science — including investigator-initiated grants, the intramural research program, and research training, among others. These decisions are governed by the Institute's research objectives.

Each Institute also decides which specific research grant applications to fund among those proposed by researchers working at universities or other research centers and whether to emphasize certain research topics within its domain.

The net effect of these decisions determines how much of the entire NIH budget is devoted to work in certain scientific disciplines (e.g., neurosciences, microbiology, genetics) or on certain diseases.

It is also important to note that past decisions — for example, the creation of an Institute, the establishment of research centers, and the awarding of grants to individual investigators (averaging four years) — have longer lives than the annual appropriations. This leaves only a part of the entire budget available each year for new opportunities.

Assessing research according to money spent on specific diseases is imprecise. Public and congressional inquiries about how the NIH spends its money often focus on the amounts given to certain Institutes or devoted to research on a specific disease.

- Research on any disease is not confined to one Institute. Research into many diseases is often carried on in several Institutes simultaneously, e.g., several Institutes are supporting research on Alzheimer's disease. An Institute's budget is an inadequate measure of support for research on specific diseases.

- It is also extremely difficult to assign the large investments in basic research to any one disease. For example, the number of grants specifically devoted to heart attacks is smaller than the number of grants awarded for research on cardiac muscle biology and lipid metabolism, which have obvious and promising implications for understanding, preventing, and treating heart attacks.

- From long experience, we know that research aimed at one target often hits another, e.g., a gene causing breast cancer in mice plays a role in the development of brain tissue. It is impossible to attribute research and discoveries like this to one disease.

There is, consequently, no "right" amount of money, percentage of the budget, or number of projects for any disease.

There are limits to planning science

Science, dealing with the unknown, is inherently unpredictable. . . . Moreover, unforeseen crises and opportunities may require the NIH and individual scientists to abandon their plans or change the direction and focus of their research. Consider two examples:

- The emergence of new diseases (AIDS or West Nile Virus), the rise of importance of others as our society changes (Alzheimer's disease), and the resurgence of old ones (tuberculosis, malaria), all require urgent attention. The expense of supporting new and unforeseen research, however, does not displace the need to continue investigations into heart disease, muscular dystrophy, arthritis, diabetes, or asthma.

- Unplanned and untargeted basic research on DNA in the 1960s and 1970s permanently changed the way medical research is done. These studies furnished the ground for the biotechnology industry that provides important therapeutic products, which we would otherwise not have, and set the stage for the Human Genome Project that has now given us a map of human genes and has revolutionized our research into virtually all diseases and disorders.

... It is also true, however, that a decision to increase support of one area of medical science — by design, according to a directive, or in response to a critical opportunity — now usually comes at the expense of something else and affects the planning of future research. . . .

The NIH must continue to support the human capital and material assets of science. To this end, the NIH's budget supports research training, acquisition of equipment and instruments, some limited construction projects, and grantee institutions' costs of enabling the research programs. . . .

Assessing scientific opportunities

... [T]he NIH places great reliance on investigator-initiated research — projects conceived by individual scientists and submitted to the NIH to undergo review by other scientists and be considered for funding. . . . Review for scientific merit is conducted by groups of predominantly non-government scientists (with knowledge in a relevant area) convened as panels called study sections. Currently, there are about 125 study sections, which normally meet three times a year to review grant applications.

The merit of a research proposal is assessed by several criteria, including: the importance of the problem or question; the innovation employed in approaching the problem; the adequacy of the methodology proposed; the qualifications and experience of the investigator; and the scientific environment in which the work will be done. Currently, slightly more than one in three grant applications received by the NIH is ultimately funded.

In addition to judging the scientific merit of individual research grant applications, the study sections, in aggregate, have another important effect on the science supported by the NIH. After each study section reviews and rates the grant applications assigned to it by NIH staff, the relative ratings of applications from all study sections are then integrated. Because, for the most part, grants are funded in order of their rating relative to other applications in the same field, the fact that a study section has been constituted in a particular area usually guarantees that at least some applications in that area of science will be funded. Because of this effect, the NIH must monitor changes occurring in science to ensure that study sections, as groups, are appropriately constituted so that they can assess the research applications in all areas of scientific endeavor.

NOTES AND QUESTIONS

1. In FY 2002, more than 30,000 applications for research projects were reviewed by the NIH, and 31 percent were funded. *See* AN INTRODUCTION TO EXTRAMURAL RESEARCH AT NIH, available at http://grants1.nih.gov/grants/intro2oer.htm. For a discussion of the current trends and outcomes of peer review of grant applications to NIH, see Theodore A. Kotchen et al., *NIH Peer Review of Grant Applications for Clinical Research*, 291 JAMA 836 (2004).

2. The process for research and development contracts is somewhat different from that applicable to grants, in that applicants are responding to an Institute-defined statement of work contained in a Request for Proposal (RFP). Typically, Institute staff develop the idea for a project, an outside advisory panel then clears it, and the staff then turn it into the RFP. Separate peer review and NIH staff review lead to discussions with the offerors who appear competitive, and an award is made to the "best final offer" that is judged to be most advantageous to the Institute. *See id.*

WHEN SCIENCE OFFERS SALVATION
REBECCA DRESSER
75-80, 83-84 (2001)

FAIRNESS IN ALLOCATING GOVERNMENT RESEARCH FUNDS

Criteria for Research Priority Setting

. . . The NIH relies on a variety of considerations in allocating research funds. According to the NIH document, *Setting Research Priorities,* the agency's resource allocations are shaped by the following criteria: 1) public health needs; 2) scientific merit of research proposals; 3) level of scientific opportunity in various areas (i.e., whether major advances appear imminent); 4) breadth and diversity of topics and approaches ("[b]ecause we cannot predict discoveries or anticipate the opportunities fresh discoveries will produce"); and 5) training and infrastructure necessary to support current and future research demands. These criteria are not ranked in significance.

Setting Research Priorities also elaborates on the first criterion, public health needs. According to the document, the nation's health needs are evaluated in light of the following considerations:

• The number of people who have a particular disease.

- The number of deaths produced by a disease.

- The degree of disability produced by a disease.

- The degree to which a disease cuts short a normal, productive, comfortable lifetime.

- The economic and social costs of a disease.

- The need to act rapidly to control the spread of a disease.

Setting Research Priorities again takes the position that all these considerations are important and does not rank them in significance. The document notes that exclusive reliance on any one consideration would produce dramatically different priorities. For example, "[f]unding according to the number of deaths would neglect chronic diseases that produce long-term disabilities and high costs to society. . . ."

Setting Research Priorities presents explicit criteria that affect NIH priority setting. Priorities may reflect other criteria as well. Former NIH Director Harold Varmus acknowledged that priority setting may be influenced by desires to 1) preserve the nation's leadership position in science, 2) contribute to economic activities in the private sector, and 3) elevate the public image of science. . . .

The Priority-Setting Process

The NIH applies its substantive priority-setting criteria in a lengthy and intricate process. After consulting with institute and center directors (who have previously met with scientists and other interest group representatives), the NIH director submits budget recommendations to the president. Once Congress establishes the final budget figures, officials at each of the institutes and centers have primary control over the division of their funds. . . .

Research proposals are selected for funding according to their merit, which is initially assessed by review panels composed of experts in relevant fields. Five criteria affect merit evaluations: 1) the importance of the problem or question the proposal addresses, 2) the level of innovation in the proposed approach, 3) the adequacy of the proposed research methods to investigate the problem, 4) the investigators' qualifications and experience, and 5) the quality of the research environment.

Funding choices are also made by a second group, the advisory council of each NIH institute and center. Advisory councils are usually composed of two-thirds scientist and one-third public members. After consultation with their advisory councils, institute and center directors may fund proposals that received lower initial merit scores if they think the research is unusually promising or fills gaps in their research portfolios.

NIH officials also have mechanisms to guide the types of proposals they receive. Officials participate in conferences to keep abreast of the problems that preoccupy scientists, clinicians, and advocates. Institutes and centers conduct meetings at which researchers, clinicians, and advocates discuss areas they perceive as underfunded. Based on this information, NIH officials decide when affirmative steps are needed to encourage research interest in a particular area. Agency officials may then sponsor conferences or issue requests for proposals in that area. Finally, the NIH director is authorized to use discretionary funds to support studies in areas identified as especially significant.

This process gives scientists who submit and review proposals a substantial role in determining the direction of biomedical research, which in turn affects how the government invests its research dollars. At the same time, the review process gives NIH officials, advocates, and other nonscientists opportunities to promote funding for particular health or scientific areas.

Problems with Priority Setting

With the increased focus on priority setting have come challenges to the NIH system. One common criticism is that the articulated priority-setting criteria are so general that NIH officials have almost total freedom in their allocation choices. As a result, it is claimed, the curiosity and career interests of the agency's scientist-administrators and their academic research colleagues assume the highest priority in funding decisions. For example, at a Senate hearing on setting research priorities, a representative of the Parkinson's Action Network said NIH had adopted a "laissez-faire" approach that allowed scientific imagination to be the dominant force in shaping research. The speaker claimed this approach had led to relatively low levels of funding for Parkinson's disease research, even though such research would merit substantially higher amounts if the formal NIH criteria were strictly applied.

Another common complaint is that the vagueness of the NIH criteria allows officials to direct disproportionately large sums to disorders represented by highly visible and sophisticated advocacy groups. As a congressional analyst reported, critics believe "NIH spending often follows current politics and political correctness" rather than the articulated public health considerations. . . .

NIH officials concede that weaknesses exist in their public health needs assessments and their data on spending by disease. In 1999 testimony to Congress, former Director Varmus attributed the deficiencies in NIH figures to the absence of "a common or accepted measure former disease burden," and to difficulties inherent in attempting to assign basic research to specific disease categories. But critics suspect that the lack of solid data provides a convenient excuse when officials are charged with failing to allocate sufficient funds to certain health problems. Moreover, though critics acknowledge that it is impossible to know the precise applications of research, they think NIH officials could do a much better job classifying studies according to their potential relevance to particular medical conditions.

Other critics seek more drastic changes in NIH priority setting. For example, analyst Tammy Tengs challenges the agency's current failure to rank its priority-setting criteria. In her view, "Congress and the Administration should revise

NIH's mission statement to clarify that its primary goal should be to produce the greatest possible reduction in the future burden of disease and injury. Moreover Tengs believes that NIH institute and center budgets should be closely tied to the predicted future burden of disease in their mission areas. She also contends that the agency should do more to create scientific opportunity in the most burdensome disease areas by channeling funds to those areas.

Additional criticism comes from Daniel Callahan, who thinks the existing criteria implicitly envision "progress without end in the improvement of health." He would like to see them replaced with more precise and realistic goals, such as "relief of pain, suffering and disability to the level that the majority of those liable to suffer from them are able to function effectively as persons, citizens, and workers." He argues that too heavy an emphasis is placed on research to extend the average life span, and not enough on studies relevant to disease prevention, public health, symptom relief, and amelioration of disabilities.

Distributive Justice Considerations

. . . Resource allocation in the research context is also especially troublesome because it requires numerous trade-offs between benefits to people who will experience the burdens of disease in the near future and people expected to suffer health problems in the more distant future. For example, officials would face such a trade-off in choosing between funding a late-phase clinical trial of a new cancer treatment and funding a gene sequencing project whose health benefits will not materialize for many years. Additional complexity is introduced by foundation and industry funding for research. The presence of other funding sources requires government officials to take into account the private sector's contributions to specific research areas.

Difficulties in Evaluating the Fairness of NIH Allocation: An Illustration

Data from an empirical study of NIH disease-specific funding reveal how morally and practically complicated it is to apply distributive justice criteria to research funding decisions. In the study, health policy analysts looked at the disease burden associated with 29 health conditions. Using six different measures of disease burden, analysts compared the disease burden scores for each of the 29 conditions to the amount the NIH spent for research on those conditions.

For three disease burden measures — the total number of people with the condition, the frequency of new cases, and the number of days people with the condition were hospitalized — the analysts found no relation between severity of disease burden and amount of NIH funding. They found a weak association between level of NIH funding and number of deaths caused by the condition. Funding levels were also weakly associated with years of life lost from the condition. NIH funding was strongly associated with another measure of disease burden known as the disability-adjusted life-year. This measure is based on the number of years of healthy life lost due to disability or death from illness or injury.

The study authors then took the number of deaths caused, years of life lost, and disability-adjusted life-years scores for the 29 conditions and used the figures to estimate the level of research funding specific conditions ought to receive. NIH funds for research on AIDS, breast cancer, dementia, and diabetes exceeded what their disease burdens would justify. Research on other conditions, such as chronic obstructive pulmonary disease, perinatal conditions, and peptic ulcers, was underfunded relative to the burdens these diseases impose. The appropriateness of NIH funding for some conditions varied with the measure of disease burden applied. For example, when number of lives lost or number of years of life lost was applied, NIH funds for schizophrenia and depression research went beyond what the level of burden would justify. But when number of disability-adjusted life-years lost was the basis for evaluating disease burden, these two conditions received less than they should have.

NOTES AND QUESTIONS

1. What conclusions do you draw from the study just described? Is NIH distributing its resources unfairly? Is NIH's behavior irrational?

2. The NIH's materials excerpted earlier in this section seem to suggest that there is no realistic way to assess how much money is being spent on particular diseases, let alone on particular scientific disciplines. Yet, as the criticisms voiced in the excerpt from Dresser indicate, knowledgeable individuals believe that such assessments can and should be made. Who do you think is correct?

3. In *Setting Research Priorities,* the NIH lists a variety of "considerations" to be taken into account in determining what types of research to support. These considerations do not include many broader questions that, arguably, should also be relevant to allocating research funding. Which of the following questions do you think ought to be asked, and how would you answer them?

    a. What is the appropriate priority to be assigned to the "worst off" individuals, i.e., people most in need of improved health? Should the highest priority go to disorders and injuries that cause death or significant disability?

    b. When should NIH support studies involving less serious health problems? What if such studies have a very high likelihood of benefiting those at risk for that type of condition?

    c. Should a limited resource go to all who might benefit or those with the greatest chance of benefit? When do lesser benefits to many outweigh greater benefits to a few?

    d. What about a type of "affirmative action" approach to funding, under which greater resources would be allocated to areas in which the agency had previously failed to give sufficient attention? *See* Dresser, *supra*, at 81-82.

[B] The Role of Advocacy

Throughout most of the history of research in the United States, members of the public seemed largely oblivious to their potential roles in the process of setting priorities or in influencing the ways in which research would be conducted. Beginning with the early 1990s, that situation changed dramatically.

WHEN SCIENCE OFFERS SALVATION
REBECCA DRESSER
75, 7 (2001)

Philosopher Daniel Callahan describes the prevailing attitude as follows: "we like what [the NIH] is doing, we trust its leadership to make good priority decisions, and we see no good reason to shake the faith of the Congress or the general public about the way NIH goes about carrying out its mission." Traditional neglect of this issue [what is a just allocation of resources for biomedical research] may reflect another common attitude, here expressed by law professor Roger Dworkin:

> The questions of how much money to spend on research and what kinds of research to support are, quite properly, political questions. We elect representatives to decide questions that have no inherently right answers, like. . . how much to spend on basic and how much on applied research; and how much to spend on each of an almost infinite number of worthy ends — cure versus prevention, AIDS versus birth defects, and so forth.

[The excerpt that follows appears earlier in the book.]

When advocates help design and conduct studies, they influence what study participants experience and the value of the data that are produced. What role should advocates play in representing the interests of prospective study participants and the interests of the current and future patients who stand to benefit from a study? How much control should advocates exercise in study planning and interpretation?

When advocates work to expand constituents' opportunities to participate in research and to try experimental interventions outside the research setting, they influence what people expect to gain from such interventions. Do advocates' hopes for research advances make them too willing to accept the risks of study participation? Do their positive views of research promote the mistaken belief that participating in a study is equivalent to receiving the best therapy?

When advocates make the case for more research funding for particular health problems, they influence how scarce research resources are distributed. Can lobbying produce a more just allocation of limited research dollars? What gets left out when researchers and officials rely on advocates to provide the "public perspective"?

Embedded in these questions are classic research ethics problems involving the protection of human study participants, the protection of patients from harmful and ineffective treatments, and the just distribution of benefits and burdens produced by biomedical research. Research advocacy presents these questions in novel and subtle ways, however. Many issues remain below the surface, and few have been subjected to explicit analysis.

Research advocacy also brings interest group politics to biomedical research policy. As advocates lobby for funding and policy actions, will biomedical research be increasingly governed by considerations similar to those that govern highway construction and the dairy industry? Will research be diverted from general public health needs and toward the health problems of the wealthy and powerful? If advocacy becomes a major factor in research decision making, can the process be designed to ensure that the interests of disadvantaged groups and individuals are represented?

[1] Legislative Advocacy

In 1991, a number of breast cancer advocates formed the National Breast Cancer Coalition (NBCC), which actively lobbied through letter-writing campaigns and testimony before Congress, demanding increased support for research on that disease. The group concluded that it needed $300 million above the then-existing allocation of $155 million for a reasonable research program. They allied themselves with those like Senator Tom Harkin of Iowa, who was seeking to shift money from the Department of Defense (DOD) to domestic social programs that would benefit women and children. NBCC initially was unsuccessful in arranging a transfer of funding from the DOD to NIH, because of a regulation that prohibited transfers from defense to domestic programs without a two-thirds Congressional majority vote. When it became apparent that Congressional support existed for additional breast cancer research, a different approach was taken. Because the army had spent $25 million in 1992 on mammography, as part of its health care program for enlisted men and women and their dependents, the advocates succeeded in amending the DOD budget to appropriate $210 million for a "war" on breast cancer — something that needed only a simple majority to pass. Together with an $80 million increase in the NIH budget for breast cancer research, NBCC succeeded in obtaining the funding they wanted for fiscal year 1993. By 1996, funding levels had increased to more than $550 million. *See* KAREN STABINER, DANCING WITH THE DEVIL: THE NEW WAR ON BREAST CANCER 60-63 (1997); BARRON H. LERNER, THE BREAST CANCER WARS 259 (2001).

As groups such as these proved to be successful in obtaining additional funding, advocates for people with various other diseases began to embrace similar strategies. The result was the development of a situation aptly described in the following article.

Patients Lobby for Cash in Research for Illness
Sheryl Gay Stolberg
N.Y. TIMES, Apr. 14, 1999, at A18

In the official Government record, the hearing that began today in Room 2358 of the Rayburn House Office Building will be listed as "public witness testimony." Unofficially, Room 2358 was long ago called Mother Teresa's Waiting Room, a name that could not be more apt.

Here, for three days this week and two days next week, the sick and afflicted and their lobbyists are gathering in an annual telethon of sorts: the competition for research financing to cure disease. Hundreds of ailments are represented, from the most common cancer to the rarest genetic disorder. Even erectile dysfunction received a mention. So many people asked to testify before the subcommittee that holds the purse strings to the National Institutes of Health that two-thirds of them were turned down. The rest were selected by lottery for the privilege of delivering a five-minute talk — time limits strictly enforced — to the 15 members of the panel, most of whom did not show up.

The competition is a rite of springtime in Washington, as certain as the blooming of the cherry blossoms, and in recent years it has hardly been polite. But with advances in biomedical research spilling out of laboratories at an unprecedented pace, and talk among lawmakers of doubling the budget for the National Institutes of Health over the next five years, the faithful of Mother Teresa's Waiting Room have cause for optimism as well as congeniality.

"People are no longer fighting amongst themselves," said Mary Woolley, president of Research America, a nonprofit advocacy group that lobbies for more money for research. "The disease groups are not pitted against each other. This concept of robbing Peter to pay Paul is one that I hope has been banished forever."

Or if not forever, then at least under the current budget. For 1999, Congress gave the institutes a $2 billion budget increase, bringing the total budget to $15.6 billion. Though President Clinton has suggested a more modest increase for 2000, of $320 million, members of both parties in Congress say they are hoping for more.

"My sense is that everyone feels that we are doing well and all ships are rising with the incoming tide," said Dr. Harold E. Varmus, the institutes' director.

Yet as today's hearing reveals, there are still many patients with real need and scientists eager to help them. Doctors pleaded with the panel for more money for research in general, and their interests in particular. "In the vernacular of 'Jerry Maguire,' the movie, 'More money, more money, more money for N.I.H.,'" Dr. A. Paul Kelly, president of the Association of Professors of Dermatology, told the panel.

There is no similar testimony in the Senate, so the hearings before the House Appropriations Subcommittee on Labor, Health and Human Services and Education are the only chance patients have to talk to appropriators in a public forum.

The session was laden with stories that were heartbreaking, albeit carefully orchestrated to grab the attention of the press and, more important, Representative John Edward Porter, Republican of Illinois, who heads the subcommittee and was the only member to sit through the entire hearing.

Judy Kimmitt Rainey, a Senate aide, testified about the devastating loss of her son to Sudden Infant Death Syndrome in 1996. As she spoke, her new baby, a girl, squirmed in the stroller beside her.

"I know that my personal story touched Chairman Porter," Mrs. Rainey said later. "I could see it in his eyes."

Christopher Reeve, the actor who was paralyzed when he fell off a horse, is on the docket for Wednesday. Doug Flutie, the football player whose son is autistic, is also scheduled to appear. Jim Kelly, the retired quarterback for the Buffalo Bills, testified today, describing in wrenching detail the life of his 2-year-old son, Hunter, who suffers from Krabbe disease, a rare neurological disorder. The child cannot move any part of his body on his own. He has never smiled.

"I have been surrounded by tough individuals throughout my entire career," Mr. Kelly said. "But never have I witnessed more strength and toughness than that of my son."

Celebrity counts in the quest for research financing, but equally important are poignant messages from average citizens, lobbyists say.

"I'll take my SIDS lady over any celebrity," said Dale P. Dirks, the lobbyist who accompanied Mrs. Rainey. "Because she's got a compelling story to tell and she's a real person. And all of us have kids."

Mr. Porter listened intently. To Mrs. Rainey, Mr. Porter confided that, as a new grandfather, he worried about Sudden Infant Death Syndrome. When a doctor asked for more money for vision research, Mr. Porter mentioned that his mother-in-law had retinitis pigmentosa. He told a representative from the Asthma and Allergy Foundation of America that his sister had asthma.

Because Congress does not appropriate money on a disease-by-disease basis, the patient advocates are angling for a brass ring with a more subtle effect: a mention in the report that accompanies the subcommittee's bill. The National Institutes of Health pays close attention to the report, and how the committee parses its language.

"There is a code in the words," said Michael Stephens, a former staff director for the subcommittee. "They might say, 'The committee is aware of X disease. The committee urges that the importance of this disease be reflected.' And then, the most that anybody ever gets: 'Within the increase provided, X should be set aside for this disease.' "

Over the years, the hearings have taken on the tenor of a family reunion. Committee staff members tell the story of a boy with a disfiguring port wine stain on his face; one year, the boy showed up with a clear complexion from laser surgery. For a time, an AIDS patient came with his wife; when she did not show up a few years ago, nobody had to ask why.

Today, 17-year-old Erin Bosch, who suffers from a congenital heart defect, appeared for the third time. She recently had surgery to reduce the size of her enlarged heart, a procedure, she hastened to tell Mr. Porter, that was pioneered with Federal money. The Congressman brightened when he saw her; she took that as a good sign.

"I feel like I make an impact," Erin said, "when he remembers me from year to year."

When Science Offers Salvation
Rebecca Dresser
76 (2001)

If members of Congress think the president's budget devotes an inadequate amount to studies on a particular health problem, they exercise their authority to set aside a specific sum for research on that problem (a process called "earmarking"). Sometimes they adopt a less intrusive strategy and simply encourage NIH to give heightened attention to the areas seen as neglected.

Congressional priority setting seems to rely on factors that typically influence the political process, including constituents' personal interests and the economic welfare of the senators' and representatives' home districts. Self-interest may play a role as well. In the late 1980s, for example, "Washington watchers" attributed legislative earmarks for prostate cancer research to "the large number of politically powerful but aging men who were themselves suffering from prostate problems." Observers also claim that "politicians frequently support additional investments in research on a particular disease after a grandchild or spouse has contracted it."

Recognizing their foibles, a number of House and Senate leaders want to discourage specific congressional directives for biomedical research funding. They believe that NIH officials overseeing the institutes and centers are more qualified to determine how much funding should go to each research area. Advocates of reduced congressional interference see increased NIH accountability as an avenue to their goal. The theory is that if NIH officials offer the public better explanations of their funding decisions and more opportunities to participate in priority setting, Congress will face less pressure to intervene.

[2] Advocacy Regarding the Manner in Which Research Is Conducted

WHEN SCIENCE OFFERS SALVATION
REBECCA DRESSER
23-25, 48-49, 51 (2001)

ADVOCATES ON THE RESEARCH TEAM — SHAPING AND ASSESSING SCIENCE

Advocates want a say in the way biomedical research is conducted. In the United States, HIV/AIDS and breast cancer advocates were the first to make this demand. . . . By the late 1990s, advocates representing a multitude of patient and community groups wanted research to reflect their judgments on which conditions should be studied and which study methods adopted. They wanted a role in interpreting, publicizing, and applying study results. And they wanted to help decide which research proposals merited government funding.

Ethical and scientific aims can be advanced by integrating advocacy views into decisions about study design, procedures, and merit. Achieving genuine integration is no simple matter, however. Attempts to make advocates part of the research team often collide with scientific tradition and the research establishment. Moreover, although the approach offers benefits to patients and society, when advocates join the research team, new risks and complications arise both for advocates and for their constituents.

Origins

A look at advocacy activities in three contexts illustrates how advocates can change research practices. In the United States, HIV/AIDS activists were leaders in challenging the research status quo. During the 1980s, as gay men sought to cope with a growing epidemic, they looked to medicine for assistance. Because physicians and scientists could tell them little about the new disease, the need for research was obvious. Activists initially campaigned for more resources and a heightened national commitment to study the condition. Once funding was secured and research under way, however, advocates rebelled against much of what they saw.

The focus of activist discontent was the randomized clinical trial (RCT). . . .

Often, one group in an RCT is assigned to receive a placebo, an agent believed to have no direct effect on the condition being studied. Sometimes, health improvements occur simply because study participants believe they are receiving something more effective for their disease — the so-called placebo effect. Adding a placebo group allows scientists to separate the improvements produced by the experimental and other active agents under study from any improvements caused by the placebo effect.

To the HIV/AIDS activists, many of the RCT conventions seemed shockingly inhumane. In their eyes, it was unethical to give anyone with a life-threatening disease an inactive agent or a relatively ineffective standard treatment instead of a promising new experimental agent. They attacked other dimensions of the RCT as well. People with HIV/AIDS often were told that during clinical trial participation they would have to refrain from taking other medications, including drugs designed to relieve symptoms unrelated to the study. Others were excluded from trials because their past medication use might improperly influence study findings. Scientists claimed that excluding these individuals would make it easier to isolate the effects of the test drugs.

Activists discovered that they had to become familiar with scientific concepts to argue effectively against the RCT's rigid rules. Lay advocates proceeded to learn "the language of the journal article and the conference hall." They became sufficiently knowledgeable to question what they saw as unnecessarily restrictive research methods and to invoke the arguments of mainstream scientists dubious about the need for such methods. Lay advocates were joined by clinicians from the gay community, who added credibility to the challenge. . . .

Practical impediments to conducting HIV/AIDS research also lent authority to the activists' claims. Many HIV-positive people refused to participate in studies if there was a chance they would receive a placebo or a standard therapy they deemed unsatisfactory. Many also were unwilling to stop taking other drugs while they participated in research. Some people entering studies later became "noncompliant" — a term activists rejected because it implied that participants should be subservient to the wishes of the scientists conducting a trial. "Noncompliant" participants gave inaccurate reports of past medication use, continued to take other drugs during a trial, dropped out of studies if they perceived no improvement in their conditions, and shared what they guessed was the promising experimental agent with other study participants who believed they were receiving only placebos. Thus, activists could make a compelling case that trials would be impossible to conduct unless RCT rules were modified.

Ultimately, advocates for people with HIV/AIDS changed conventional clinical trial practices and, in the process, taught scientists to see them as essential research contributors. Sociologist Steven Epstein summed up the activists' achievements as follows:

> The arguments of AIDS activists have been published in scientific journals and presented at scientific conferences. . . . Their arguments have brought about shifts of power between competing visions of how clinical trials should be conducted. Their close scrutiny has encouraged basic scientists to move compounds more rapidly into clinical trials. And their networking has brought different communities of scientists into cooperative relationships with one another. . . .

HOPE VERSUS HYPOTHESIS TESTING: EXPANDED ACCESS TO EXPERIMENTAL INTER-
VENTIONS

The Path to Expanded Access

During the 1980s, advocates for people with HIV/AIDS mounted a vigorous attack on the rules governing access to unproven interventions. Faced with a lethal epidemic and no effective treatments, activists were intensely committed to the search for new drugs to reduce death and suffering. As they embarked on this urgent mission, however, they collided with a drug development system that was slow, inflexible, and highly risk-averse. People with no time to spare were shocked to learn that it took about ten years for new drugs and other medical products to undergo the human testing that was a prerequisite to approval for clinical use.

Displaying banners proclaiming "Red Tape Is Killing Us" and "Release the Drugs Now," HIV/AIDS activists took to the streets and conference halls to protest Food and Drug Administration (FDA) rules on drug testing. With these actions, they joined drug manufacturers and conservative policy groups already lobbying the agency to loosen its approach. By becoming part of this unusual coalition, activists helped set in motion . . . FDA actions making experimental agents more available to people with HIV/AIDS and other serious illnesses. . . .

Another FDA initiative came in 1992. This was the accelerated approval rule, which allows the FDA to rely on so-called surrogate endpoint data in approving new drugs for serious diseases. Before then, drug manufacturers seeking FDA approval had to show that an investigational agent safely and effectively produced "a clinically meaningful endpoint that is a direct measure of how a patient feels, functions, or survives." But waiting for clinical endpoint data slowed the study process. For example, an HIV/AIDS drug study had to continue long enough to allow researchers to assess whether the new agent postponed death or prevented opportunistic infections. Activists and community physicians argued that earlier indicators of improvement, such as cell counts associated with stronger immune system function, could be substituted for clinical endpoints. The FDA accepted this argument when it adopted the accelerated approval rule, which permits approval if the experimental agent is safe and effective in producing surrogate endpoints reasonably linked with actual clinical improvement. . . .

Activists were enthusiastic partners in the campaign to publicize clinical trial availability and increase insurance coverage for trial participants. These programs were consistent with the advocacy view that "increasing patient participation in research . . . is the only means to test newer and better treatments, and thus, save lives." Expanded access has become a motto for advocates, researchers, and federal officials. But it is not clear that advocates should be entirely happy with the consequences.

NOTES AND QUESTIONS

1. On balance, do you view the role of activists in setting the research agenda as positive or negative? What else would you like to know before answering this question?

2. As you learn more about the existing system for protecting human subjects, consider the implications of the changes in the world of research you have read about in this chapter. If the climate in which research is conducted has changed so dramatically since the existing oversight structure was first created, should the system be redesigned to reflect this fact? If so, what elements might you change and which would you keep the same?

Chapter 3

THE FEDERAL AND STATE REGULATORY STRUCTURE

In the two preceding chapters, we took a largely historical approach, examining the events that shaped the current system for regulating human subjects research. With this chapter, we now turn to the task that will occupy the remainder of this book: explaining how that current system functions. In particular, this chapter concentrates on the key aspects of the federal regulations that form the core of that regulatory system, and on the two federal agencies that play the greatest role in enforcing those regulations. We also explain the more limited role of state law.

§ 3.01 OVERVIEW OF THE LEGAL STRUCTURE

Most of the law relating to human subject research exists on the federal level. As with most types of law, it comes primarily from three sources: legislatures, administrative agencies, and courts. The most important piece of legislation for our purposes is the National Research Act of 1974. As discussed in Chapter 2, that Act led to the creation of the National Commission for the Protection of Human Subjects of Biomedical and Behavioral Research, and eventually to the current regulations governing human subject research in the United States.

Statutes often provide only a broad outline of what the law requires. Fleshing out the details of the law, together with performing the day-to-day implementation of what a particular statute requires, is often left to administrative agencies. There are two administrative agencies that play major roles in regulating research with human subjects. The most important agency is the Office for Human Research Protections, or OHRP (previously known as the Office for Protection from Research Risks, or OPRR), which is located within the Department of Health and Human Services (DHHS). OHRP has authority to regulate the great bulk of the human subject research that takes place in this country. The other important administrative agency is the Food and Drug Administration (FDA), which has a somewhat narrower jurisdiction: it is concerned only with research related to the products that it is authorized to regulate.

In both instances, the agencies have promulgated specific sets of regulations that describe how to conduct research with human subjects. As we shall see, while the two sets of regulations are very similar, they are not identical. Sometimes a particular study will come within the jurisdiction of both of these agencies. In that circumstance, *researchers have to be careful to meet the requirements of both sets of regulations.*

While most of the law relating to human subject research is embodied in these federal regulations, there are also relevant laws at the state level. In some instances — such as the conditions for enrolling an incompetent person in a research study — the federal regulations have the effect of deferring to state law for the resolution of an important issue. In addition, the federal regulations do not override state laws that "provide additional protections for human subjects." 45 C.F.R. § 101(f). A growing number of states are passing their own laws that regulate one or another aspect of research.

Controversies often occur over how to interpret either the state or federal laws, and in those instances the courts may end up resolving the dispute. Until recently, there have been relatively few court cases involving research studies, but that has been changing in the past few years. It is likely that the courts will play a growing role in the future evolution of the law relating to research. The role of litigation in human subject research is discussed more extensively in Chapter 12, at page 496.

Finally, it is worth mentioning the role of legally binding obligations created by private agreements. Modern-day research often involves complicated contractual arrangements among the sponsors of studies (such as pharmaceutical manufacturers), the institutions where studies take place, and, in some cases, individual researchers. And there is a growing recognition that the consent forms signed by research subjects may themselves create legal obligations on the part of researchers, their institutions, and study sponsors.

§ 3.02 DEPARTMENT OF HEALTH AND HUMAN SERVICES REGULATIONS

The most important set of federal regulations for protecting human subjects is the so-called "Common Rule." It establishes the basic structure by which human subjects are protected in the United States. Although, as discussed below, the same set of regulations is duplicated by several federal agencies, the version most frequently cited is the one that appears at 45 C.F.R. Part 46. That set of regulations is administered by DHHS, and more specifically by OHRP, which is located within DHHS. Formally speaking, the "Common Rule" only refers to Subpart A of these regulations, which establishes the basic structure of the system under which institutional review boards (IRBs) review research. Subparts B, C, and D, which provide the rules for studies involving certain classes of "vulnerable" subjects, are not technically part of the Common Rule, although it is not uncommon for people to refer to all of the regulations under 45 C.F.R. Part 46 as the Common Rule.

[A] The Common Rule

In order for the Common Rule to apply to a particular study, the study must (1) meet certain jurisdictional requirements of the Rule, (2) involve "research," and (3) involve the use of "human subjects." These three key criteria are discussed below.

[1] Scope of Coverage

The primary way in which a human research study becomes subject to the Common Rule is that the study is either directly conducted by the federal government, or it is funded by the federal government. As discussed below, a key element of enforcing these regulations involves requiring institutions where federally funded research takes place to enter into contractual agreements with the federal government. *See infra*, page 137. These contracts (formally called "assurances") contain a commitment that all federally funded research at the institution will comply with the Common Rule. With regard to research that is not federally funded, the federal government merely requires a commitment that the institution comply with the general principles contained in the Belmont Report. Many such institutions, however, also include in these contracts a specific commitment to apply the requirements of the Common Rule (and often also Subparts B, C and D) to all research they conduct, regardless of whether it is federally funded. In this way, the impact of the Common Rule regulations becomes far broader than might otherwise have been the case.

45 C.F.R. §46.101(a): To What Does This Policy Apply?

This provision is reproduced in Appendix A, at page A-1. Please review it before proceeding.

[2] Definition of Research

Although the Common Rule includes a relatively specific definition of what constitutes research, the line between research and certain other activities remains somewhat blurry. The areas in which the greatest controversy exists are (1) providing a patient with "innovative" or "experimental" care, (2) conducting quality assurance or quality improvement activities, and (3) undertaking public health initiatives.

45 C.F.R. § 46.102(d): Definition of Research

This provision is reproduced in Appendix A, at page A-4. Please review it before proceeding.

NOTES AND QUESTIONS

1. One of the key terms in this definition is the word "generalizable." It is included to embody the concept that, if information is being collected that is not

useful to anyone other than the persons who are collecting it, or a small group with whom they are working (such as other people at their institution), then what is being done is not research. This concept plays an important role in distinguishing research from quality improvement, an issue discussed below, at page 115. Can you think of examples of information that someone might collect that would *not* be considered "generalizable"? Would the reasons we want to protect research subjects also apply to someone who is a subject in such an endeavor? If so, should the word "generalizable" be eliminated from the regulatory definition of research?

2. Another key term is the word "systematic." How does the inclusion of this word alter the coverage of the definition? What additional activities might be considered research if it were not part of the definition?

3. Occasionally something noteworthy may happen to a particular patient — for example, the patient may have a common disease but also develop symptoms never before seen with that disease. Doctors often write up these interesting events as "case studies" and try to publish them in journals so that their colleagues can be aware of them. Does a case study meet the definition of research? What if the doctor prepares a write-up in which he or she compares four patients who all showed the same unusual symptoms? Does the answer to these questions turn on *when* the doctor decided to write the case study — i.e., before or after the patient's treatment was finished?

4. A scholar who studies changes in the doctor-patient relationship over time intends to collect the names of people who have lived in a particular community all their lives and are now at least eighty years old. He will then, with their consent, interview them and try to develop an understanding of how they interacted with their physicians when they were in their twenties. Is this research? Why or why not? *See* Jeffrey Brainard, *Federal Agency Says Oral History Is Not Subject to Rules on Human Research Volunteers*, CHRONICLE HIGHER EDUC., October 21, 2003.

[a] What Is a Research Protocol?

At the heart of any research study is its protocol. The protocol is the written document that spells out what will happen in the study. It should describe the question that the study is attempting to answer, and should go on to provide a detailed description of what the researchers intend to do in trying to answer that question. Thus, the protocol will indicate, among other things, which people are eligible to participate in the study, what will happen to them in the study, how the study will be monitored while it is taking place, and what types of statistical analyses will be performed.

The protocol plays a special role in the determining whether a study is in conformity with the applicable regulations. As will be discussed in the following chapter, an IRB, in evaluating a proposed study, will base its review in large part on the written protocol that it is submitted to it. That document, together with the researcher's answers to an application form that poses a variety of questions about the study, will be evaluated to determine whether the study is well-designed, and whether it provides appropriate protections for the well-being of subjects.

[b] Research versus Clinical Innovation

THE BELMONT REPORT: ETHICAL PRINCIPLES AND GUIDELINES FOR THE PROTECTION OF HUMAN SUBJECTS NATIONAL COMMISSION FOR THE PROTECTION OF HUMAN SUBJECTS OF BIOMEDICAL AND BEHAVIORAL RESEARCH
(1979)

It is important to distinguish between biomedical and behavioral research, on the one hand, and the practice of accepted therapy on the other, in order to know what activities ought to undergo review for the protection of human subjects of research. The distinction between research and practice is blurred partly because both often occur together (as in research designed to evaluate a therapy) and partly because notable departures from standard practice are often called "experimental" when the terms "experimental" and "research" are not carefully defined.

For the most part, the term "practice" refers to interventions that are designed solely to enhance the well-being of an individual patient or client and that have a reasonable expectation of success. The purpose of medical or behavioral practice is to provide diagnosis, preventive treatment or therapy to particular individuals. By contrast, the term "research" designates an activity designed to test an hypothesis, permit conclusions to be drawn, and thereby to develop or contribute to generalizable knowledge (expressed, for example, in theories, principles, and statements of relationships). Research is usually described in a formal protocol that sets forth an objective and a set of procedures designed to reach that objective.

When a clinician departs in a significant way from standard or accepted practice, the innovation does not, in and of itself, constitute research. The fact that a procedure is "experimental," in the sense of new, untested or different, does not automatically place it in the category of research. Radically new procedures of this description should, however, be made the object of formal research at an early stage in order to determine whether they are safe and effective. Thus, it is the responsibility of medical practice committees, for example, to insist that a major innovation be incorporated into a formal research project.

Research and practice may be carried on together when research is designed to evaluate the safety and efficacy of a therapy. This need not cause any confusion regarding whether or not the activity requires review; the general rule is that if there is any element of research in an activity, that activity should undergo review for the protection of human subjects.

ANCHEFF v. HARTFORD HOSPITAL

Supreme Court of Connecticut, 799 A.2d 1067 (Conn. 2002)

The principal issue . . . is whether the trial court properly excluded from evidence a certain report of a federal commission regarding the protection of human subjects of biomedical and behavioral research. . . . The plaintiff claims that the trial court improperly: (1) excluded from evidence the Belmont Report; (2) excluded from evidence a certain medical consent form; and (3) instructed the jury on the question of the meaning of medical research. We affirm the judgment of the trial court.

The plaintiff brought this medical malpractice action against the hospital for injuries he allegedly had suffered arising out of an improperly administered program involving a drug known as Gentamicin. Insofar as is relevant to the issues on appeal, the plaintiff claimed that the hospital had improperly: conducted clinical trials and study procedures regarding Gentamicin; failed to inform the plaintiff that he was a participant in such a trial or procedure; failed to obtain his informed consent for such participation; and failed to disclose to him the experimental nature of his course of treatment with the drug. After a trial to the jury, a verdict was returned in favor of the hospital. The plaintiff then moved to set aside the verdict, which the trial court denied. This appeal followed.

The jury reasonably could have found the following facts. In January, 1993, the plaintiff underwent back surgery, after which he developed a deep wound infection reaching his spinal column. He was admitted to the hospital on February 5, 1993, where [Dr.] Tress was consulted as a specialist in infectious diseases. Cultures disclosed the presence of enterococcus, a difficult bacteria to eradicate. Because Tress suspected enterococcal osteomyelitis, a potentially life-threatening form of bone infection, he ordered a course of combined antibiotic therapy of Gentamicin and Unasyn. Gentamicin has known [harmful effects to kidney and hearing function] regardless of how it is administered.

Initially, Tress ordered Gentamicin to be administered once a day in a dose of 480 milligrams. Pursuant to an inpatient dosing program previously enacted by the hospital, the hospital pharmacy increased the daily dosage to 615 milligrams. Thereafter, Tress examined the plaintiff's condition, and determined that the increased dosage was appropriate. The plaintiff received this combined dosage of drug therapy for approximately twelve days in the hospital. During that time, his kidney clearance and serum levels were monitored for signs of impaired kidney clearance and drug accumulation, with negative results during the plaintiff's stay in the hospital. The plaintiff was discharged from the hospital on February 24, 1993.

Tress prescribed a course of home intravenous antibiotic therapy of Gentamicin and Unasyn at the same levels, in order to eradicate the infection. Although the infection was successfully treated, on March 17, 1993, the plaintiff developed side effects from the Gentamicin, namely, vestibular toxicity, or poisonous effects to the inner ear, which resulted in the loss of the functioning of his inner ear, including his sense of balance. The plaintiff claimed at trial that he suffered total and permanent destruction of the functioning of his inner ear due to an excessive administration of Gentamicin. . . .

The plaintiff first claims that the trial court improperly excluded from evidence the Belmont Report. Specifically, he claims that he sought to establish at trial that the hospital's program of administering Gentamicin constituted medical research, and that, therefore, the hospital was required to have that program reviewed by an institutional review board and to provide the plaintiff with a detailed written consent form outlining the risks, benefits and alternatives, as well as the experimental nature, of the program. The Belmont Report, he claims, supported this claim. We conclude that, as the question was presented to the trial court, the court did not abuse its discretion in excluding the Belmont Report from evidence.

In order to analyze this claim, it is necessary to recount, first, the role that the question of medical research played in the trial. At the heart of the plaintiff's case, insofar as this appeal is concerned, was his claim that the hospital's program for administering Gentamicin, known as the once-daily aminoglycoside regimen, constituted engaging in medical research. . . .

The plaintiff produced the following evidence tending to prove that the hospital's Gentamicin program constituted medical research. The hospital's program provided for a level dose of seven milligrams per kilogram of body weight (7 mg/kg), a dosage that previously had not been tested on humans. In 1993, the hospital was the only one in the country that prescribed that dosage to entire classes of patients. This dosage departed from the conventional dosage of 3 mg/kg approved by the federal Food and Drug Administration. The hospital had described both the dosage of 7 mg/kg and its method of administration, namely, one daily injection as opposed to the conventional administration of three injections per day, as "radical." In addition, the hospital administered the drug to a class of patients pursuant to a "protocol," which meant that, if a physician failed to prescribe the dosage of 7 mg/kg called for in the protocol, the hospital pharmacist would change the dosage automatically.

In publications to the medical community, the hospital had stated that the Gentamicin program was "a radical change from standard aminoglycoside administration schedules," and that "the [Gentamicin] program was unlike most other hospital-wide programs because it was not a conversion to a therapeutic alternative but, rather, a radical change in both the conventional dosing and administration of the aminoglycosides." Data was collected by the hospital on each patient apart from what was kept in the patient's medical record. In addition, the physicians responsible for enacting the Gentamicin program at the hospital, namely, Charles Nightingale, David Nicolau and Richard Quintilliani, lectured to the medical community on the findings of the program. . . .

The hospital, to the contrary, offered the following evidence tending to prove that the Gentamicin program did not constitute medical research. Before the program was enacted by the hospital in August, 1992, the physicians in the hospital's department of infectious diseases, pharmacy and therapeutics committee, antibiotic subcommittee, and medical executive committee approved it. On the basis of the voluminous data and known principles of pharmacokinetics, these committees and the physicians on them determined that the program embodied sound policy for the well-being of patients and did not constitute medical research.

In addition, the hospital introduced evidence to establish the following. The Gentamicin program had been widely studied for many years before the hospital implemented it, and it was not implemented to test the safety of Gentamicin. The program was not a clinical trial, and its implementation did not involve control groups, randomization or double blinding, which are some hallmarks of research. . . . On the basis of the scientific data, the program was implemented for inpatients at the hospital to maximize the killing of bacteria and discourage the accumulation of the drug in the patient's body. It permitted a greater drug-free interval than the conventional method of administration, and therefore resulted in less accumulation of the drug, and was at least as safe and more effective than multiple daily dosing. In addition, the hospital presented evidence that the Gentamicin program is now employed in approximately 80 percent of the hospitals in the United States. . . .

[With regard to admitting the Belmont Report into evidence, the trial] court stated: ". . . [The Report] refers to the Nuremberg War Crime trials, Nuremberg Code, judging physicians, scientists who conducted biomedical experiments on concentration camp prisoners. It also references the exploitation of unwilling prisoners as research subjects in Nazi concentration camps was [sic] condemned as a particularly flagrant injustice. In this country in the 1940s [the] Tuskegee syphilis study used rural black men to study the untreated course of a disease. It also talks about justice arrives from social, racial, sexual and cultural biases, institutionalized in society. Its prejudicial effect greatly outweighs its very limited evidentiary value." . . .

It is clear from the trial court's articulation that the basis of its ruling was that the Belmont Report's probative value was outweighed by its likely unfair prejudicial effect. The court acted in accord with [Connecticut law].

NOTES AND QUESTIONS

1. Imagine that you were a member of the jury that heard the *Ancheff* case. Would you have concluded that John Ancheff was in a research study? What pieces of information would have been most important in reaching your deci-

sion? What is the relevance of the fact that the hospital was continuing to collect information on each patient who got the higher dose of the drug and putting that information in a file separate from the patient's medical records?

2. One of the claims made by John Ancheff is that the hospital failed to tell him of "the experimental nature of his treatment with the drug." Is this a separate question from determining whether or not he was in a research study? Is it possible that he was not in a research study but was nonetheless getting experimental treatment? (As is discussed later in this chapter, once a drug is approved by the Food and Drug Administration for treating one particular medical problem, federal law does not prevent doctors from using the drug in different ways, such as altering the dose or using it to treat other problems.) If so, how would you determine whether the treatment was experimental? *See*, e.g., *Estrada v. Jacques*, 321 S.E.2d 240 (1984) (discussing informed consent issues regarding experimental treatments).

3. In the summer of 2003, Iranian sisters Ladan and Laleh Bijani, who were joined at the head, underwent a surgical procedure in Singapore to separate them. While similar procedures had been performed (though rarely) on other sets of conjoined twins, they had always been done while the twins were still children. This was the first time such a procedure was performed on adults. The doctors indicated that there was a 50 percent chance that the twins would die. The twins chose to go ahead with the procedure, and the worst did happen—they both died. *See* Denise Grady, *2 Women, 2 Deaths and an Ethical Quandary*, N.Y. TIMES, July 15, 2003, at D1. Had this operation taken place at a major university medical center in the United States, would IRB approval have been required prior to the operation? What additional information might you want to know to help answer that question?

4. Sometimes the abdomen of a developing fetus allows portions of the intestines to squeeze outside of the fetus's body. The blood supply is cut off, and the intestines die. When the child is born, it doesn't have enough small intestines to absorb nutrients. One way of treating this condition involves a complicated surgical procedure to lengthen the small intestine. Dr. Heung Bae Kim, while he was still a medical student, thought of a new way to do the surgery that was much simpler. His attending physician at the time told him it would never work. A decade later, while completing a fellowship in pediatric surgery at Children's Hospital in Boston, he again mentioned his idea, and the surgeon he was working with thought it was ingenious. The procedure was successfully performed on one child, after being reviewed by the hospital's IRB under "a special consent process for innovative procedures." Denise Grady, *Brainstorm to Breakthrough: A Surgical Procedure is Born*, N.Y. TIMES, August 4, 2003, at A1. Should physicians routinely seek IRB review of "innovative procedures" that do not technically constitute research? What should physicians do if they do not practice in institutions that have IRBs?

5. The standard way to perform a corneal transplant involves sewing the new cornea into the patient's eye. It can take one to two hours to perform this deli-

cate sewing, and over the several months following the operation, the patient's vision may be blurry as sutures are cut to help adjust uneven tension on the cornea. Dr. James Rowsey, head of the ophthalmology department at the University of South Florida, came up with the idea of cutting the donor cornea so that it has little tabs on it, which could be slipped into pockets cut into the patient's cornea, thus eliminating the need for sutures. This could dramatically shorten the length of the operation and allow the patient's vision to improve more quickly following the surgery. After performing the operation on cats, he moved on to doing it on people. When he was later accused of violating the federal research regulations, because he had not filed for approval of a research study, his defense was that his surgical technique was so very similar to the standard one that he was not doing anything experimental. Did he need to file for IRB approval? What additional information might you want to know? What parts of the definition of research would be most relevant to answering this question? *See* Determination Letter from Compliance Oversight Branch, OHRP, to University of South Florida, dated September 28, 2000, available at http://www.hhs.gov/ohrp/detrm_letrs/sep00f.pdf.

6. The examples in notes 3 through 5 all involve alterations in surgical procedures. Surgeons have often claimed that because each patient is different — everyone, to some extent, has a unique anatomy — there is always a bit of experimentation involved in any surgical procedure. This argument has led some to conclude that a great deal of surgical innovation does not come within the purview of the research regulations, because it is usually not systematic, but rather represents the accumulation of innovative changes gradually made to reflect the challenges presented by each patient's unique problem. Do you agree with that conclusion?

7. One of the more recent new technologies for dealing with certain cases of male infertility is intracytoplasmic sperm injection, or ICSI. This technique involves directly injecting a single sperm into an egg, thus creating a fertilized egg. The first successful use of this technology was in 1992 in Belgium, and within a year it was being used in clinical care in the United States. How should a determination be made that such a new technology is sufficiently safe and will not, for example, lead to the creation of fetuses with serious abnormalities? In determining whether patients receiving ICSI were research subjects, is it relevant that the U.S. physicians performing ICSI for the first time were unable to duplicate the high success rates of their more experienced Belgium counterparts? *See* NEW YORK TASK FORCE ON LIFE AND THE LAW, ASSISTED REPRODUCTIVE TECHNOLOGIES: ANALYSIS AND RECOMMENDATIONS FOR PUBLIC POLICY 162-64 (1998).

8. As the *Ancheff* case and the examples above indicate, there is a difference between how the legal system deals with a doctor who provides "innovative" care directly to a patient (outside of the research setting), and a researcher who provides such care to a subject participating in research. Some have suggested that the current rules provide inadequate protection to patients who are given

innovative care outside of research, and that the regulations governing research should be revised to also apply to that situation. *See, e.g.*, Jon Tyson, *Dubious Distinctions Between Research and Clinical Practice Using Experimental Therapies: Have Patients Been Well Served?* In AMNON GOLDWORTH ET AL. (EDS.), ETHICS AND PERINATOLOGY 214 (1995). Is that a good suggestion? Are subjects who get innovative care from a doctor inadequately protected under the existing rules? For a discussion of how tort law currently views innovative therapy, see Chapter 1, at page 16 and Chapter 7, at page 304.

9. For additional discussion of these issues, see, e.g., Nancy M.P. King, *The Line Between Clinical Innovation and Human Experimentation*, 32 SETON HALL L. REV. 573 (2002); Nancy M.P. King, *Experimental Treatment: Oxymoron or Aspiration?* 25 HASTINGS CENTER REP., July-Aug. 1995, at 6; John Lantos, *How Can We Distinguish Clinical Research from Innovative Therapy?* 16 AM. J. PEDIATRIC HEMATOLOGY/ONCOLOGY 72 (1994); Iain Chalmers & Richard I. Lindley, *Double Standards on Informed Consent to Treatment*, in LEN DOYAL & JEFFREY S. TOBIAS (eds.), INFORMED CONSENT IN MEDICAL RESEARCH 266 (2001).

[c] Research versus Quality Improvement

The Quality Improvement-Research Divide and the Need for External Oversight
Eran Bellin & Nancy Neveloff Dubler
91 AM. J. PUB. HEALTH 1512 (2001)

Federal regulations intended to protect human research subjects require institutional review boards (IRBs) to review and approve the design and process of research to enhance subjects' understanding, protect autonomy, and minimize risk. In contrast, hospital quality assurance studies have been conducted in private settings, often explicitly shielded by state law, to encourage honest exploration of mistakes by physician reviewers. Since their goal of improving patient care seems morally unambiguous, quality assurance studies have received scant ethical attention, and there has been no call for supervision external to the participants. Historically, quality assurance has consisted primarily of retrospective reviews of physician practice triggered by alarming outcomes. However, the public's perception of the frequency of errors in medical practice is evolving. Oversight agencies and the public are demanding a transition to an active process of continuous quality improvement. . . .

In an implicit modern reflection of the social contract, the patient consents to and pays for treatment and the medical community obligates itself to prevent errors, identify them when they occur, learn from them, and preclude their repetition. Unlike research, an optional external activity imposed on the physician-patient relationship, continuous quality improvement is ethically intrinsic to providing care. The notion of a formal consent process has thus been considered irrelevant, although the issue has never been debated formally. . . .

The continuous quality improvement process is embedded in an organizational matrix committed to using the results of the study to inform immediately the process of care. It is this feedback loop, with its expectation of responsiveness, that motivates and legitimates continuous quality improvement reviews. . . .

Quality improvement projects can be of 2 distinct types: retrospective review or prospective interventional. For the retrospective review of records, the critical determinant of nonresearch status is the commitment, in advance of data collection, to a corrective action plan given any one of a number of possible outcomes. The sponsor of this review must have both clinical supervisory responsibility and the authority to impose change. Even the creation of pseudocohorts by the random review of charts with specific characteristics, the use of advanced statistical models, or the extraction of generalizable knowledge for publication does not change the essential character of the work. However, the same record review performed without this commitment is research and subject to external review by an IRB.

Prospective interventional studies, even when sponsored by the clinical authority responsible for quality improvement, require external scrutiny. We present 3 examples.

Example 1

A health maintenance organization (HMO) would like to test the efficacy and cost of 2 established therapies for hypertension. Under present practice standards, the HMO can differentially reimburse patients or reward physicians for compliance with the cost saving standard. Suppose the HMO wished to rigorously evaluate its approach to care by randomizing patients to 1 of 2 strategies. It is clear that such a study requires review by an IRB and informed consent. Even though the primary endpoint, hypertension control, can be achieved through either therapy, the side effect profiles are different. Patients have a right to expect that their physicians will optimize their treatment both for the primary endpoint and with consideration for their preferences for side effects. At the very least, patients expect an honest relationship with the physician and expect to be told if some motivation other than their best interest is driving the decision. The fact that the HMO can virtually order the use of a particular regimen by restricting its formulary is immaterial. If it differentially assigns therapy to explore outcomes, it engages in research. . . .

Example 3

A continuous quality improvement department is trying to decide whether investing the resources for the ongoing review of care of AIDS patients is worth the effort. It has the technical computer capability to review automatically, on a monthly basis, the CD4 counts, viral loads, and medications of all of its patients. The costly part of the intervention would be convening case reviews and patient interviews to attempt to improve the outcome of care. To answer the question rigorously, the study design must create 2 de facto standards of care in the clinic. Were the clinic to prospectively assign intervention differentially, there would be no question that this would be research and IRB review would be required. In a clever manipulation, however, the continuous quality improvement department randomizes one half of the patients to monthly computer quality improvement review. The restriction of quality improvement review to a randomly selected subset is clearly within the quality improvement tradition. Those randomized to surveillance who are found to be failing their therapies are reported to the medical director.

Once presented with evidence that individuals are not achieving desired endpoints, the director of the AIDS clinic decides to convene 3 senior physicians to discuss those patients. The team reviews the charts for evidence of medical errors, examining the appointment log and prescription pickup record for evidence of noncompliance. The director then develops a program to ensure improved compliance or improved attention to standards of care by physicians for the identified patients.

The intervention is generated by the clinical director independently of the randomization. The collection of data morally compels the director to provide "the best standard of care" but does not formally assign the rest of the clinic to an inferior standard. The standard care of the other patients in the clinic is not functionally interfered with by the medical director, who is ignorant of any flaws in their care. After a year of this creative manipulation, the computer system is asked to review the clinical outcomes of both groups.

At no point in this process has there been a formal violation of continuous quality improvement procedure or practice, nor has there been specific assignment of intervention; however, this is clearly a technical manipulation to avoid the designation of research and to sidestep external review. While the study itself might be legitimate, the manipulation makes it a potentially dangerous model. In addition, the lack of a formal review process and of an honest design precludes the use of interim statistical analyses, through which the department might find benefit early, end the "trial," and provide the intervention to the "control group." . . .

The line between quality improvement and research is rapidly being effaced. With new medical information systems that can identify patients with particular medical problems, characterize the intervention, and evaluate the care delivered against an agreed upon standard, there is a clear ethical imperative to advance the quality improvement process to lessen mistakes and prevent substandard care. The relevant ethical issue is whether there is a need for some oversight mechanism, external to the quality improvement process, to protect patients. We say that there is.

In the history of research, the abuse of human subjects led to the creation of clear guidelines for the review of research protocols. IRBs examine the possible risks and benefits for the subjects and approve the informed consent process that is designed to educate and empower prospective subjects. This review is necessitated by the experience that research protocols can either provide benefit or actually harm subjects and on the ethical premise that voluntary informed consent must precede assumption of risk.

Prospective quality improvement evaluations that allocate treatment with or without randomization to different cohorts generally to identify the most cost-effective care but sometimes to identify best practice should, like research, be subject to review and should trigger considerations of informed consent. This rule should apply whether or not generalizable information is created for public presentation or dissemination.

NOTES AND QUESTIONS

1. What are the dividing lines that Bellin and Dubler suggest for determining which quality improvement projects should be considered research? How do those dividing lines compare to the definition of research in the Common Rule? Do you agree with the conclusions of the authors? Why or why not?

2. Another group of commentators proposed a two-part test for separating quality improvement from research. Under their test, a quality improvement initiative should be considered research if "(1) the majority of patients involved are not expected to benefit directly from the knowledge to be gained, or (2) if additional risks or burdens are imposed to make the results generalizable." David Casarett et al., *Determining When Quality Improvement Initiatives Should Be Considered Research: Proposed Criteria and Potential Implications*, 283 JAMA 2275 (2000). Can this rule be derived from the definition in the regulations? What are the differences between the results produced by it and the rule proposed by Bellin and Dubler? Does one of the rules seem better to you, and if so, why? For a case study applying the Casarett rule to a controversy about the best way to test women for reproductive tract infections with the organism Chlamydia trachomatis, see David Doezema and Mark Hauswald, *Quality Improvement or Research: Distinction Without a Difference?* 24 IRB, July-Aug. 2002, at 9.

3. A hospital asks all its patients to complete a post-discharge satisfaction survey. A clinic randomizes patients to receive (or not receive) reminders of their appointments, and then measures the no-show rate. In each case, is this research under the Casarett rule? Under the Bellin-Dubler rule?

[d] Research versus Public Health Initiatives

GUIDELINES FOR DEFINING PUBLIC HEALTH RESEARCH AND PUBLIC HEALTH NON-RESEARCH CENTERS FOR DISEASE CONTROL AND PREVENTION
(1999)

The practice of public health poses several challenges in implementing 45 CFR 46. Although some public health activities can unambiguously be classified as either research or non-research, for other activities the classification is more difficult. The difficulty in classifying some public health activities as research or non-research stems either from traditionally held views about what constitutes public health practice or from the fact that 45 CFR 46 does not directly address many public health activities. In addition, the statutory authority of state and local health departments to conduct public health activities using methods similar to those used by researchers is not recognized in the regulations. Human subject protections applicable for activities occurring at the boundary between public health non-research and public health research are not readily interpretable from the regulations.

The regulations state that "research means a systematic investigation, including research development, testing and evaluation, designed to develop or contribute to generalizable knowledge." Obtaining and analyzing data are essential to the usual practice of public health. For many public health activities, data are systematically collected and analyzed, blurring the distinction between research and non-research. Scientific methodology is used both in non-research and research activities that comprise the practice of public health. Because scientific principles and methodology are applied to both non-research and research activities, knowledge is generated in both cases. Furthermore, at times the extent to which that knowledge is generalizable may not differ greatly in research and non-research. Thus, non-research and research activities cannot be easily defined by the methods they employ. Three public health activities — surveillance, emergency responses, and evaluation — are particularly susceptible to the quandary over whether the activity is research or non-research.

The key word in the regulations' definition of research for the purpose of classifying public health activities as either research or non-research is "designed." The major difference between research and non-research lies in the primary intent of the activity. The primary intent of research is to generate or contribute to generalizable knowledge. The primary intent of non-research in public health is to prevent or control disease or injury and improve health, or to improve a public health program or service. Knowledge may be gained in any public health endeavor designed to prevent disease or injury or improve a program or service. In some cases, that knowledge may be generalizable, but the primary intention of the endeavor is to benefit clients participating in a public health program or a population by controlling a health problem in the population from which the information is gathered. . . .

Examples of CDC surveillance, emergency responses, and evaluation activities that are non-research and research.

SURVEILLANCE:

Non-research —

> National Notifiable Diseases Surveillance System (NNDSS) — States and territories have asked CDC to act as a common data collection point for data on nationally notifiable diseases. A notifiable disease is considered by the Council of State and Territorial Epidemiologists to be a condition for which regular, frequent, and timely information about individual cases is necessary at the national level for the prevention and control of disease. NNDSS data are collected and published weekly in the Morbidity and Mortality Weekly Report and annually in the Summary of Notifiable Diseases, United States. The NNDSS is essential to the day-to-day practice of public health. The primary intent of the surveillance system is to provide CDC and state and local health officials with information to detect and control outbreaks of disease. The NNDSS is also used to measure the impact of programs such as immunization. The intended benefits resulting from the NNDSS are for the residents of the states and local areas who contribute data to the system.

> Diabetes Surveillance Report — Using public use data from several national surveys, a national diabetes surveillance system is produced. Data from the surveillance system are used to describe the burden of diabetes and its complications on a national and state level. The primary intent of the surveillance system is to provide information for the development of national and state public health priorities and policies regarding the prevention and control of diabetes. The intended benefits are for those who have diabetes or those who are at risk of developing diabetes.

Research —

> A Sentinel Surveillance System for Lassa Fever in the Republic of Guinea — Four study sites were selected to identify and describe cases of Lassa fever. Cases were identified from hospital and outpatient admissions. The purpose of the project was to generate baseline information on the Lassa virus and human clinical Lassa fever in the Republic of Guinea. No public health interventions were planned as part of this project; there were no direct benefits for study participants. Thus, the primary intent was to contribute to the knowledge of Lassa fever.

NOTES AND QUESTIONS

1. The CDC comments suggest that the primary purpose of an activity should determine whether the activity is research. Contrast that approach to the last sentence of the excerpt from the Belmont Report, noting that if there is *any* element of research in an activity, it should undergo IRB review. Are these two views compatible? Does the definition of research in the regulations adopt one or the other of these positions?

2. "As part of the evaluation of the school-based HIV prevention program in Denver public schools, principals, teachers, student contact staff, students, and parents were interviewed. HIV program efforts in policy awareness, staff development, curriculum implementation, and status of students receiving HIV prevention education were assessed." Was this research? Why or why not? *See* CDC, GUIDELINES FOR DEFINING PUBLIC HEALTH RESEARCH AND PUBLIC HEALTH NON-RESEARCH (1999), available at http://www.cdc.gov/od/ads/opspoll1.htm.

3. For further discussion of this issue, including a proposed checklist for public health practitioners to use in determining whether they are doing research, see COUNCIL OF STATE AND TERRITORIAL EPIDEMIOLOGISTS, PUBLIC HEALTH PRACTICE VS. RESEARCH: A REPORT FOR PUBLIC HEALTH PRACTITIONERS INCLUDING CASES AND GUIDANCE FOR MAKING DISTINCTIONS (2004), available at http://www.cste.org.

[3] Definition of Human Subject

There are two very different ways a study can involve the use of human subjects: the researchers may be directly interacting with human beings, or they may be obtaining access to identifiable private information about people. If *either* of these criteria is met, then the study involves human subjects.

45 C.F.R. § 46.102(f): DEFINITION OF HUMAN SUBJECT

This provision is reproduced in Appendix A, at page A-4. Please review it before proceeding.

NOTES AND QUESTIONS

1. OHRP provides a number of decision charts intended to help people work through various aspects of the regulations, including one that examines whether a particular activity constitutes research and involves the use of human subjects. *See* OFFICE FOR HUMAN RESEARCH PROTECTIONS, CHART 1: IS AN ACTIVITY RESEARCH INVOLVING HUMAN SUBJECTS COVERED BY 45 CFR PART 46? available at http://www.hhs.gov/ohrp/humansubjects/guidance/decisioncharts.htm.

2. A researcher sits in the waiting room of an oncologist, recording information about the behavior of the patients (e.g., do they come alone, do they appear nervous, do they read magazines, and if so, for how long), to determine how patients deal with a diagnosis of cancer. The researcher never has access to the names or other identifying information of any of the patients. Are human subjects involved in the study?

3. In the mid-1970s, a group of researchers

> observed men urinating in a public lavatory in order to test their hypothesis that close proximity to another man produces arousal which, in turn, would influence the rate and volume of [urination.] . . . In order to do this, they placed signs over urinals that they did not wish to have the subject use indicating that they were out of order. The urinary stream was observed by a colleague in an adjacent toilet stall with the aid of a prism periscope hidden in a stack of books. To create the condition of crowding, another investigator pretended to use an adjacent urinal.

ROBERT J. LEVINE, ETHICS AND REGULATION OF CLINICAL RESEARCH 220 (2d ed. 1988). Did this study involve human subjects? If your answer is different from the one you gave for note (2), what aspects of this study led you to that different conclusion? Would your answer be any different for a similar study that still involved a researcher using the periscope, but did not involve using "out of order" signs or having members of the research team "crowding" the subjects?

4. A researcher goes to the medical records department and asks to be given the charts of the last 50 patients who suffered fatal heart attacks while in the hospital. The researcher will photocopy these charts, and will then take the photocopies to his office and analyze them to determine if the hospital is providing appropriate treatment to in-patients who suffer heart attacks. Are human subjects involved in the study?

5. A researcher wants to conduct a study using a modified virus as a method to treat a type of cancer. For the first part of her study, she needs to determine where in a patient's body the virus tends to accumulate. This requires injecting the virus into a person's body, and then biopsying multiple organs within a few hours. Because very few people would consent to such an experiment, she has proposed two possible groups of subjects. The first group would include people who are in the hospital dying, and likely to live only a few more hours (because, for example, a decision has been made to stop life support). These subjects would be given the virus while they are still alive, and the biopsies would be performed after they died. A second group of possible subjects would be people who are brain dead — i.e., people who are legally dead but whose hearts are still beating because ventilator support has not yet been removed. What issues are raised in considering which group of subjects to enroll? *See, e.g.,* Rebecca D. Pentz et al., *Revisiting Ethical Guidelines for Research with Terminal Wean and Brain-Dead Participants,* 33 HASTINGS CENTER REP., Jan.-Feb. 2003, at 20; Mark

R. Wicclair & Michael DeVita, *Oversight of Research Involving the Dead*, 14 KENNEDY INST. ETHICS J. 143 (2004); Jennifer Couzin, *Crossing a Frontier: Research on the Dead*, 299 SCIENCE 29 (2003). If persons who are brain dead do not constitute human subjects under the federal regulations, does that mean that researchers need not seek IRB approval for studies involving brain-dead subjects? Should institutions require some sort of approval process for research involving brain-dead subjects even if such a process is not required by the Common Rule?

[4] Exempt Studies

There is a special category of studies that are "exempt" from the Common Rule's requirements. A list of these types of studies appears at the very beginning of the Common Rule. In general, these studies would otherwise be subject to the requirements of the Common Rule, but due to their low risk level, the government has determined that it is not worth the effort to subject them to the administrative burdens imposed by the regulations.

Although there are six categories of exempt studies, three of these categories are most commonly encountered: educational research, 45 C.F.R. § 101(b)(1); surveys, interviews, and observation of public behavior, § 101(b)(2); and studies involving the use of existing data or specimens, § 101(b)(4).

45 C.F.R. § 46.101(b): CATEGORIES OF EXEMPT RESEARCH

This provision is reproduced in Appendix A, at page A-1. Please review it before proceeding. Pay particular attention to subsections (1), (2), and (4).

NOTES AND QUESTIONS

1. OHRP provides several decision charts to help people understand the exemption categories. *See* OFFICE FOR HUMAN RESEARCH PROTECTIONS, CHARTS 2 THROUGH 7, available at http://www.hhs.gov/ohrp/humansubjects/guidance/decisioncharts.htm. For a discussion of the exempt categories, including more decision charts, see Ivor A. Pritchard, *Searching for "Research Involving Human Subjects": What is Examined? What is Exempt? What is Exasperating?* 23 IRB, May-June 2001, at 5.

2. It is important to remember that, just because a study might be exempt, the researchers are not free to ignore the IRB at their institution. Most institutions have adopted policies that require researchers who want to conduct potentially exempt studies to file documents with the IRB, so that the IRB can make its own determination that the study is exempt. In fact, the federal government encourages institutions to adopt this type of policy. The rules about determining when a study is or is not exempt are far from straightforward,

and allowing investigators to make their own determinations that a study is exempt would likely lead to some studies inappropriately escaping IRB oversight.

3. While meeting the requirements for an exemption means that the study need not comply with all of the detailed requirements of the Common Rule — including the risk-benefit review by an IRB, the use of written consent forms, and the requirement for annual recertification by an IRB — it does not mean that the researcher can ignore basic ethical guidelines. The federal government requires, as a provision in the "assurance" with the federal government that institutions conducting federally funded research must sign, that even exempt studies conform to the general guidelines contained in the Belmont Report. *See* OFFICE FOR HUMAN RESEARCH PROTECTIONS, FEDERALWIDE ASSURANCE OF PROTECTION FOR HUMAN SUBJECTS § A(1), available at http://www.hhs.gov/ohrp/humansubjects/assurance/filasurt.htm.

4. Make sure you read the important footnote relating to the exempt categories at page A-3, which specifies that none of the exemptions apply to studies on the "vulnerable populations" described in Subparts B and C of 45 C.F.R. Part 46, and that the Category 2 exemption does not generally apply to research involving minors. What are some of the consequences of this footnote?

5. An elementary school teacher wants to change the way she teaches a particular session by organizing the material in an innovative way. She proposes to also give the students a post-session not-for-credit quiz to see how well the session worked. She intends to write up the results and submit it to a journal for teachers. She wants to require the students to take the quiz, and she does not want to tell their parents about the quiz. Can she do this without obtaining the approval of the IRB at her institution? (Assume that her school does have an IRB and has agreed to comply with the federal regulations with regard to any research at the school.)

6. A researcher proposes to give patients in the waiting room of an AIDS clinic a questionnaire asking them for detailed information about their sexual practices. Some of the answers might indicate that the subjects had committed a crime. The researcher will not record the name of the person, or any other information that would enable her to identify any subject. Is the study exempt?

7. A researcher who is studying trends in popular culture hands out questionnaires to preteens leaving a movie theater after a Saturday matinee. The questionnaires, which are anonymous, ask the children what sorts of movies they enjoy. Is the study exempt?

8. A researcher proposes to collect information on the next 100 patients who are treated for heart attacks at his institution. He wants to record only the patients' ages, the length of the period between when the patients had symptoms and when they arrived at the hospital, and the length of time they stayed in the hospital. In each case he will collect this information from the patients' medical records the day after they are discharged. He will not write down any-

thing other than the above information (such as the patient's name or medical record number) in his research records. Is his study exempt?

9. Assume the same researcher modified the study somewhat, so that he was using the records of the last 100 patients who had heart attacks. He is again going to record only the information described above. Because he is concerned that he might discover that he left out a piece of information on one or more of his subjects, when he leaves the medical records room after writing down the information he wanted on all of the subjects, he will keep a list that has the subject number he has assigned to each person in the study, and next to that number that patient's medical record number. He will keep that list in a locked drawer in his office, not show it to anyone, and use it only if he discovers that he is missing a piece of data on one or another of the subjects. Is his study exempt?

[B] Additional DHHS Regulations Governing Vulnerable Populations

An important aspect of the federal regulations is the recognition that certain categories of people are "vulnerable," and thus they need to be accorded special protections to make sure that researchers do not take advantage of them. This problem is considered so important that of the four "sub-parts" of the federal regulations, three of them — B, C, and D — are wholly concerned with issues relating to vulnerable populations.

45 C.F.R. § 46.111(b), AND PART 46, SUBPARTS B, C, AND D: VULNERABLE POPULATIONS

These provisions are reproduced in Appendix A, beginning on page A-18. Please skim them before proceeding.

The Invisible Vulnerable: The Economically and Educationally Disadvantaged Subjects of Clinical Research
T. Howard Stone
31 J.L. MED. & ETHICS 149 (2003)

[The federal regulations] refer to the need for special precautions when persons characterized as vulnerable are used as human research subjects. Under the Common Rule, persons considered "vulnerable" are those who are likely to be susceptible to coercive or undue influence; the term "vulnerable" includes "children, prisoners, pregnant women, mentally disabled persons," or those who are "economically or educationally disadvantaged." The need for special precautions with some of these vulnerable persons in the context of research has long been addressed by both mandatory additional protections found in Subparts B through D of 45 C.F.R. pt. 46 (that are not, coincidentally, part of the Common Rule) and additional detailed guidance documents provided by HHS or its components to investigators and their respective institutions. . . .

The vulnerability of subjects of research is inextricably tied to the efficacy of their consent to participate in a given research protocol. A person's individual circumstances, together with the particulars of a specific research project — both of which may be continuously variable — may therefore at any given time render such person more or less vulnerable as a subject of research. This suggests that prior to and while any person serves as a subject of research, consent be individualized to take into account a person's circumstances with respect to the research project. Regardless of individualized vulnerability, some persons are grouped into categories considered especially vulnerable, and for some categories public policy requires additional protections.

For example, persons who are incarcerated or institutionalized, such as prisoners, have at times been considered inappropriate subjects of either all or many types of research, owing to the authoritarian, punitive setting in which prisoners must live. The ability of prisoners to "make truly voluntary and uncoerced decisions" about taking part as a research subject is explicitly suspect. The authors of *The Belmont Report* state that, as a "matter of social justice . . . prisoners may be involved as research subjects, if at all, only on certain conditions." To address these and related concerns, the additional protections found at Subpart C of 45 C.F.R. pt. 46 are invoked whenever a human subject happens to be a prisoner. Subpart C essentially "raises the bar" for research involving the use of prisoners as subjects, and primarily serves to limit the risks to which prisoners might be exposed as subjects as well as impose additional duties upon an institutional review board (IRB) when reviewing and approving such research. As an adjunct to Subpart C, the National Institutes of Health's Office for Protection from Research Risks (OPRR, now the HHS Office for Human Research Protection, or OHRP) provides somewhat more detailed guidance regarding prisoners as subjects to researchers, research institutions, and research sponsors, including information in the OPRR Institutional Review Board Guidebook and the OPRR May 2000 guidance letter.

Children are also considered inappropriate as subjects of certain types of research, largely owing to their obvious lack of decisional capacity or maturity. Like prisoners, children are also considered unable to make voluntary and uncoerced decisions about taking part in research, especially in light of the generally dependent and authoritarian nature of a child's relationships with adults. In response to these concerns, the additional protections found at Subpart D of 45 C.F.R. pt. 46 are triggered whenever children are used as human subjects, and generally serve to significantly limit the risks to which children may be exposed as human subjects. As with prisoners, HHS provides researchers, research institutions, and research sponsors with specific guidance and policy regarding children as subjects, including the requirement that children not be improperly excluded from research participation. Determining when prisoners or children are no longer in need of additional protection is — at least within the context of 45 C.F.R. pt. 46, Subparts C and D, respectively — straightforward: Subpart C no longer applies to a person who is released from prison, and Subpart D no longer applies to a person who reaches the legal age of consent.

Like prisoners and children, persons who are economically or educationally disadvantaged are also specifically identified as a "vulnerable population." In carrying out their responsibilities under the Common Rule, IRBs are required to make sure that applicable criteria for approval of research are satisfied. One of these criteria is to ensure that the selection of subjects is equitable. In making this determination, IRBs are exhorted to be "particularly cognizant of the special problems of research involving vulnerable populations, such as . . . economically or educationally disadvantaged persons." As an additional criterion for approval of research involving economically or educationally disadvantaged persons, IRBs must ensure that "additional safeguards have been included in the study to protect the rights and welfare of these subjects."

However, unlike prisoners and children, or other groups of persons designated as vulnerable under the Common Rule — and for reasons that are not clear — persons who are economically or educationally disadvantaged are not the focus of any specific additional protections under 45 C.F.R. pt. 46 or supplementary HHS guidance. There are no subparts of 45 C.F.R. pt. 46 or any guidance materials that might serve to elucidate how IRBs are to discharge their responsibility for ensuring that additional safeguards have been included in studies involving economically or educationally disadvantaged persons. Moreover, unlike for other vulnerable populations, and with the exception of articles pertaining to the readability of consent documents, there is a dearth of literature addressing how IRBs should approach the review of research involving persons who are economically or educationally disadvantaged. In effect, IRBs are left on their own to make these determinations. As a result, persons who are economically or educationally disadvantaged and who serve as human research subjects remain unduly vulnerable to clinical research risks, and they have become the "invisible vulnerable."

Regulating Research on the Terminally Ill: A Proposal for Heightened Safeguards
Christian Addicott
15 J. CONTEMP. HEALTH L. & POL'Y 479 (1999)

Many factors contribute to the vulnerability of the terminally ill. Individuals' psychological responses to terminal illness vary widely. Some employ healthy coping mechanisms, but many suffer from a variety of psychological problems — such as acute anxiety, depression, anger, and dependency — that can make it difficult, if not impossible, to rationally evaluate the pros and cons of participating in potentially life-threatening research. In addition, tremendous financial and professional rewards for discovering new treatments and publishing the results provide a strong incentive for researchers to bend or break the rules. As a result, the terminally ill patient considering whether to participate as a research subject is highly vulnerable to coercion and undue influence.

Federal regulations governing human research provide special protections to "vulnerable" populations such as children and prisoners who may be incapable of giving their voluntary informed consent to participate as research subjects. No such protections are extended to the terminally ill. Indeed, over the past fifteen years AIDS activists have fought for deregulation, and the terminally ill now have earlier access to experimental drugs when there are no adequate therapies available, and promising new drugs for the terminally ill are put on a fast track for regulatory approval. The terminally ill have come to be seen by researchers and regulators alike not as passive and weak, but as autonomous agents with the right to evaluate information and make their own decisions. These important gains, however, have tended to obfuscate the fact that the terminally ill are highly vulnerable to coercion and undue influence by inattentive or unethical researchers.

A confluence of factors works together to make the terminally ill vulnerable to research abuse. The terminally ill are desperate for a cure and often suffer from depression, anxiety, or other psychological disorders that may be exacerbated by the physiological symptoms of their illnesses. These psychological symptoms make rational decision-making extremely difficult. Also, the terminally ill are often hospitalized, feel dependent on the researchers in whose hands they have placed their lives, and as a result may be reluctant to ask difficult questions — wanting instead to play the good patient to curry favor and to avoid reprisals. Often, patients simply presume that whatever their doctor recommends is in their best interest, and fail to understand the dual roles of the physician/researcher. Moreover, researchers are under tremendous financial and professional pressures to complete their studies quickly and publish the results, and thus may be reluctant to say or do things that will decrease the likelihood of enrolling eligible subjects.

[The excerpt that follows is from earlier in the article.]

[T]he following regulatory reforms should be adopted:

(1) The terminally ill should be classified under the regulations as a vulnerable population;

(2) Institutional Review Boards (IRBs) that approve research involving the terminally ill should be required to include or consult with at least one member who would represent the interests of the terminally ill;

(3) Researchers who involve the terminally ill as subjects should be trained to recognize the psychological difficulties that the terminally ill face;

(4) With a few exceptions, research on the terminally ill should be prohibited unless it is intended to provide a therapeutic benefit to the subjects;

(5) Terminally ill patients should receive psychological evaluations before participating in research studies; and

(6) Subject advocates should be available to assist the terminally ill during the informed consent process.

NOTES AND QUESTIONS

1. While these excerpts focus on the economically or educationally disadvantaged and the terminally ill, they are not the only groups that might be considered to be "shortchanged" by the regulations. "Adults lacking decision-making capacity" is a group that, although specifically designated as requiring special protections, does not have a separate Subpart of the regulations explaining what those special protections should be. Some guidance is proved in Chapter 6D, Cognitively Impaired Persons, of the *Institutional Review Board Guidebook*, available at http://www.hhs.gov/ohrp/irb/irb_chapter6.htm.

2. Why do you think there are no specific regulations dealing with the economically or educationally disadvantaged, the terminally ill, or those who lack decision-making capacity? With regard to the latter group, regulations have been proposed a number of times at both the federal and state levels, but have never been approved.

3. If you were asked to draft a set of regulations that specified the special protections to be accorded economically or educationally disadvantaged subjects, what types of rules would you include? For the former group, for example, should special attention be paid to studies that offer free medical care or other types of financial inducements to enroll in a study? For the latter group, should special attention be paid to the reading level of the consent form?

1 ETHICAL AND POLICY ISSUES IN RESEARCH INVOLVING HUMAN PARTICIPANTS
NATIONAL BIOETHICS ADVISORY COMMISSION
85-92 (2001)

The current DHHS regulations regarding vulnerable individuals are beset with various conceptual and practical difficulties. For example, the subparts offer no definition of vulnerability and no analysis of the types of characteristics that render persons vulnerable. The list of vulnerable groups (children, prisoners, pregnant women, fetuses, mentally disabled persons, and economically and educationally disadvantaged persons) provided in Subpart A, 45 CFR 46.111 and 21 CFR 56.111 is incomplete on the one hand and overly broad on the other. For example, injection drug users, the seriously ill, the elderly, and undocumented immigrants could, in particular circumstances, also be considered vulnerable. On the other hand, vulnerability is sensitive to context, and individuals may be vulnerable in one situation but not in another. For example, people of low income are rendered vulnerable in studies offering large financial incentives to take on research risk. In addition, the regulations provide inadequate guidance about the types of safeguards that would be appropriate to protect against the risks associated with vulnerability. Subpart A of the regulations requires IRBs to ensure that such individuals are protected, but it does not describe how to achieve such protection. In addition to the shortcomings in the regulations, at least two aspects of the current research enterprise suggest a need to evaluate the protections for vulnerable research participants. Increases in research funding are leading to more research involving human participants, and as more people become research participants, more individuals with vulnerabilities are likely to be included. Moreover, because clinical research often holds the prospect of direct benefit and may be perceived as a means of access to health care, serious illness or lack of health insurance may significantly intensify a person's desire to be involved in research.

Although the use of subparts in the DHHS regulations makes it clear which groups should be considered vulnerable, this advantage is outweighed by several disadvantages. Given the limited required safeguards, the current regulations provide insufficient respect for persons and are not sufficiently responsive to the full array of vulnerability experienced by prospective participants. The use of regulatory subparts is not the optimal means by which to protect vulnerable individuals for the following reasons:

- Providing protections for all potentially vulnerable groups would require developing an unwieldy list of additional subparts.

- To the extent that different groups may require the same types of protection, the addition of a long list of subparts may introduce unnecessary duplication in the regulations.

- A group-based approach to vulnerability leaves unanswered questions about how to safeguard persons with multiple vulnerabilities.

- The status of particular groups may change. For example, as members of a particular group become increasingly less subjected to stereotypes, they become increasingly less prone to social vulnerability. Although IRBs and investigators should remain concerned about this general category of vulnerability, their treatment of this particular group should reflect its changing social status. Accommodating such a changing social reality would require regulatory change to a group-based subpart approach to vulnerability, but not to an analytical approach. In order to improve the protections found in the current subparts, each subpart would have to be revised based on an analytical understanding of vulnerability in order to fully reflect its nature and variability and to contain appropriate safeguards.

- Group-based subparts classify certain persons as vulnerable, rather than classifying situations in which individuals might be considered vulnerable. For example, persons with severe illnesses for which there are no acceptable treatments may be medically vulnerable in certain kinds of clinical trials, but not vulnerable at all in many other types of research (e.g., survey research).

An analytic approach provides a context-sensitive understanding of vulnerability that avoids the implementation of unnecessary protections, which not only impede the progress of research, but also fail to respect the personhood of the potential participants. Thus, an analytical approach not only provides for greater regulatory efficiency than group-based categorization, but it provides more appropriate safeguards. Further discussion is needed regarding the issue of whether a subpart approach to regulation provides appropriate safeguards. . . .

Cognitive or Communicative Vulnerability

. . . [T]hose with a *communicative vulnerability*, such as participants who speak or read different languages than do investigators, do not lack capacity, but are in situations that do not allow them to exercise their capacities effectively. This type of vulnerability heightens the risk that investigators will not fully respect the prospective participants because standard informed consent procedures will not suffice. . . .

Every effort must be made to enable prospective research participants to exercise autonomous choice, and investigators should make every effort to reduce situational barriers that impinge on the ability of prospective participants to exercise their authority. Sometimes, when a situational barrier is temporary, it might be possible to delay enrollment of prospective participants until the situation has passed. In other cases, it might be best to obtain informed consent from participants before exposure to the situation that limits autonomy, for example, obtaining consent from pregnant women who will be studied during labor and delivery. Sometimes such situations are structural. For example, sometimes investigators and prospective participants speak different languages. Language barriers can be reduced by using translators or translating consent forms.

Institutional Vulnerability

Prospective participants may have an institutional vulnerability when they have the cognitive capacity to consent but are subject to the formal authority of others who may have independent interests in whether the prospective participant agrees to enroll in the research study. The most commonly cited examples of individuals facing such institutional influences are prisoners and enlistees in the military, but the category also includes college students when they are required to be research participants for course credit or when such participation could affect their grades. This type of vulnerability increases the risk that one's decision concerning participation will not be truly voluntary, consequently increasing the risk that one's personhood will not be fully respected. In addition, it presents the risk that the subordinated status of these individuals will be exploited.

To safeguard against the ethically inappropriate enrollment of institutionally vulnerable persons, special attention should be paid to both participant selection and the voluntariness of the choice of prospective participants. Ways to reduce vulnerability might include working with institutional officials before initiating the research study to ensure that there are no inappropriate incentives or pressures to enroll, and when possible, not informing institutional staff about which individuals are participating. For example, if study participation takes one hour, those who refuse could be offered the option of staying in the study area for an hour. In this way, institutional staff would not know who participated and who did not.

Selection of participants from within the institutional setting should be fair and immune from the influence of institutional authorities. For example, in the informed consent process, investigators should emphasize that participation is voluntary, and protections should be in place to protect prospective participants from possible retaliation for their decisions (e.g., no effect on parole status or grades). In addition, during the informed consent process, no institutional authority should be present, except for possibly an ombudsperson.

Deferential Vulnerability

Prospective participants might have a deferential vulnerability when they have the cognitive capacity to consent but are subject to the authority of others who might have independent interests in whether prospective participants agree to enroll in the research study. This category raises the concern that the interests of the prospective participants could be subordinated to those of others. However, with deferential vulnerability, the subordination is affected not by *formal hierarchies* (as it is with institutional vulnerability), but instead by *informal* ones. Such informal power relationships can be socially constructed (e.g., based on gender, race, or class inequalities, or they can be inequalities of power and knowledge of the kind that occur in doctor-patient relationships), or they can be more subjective in nature (e.g., parents who regularly defer to the wishes of their adult children regardless of their own concerns). In any case, deferential vulnerability may be subtle. Like institutional vulnerability, deferential vulnerability heightens the risk that the prospective participant's decisions will not be truly voluntary. In addition, it presents the special risk that the subordinated status of these individuals will be used to someone else's advantage, resulting in their exploitation.

It should be noted that not all deferential behavior is subordinating. For example, some individuals might so trust their physicians' expertise that they defer to them about enrolling in a research study. Physician-investigators should be especially aware of this vulnerability, because when they approach their patients about enrolling in a research study, they could be concerned that refusing will negatively affect attitudes toward them or the quality of care they will receive. Here, as with institutional vulnerability, care must be taken to design the research study to ensure that the informed consent process is truly voluntary and that investigators do not take advantage of the subordinated status of prospective participants. Safeguards might include employing research staff who are sensitive to such deference and who can assess whether the participant is truly exercising autonomy and who can adjust the informed consent process to the prospective participant. Investigators should consider whether to have discussions with the prospective participant with or without the presence of the party to whom he or she ordinarily defers.

Medical Vulnerability

This category concerns potential participants who have serious health conditions for which there are no satisfactory standard treatments (e.g., metastatic cancer or rare disorders). Seriously ill individuals are often drawn to research because they or their physicians believe it is the best alternative to standard treatment. In these dire circumstances it can be difficult for prospective participants to weigh the risks and potential benefits associated with the research. This type of vulnerability increases the risk that informed consent might be based on misunderstanding potential benefits or might be motivated by a desire to find a treatment. It also increases the risk that these participants will be exploited, because either they have unreasonable expectations about the potential benefits or investigators mislead them about risks and potential benefits, and the risks are not reasonable in relation to the potential benefits. In research involving the medically vulnerable, every effort must be made to ensure that prospective participants are presented with accurate information (to avoid exploitation) and that they comprehend that information. Assuring appropriate comprehension might require more than attending to the clarity of information provided. Because physician-investigators might harbor unrealistic expectations for their patients-participants, and because patients-participants too easily blur the roles played by physician-investigators, these situations can lead to what has been called the *therapeutic misconception*. In these cases, medical vulnerability could be reduced by having an impartial third party approach prospective participants about enrollment and conduct the informed consent process or by having investigators make third parties available to discuss the research. Prospective participants could also be given time to consider the risks and potential benefits of the study and make a decision about participation. As much as possible, individuals should not learn of a diagnosis or that a standard treatment has failed at the same time that they are being asked to participate in a research study. . . .

Economic Vulnerability

Prospective participants might have an economic vulnerability when they have the cognitive capacity to consent but are disadvantaged in the distribution of social goods and services such as income, housing, or health care. This type of vulnerability heightens the risk that the potential benefits from participation in the research study might constitute undue inducements to enroll, threatening the voluntary nature of the choice and raising the danger that the potential participant's distributional disadvantage could be exploited. For example, offers of large sums of money as payment for participation or access to free health care services (for conditions not related to the research) could lead some prospective participants to enroll in a research study when it might be against their better judgment and when otherwise they would not do so. To safeguard against this vulnerability, IRBs should make certain that research offers a "reasonable choice" to prospective participants. This might be an easy assessment for the IRB reviewing a research study in which payment is involved, and the amount of payment could be reduced. However, it can be more difficult for the IRB when the potential benefits include access to free medical care or social or other services.

Social Vulnerability

Prospective participants might have a social vulnerability when they have the cognitive capacity to consent but belong to undervalued social groups. The treatment of members of such groups is not simply attributable to their economic vulnerability, although it is true that members of undervalued groups often lack financial resources. Social vulnerability is a function of the social perception of certain groups, which includes stereotyping and can lead to discrimination. In any case, the perceptions devalue members of such groups, their interests, their welfare, or their contributions to society.

These social perceptions are pervasive and often insidious and can affect persons' conceptions of certain groups. Thus, investigators, IRB members, and research sponsors should be sensitive to such social perceptions and their effects, and efforts should be made to allow members of such groups to participate in decisionmaking and oversight processes. Involving the community in the various stages of the research process, especially in study planning, can be helpful in reducing stereotyping and stigmatization. Also, investigators and IRBs should consider whether studies can be designed to include participants from all segments of society, rather than only or primarily from socially undervalued segments.

Aligning Protections with Vulnerabilities

Although there may be some overlap among the six distinct, ethically relevant types of vulnerability described above, each depicts a particular susceptibility to be used in ethically inappropriate ways in research. Moreover, many individuals might experience more than one of these vulnerabilities. For example, prospective participants might be poor, seriously ill, and not conversant in English. When multiple vulnerabilities exist, appropriate safeguards to address each vulnerability should be in place.

This model improves on the current DHHS regulations, which focus on groups of vulnerable people rather than on types of vulnerability, in three ways. First, it recognizes a fuller array of vulnerabilities that might be experienced by members of a particular group, while current regulations often fail to recognize that members of a vulnerable group might be vulnerable in more than one way. For example, current regulations recognize the institutional vulnerability of prisoners, but not their economic or social vulnerability. Second, the model portrays certain individuals as vulnerable in certain circumstances, while the current regulations classify entire groups as vulnerable. For example, current regulations classify all pregnant women as vulnerable, even though women are seldom vulnerable because of the pregnancy itself. Rather, pregnant women might at certain times be medically vulnerable (e.g., during labor). In addition, the current regulations classify economically disadvantaged persons as vulnerable, but, in certain situations, they would not be (e.g., certain types of survey research involving no remuneration).

The proposed model better expresses respect for persons by allowing people to be treated as individuals rather than as members of a group. Such an analytical model both challenges investigators and enables them and IRBs to extend their consideration of vulnerability beyond the incomplete list of vulnerable groups provided in the current regulations and to account for variations among prospective participants.

Third, the model also suggests appropriate safeguards for each type of vulnerability. The current system proposes two general sorts of safeguards: limiting the risk to which participants may be exposed and implementing stricter consent requirements. Given the limited variety of substantive safeguards required, current regulations are not sufficiently responsive to the full array of vulnerabilities. Safeguards must be tailored to respond to particular types and should avoid the exclusively protectionistic attitude toward vulnerability inherent in the current regulations. In general, the suggested safeguards have been designed to strike a balance between protecting vulnerable persons from harm and allowing them to reap the potential benefits of participation in research.

For *all* types of vulnerability, IRBs should ensure that the risks to which vulnerable persons are exposed would be acceptable to all prospective participants, i.e., those who are vulnerable as well as those who are not. Because the perspectives and experiences of vulnerable persons can differ considerably from those who are not vulnerable, vulnerable persons should be encouraged to participate in the study design and oversight processes. Such participatory processes serve as important safeguards in research involving vulnerable persons and can help to build trust in the research enterprise.

In designing a research study, investigators should consider how they would handle prospective participants who are vulnerable. To the extent possible, investigators and IRBs should try to identify, at the time of the IRB's initial review of a research study, the types of vulnerabilities of individuals who might be enrolled. In many studies, enrolling prospective participants who might be vulnerable can be anticipated by its stated purpose and design or by the inclusion criteria. When such individuals can be identified up front, IRBs can require that appropriate safeguards be in place before the initiation of the study. However, in some studies, it might not be possible to anticipate the inclusion of prospective participants with vulnerabilities until enrollment. In general, such prospective participants should not be enrolled until the protocol has been discussed with the IRB and then potentially revised and approved. IRBs should not halt the study, but should consider delaying enrollment of these individuals. In addition, IRBs should develop mechanisms for reviewing such protocols.

Finally, unless the particular research study requires such an approach (e.g., a research study of the efficacy of a particular drug when used in children), as a matter of justice, it is never appropriate to target persons with vulnerabilities for disproportionate inclusion or exclusion in research.

NOTES AND QUESTIONS

1. The NBAC position, as expressed in the excerpt quoted above, suggests that the entire approach taken by the federal regulations with respect to research on "special populations" is analytically unwise. Do you agree with that criticism? What might be the drawbacks of replacing the existing subparts with NBAC's analytical framework? For another critical look at the concept of vulnerability, see Carol Levine et al., *The Limitations of "Vulnerability" as a Protection for Human Research Participants*, 4 AM. J. BIOETHICS, Summer 2004, at 44 (and responses to that article in the same issue).

2. Imagine that you have been asked to revise the regulations according to the framework suggested by NBAC. What might an outline of the subheadings of the revised regulations look like?

3. Based on the excerpts that you read earlier in this section, how might Stone and Addicott react to the changes proposed by NBAC? Do you think they would view them as a step in the right direction? Which, if any, of Addicott's six specific recommendations would likely become a reality if the NBAC recommendations were implemented?

[C] The DHHS Office for Human Research Protections

The DHHS Office for Human Research Protections (OHRP) is the agency with the primary responsibility for enforcing the Common Rule. That enforcement takes place by means of two distinct activities: first, by making sure that institutions conducting federally funded research enter into the appropriate contractual agreements with the federal government; and second, by having staff of the agency conduct "site visits," either randomly or in response to a specific complaint, to see how well institutions are following the requirements of the regulations.

45 C.F.R. § 46.103: ASSURING COMPLIANCE WITH THIS POLICY

This provision is reproduced in Appendix A, at page A-5. Please review it before proceeding.

Who's Watching the Watchdogs? Responding to the Erosion of Research Ethics by Enforcing Promises
Lori A. Alvino
103 COLUM. L. REV. 893 (2003)

The Office for Human Research Protections (OHRP) is responsible for implementing the Common Rule and for providing guidance on ethical issues in all federally sponsored or federally affiliated biomedical research. The Common Rule currently requires that any institution that conducts federally funded human-subject research submit to the department or agency sponsoring that research a written assurance that its researchers will comply with all of the requirements of the Common Rule. Until December 2001, the OHRP approved three types of assurances: Single Project Assurances (SPAs), which apply to a single research activity at a single location; Multiple Project Assurances (MPAs), which cover multiple — often unrelated — research activities at a single location; and Cooperative Project Assurances (CPAs), which cover multiple research activities at multiple locations. Beginning in December 2001, however, the OHRP made available a new type of assurance: the Federal Wide Assurance (FWA). FWAs are designed to streamline the research-approval process by allowing a research institution with a valid FWA on file with the OHRP to receive funds from any department or agency that subscribes to the Common Rule without filing any additional assurances. SPAs, MPAs, and CPAs are replaced with FWAs as the former expire; all existing assurances must be superseded by FWAs no later than December 31, 2003.

The Common Rule specifies the elements of a valid assurance. Each research institution must develop and promise to follow a "statement of principles . . . in the discharge of its responsibilities for protecting the rights and welfare of human subjects of research conducted at or sponsored by the institution, regardless of whether the research is subject to federal regulation." Thus, in exchange for receiving federal funds for some of its research, an institution agrees to comply with the ethical requirements of either the Belmont Report or a similar set of ethical principles acceptable to OHRP for all of its research — whether privately or federally funded.

NOTES AND QUESTIONS

1. OHRP provides the full text of an FWA "contract," with instructions on how to obtain an FWA, at its Web site: http://www.hhs.gov/ohrp/assurances/assurances_index.html.

2. The creation of the FWA system has itself generated some controversy. Some officials in the White House questioned whether OHRP had the authority to accomplish such a substantial change without a formal amendment to the federal regulations governing human subject research. Changing the regulations is a complicated process, requiring publication of the proposed changes and solicitation of public comment on those changes. If the FWA system was not validly adopted, this might mean that the FWA agreements between OHRP and more than a thousand institutions conducting research might not be enforceable by the government. *See* Jeffrey Brainard, *White House Weighs Changes to Policies on Human Subjects*, CHRONICLE HIGHER EDUC., November 1, 2002, at A23.

3. What are the advantages and disadvantages of having institutions where research is conducted enter into contracts with the federal government agreeing to follow the rules set forth in the regulations? What alternative approaches might there be, assuming you had the power to rewrite the regulations and create a framework different from the FWA approach?

4. Why do you think so many institutions elect to voluntarily apply the requirements of the Common Rule to all the research they conduct, and not just to federally funded research? Are there benefits to the institution from making such a choice? What considerations might lead an institution *not* to make such a choice?

5. Assume that you are at an institution that chose not to apply the Common Rule requirements to non-federally funded research, and instead wrote into its FWA a commitment to merely follow the Belmont Report requirements. In terms of research ethics rules, in what ways might the non-federally funded studies be conducted differently from the federally funded studies? Consider, for example, an internally funded randomized study that compares two different surgical procedures for removing an inflamed appendix (standard care versus use of a proposed smaller incision). What specific aspects of the federal regulations might this researcher be able to avoid complying with?

MEMORANDUM FROM DIRECTOR, OHRP, TO OHRP STAFF, REGARDING COMPLIANCE OVERSIGHT PROCEDURES
(December 4, 2000)

As you know, the Office for Human Research Protections (OHRP) is responsible for oversight of compliance by awardee institutions with the Department of Health and Human Services (HHS) Regulations for Protection of Human

Subjects (45 CFR Part 46). This memorandum summarizes the procedures utilized by OHRP staff in conducting compliance oversight activities. These procedures have been developed over a period of years, and their effectiveness has been demonstrated in a number of investigations. Deviations from these procedures should occur only in extraordinary circumstances and must be approved by the Director, OHRP.

Background

Institutions engaged in human subject research that is conducted or supported by HHS, must provide written Assurances of Compliance to HHS describing the means they will employ to comply with the HHS Regulations. OHRP negotiates and approves these Assurances on behalf of the Secretary, HHS. An Assurance approved by OHRP commits the institution(s) and its personnel to full compliance with the Regulations.

In carrying out its oversight responsibility, OHRP evaluates all written allegations or indications of noncompliance with the HHS Regulations derived from any source. All compliance oversight evaluations are predicated on the HHS Regulations and the institution's Assurance of Compliance.

OHRP holds accountable and depends upon institutional officials, committees, research investigators, and other agents of the institution to assure conformance with the institution's Assurance and thus with the Regulations. Only through the partnership established by the Assurance can the shared responsibility to protect the rights and welfare of human subjects be discharged in accordance with Section 491 of the Public Health Service Act.

Compliance Oversight Evaluations

When OHRP initiates a compliance oversight evaluation, appropriate institutional officials are so advised in writing, and they are informed as to the likely administrative course of events. Activities expected of the institution are explained in writing initially and at appropriate times during the course of the evaluation. Except in rare circumstances when sound ethics dictates the need to act immediately, OHRP takes no action against any institution without first affording the institution an opportunity to offer information which might refute indications of noncompliance. . . .

Possible Outcomes

Corrective actions based on compliance oversight evaluations are intended to remedy identified noncompliance with the HHS Regulations and to prevent reoccurrence. Because each case is different, OHRP tailors its corrective actions to foster the best interests of human research subjects, and to the extent possible, the institution, the research community, and HHS. Most compliance oversight evaluations and resultant corrective actions are resolved at the OHRP level. In some instances, however, OHRP recommends actions to be taken by other HHS officials.

OHRP's compliance oversight evaluations may result in one or more of the following outcomes:

(1) OHRP may determine that protections under an institution's Assurance of Compliance are in compliance with the HHS Regulations.

(2) OHRP may determine that protections under an institution's Assurance of Compliance are in compliance with the HHS Regulations but that recommended improvements to those protections have been identified.

(3) OHRP may determine that protections under an institution's Assurance of Compliance are not in compliance with the HHS Regulations and require that an institution develop and implement corrective actions.

(4) OHRP may restrict its approval of an institution's Assurance of Compliance. Affected research projects continue to be supported by HHS only if the terms of the restriction are being satisfied. . . .

(5) OHRP may withdraw its approval of an institution's Assurance of Compliance. The institution's research projects cannot be supported by any HHS component until an appropriate Assurance is approved by OHRP.

(6) OHRP may recommend to appropriate HHS officials

(a) that an institution or an investigator be temporarily suspended or permanently removed from participation in specific projects, and/or

(b) that peer review groups be notified of an institution's or an investigator's past noncompliance prior to review of new projects.

(7) OHRP may recommend to HHS that institutions or investigators be declared ineligible to participate in HHS supported research (Debarment). . . . Any Debarment is Government wide, and not just applicable to HHS funding.

Sequence of Events

The typical sequence of events to be followed in an OHRP compliance oversight evaluation is as follows:

(1) OHRP discovers or receives a written allegation or indication of noncompliance with the HHS Regulations (45 CFR Part 46). OHRP may receive such allegations or indications from a variety of sources, including the institution itself. (Under the HHS Regulations, institutions are required to report any serious or continuing noncompliance to OHRP.)

(2) OHRP determines that it has jurisdiction in the matter on the basis of HHS support and/or an applicable Assurance of Compliance . . . .

(3) OHRP either (i) acknowledges the institution's report of noncompliance or (ii) notifies the institution's Assurance Signatory Official of the possible noncompliance and, as necessary, initiates a compliance evaluation and requests in writing that the institution investigate the matter and report to OHRP by a specified date. . . .

(4) OHRP evaluates the institution's report and any other pertinent information to which it has access. OHRP may (a) request that the institution submit additional information in writing; (b) conduct telephone interviews with institutional officials, committee members, and/or research investigators; or (c) conduct an on-site evaluation of protections under the applicable Assurance of Compliance. (NOTE: On-site evaluations of protections under an Assurance of Compliance may also be conducted in the absence of specific allegations or indications of noncompliance.)

(5) OHRP issues in writing a determination for each evaluation to the Signatory Official and other appropriate institutional officials. The determination letter to the institution summarizes (i) findings of noncompliance with the HHS Regulations, if any; and/or (ii) the corrective actions proposed and/or implemented by the institution that appropriately address the findings of noncompliance. In such circumstances, the complainant(s) are ordinarily informed in writing of OHRP's determination upon completion of its evaluation.

(6) An OHRP determination letter is made accessible on the OHRP website . . . once the document has been requested under FOIA or ten working days after the document is issued to the institution, whichever occurs first.

(7) An institution may request review by the Director of OHRP of determinations and findings resulting from a compliance oversight evaluation.

NOTES AND QUESTIONS

1. All of the determination letters issued by OHRP since mid-2000 can be viewed at http://www.hhs.gov/ohrp/compliance/letters/index.html.

2. OHRP has also produced a list of common and not-so-common findings it makes when reviewing an institution's compliance program: http://www.hhs.gov/ohrp/compliance/findings.pdf. This list is very useful for an institution that wants to conduct an internal review of the adequacy of its system for protecting human subjects.

3. A somewhat dated but nonetheless very helpful source of guidance regarding OHRP's interpretation of 45 C.F.R. Part 46 is a document its predecessor agency (OPRR) commissioned, titled PROTECTING HUMAN RESEARCH SUBJECTS: INSTITUTIONAL REVIEW BOARD GUIDEBOOK (1993), which is available at http://www.hhs.gov/ohrp/irb/irb_guidebook.htm. As its title indicates, this book is specifically intended to help IRBs navigate their way through the regulations. While the document is not legally binding on OHRP, it nonetheless in most instances accurately represents the agency's views.

4. Are the sanctions available to OHRP adequate? In recent years, there has been a great deal of debate about that issue, with the government proposing, among other things, allowing fines (up to the million dollar range) to be imposed on those who violate research integrity rules. *See, e.g.*, Donna Shalala, *Protecting Research Subjects — What Must Be Done*, 343 NEW ENG. J. MED. 808 (2000).Would that be a good change?

5. OHRP remains a relatively small agency, and certainly is not in a position to be doing a hands-on review of anything more than a small percentage of IRB activity in this country. That may explain why OHRP officials have recently been encouraging the development of private arrangements for "accrediting" IRBs. This phenomenon is discussed in the next chapter. *See* Chapter 4, at page 202.

§ 3.03 FOOD AND DRUG ADMINISTRATION REGULATIONS

The Food and Drug Administration plays an important role in research. It is assigned by Congress the primary responsibility for determining when certain types of treatments — in particular drugs, devices, and biologics — can be marketed in the United States. As part of that authority, it determines what types of studies need to be conducted in order to prove that a particular new treatment is safe and effective for treating a particular medical problem. That aspect of the FDA's role therefore has a major impact on the types of research that take place in the United States. In addition, as was noted earlier, the FDA has its own set of regulations relating to the specific topic of protecting research subjects, which is slightly different from the Common Rule.

The results of the studies that the FDA has approved must be presented to an expert panel, which makes a recommendation to the FDA regarding whether the studies have demonstrated that the drug, device, or biologic is "safe and effective." Note that neither the government nor the expert panel does any comparative analysis. The drug must merely be safe and effective. It need not be better than another previously approved drug. As you read this section, think about the ramifications of this review structure for the American drug industry and for patients.

[A] Human Subject Protections

The FDA's version of the Common Rule appears in two pieces, at 21 C.F.R. Part 56 (the rules for IRBs) and at 21 C.F.R. Part 50 (the rules for informed consent). The FDA has conveniently provided a list of the differences between its regulations and the DHHS regulations.

INFORMATION SHEETS: GUIDANCE FOR INSTITUTIONAL REVIEW BOARDS AND CLINICAL INVESTIGATORS, *Appendix E,* *Significant Differences in FDA and HHS Regulations* *for Protection of Human Subjects* FOOD AND DRUG ADMINISTRATION (1998)

This document is reproduced in Appendix C. Please skim it before proceeding.

NOTES AND QUESTIONS

1. The FDA Information Sheets are a series of pronouncements by the FDA on numerous issues related to the protection of human subjects. This document, which is published by the FDA as a paperback book, is also available at http://www.fda.gov/oc/ohrt/irbs/default.htm. Although the Information Sheets are only advisory in nature, they are a very good indication of the agency's official position on many issues.

2. Perhaps the most significant difference between the two sets of regulations relates to the circumstances that bring a study under federal jurisdiction. While the DHHS regulations usually look to whether a study is federally funded, the funding source is irrelevant under the FDA regulations. On the other hand, while the DHHS regulations (assuming the funding requirement is met) apply to all activities that meet the definition of "research" with "human subjects," the FDA regulations have a somewhat narrower scope. Specifically, under the FDA regulations, IRB review is required only for "clinical investigations," defined as "any experiment that involves a test article and one or more human subjects." 21 C.F.R. § 56.102(c). A test article, for most purposes, will be either a drug, biologic product, or device that is intended for "human use." 21 C.F.R. § 56.102(l).

3. For each of the following studies, determine if it would be subject to (a) only the DHHS regulations, (b) only the FDA regulations, or (c) both sets of regulations: (i) a private doctor, not affiliated with a university, conducts a study, using his own funds, that involves using an FDA-approved drug in subjects who have a disease different from the one that the drug is approved to treat; (ii) the doctor conducts that same study, but uses federal funds; (iii) the same study is conducted by a doctor affiliated with a major university, using his own funds; (iv) the same study is conducted by the university-affiliated doctor, but

in this case it has federal funding; (v) a private doctor, in his own office, using his own funds, compares two differently-shaped incisions for removing pre-cancerous moles from a subject's arm.

4. What is the status of exempt studies (as defined in the DHHS regulations) under the FDA regulations?

5. In addition to the federal regulations, there is a set of international standards for "good clinical practice" in designing and conducting research studies. These standards have been created by the International Conference on Harmonisation of Technical Requirements for Registration of Pharmaceuticals for Human Use, commonly referred to as the ICH. The purpose of these rules is "to provide a unified standard for the European Union (EU), Japan, and the United States to facilitate the mutual acceptance of clinical data by the regulatory authorities in these jurisdictions." Although the FDA has stated that these standards are not binding on either itself or the public, it is one of the sponsors of the ICH, and it played a role in creating the standards. These rules have been published in the federal register, 62 FED. REG. 25,692 (1997), and the FDA notes that they represent its "current thinking on good clinical practices." *Guidance for Industry, E6 Good Clinical Practice Consolidated Guidance*, available at http://www.fda.gov/cder/guidance/959fnl.pdf. In a variety of respects (such as the details of IRB operation and the rules for obtaining informed consent), the ICH guidelines are more specific than the federal regulations. Compliance with these additional details would appear to be especially important for companies that are either conducting research or seeking marketing approval outside the United States.

[B] The Drug Approval Process

UNITED STATES v. RUTHERFORD
Supreme Court of the United States, 442 U.S. 544 (1979)

[T]he Federal Food, Drug, and Cosmetic Act prohibits interstate distribution of any "new drug" unless the Secretary of Health, Education, and Welfare approves an application supported by substantial evidence of the drug's safety and effectiveness. As defined in the Act, the term "new drug" includes

> [any] drug . . . not generally recognized, among experts qualified by scientific training and experience to evaluate the safety and effectiveness of drugs, as safe and effective for use under the conditions prescribed, recommended, or suggested in the labeling. . . .

Exemptions from premarketing approval procedures are available for drugs intended solely for investigative use and drugs qualifying under either of the Act's two grandfather provisions.

In 1975, terminally ill cancer patients and their spouses brought this action to enjoin the Government from interfering with the interstate shipment and sale of Laetrile, a drug not approved for distribution under the Act. . . .

After completion of administrative hearings, the Commissioner issued his opinion on July 29, 1977. He determined first that no uniform definition of Laetrile exists; rather, the term has been used generically for chemical compounds similar to, or consisting at least in part of, amygdalin, a glucoside present in the kernels or seeds of most fruits. The Commissioner further found that Laetrile in its various forms constituted a "new drug" as defined in § 201 (p)(1) of the Act because it was not generally recognized among experts as safe and effective for its prescribed use. . . .

Having determined that Laetrile was a new drug, the Commissioner proceeded to consider whether it was exempt from premarketing approval under the 1938 or 1962 grandfather provisions. On the facts presented, the Commissioner found that Laetrile qualified under neither clause. . . .

The Court of Appeals [reversed the Commissioner's determination and instead] held that "the 'safety' and 'effectiveness' terms used in the statute have no reasonable application to terminally ill cancer patients." Since those patients, by definition, would "die of cancer regardless of what may be done," the court concluded that there were no realistic standards against which to measure the safety and effectiveness of a drug for that class of individuals. The Court of Appeals therefore approved the District Court's injunction permitting use of Laetrile by cancer patients certified as terminally ill. . . . In addition, the court directed the FDA to promulgate regulations "as if" the drug had been found " 'safe' and 'effective' " for terminally ill cancer patients.

We . . . now reverse.

The Federal Food, Drug, and Cosmetic Act makes no special provision for drugs used to treat terminally ill patients. By its terms, § 505 of the Act requires premarketing approval for "any new drug" unless it is intended solely for investigative use or is exempt under one of the Act's grandfather provisions. . . .

Nothing in the history of the 1938 Food, Drug, and Cosmetic Act, which first established procedures for review of drug safety, or of the 1962 Amendments, which added the current safety and effectiveness standards in § 201 (p)(1), suggests that Congress intended protection only for persons suffering from curable diseases. To the contrary, in deliberations preceding the 1938 Act, Congress expressed concern that individuals with fatal illnesses, such as cancer, should be shielded from fraudulent cures. . . .

A drug is effective within the meaning of § 201 (p)(1) if there is general recognition among experts, founded on substantial evidence, that the drug in fact produces the results claimed for it under prescribed conditions. Contrary to the Court of Appeals' apparent assumption, effectiveness does not necessarily denote capacity to cure. In the treatment of any illness, terminal or otherwise, a drug is effective if it fulfills, by objective indices, its sponsor's claims of prolonged life, improved physical condition, or reduced pain.

So too, the concept of safety under § 201 (p)(1) is not without meaning for terminal patients. Few if any drugs are completely safe in the sense that they may be taken by all persons in all circumstances without risk. Thus, the Commissioner generally considers a drug safe when the expected therapeutic gain justifies the risk entailed by its use. For the terminally ill, as for anyone else, a drug is unsafe if its potential for inflicting death or physical injury is not offset by the possibility of therapeutic benefit. Indeed, the Court of Appeals implicitly acknowledged that safety considerations have relevance for terminal cancer patients by restricting authorized use of Laetrile to intravenous injections for persons under a doctor's supervision.

Moreover, there is a special sense in which the relationship between drug effectiveness and safety has meaning in the context of incurable illnesses. An otherwise harmless drug can be dangerous to any patient if it does not produce its purported therapeutic effect. But if an individual suffering from a potentially fatal disease rejects conventional therapy in favor of a drug with no demonstrable curative properties, the consequences can be irreversible. For this reason, even before the 1962 Amendments incorporated an efficacy standard into new drug application procedures, the FDA considered effectiveness when reviewing the safety of drugs used to treat terminal illness. The FDA's practice also reflects the recognition, amply supported by expert medical testimony in this case, that with diseases such as cancer it is often impossible to identify a patient as terminally ill except in retrospect. Cancers vary considerably in behavior and in responsiveness to different forms of therapy. Even critically ill individuals may have unexpected remissions and may respond to conventional treatment. Thus, as the Commissioner concluded, to exempt from the Act drugs with no proved effectiveness in the treatment of cancer "would lead to needless deaths and suffering among . . . patients characterized as 'terminal' who could actually be helped by legitimate therapy."

It bears emphasis that although the Court of Appeals' ruling was limited to Laetrile, its reasoning cannot be so readily confined. To accept the proposition that the safety and efficacy standards of the Act have no relevance for terminal patients is to deny the Commissioner's authority over all drugs, however toxic or ineffectual, for such individuals. If history is any guide, this new market would not be long overlooked. Since the turn of the century, resourceful entrepreneurs have advertised a wide variety of purportedly simple and painless cures for cancer, including liniments of turpentine, mustard, oil, eggs, and ammonia; peat moss; arrangements of colored floodlamps; pastes made from glycerin and limburger cheese; mineral tablets; and "Fountain of Youth" mixtures of spices, oil, and suet. In citing these examples, we do not, of course, intend to deprecate the sincerity of Laetrile's current proponents, or to imply any opinion on whether that drug may ultimately prove safe and effective for cancer treatment. But this historical experience does suggest why Congress could reasonably have determined to protect the terminally ill, no less than other patients, from the vast range of self-styled panaceas that inventive minds can devise.

We note finally that construing § 201 (p)(1) to encompass treatments for terminal diseases does not foreclose all resort to experimental cancer drugs by patients for whom conventional therapy is unavailing. Section 505 (i) of the Act exempts from premarketing approval drugs intended solely for investigative use if they satisfy certain preclinical testing and other criteria. An application for clinical testing of Laetrile by the National Cancer Institute is now pending before the Commissioner. That the Act makes explicit provision for carefully regulated use of certain drugs not yet demonstrated safe and effective reinforces our conclusion that no exception for terminal patients may be judicially implied. Whether, as a policy matter, an exemption should be created is a question for legislative judgment, not judicial inference.

NOTES AND QUESTIONS

1. In *Rutherford*, the Supreme Court resolved only the narrow question of whether the rules applied by the federal government in preventing the sale of Laetrile were consistent with what Congress said in passing the Food, Drug and Cosmetic Act. There is a separate question that it did not address — i.e., whether laws limiting dying people's access to drugs such as Laetrile violate the constitutional rights of terminally ill patients. Lower federal courts in somewhat similar cases have generally determined that individuals do not have a constitutionally protected right to receive the medical care they want. *See, e.g.,* Abigail Alliance v. McClellan, No. 03-1601 (RMU) (D.D.C. Aug. 30, 2004). The Supreme Court has never directly spoken on this issue. However, in her concurrence in *Washington v. Glucksberg*, 521 U.S. 702 (1997), a case upholding a state statute prohibiting physician-assisted suicide, Justice O'Connor suggested that terminally ill patients who are "experiencing great pain" might have a constitutionally cognizable interest in obtaining medical treatment necessary to control that pain. *See* Glucksberg, 521 U.S. at 736-37 (O'Connor, J., concurring).

2. As the Supreme Court noted in *Rutherford*, the usual way for someone to obtain a drug that has not yet been approved by the FDA for any use is to participate in a research study. But the FDA has also created several additional ways for a doctor to give a patient an unapproved drug: (a) The drug manufacturer may file with the FDA a protocol known as a "treatment IND" (sometimes informally called "compassionate use"), which, if approved, will allow the drug to be given to patients outside of a study. This can be done only if the drug is intended for "the treatment of serious and life-threatening illnesses for which there are no satisfactory alternative treatments." (b) In an emergency, where there is no time for a protocol to be approved, the FDA may authorize the drug to be used for a patient who is in a life-threatening situation and there is

no standard acceptable treatment. (c) Cancer drugs that are being evaluated in Phase 3 studies (described later in this chapter) can be given to patients after FDA approval of a protocol filed under a process called a "Group C Treatment IND." (d) Finally, a special procedure has been created for allowing access to promising drugs that are being studied to treat AIDS/HIV and related diseases. This procedure, known as a "parallel track," allows individuals to obtain the new drug outside of a study in certain circumstances. For more information on all of these options, *see,* e.g., FDA INFORMATION SHEETS AT 54, TREATMENT USE OF INVESTIGATIONAL DRUGS (1998); Steven R. Salbu, *The FDA and Public Access to New Drugs: Appropriate Levels of Scrutiny in the Wake of HIV, AIDS, and the Diet Drug Debacle*, 79 B.U. L. REV. 93 (1999). Note how expanding access to unapproved drugs can create a dilemma for both drug companies and society in general. By allowing access to the drug outside of a study, people may be discouraged from participating in the study, and thus we may delay finding out whether the drug works or whether it has unacceptable risks. Moreover, participants in the study, half of whom will not get the drug, may think it unfair that others can directly get the drug.

The Architecture of Government Regulation of Medical Products
Richard A. Merrill
82 VA. L. REV. 1753 (1996)

As amended in 1962, the [Food, Drug, and Cosmetic] Act prohibits the shipment in interstate commerce of any new drug for which FDA has not approved [a New Drug Application, known as an] NDA. Approval, however, requires the submission of data from clinical studies designed to demonstrate safety and effectiveness, so Congress had to provide a mechanism to allow shipment of unapproved drugs to the investigators who actually conduct such trials. Accordingly, the Act empowers FDA to grant exemptions for investigational drugs. This generous authority has been the source of two progressively more elaborate sets of requirements governing clinical studies of therapeutic drugs.

One set consists of requirements designed to assure the ethical integrity of clinical studies. The core of this set is the requirement that investigators, with rare exceptions, must secure and document the informed consent of every participant. FDA has supplemented this requirement with a mandate that proposed studies be approved by a local institutional review board ("IRB"). To facilitate its own monitoring of compliance with these requirements, the agency has also promulgated specifications for IRB operations and recordkeeping.

The second and, from the standpoint of medical innovation, probably more important set of FDA requirements address the design and recordkeeping for clinical studies. These requirements aim to assure that such studies will produce useful evidence of a drug's safety and, particularly, its effectiveness. These requirements are embodied in general provisions elaborating the Act's demand for adequate and well-controlled clinical studies; in agency testing guidelines for specific classes or types of drugs; and in reviewer critiques of individual clinical protocols, elicited in advance by sponsors or offered in the context of reviewers' analyses of applications for marketing approval.

These multiple instructions to drug sponsors and clinical investigators constitute a continually expanding body of FDA "law" governing drug trials. FDA officials believe that they embody what objective experts would consider sound experimental design; sponsors and some clinicians believe that agency reviewers are prone to demand more, and more extensive, studies than are needed to support sound judgments about effectiveness. This exposes an important issue: To what degree do FDA's expectations for clinical trials exceed the measures that drug sponsors would undertake if they did not have to obtain agency approval? Drug sponsors would surely do some testing of their product in order to minimize their risk of liability and to defend against charges of misbranding. In an increasingly cost-sensitive market for medical care, sponsors would have incentives to generate evidence that their drugs worked, perhaps even evidence that they worked better than others. Furthermore, FDA's standards reflect the influence of the academic literature on the design and evaluation of clinical trials, which unquestionably has increased rigor and added complexity. The question, then, is whether FDA's expectations place additional burdens on those who develop and test drugs — burdens that could be attributed to the form of regulation Congress has prescribed.

It may not be possible to answer this question with assurance. What can safely be said is that FDA's current standards for clinical studies are considerably more elaborate, and compliance with them considerably more expensive, than the requirements it was enforcing two decades ago. And, it is undeniable that a drug sponsor must satisfy them or it will never see its drug approved. The disincentives to challenging FDA's views are formidable; sponsors almost invariably engage the agency on its own terms. Moreover, even if it were easier to challenge reviewer demands for further tests — the most common sort of dispute between sponsors and the agency — the time lost doing so would represent a major disincentive. It is often easier, and usually less expensive, to conduct and submit the results of a study that a reviewer "suggests," but that the sponsor considers unnecessary.

In sum, in the new drug approval process — as in most administrative licensing regimes — FDA exercises effectively unchallengeable authority to dictate the number and kinds of studies required to support approval and nearly unreviewable discretion to interpret the results.

ELI LILLY & CO. v. COMMISSIONER

United States Tax Court
84 T.C. 996 (1985), aff'd in part and rev'd in part, 856 F.2d 855
(7th Cir. 1988)

The Federal Food, Drug, and Cosmetic Act requires the submission and FDA approval of [a New Drug Application, or] NDA prior to the introduction into interstate commerce of any new drug, including patented drugs. Subsequent to 1962 . . . the process for obtaining an NDA involved as a prior step the filing of a document known as an Investigatory New Drug Application (hereinafter IND).

An IND contained the background of the new drug at the point in time at which it was filed. It described the method and chemistry of synthesizing the new drug; the procedures and tests for controlling the quality of the drug; summaries of animal pharmacology tests performed to assess the drug's therapeutic potential; results of animal toxicology studies performed to assess the safety of the drug; the labeling the developer intended to use to ship the drug in interstate commerce; the names of the investigators who would be conducting the clinical studies in humans; and the plans or protocols to be used in those studies. Petitioner's INDs were prepared by the regulatory affairs department of Lilly Research Laboratories' medical research division. During the years in issue, the regulatory affairs department had approximately 60 employees. The preparation of an IND was largely a process of collating finished packages of materials received from other areas of Lilly Research Laboratories. It took two or three of the clerical personnel in that department approximately 2 to 3 days to collate and duplicate an IND.

Assuming that the FDA did not have serious objections with respect to the IND, the pharmaceutical company was free to begin clinical studies in humans after a 30-day waiting period. The clinical studies for a new drug generally were divided into three phases referred to as phase I, phase II, and phase III. Although there were qualitative distinctions in the nature of the clinical studies performed in each phase, the three phases were not performed in strict chronological order and often overlapped in time.

Phase I clinical studies consisted largely of dose ranging studies in normal human subjects. During the years in issue, phase I clinical studies usually involved 20 to 50 subjects and took from 3 to 6 months to complete, depending upon the new drug being tested. Petitioner's phase I studies ordinarily were performed in the Lilly Clinic.

Phase II clinical studies were the initial efficacy studies for the new drug. The purpose of those studies was to demonstrate that the drug had some valuable, therapeutic activity. In those studies, the new drug was given to a small number of patients who had the disease or medical condition that the new drug was intended to treat.

At some point during phase II, sufficient information with respect to the efficacy and toxicity of the new drug was accumulated to permit a decision as to whether the new drug would be able to complete successfully the FDA approval process or whether the testing of the new drug should be abandoned. That point in a new drug's development was referred to as the NDA decision point. The NDA decision point was important because it was at that time that it was decided whether to commit the considerable resources necessary to complete the phase II and phase III clinical studies for the new drug. The amount of time between the end of phase I and the NDA decision point varied greatly depending upon the new drug being tested, but generally ranged between 1 and 2 years.

Phase III studies were similar to and essentially a continuation of phase II studies. Phase III studies, however, were more extensive. They involved more patients than were involved in phase II studies, and more attributes of a new drug were assessed. The drug was tested under various dosage schedules and in conjunction with other drugs. A major objective of phase III studies was to expose large numbers of patients to the new drug to collect information with respect to potential side effects or abnormalities in the patients and for the large body of safety data necessary to support an NDA.

Petitioner generally attempted to have its new drugs investigated by well-known clinical investigators, outside physicians who were paid by petitioner to study the new drugs. The testing usually was done at large teaching hospitals in various locations around the country to provide test data under various conditions. Petitioner contracted with those clinical investigators and provided them with case report forms on which to report the data produced by the clinical studies. The case report forms completed by the clinical investigators were forwarded to petitioner's regulatory affairs department where they were entered into a computer. The regulatory affairs department worked with petitioner's computer analysts and statisticians to devise computer-generated tables summarizing the clinical data, which tables eventually became part of the applicable NDAs. The time from the NDA decision point to the completion of phase III clinical studies varied greatly depending on the drug being tested but generally ranged between 2 and 3 years.

The NDA was in large part a duplication and elaboration of the material included in an IND. The NDA included the information originally submitted in the IND and all additional information the applicant had collected relative to the new drug, including but not limited to: (1) Detailed descriptions of the manufacturing and quality control procedures; (2) any animal pharmacology studies done subsequent to the filing of the IND; (3) any animal toxicology studies done subsequent to the filing of the IND; (4) all information relative to phases I, II, and III clinical studies on humans during the IND process, including the names of the investigators and the results of their research; (5) the labels and labeling information; and (6) the package insert for the new drug. The NDA material submitted to the FDA generally was voluminous.

By regulation, the FDA had 180 days from the filing of an NDA within which to respond. The FDA could and often did ask questions with regard to the clinical, toxicology, and pharmacology studies reported in the NDA. When such questions were raised with respect to NDAs filed by petitioner, personnel of petitioner's regulatory affairs department or the individuals in Lilly Research Laboratories who prepared the data submitted with the NDA discussed those questions with the FDA. If necessary, petitioner supplied additional information to the FDA. During that interaction period, a regional office of the FDA conducted an inspection of the manufacturing facilities to be used to produce the new drug. . . .

When the FDA completed its review of the NDA, and if the FDA was satisfied, it issued a letter stating that the new drug was approvable contingent upon a review of final printed labeling and package inserts. When petitioner received an approvable letter from the FDA, it printed final labeling and package inserts for the new drug and submitted those materials to the FDA. At that point, petitioner also submitted to the FDA the promotional materials it planned to use to market the drug. If the FDA found those materials satisfactory, it issued a letter to petitioner approving the NDA and giving petitioner the right to market the new drug.

During the years 1971 through 1973, the average period from the filing of an NDA to its final approval by the FDA was approximately 2 years. Only 1 in every 10 new drugs for which an IND was filed, successfully completed the process and received FDA approval. While the time frame leading to an NDA varied extensively, the entire procedure from the initial chemical synthesis and identification of a new drug to the approval of an NDA for the new drug ranged from approximately 7 years to 13 years.

The approval letters issued by the FDA contained specific provisions and conditions relative to the maintenance of that approval. The pharmaceutical companies were required to maintain certain records and to make certain periodic reports to the FDA. The companies were required to report every 3 months for the first year, every 6 months the second year, and annually thereafter. In addition, the pharmaceutical companies were required to submit to the FDA any information concerning accidents or certain complaints relative to a drug on a priority basis. Immediate notification was required of labeling mix-ups, bacteriological contamination, or chemical degradation; notification was required within 15 days of receiving complaints or learning of serious, unexpected side effects of a drug.

If a pharmaceutical company desired to make any major change in the manufacturing or marketing of a drug, such as the addition of a new indication for the drug or a change in its dosage schedule, additional materials were submitted to the FDA in the form of a supplemental NDA. The supplemental NDA described the desired change and included data supporting that change.

FDA-approved NDAs cannot be assigned or transferred by pharmaceutical companies. The approved NDA is peculiar to the pharmaceutical company that obtained it because it contains information specific to that company. A second pharmaceutical company desiring to market the same drug would be required to file and obtain approval of its own NDA for the drug. If the pharmaceutical company that originally obtained FDA approval to market the drug granted the second pharmaceutical company the right to refer to the information in the first company's NDA file, the second company could obtain FDA approval of an NDA simply by submitting to the FDA the appropriate labeling, manufacturing, and quality control information.

NOTES AND QUESTIONS

1. According to the FDA regulations, a Phase 1 study should usually involve about 20 to 80 subjects, a Phase 2 study no more than several hundred subjects, and a Phase 3 study anywhere from several hundred to several thousand subjects. *See* 21 C.F.R. § 312.21.

2. The definitions of Phase 1, 2, and 3 studies are rather vague, and it sometimes will not matter whether a particular study fits into one category or another. Thus, for example, studies will often be labeled Phase 1/2 or Phase 2/3. Moreover, there can be a great deal of variation in the types of studies that might be considered to fit under a particular category. For example, some Phase 2 studies might involve giving all of the subjects a new drug, while a study in which subjects are randomized between the new drug and a placebo might also be considered a Phase 2 study. For an example of the types of studies one particular drug went through, see In re Synergen, Inc., 863 F. Supp. 1409 (D. Colo. 1994).

3. There are also Phase 4 studies, which in general are studies of an approved drug relating to using the drug for its approved purpose. Sometimes the FDA may approve a drug but still have some concerns about safety or efficacy, and thus may require that these additional studies be conducted by the drug manufacturer. Not infrequently, drug manufacturers design something that vaguely looks like it is a study, but their actual purpose is not to collect information about the drug but rather to promote use of the new drug by encouraging doctors and patients to become familiar with it. A tip-off that this is occurring is when the study design seems to make no sense: for example, even though the disease being treated is a common one, and large numbers of subjects could be recruited at a small number of medical centers, the study might involve 500 study sites with 5 subjects being enrolled at each site. While there is nothing necessarily inappropriate about such studies, IRBs may wish to pay special attention to them, and perhaps to make sure that the consent process makes clear to subjects the likely true purpose of the study.

4. Phase 1 studies, which primarily involve giving one subject after another higher and higher doses of a drug to determine the dose at which significant side

effects begin to be seen, pose special ethical problems when they are conducted on subjects with cancer or other life-threatening diseases. Such subjects often fail to appreciate how unlikely it is that being in the study will benefit them. Only about five percent of the people participating in these trials have any response to the drug, and the very small percentage of people who have a complete response (cancer being temporarily put into remission) may be balanced by an equal percentage of people who suffer or die from the drug's side effects. The failure in understanding may in large part be due to inadequacies in the consent forms used in such studies. This issue is discussed in greater detail in Chapter 7.

5. One type of pill that millions of people take — so-called "dietary supplements," which used to be found only on the counters of specialized nutrition stores and now are ubiquitous — is to a large extent beyond the regulatory authority of the FDA. As a result of lobbying by the manufacturers of these products, Congress passed the Dietary Supplement Health and Education Act, which since 1994 has prevented the FDA from requiring these pills to undergo the usual safety and efficacy testing required of drugs. In effect, the burden of proof has been flipped: the FDA can prevent marketing of a dietary supplement only if it can demonstrate a "significant and unreasonable risk" to users. Given the agency's limited resources, this rarely happens, although it did act in 2004 in banning the sale of the herbal product ephedra, which had been marketed for use in weight loss. *See, e.g.*, Amy M. Ling, *FDA to Ban Sales of Dietary Supplements Containing Ephedra*, 32 J.L. MED. & ETHICS 184 (2004); Margaret Gilhooley, *Herbal Remedies and Dietary Supplements: The Boundaries of Drug Claims and Freedom of Choice*, 49 FLA. L. REV. 669 (1997); Steven R. Salbu, *The FDA and Public Access to New Drugs: Appropriate Levels of Scrutiny in the Wake of HIV, AIDS, and the Diet Drug Debacle*, 79 B.U. L. REV. 93 (1999).

INFORMATION SHEETS: GUIDANCE FOR INSTITUTIONAL REVIEW BOARDS AND CLINICAL INVESTIGATORS, "OFF-LABEL" AND INVESTIGATIONAL USE OF MARKETED DRUGS, BIOLOGICS AND DEVICES
FOOD AND DRUG ADMINISTRATION
49 (1998)

"Off-Label" Use of Marketed Drugs, Biologics and Medical Devices

Good medical practice and the best interests of the patient require that physicians use legally available drugs, biologics and devices according to their best knowledge and judgment. If physicians use a product for an indication not in the approved labeling, they have the responsibility to be well informed about the product, to base its use on firm scientific rationale and on sound medical evidence, and to maintain records of the product's use and effects. Use of a marketed product in this manner when the intent is the "practice of medicine" does not require the submission of an Investigational New Drug Application (IND), Investigational Device Exemption (IDE) or review by an Institutional Review Board (IRB). However, the institution at which the product will be used may, under its own authority, require IRB review or other institutional oversight.

Investigational Use of Marketed Drugs, Biologics and Medical Devices

The investigational use of approved, marketed products differs from the situation described above. "Investigational use" suggests the use of an approved product in the context of a clinical study protocol [see 21 CFR 312.3(b)]. When the principal intent of the investigational use of a test article is to develop information about the product's safety or efficacy, submission of an IND or IDE may be required. However, according to 21 CFR 312.2(b)(1), the clinical investigation of a marketed drug or biologic does not require submission of an IND if all six of the following conditions are met:

(i)   it is not intended to be reported to FDA in support of a new indication for use or to support any other significant change in the labeling for the drug;

(ii) it is not intended to support a significant change in the advertising for the product;

(iii) it does not involve a route of administration or dosage level, use in a subject population, or other factor that significantly increases the risks (or decreases the acceptability of the risks) associated with the use of the drug product;

(iv) it is conducted in compliance with the requirements for IRB review and informed consent [21 CFR parts 56 and 50, respectively];

(v)   it is conducted in compliance with the requirements concerning the promotion and sale of drugs [21 CFR 312.7]; and

(vi) it does not intend to invoke 21 CFR 50.24 [which deals with emergency research].

NOTES AND QUESTIONS

1. As the FDA acknowledges in these comments, Congress has not given it any authority to control how doctors use a drug once it has been approved for at least one use. Thus, for example, had Laetrile been approved as a treatment for epilepsy, the patients in the *Rutherford* case would have been able to get the drug, so long as they were able to talk a doctor into writing a prescription for it. Is the ability of doctors to prescribe drugs in such an off-label manner consistent with the basic rationale behind the Food, Drug and Cosmetic Act, as discussed in the *Rutherford* case?

2. Off-label use of medications is very common. Some estimates suggest that somewhere between twenty and sixty percent of the prescriptions written in this country may be for off-label uses. *See, e.g.*, Michael I. Krauss, *Loosening the FDA's Drug Certification Monopoly: Implications for Tort Law and Consumer Welfare*, 4 GEO. MASON L. REV. 457, 472 (1996). In many instances, drug manufacturers have no interest in doing the millions of dollars worth of testing that would be required to meet the FDA's rigorous criteria for having a new use approved, because doctors may end up using the drug following one or two studies that seem to show effectiveness.

3. Although the FDA cannot directly prevent doctors from using drugs on an off-label basis, federal law prohibits drug manufacturers from advertising off-label uses. *See* Washington Legal Foundation v. Henney, 202 F.3d 331, 333 (D.C. Cir. 2000). In 1996, the FDA issued guidance statements designed to impose additional restrictions on manufacturers' promotion of off-label uses. The guidances limited manufacturers' ability to send physicians medical journal articles or textbooks regarding off-label uses of drugs or to support continuing medical education programs promoting such uses. However, in 1998, a federal district court struck down those guidance statements as a violation of the First Amendment. In essence, the court held that manufacturers have a right to publicize truthful information, such as the results of a study tentatively showing that a drug may be effective for a particular use, even if that study would not meet the FDA's standards for demonstrating effectiveness and changing the labeling on the drug. *See* Washington Legal Foundation v. Friedman, 13 F. Supp. 2d 51 (D.D.C. 1998). That decision was vacated on appeal for technical reasons unrelated to the court's constitutional analysis. *See* Henney, *supra*. The FDA ultimately withdrew the challenged guidances. *See* Margaret Gilhooley, *Drug Regulation and the Constitution after* Western States, 37 U. RICH. L. REV. 901 (2003).

4. The majority of drugs used for treating children have traditionally been used on an off-label basis, because manufacturers rarely tested drugs on children after they had received approval for using them in adults. That has changed in recent years, due in large part to incentives and penalties imposed by federal law. This issue is discussed further in Chapter 13, at page 531.

5. Imagine that a researcher is studying a chemical compound, one never previously approved by the FDA for any use, because it causes changes in lung functioning that are similar to what happens during an asthma attack. The researcher's goal is to better understand how the lungs work, not to generate data related to the risks and benefits of using the compound to treat or diagnose medical problems. (This hypothetical is a variation on what happened in the study that led to the death of Ellen Roche, discussed in Chapter 4 at page 182.) Would a researcher be required to obtain FDA approval to conduct this study? Note that the Food, Drug and Cosmetic Act gives the FDA broad authority to regulate drugs, and the definition of drugs includes articles "intended to affect the structure or any function of the body of man." 21 U.S.C.A. § 321(g)(1)(C). *See*

M. Alexander Otto, *FDA Warning Letter Hints at Crackdown on Unregulated Research, IND Enforcement*, 2 MED. RESEARCH L. & POL'Y REP. (BNA) 339 (2003).

[C] The Device Approval Process

MEDTRONIC, INC. v. LOHR

Supreme Court of the United States, 518 U.S. 470 (1996)

Despite the prominence of the States in matters of public health and safety, in recent decades the Federal Government has played an increasingly significant role in the protection of the health of our people. Congress' first significant enactment in the field of public health was the Food and Drug Act of 1906, a broad prohibition against the manufacture or shipment in interstate commerce of any adulterated or misbranded food or drug. Partly in response to an ongoing concern about radio and newspaper advertising making false therapeutic claims for both "quack machines" and legitimate devices such as surgical instruments and orthopedic shoes, in 1938 Congress broadened the coverage of the 1906 Act to include misbranded or adulterated medical devices and cosmetics.

While the [Food, Drug and Cosmetic Act] provided for premarket approval of new drugs, it did not authorize any control over the introduction of new medical devices. As technologies advanced and medicine relied to an increasing degree on a vast array of medical equipment "from bedpans to brainscans," including kidney dialysis units, artificial heart valves, and heart pacemakers, policymakers and the public became concerned about the increasingly severe injuries that resulted from the failure of such devices.

In 1970, for example, the Dalkon Shield, an intrauterine contraceptive device, was introduced to the American public and throughout the world. Touted as a safe and effective contraceptive, the Dalkon Shield resulted in a disturbingly high percentage of inadvertent pregnancies, serious infections, and even, in a few cases, death. In the early 1970s, several other devices, including catheters, artificial heart valves, defibrillators, and pacemakers (including pacemakers manufactured by petitioner Medtronic), attracted the attention of consumers, the Food and Drug Administration (FDA), and Congress as possible health risks.

In response to the mounting consumer and regulatory concern, Congress enacted the statute at issue here: the Medical Device Amendments of 1976. The Act classifies medical devices in three categories based on the risk that they pose to the public. Devices that present no unreasonable risk of illness or injury [such as crutches and band aids] are designated Class I and are subject only to minimal regulation by "general controls." Devices that are potentially more harmful [such as wheelchairs and tampons] are designated Class II; although they may be marketed without advance approval, manufacturers of such devices must comply with federal performance regulations known as "special controls."

Finally, devices that either "present a potential unreasonable risk of illness or injury," or which are "purported or represented to be for a use in supporting or sustaining human life or for a use which is of substantial importance in preventing impairment of human health," are designated Class III. Pacemakers are Class III devices.

Before a new Class III device may be introduced to the market, the manufacturer must provide the FDA with a "reasonable assurance" that the device is both safe and effective. Despite its relatively innocuous phrasing, the process of establishing this "reasonable assurance," which is known as the "premarket approval," or "PMA" process, is a rigorous one. Manufacturers must submit detailed information regarding the safety and efficacy of their devices, which the FDA then reviews, spending an average of 1,200 hours on each submission.

Not all, nor even most, Class III devices on the market today have received premarket approval because of two important exceptions to the PMA requirement. First, Congress realized that existing medical devices could not be withdrawn from the market while the FDA completed its PMA analysis for those devices. The statute therefore includes a "grandfathering" provision which allows pre-1976 devices to remain on the market without FDA approval until such time as the FDA initiates and completes the requisite PMA. Second, to prevent manufacturers of grandfathered devices from monopolizing the market while new devices clear the PMA hurdle, and to ensure that improvements to existing devices can be rapidly introduced into the market, the Act also permits devices that are "substantially equivalent" to pre-existing devices to avoid the PMA process.

Although "substantially equivalent" Class III devices may be marketed without the rigorous PMA review, such new devices, as well as all new Class I and Class II devices, are subject to the requirements of § 360(k). That section imposes a limited form of review on every manufacturer intending to market a new device by requiring it to submit a "premarket notification" to the FDA (the process is also known as a "§ 510(k) process," after the number of the section in the original Act). If the FDA concludes on the basis of the § 510(k) notification that the device is "substantially equivalent" to a pre-existing device, it can be marketed without further regulatory analysis (at least until the FDA initiates the PMA process for the underlying pre-1976 device to which the new device is "substantially equivalent"). The § 510(k) notification process is by no means comparable to the PMA process; in contrast to the 1,200 hours necessary to complete a PMA review, the § 510(k) review is completed in an average of only 20 hours. As one commentator noted, "the attraction of substantial equivalence to manufacturers is clear. [Section] 510(k) notification requires little information, rarely elicits a negative response from the FDA, and gets processed very quickly."

Congress anticipated that the FDA would complete the PMA process for Class III devices relatively swiftly. But because of the substantial investment of time and energy necessary for the resolution of each PMA application, the ever-increasing numbers of medical devices, and internal administrative and resource difficulties, the FDA simply could not keep up with the rigorous PMA process. As a result, the § 510(k) premarket notification process became the means by which most new medical devices — including Class III devices — were approved for the market. In 1983, for instance, a House Report concluded that nearly 1,000 of approximately 1,100 Class III devices that had been introduced to the market since 1976 were admitted as "substantial equivalents" and without any PMA review. This lopsidedness has apparently not evened out; despite an increasing effort by the FDA to consider the safety and efficacy of substantially equivalent devices, the House reported in 1990 that 80% of new Class III devices were being introduced to the market through the § 510(k) process and without PMA review.

INFORMATION SHEETS: GUIDANCE FOR INSTITUTIONAL REVIEW BOARDS AND CLINICAL INVESTIGATORS, MEDICAL DEVICES FOOD AND DRUG ADMINISTRATION
62-63, 66 (1998)

A medical device is defined, in part, as any health care product that does not achieve its primary intended purposes by chemical action or by being metabolized. Medical devices include, among other things, surgical lasers, wheelchairs, sutures, pacemakers, vascular grafts, intraocular lenses, and orthopedic pins. Medical devices also include diagnostic aids such as reagents and test kits for in vitro diagnosis (IVD) of disease and other medical conditions such as pregnancy.

Clinical investigations of medical devices must comply with the Food and Drug Administration (FDA) informed consent and Institutional Review Board (IRB) regulations [21 CFR parts 50 and 56, respectively]. . . .

Except for certain low risk devices, each manufacturer who wishes to introduce a new medical device to the market must submit a premarket notification to FDA. FDA reviews these notifications to determine if the new device is "substantially equivalent" to a device that was marketed prior to passage of the Amendments (i.e., a "pre-amendments device"). If the new device is deemed substantially equivalent to a pre-amendments device, it may be marketed immediately and is regulated in the same regulatory class as the pre-amendments device to which it is equivalent. . . . If the new device is deemed not to be substantially equivalent to a pre-amendments device, it must undergo clinical testing and premarket approval before it can be marketed unless it is reclassified into a lower regulatory class.

Investigational Device Exemption (IDE)

An investigational device is a medical device which is the subject of a clinical study designed to evaluate the effectiveness and/or safety of the device. Clinical investigations undertaken to develop safety and effectiveness data for medical devices must be conducted according to the requirements of the IDE regulations. . . . Certain clinical investigations of devices (e.g., certain studies of lawfully marketed devices) may be exempt from the IDE regulations. Unless exempt from the IDE regulations, an investigational device must be catego-rized as either "significant risk" (SR) or "nonsignificant risk" (NSR). The deter-mination that a device presents a nonsignificant or significant risk is initially made by the sponsor. The proposed study is then submitted either to FDA (for SR studies) or to an IRB (for NSR studies). . . .

Distinguishing Between SR and NSR Device Studies

The effect of the SR/NSR decision is very important to research sponsors and investigators. SR device studies are governed by the IDE regulations. NSR device studies have fewer regulatory controls than SR studies and are gov-erned by the abbreviated requirements. The major differences are in the approval process and in the record keeping and reporting requirements. The SR/NSR decision is also important to FDA because the IRB serves, in a sense, as the Agency's surrogate with respect to review and approval of NSR studies. FDA is usually not apprised of the existence of approved NSR studies because sponsors and IRBs are not required to report NSR device study approvals to FDA. If an investigator or a sponsor proposes the initiation of a claimed NSR investigation to an IRB, and if the IRB agrees that the device study is NSR and approves the study, the investigation may begin at that institution immedi-ately, without submission of an IDE application to FDA.

NOTES AND QUESTIONS

1. The FDA has stated that the term "minimal risk," as used in the Common Rule (*see* 45 C.F.R. § 46.102(i)), refers to a different concept than the term "no significant risk" as used in the device regulations. What is the relationship between these two concepts? Does one refer to a risk level that is lower than the other (and if so, which is which)? Or, if not, is the relationship more compli-cated? What reasons might there be for the differences between these two con-cepts?

2. Are the differences in the processes by which drugs and devices are approved justified? Why or why not?

[D] The FDA Office for Good Clinical Practice

The FDA does not have a direct counterpart to DHHS's OHRP: there is no subdivision in the FDA whose sole purpose relates to the ethics of human sub-jects research. However, that task is part of a somewhat broader mandate that the FDA has assigned to a recently created unit, called the Office for Good Clinical Practice.

FDA and the Quality and Integrity of Research
FDA CONSUMER, January-February 2002

The FDA has established an office to help ensure that research studies involving humans are conducted according to good clinical practice.

Good clinical practice (GCP) is a standard for the total research process: designing studies, conducting and monitoring them, recording data, analyzing results, and reporting and submitting these results to support product applications to the FDA.

The FDA's newly established office for good clinical practice (OGCP) requires that FDA-regulated medical research conform to the GCP standard. Compliance with this standard assures that the data and reported results are credible and accurate and that the rights, safety, and well-being of people in studies are protected. "Poor quality data has an impact on the accuracy of product labels and advertising that will be used by the public — and may lead to inappropriate decision-making on product approvals," says David Lepay, M.D., Ph.D., director of the OGCP. "Our office is out to ensure FDA's broad public protection role of high-quality decision-making on product approvals and labeling. We also want to protect subjects participating in clinical research that is critical to FDA decision-making."

To help make sure that the GCP standard is followed, the FDA conducts more than 1,000 inspections of clinical trials each year.

The OGCP, established in October and located within the office of the FDA commissioner, works closely with the FDA centers, the FDA's office of regulatory affairs, and the Department of Health and Human Services' office for human research protections. The OGCP staff also works with international colleagues to implement GCP standards globally.

§ 3.04 RESEARCH NOT COVERED BY THE FEDERAL REGULATIONS

There are three ways in which a study might be subject to the federal regulations governing human subject protection: (1) the study is conducted or funded by the federal government; (2) the study is conducted at an institution that has agreed, in the assurance it entered into with the federal government, to apply the Common Rule to all research taking place at that institution; or (3) the study concerns something that brings it within the jurisdiction of the FDA (a drug, device, or a biologic). While one or another of these three rules will apply to most of the human subject research in this country, there are nonetheless studies that do not fall under any of them, and thus are not subject to the Common Rule. For that to happen, it must be the case that (1) the study is *not* conducted or funded by the federal government; (2) it is *not* being conducted at an institution that has contractually committed itself to apply the Common Rule to all research taking place there; and (3) the study does *not* come within the jurisdiction of the FDA. (It should be noted that some states also have enacted their own laws that impose requirements similar to those of the Common Rule on some studies that take place within their borders. Those laws are discussed in the next section of this chapter.)

There are many types of research that, if conducted without federal funding and not otherwise subject to FDA regulation, might therefore be beyond the scope of federal regulation. The National Bioethics Advisory Commission (NBAC) listed research taking place in the following settings as possibly fitting into that situation: colleges and universities not receiving federal research funds; in vitro fertilization clinics; weigh-loss or diet clinics; offices of some physicians, dentists, and psychotherapists; and legal clinic offices. *See* NATIONAL BIOETHICS ADVISORY COMMISSION, *supra*, at 29.

For a researcher or study sponsor, there obviously can be advantages to not being subject to the Common Rule. Some types of studies might not be permissible at all under the regulations: for example, a study on children that does not fall into one of the required risk categories specified in 45 C.F.R. 46 Subpart D, or a study on fetuses that does not meet the criteria of Subpart B.

NOTES AND QUESTIONS

1. A doctor at a small community hospital decides to conduct a study about how best to make the first incision when performing an operation to remove a patient's gall bladder: half of the subjects will get the standard horizontal incision, and the other half will be given a crisscross incision. Will this study be subject to the Common Rule?

2. In 1998, the *New York Times* reported that doctors in Manhattan had conducted a study in which they performed two different facelift operations on 21 patients — one on each half of each patient's face — to see which came out better. One procedure was far more aggressive than the other and carried a higher risk of cutting facial nerves and partially paralyzing the face, but it was likely to be more effective in the long term. The study was published in a medical journal in 1996. No IRB approval was sought for the study, and patients allegedly were not given consent documents explaining the procedures and risks. The surgeons claimed that this was not experimentation because both techniques were well established. A number of commentators quoted in the article claimed that the research should have been reviewed. Federal authorities concluded that the study was indeed human experimentation, but that because no federal funds were used to conduct it, the agency had no jurisdiction to investigate further. *See* Phillip J. Hilts, *Study or Human Experiment? Face-Lift Project Stirs Ethical Concerns*, N.Y. TIMES, June 21, 1998, at 25.

3. Is it a good thing that only some research is subject to the Common Rule? How do you think the current system came about? There have been a variety of reform proposals in recent years, most of them recommending that the Common

Rule be modified to apply to all research. *See, e.g.*, NATIONAL BIOETHICS ADVISORY COMMISSION, *supra*, at 12. These suggestions have reached the ears of some members of Congress, who have occasionally introduced bills that would change this state of affairs. For example, in 2002, Senator Edward M. Kennedy was a co-sponsor of a proposed "Research Revitalization Act," which would have broadened the scope of the federal regulations so that they applied to all research with human subjects that takes place in this country, regardless of the source of funding and regardless of whether it involved FDA-regulated products. S. 3060, 107th Cong., 2d Sess. (2002). Does Congress have the authority under the Constitution to regulate research that is not funded by the government and does not concern a federally regulated product? *See*, e.g., William H. Carlile, *Attorney Questions Applying Common Rule to Private Studies Not Regulated by the FDA*, 1 MED. RES. L. & POL'Y REP. (BNA) 12 (2002).

§ 3.05 STATE LAWS

There are laws regulating human subject research at both the state and federal levels. Although the federal rules usually receive the greatest attention, state laws also play an important (and likely growing) role in the day-to-day conduct of research. It is necessary to understand not only what aspects of this field are regulated by the states, but also how to resolve conflicts between what is required by state laws and what is required by federal law.

Oversight of Human Subject Research:
The Role of the States
in NATIONAL BIOETHICS ADVISORY COMMISSION
2 ETHICAL AND POLICY ISSUES IN RESEARCH INVOLVING HUMAN PARTICIPANTS
Jack Schwartz
M-1 (2001)

Federal regulations establish basic protections for human subjects that cannot be diminished by state law. That is, a researcher or institution subject to a federal requirement must comply with it. This obligation exists whether or not a comparable requirement is imposed by state law. Moreover, a researcher may not engage in an activity prohibited by federal law even if state law were to allow it. As the Supreme Court recently reiterated, "even if Congress has not occupied the field, state law is naturally preempted to the extent of any conflict with a federal statute." The same principle, grounded in the Supremacy Clause of the United States Constitution, leads to preemption of state laws that conflict with federal regulations.

Yet, state law is hardly irrelevant to the research enterprise. First, to the extent that research is not subject to federal law, pertinent state law (if any) becomes the only legally applicable regulatory regime. Second, federal law, when it does apply to research, expressly preserves any additional state protections. The Common Rule contains the following non preemption language: "This policy does not affect any State or local laws or regulations which may otherwise be applicable and which provide additional protections for human subjects." In addition to this general provision, the Common Rule more specifically recognizes additional state requirements for informed consent: "The informed consent requirements in this policy are not intended to preempt any applicable Federal, State, or local laws which require additional information to be disclosed in order for informed consent to be legally effective." Identical language appears in the regulations of the Food and Drug Administration.

This policy decision, to preserve a role for states in the regulation of the research enterprise, is unsurprising, for the protection of human subjects may be seen as an application of a state's core function, protecting its citizens against harm. As the Supreme Court observed many years ago, "The police power of a state . . . springs from the obligation of the state to protect its citizens and provide for the safety and good order of society. . . . It is the governmental power of self protection and permits reasonable regulation of rights and property in particulars essential to the preservation of the community from injury."

Yet, state regulation of research has not escaped criticism. Some contend that, especially as research increasingly involves multi-site collaborations, a regulatory system inefficiently increases compliance costs if it imposes requirements or restrictions that differ from one site to the next. These critics insist that federal regulation is sufficient and state regulation unnecessary or even harmful. . . .

Statutes and Regulations: Imposing Limits or Prerequisites Regulating All Research

One of the oft-noted voids in the current federal regulatory system is that some privately funded research is unregulated. That is, research is subject to federal regulation only if it is conducted or funded by agencies that have subscribed to the Common Rule; is the basis on which the Food and Drug Administration (FDA) will be asked to approve a drug or device; or is conducted at an institution that, as an aspect of its assurance to the Office for Protection from Research Risks (now the Office for Human Research Protections), has agreed to conduct all research at the institution in accordance with the Common Rule. Otherwise, research is free of federal regulation. Consequently, as the Commission has pointed out, "the absence of Federal jurisdiction over much privately funded research means that the U.S. government cannot know how many Americans currently are the subjects in experiments, cannot influence how they are recruited, cannot ensure that research subjects know and understand the risks they are undertaking, and cannot ascertain whether they have been harmed."

If Congress sought to assert federal jurisdiction over all privately funded research, its ability to do so would depend on the scope of its Commerce Clause power in this context. "Every law enacted by Congress must be based on one or more of its powers enumerated in the Constitution." By contrast, a state need invoke no particular grant of constitutional authority to regulate privately funded research or any other activity within its borders; state legislatures have plenary power, subject only to constitutional limitations. As the Supreme Court wrote more than a century ago, "The legislative power of a State extends to everything within the sphere of such power, except as it is restricted by the Federal Constitution or that of the State." A state legislature that deemed it appropriate to regulate research beyond the scope of existing federal regulations is unquestionably free to do so as an aspect of its sovereign power.

Hence, the concerns expressed by the Commission about the consequences of limited federal jurisdiction might be ameliorated if privately funded research were subject to state laws that provided for the twin protections of informed consent and independent review. Only two states, however, New York and Virginia, have applied these protections to biomedical research generally. A third state, California, has applied a vigorous informed consent requirement comprehensively.

The New York law, enacted in 1975, applies to "human research," defined as "any medical experiments, research, or scientific or psychological investigation, which utilizes human subjects and which involves physical or psychological intervention by the researcher upon the body of the subject and which is not required for the purposes of obtaining information for the diagnosis, prevention, or treatment of disease or the assessment of medical condition for the direct benefit of the subject." The law excludes studies limited to tissue or fluid specimens taken in the course of standard medical practice, epidemiological studies, and "human research which is subject to, and which is in compliance with, policies and regulations promulgated by any agency of the federal government for the protection of human subjects." By means of this last exclusion, the New York law avoids any additional regulatory burden on research that is already subject to the Common Rule or FDA regulations.

The New York law extends to privately funded research the core requirements of the federal scheme: informed consent and institutional oversight. "No human research may be conducted in this state," the law directs, "in the absence of the voluntary informed consent subscribed to in writing by the human subject" or, in the case of a minor or other individual "legally unable to render consent," by someone who is "legally empowered to act on behalf of the human subject." . . .

California enacted its Protection of Human Subjects in Medical Experimentation Act in 1978. The law's scope is narrower than New York's or Virginia's, for it contains no provisions for IRB review. Instead, it gives strong legal force to the informed consent requirement. . . .

The California law requires informed consent from the subject or one of several specified legally authorized representatives. If a representative provides consent, the research must be "related to maintaining, or improving the health of the human subject or related to obtaining information about a pathological condition of the human subject." Conducting a medical experiment without first obtaining informed consent subjects the principal investigator to civil damages, if the failure is negligent, or to criminal prosecution, if the failure is willful.

The elements of informed consent largely parallel those of the Common Rule. The California law also requires explicit identification of the research sponsor or funding source, or the name of the manufacturer if a drug or device is involved, and contact information for "an impartial third party not associated with the experiment, to whom the subject may address complaints about the experiment."

Conclusion

The singular title of this paper, "The Role of the States," might better have been phrased in the plural. The regulation of human subject research varies markedly from state to state, from efforts at comprehensive regulation in a few to the imposition of limited protections in others. Their regulatory styles differ as well. Some codify informed consent and independent review requirements without detailed specification of methods; others implement these protections through incorporation into state law of federal standards, sometimes augmented by useful elaboration or specification; and still others add requirements or restrictions that reflect a state's own policy choices. Indeed, in this last category are enactments that may be subject to constitutional objection — for example, restrictions on fetal research that may be worded so vaguely as to offend due process standards.

This diversity is the product of a policy environment in which an incomplete federal regulatory scheme encourages a focus on state level agendas, be it advocates pursuing restrictive regulation in particular areas or research enterprises seeking to block undesired regulation. Whether in state legislatures or the courts, and whether they turn out to be mild or draconian, sporadic state responses to controversial research practices can be anticipated unless, of course, the Commission were to recommend, and Congress were to pass, a broadly preemptive federal law.

Thus, a fundamental policy issue for the Commission is whether it is content with the prevailing relationship between federal and state law, in which federal standards are a floor, requiring compliance with both the federal standards and state law, if the state law is more protective of subjects; or whether the Commission believes that federal law should be both a floor and a ceiling, reflecting a conclusive judgment about the extent to which the research enterprise is to be subject to regulation, a judgment that should not be diminished by state-to-state variation. Were the Commission to adopt the latter position, it would need to consider carefully a federal constitutional issue beyond the scope of this paper: the extent to which Congress, exercising its power over interstate commerce, or, by delegation, an Executive Branch agency, may preempt state law in this area.

NOTES AND QUESTIONS

1. How would you answer the question Schwartz poses in the final paragraph: should the federal regulations preempt the states from imposing any stricter rules, effectively providing both a floor and ceiling? What policy arguments can you make in support of and in opposition to such extensive federal preemption?

2. For some important issues, the federal regulations in effect defer to state law. For example, if a subject is incompetent and thus someone else is needed to give consent for that person's participation in a study, the federal regulations result in having state law determine who can give consent. *See* 45 C.F.R. § 46.102(c); *see also* Chapter 14, at page 601. In effect, in such situations, the federal law is providing neither a floor nor a ceiling. What are the arguments in favor of, and against, that type of rule? Describe what a hypothetical federal rule might contain if it provided a "floor" on this consent issue. Answer the same question for a rule that served as both floor and ceiling.

MARYLAND CODE ANNOTATED, HEALTH-GENERAL

§ 13-2002. Compliance with federal regulations; scope

(a) Compliance with federal regulations. — A person may not conduct research using a human subject unless the person conducts the research in accordance with the federal regulations on the protection of human subjects.

(b) Scope to include all research. — Notwithstanding any provision in the federal regulations on the protection of human subjects that limits the applicability of the federal regulations to certain research, subsection (a) of this section applies to all research using a human subject.

NOTES AND QUESTIONS

1. This provision of the Maryland Health Code was enacted in 2002, in large part as a response to a number of high-visibility events that took place in Maryland, including the death of Ellen Roche in an experiment at Johns Hopkins (discussed in Chapter 4, at page 182) and the Maryland Court of Appeals' decision regarding a study of children living in homes with lead paint contamination (discussed in Chapter 13, at page 567). *See* David Nitkin, *Senate OKs Bill to Tighten Rules on Human Research*, BALTIMORE SUN, April 6, 2002, at 1B.

2. The Maryland law adopts the definition of "research" and "human subject" that are used in the Common Rule. *See* Maryland Code Annotated, Health-Gen. § 13-2001.

3. One of the other provisions of the new law, designed to make the regulatory process in this area more open to public scrutiny, requires that the final minutes of any IRB meeting must be released to any person who requests them. *See* Maryland Code Annotated, Health-Gen. § 13-2003.

4. What was the likely purpose of § 13-2002(b)? What types of studies are likely to be affected by the enactment of § 13-2002(a)?

5. An early version of this legislation specifically stated that the law would not apply to studies that were exempt under the federal regulations. Based on a reading of the language that was ultimately adopted, what effect should this law have on exempt studies? *See* Letter from Maryland Attorney General to Governor of Maryland reviewing House Bill 917, May 2, 2002, available at http://www.oag.state.md.us/Healthpol/hb917letter.pdf.

Chapter 4

INSTITUTIONAL REVIEW BOARDS

As noted in the previous chapter, institutional review boards, commonly referred to as IRBs, play a key role in this nation's framework for protecting the well-being of research subjects. In this chapter we further explore the rationale for the use of IRBs, the details of how they are constituted and how they operate, and the growing controversy about whether they are adequate to the task given them.

§ 4.01 PURPOSE AND DUTIES

The current system for protecting human subjects — and particularly the role given to IRBs — owes quite a bit to accidents of history, as described below. In addition, that system was developed around a belief that human subjects can best be protected by a decentralized approach, in which the views of people attuned to local values and circumstances play a major role. In recent years, the importance of local review has been subjected to challenge by a number of changes in the system. As you read the excerpts in this chapter, think about the different ways in which a system of human subject protections might be implemented, particularly with respect to the choice between a relatively centralized system and one that delegates most of the decision-making to local entities.

INSTITUTIONAL REVIEW BOARDS: A TIME FOR REFORM
OFFICE OF INSPECTOR GENERAL, DEPARTMENT
OF HEALTH AND HUMAN SERVICES
(1998)

Institutional Review Boards: The Basics

What Do They Do?

The responsibilities of IRBs fall into two main categories: initial review and continuing review of research involving human subjects.

Initial Review: IRBs review and approve a research plan before the research is carried out. This review encompasses the research protocol, the informed consent document to be signed by subjects, any advertisements to be used in recruiting subjects, and other relevant documents. In carrying out this review, the boards seek to ensure that any risks subjects may incur are warranted in relation to the anticipated benefits, that informed consent documents clearly convey the risks and the true nature of research, that advertisements are not misleading, and that the selection of subjects is equitable and justified. IRBs

focus much attention on the informed consent document because it is the vehicle for providing information to potential research subjects.

Continuing Review: The continuing review process is multifaceted and
includes required reviews "at an interval appropriate to the degree of risk but
not less than once per year." In addition to this continuing review, study amendments and reports of unexpected adverse experiences by subjects are received
periodically and reviewed to ensure that the risk-benefit ratio of the research
has not changed and remains acceptable. . . .

Where Are They Located?

An estimated 3,000 to 5,000 IRBs can be found across the country. They are
most commonly associated with hospitals and academic centers. Boards also
exist in managed care organizations, government agencies (such as the National
Institutes of Health, the Centers for Disease Control, and State governments),
or as for-profit entities that are independent of the institutions in which the
research takes place.

How Are They Organized?

Federal regulations require that boards have at least five members with
varying backgrounds. At least one member must have primarily scientific interests, one must have primarily nonscientific interests, and one must be otherwise
unaffiliated with the institution in which the IRB resides. A quorum, with at
least one member whose interests are primarily nonscientific present, is needed
for voting.

How Does the Department of Health and Human Services (HHS) Oversee Them?

Two agencies within HHS share responsibility for IRB oversight: the Office
for Protection from Research Risks (OPRR) in NIH [now known as the Office for
Human Research Protections, or OHRP] and the FDA. The OPRR's main tool for
oversight is the assurance document. Any institution that intends to conduct
HHS-funded research must have an assurance on file with OPRR. The assurance is a written statement of an institution's requirements for its IRB and
human subject protections. The OPRR also conducts a small number of site visits. The FDA's main mechanism for IRB oversight is the inspection process.
The FDA also inspects research sponsors and scientists (known as research
investigators).

Local Institutional Review Boards
in NATIONAL BIOETHICS ADVISORY COMMISSION
2 ETHICAL AND POLICY ISSUES IN RESEARCH INVOLVING HUMAN
PARTICIPANTS K-1
Steven Peckman
(2001)

It appears that the concept of local IRB review grew out of hospital based scientific peer review committees that operated on an ad hoc basis to address difficult ethical patient care issues. The "peers" were other physicians or experts within the institution. By 1953, Jack Masur, Clinical Research Center Director at the NIH, instructed each NIH institute to establish a "disinterested committee of scientists called the Clinical Research Committee" to review human research that involved "unusual hazard." The committees would review and approve intramural research conducted at the NIH, with "normal" volunteers. . . .

The implementation of policies requiring committee review of the ethics of proposed federally funded research was prompted by several crises [between 1958 and 1968, among them the Willowbrook study, the Jewish Chronic Disease Hospital study, the publication of Henry Beecher's landmark article, as discussed in chapter 1, and the transplantation into humans of a sheep heart and a chimpanzee kidney]. . . . NIH Director James Shannon, concerned about the problems, met with the National Advisory Health Council in September 1965, and proposed an impartial prospective peer review system to address the "risks of the research and of the adequacy of protections of the rights of subjects." The Council accepted his proposal. On the heels of the change in NIH policy, Surgeon General William H. Stewart issued the first comprehensive federal policy for the protection of human subjects in February 1966. The policy required institutions to create local committees to prospectively review new, renewal, supplemental, and continuing grant applications for federally funded biomedical human research. . . . The local institutions were henceforth responsible for applying "wisdom and sound professional judgment [to] determine what constitutes the rights and welfare of human subjects in research, what constitutes informed consent, and what constitutes the risks and potential medical benefits of a particular investigation." . . .

The National Research Act became law in 1974. It outlined protections for human subjects involved in biomedical and behavioral research, it required the DHEW Secretary to promulgate regulations requiring IRB review for all federally funded biomedical or behavioral research, and it impaneled the National Commission for the Protection of Human Subjects in Biomedical and Behavioral Research. The National Commission was charged to assess the state of protections for human subjects around the country and to provide guidance for institutions and investigators when confronting the ethical issues of human subject research. The Commission authored several reports including a document examining IRBs, and in 1979 it issued the definitive American declaration on the ethical conduct of human research, the Belmont Report. Following the public revelations of the syphilis study, membership requirements for IRBs were expanded again by the DHEW in regulations issued in 1974. The new regulations emphasized the importance of considering research in the context of community standards. The regulations defined the composition of an IRB as having a minimum of five members and that it should "...include persons whose primary concerns lie in the areas of legal, professional, and community acceptability rather than in the conduct of research, development, and services programs supported by the HEW." In order to ensure a diversity of opinion when considering protocols, membership on an IRB could not come from a single professional or lay group. Furthermore, the regulations now protected against an implicit institutional bias and conflict of interest by mandating that a legally convened meeting must include at least one member not otherwise affiliated with the institution.

The 1978 National Commission *Report and Recommendations: Institutional Review Boards,* outlined steps necessary to ensure the protection of the dignity and welfare of research subjects. The report defined local IRB review as the cornerstone of the national system for protections and it highlighted the importance of local IRB review:

> The Commission believes that the rights of subjects should be protected by local review committees operating pursuant to federal regulations and located in institutions where research involving human subjects is conducted. Compared to the possible alternatives of a regional or national review process, local committees have the advantage of greater familiarity with the actual conditions surrounding the conduct of research. Such committees can work closely with investigators to assure that the rights and welfare of human subjects are protected and, at the same time, that the application of policies is fair to the investigators. They can contribute to the education of the research community and the public regarding the ethical conduct of research. The committees can become resource centers for information concerning ethical standards and federal requirements and can communicate with federal officials and with other local committees about matters of common concerns.

... By 1993, the concept of local IRB review was firmly entrenched for institutions that receive federal funds. The NIH/Office for Protection from Research Risks' (OPRR's) *1993 Protecting Human Research Subjects: Institutional Review Board Guidebook* explains the concept of local review, and advises institutions that an IRB:

> must be sufficiently qualified through the experience and expertise of its members and the diversity of their backgrounds, including considerations of their racial and cultural heritage and their sensitivity to issues such as community attitudes, to promote respect for its advice and counsel in safeguarding the rights and welfare of human subjects. In

addition, possessing the professional competence necessary to review specific research activities, the IRB must be able to ascertain the acceptability of proposed research in terms of institutional commitments and regulations, applicable law, and standards of professional conduct and practice.

The federal regulations further require that "if an IRB regularly reviews research that involves a vulnerable category of subjects, such as children, prisoners, pregnant women, or handicapped or mentally disabled persons, consideration shall be given to the inclusion of one or more individuals who are knowledgeable about and experienced in working with these subjects." . . .

As outlined above, the concept of local IRB review evolved over the last 50 years from a peer review system to one of community participation. . . . In order to create a more just and representative system, the peer review model was discarded in favor of the local institutionally based IRB system, which includes nonaffiliated or community and nonscientific membership and directly engages the local research institution. . . . Ultimately, the federal government achieved sophisticated goals: predicating a research institution's receipt of research funding on a commitment to ensure both the ethical design of the research and the ethical conduct of its faculty through local IRB review. Such requirements hold an institution's proverbial "feet to the fire" regarding responsibility for the review and the ethical conduct of research.

The National Commission believed local IRB review offers a distinct advantage over regional or national committee oversight in the review of human research. The local IRB is in a superior position to interact with the institution, the investigator, and the community of potential research subjects, and to assure that the proposed research fulfills the three ethical principles of the Belmont Report: respect for persons, beneficence, and justice. Former OPRR Director Gary Ellis echoed the National Commission's recommendations and affirmed the importance of local review:

> We embrace the local IRB at the research site as the cornerstone of the American system of protection of human subjects. IRB review is both prospective and a continuing review of proposed research by a group of individuals with no formal interest in the research. It is local review by individuals who are in the best position to know the research at the site, the resources at the institution, the capabilities and the reputations of the investigators and staff, the prevailing attitudes and ethics of the community and most importantly, the likely subject population.

Implicit in Ellis' statement is the view that local IRB review provides institutions with an opportunity to demonstrate responsibility and to build a culture of trust and ethical conduct in the performance of human research. The institution's commitment to local review is manifested through its ethical obligation to provide educational opportunities for investigators, the IRB, and staff, to provide adequate personnel and resources for the IRB, and to ensure oversight of approved research with participation of both the local scientific community and the community of potential research subjects. The institution thereby demonstrates accountability for the conduct of research and the application of regulations and ethical principles that assure the protection of the rights and welfare of the human subjects.

NOTES AND QUESTIONS

1. The "local" character of IRB review is considered by many to be an important aspect of the current system. As Peckman notes, one of the primary reasons for requiring each institution to have its own IRB was to promote the development of an "institutional culture" that encourages ethical behavior. Peckman says relatively little about the potential drawbacks of this system, such as the possibility that the IRB, as part of the institution, may feel some pressure to approve research that is important to the institution. Do you think that might be a problem? Note that funded research may be an important source of revenue for many institutions. Moreover, when a researcher obtains research funding, a portion of that funding, for so-called "indirect costs," goes to support the institution as a whole. If pressure to approve studies might be a problem, is it nonetheless outweighed by the benefits described by Peckman?

2. The notions of "community standards" and "community acceptability" of research appear to be important ones for the IRB system. What, exactly, is meant by these concepts? There are certainly specific groups that, due to their views, would not find a particular type of study acceptable. Jehovah's Witnesses, whose religious views hold that receiving a blood transfusion is unacceptable, would certainly not be appropriate candidates for a study about how much blood to transfuse after certain types of blood loss. Can you think of other examples of studies where information about the local community might be relevant? Consider, for example, the general issues of recruitment practices, confidentiality, and informed consent, and how they might need to be altered in a community that has a large population of illegal aliens, many of whom do not speak English.

3. Assuming that a study does not involve a special population, such as Jehovah's Witnesses or persons who do not speak English, does the concept of community standards have any meaning? In a study involving a new type of pacemaker for people with heart problems, is an IRB supposed to determine how the community feels about this type of research? How should it determine this? Should there be, for example, different standards for approving this study in Kansas City than in New York?

4. The predecessor agency to OHRP issued guidance to institutions in 1998 explaining what measures an IRB should be taking to make sure that it has appropriate "knowledge of the local research context." OFFICE FOR PROTECTION FROM RESEARCH RISKS, KNOWLEDGE OF LOCAL RESEARCH CONTEXT (1998, updated

in 2000), available at http://www.hhs.gov/ohrp/humansubjects/guidance/local.htm. This guidance was partly motivated by the growth of "for-hire" IRBs that usually have no geographical connection to the institutions that hire them, a development that is discussed below, at page 197.

5. In 1999, after newspapers disclosed that there were research studies at the University of Nebraska involving the use of fetal tissue, the president of that university created the Nebraska Bioethics Advisory Commission. *See* Kimberly Sweet, *Bioethics Committee Being Planned to Examine U. Nebraska's Research*, DAILY NEBRASKAN, December 9, 1999. His purpose was to "improve public discussion" of research issues. The Commission would not be involved in approving specific research studies, but rather in "reviewing policies." Is it appropriate for a state to create such a commission? If so, in what way should its task differ from what an IRB is doing when it is incorporating community standards into its review?

§ 4.02 COMPOSITION

Although the regulations give a fair amount of detail about what types of members an IRB must have, there still remain a variety of unanswered questions. In light of the mandate that IRBs have been given, think about whether the regulations provide sufficient guidance to institutions about how to select IRB members.

45 C.F.R. § 46.107: IRB MEMBERSHIP

This provision is reproduced in Appendix A, at page A-7. Please review it before proceeding.

NOTES AND QUESTIONS

1. Being a member of an IRB generally is considered a somewhat thankless task. Serving on an IRB can require a substantial time commitment, with few offsetting benefits. Relatively few institutions provide any financial compensation, let alone substantial compensation, to members. Moreover, for the IRB members who are affiliated with the institution, it is rare that they are compensated in any non-financial way, such as being given a reduced teaching or research load. Given the reasons for creating the system of IRB review, is this state of affairs appropriate?

2. The membership of the IRB for a hypothetical university medical center consists of three doctors who are members of the medical staff, two nurses at the institution, and a law professor from a school in a nearby city. Is this IRB in compliance with the regulations?

3. How should it be determined whether the members of an IRB have "varying backgrounds"? If the IRB mainly reviews medical studies, is it acceptable that ninety percent of the members are doctors, but that they come from different fields of medicine (e.g., surgery, radiology, internal medicine)?

4. Although it is not specifically mentioned in the regulations, OHRP permits IRBs to use a system of "alternate" members. Under this system, two or more people may share any position on the IRB. If that position has special qualifications (for example, it is the unaffiliated member, or it is for someone knowledgeable about statistics), then each of the alternates should possess the necessary skills. Only one of the people sharing such a position can be permitted to vote at any time or be included in determining if there is a quorum, consistent with the concept that they are sharing a single position on the IRB. The use of alternate members can make it easier for an IRB to meet the quorum requirements at meetings (discussed later in this chapter).

5. The use of alternate members can also help the IRB to meet various specific membership requirements. For example, as discussed in Chapter 15, an IRB reviewing a study involving prisoners must have a member who is a prisoner or a prisoner representative. *See* Chapter 15, at page 643. For many IRBs, however, it will be relatively infrequent that the IRB reviews prisoner studies at a particular meeting. Thus, such a person might be appointed as an alternate to the non-scientific or community member, thereby satisfying the requirements for reviewing prisoner studies, yet not making it any more difficult to obtain a quorum for the typical meeting.

Local Institutional Review Boards in NATIONAL BIOETHICS ADVISORY COMMISSION 2 ETHICAL AND POLICY ISSUES IN RESEARCH INVOLVING HUMAN PARTICIPANTS Steven Peckman K-1 (2001)

In this section I will discuss the participation of the nonaffiliated community member as a nonscientist. A recent NIH IRB survey noted that most nonaffiliated members are nonscientists. The federal regulations require that an IRB include at least one member who is not affiliated with the institution, commonly known as the community member or lay member, and one nonscientific member. The nonaffiliated membership on the IRB provides a voice for the community of research subjects during the review of research. [OHRP] suggests that the nonaffiliated member should come from the local "community-at-large. . . . The person selected should be knowledgeable about the local community and be willing to discuss issues and research from that perspective." The [OHRP] guidance implies that the nonaffiliated member's charge is to represent community concerns and by extension the concerns of specific subject populations. Recognition of both the implicit scientific bias in the traditional peer review system and the need for community participation in the ethical evaluation of human research, coincides with a societal shift in emphasis from the individual to the social environment in which individuals exist. Through community representation, the IRB is able to acknowledge and address such important issues as the social context and impact of research, the heterogeneity of our society, the impact of scientific paternalism on notions of autonomy, beneficence and justice, the recognition that, in addition to physical risk, scientific inquiry includes potential social, psychological, and economic risk for subjects, and the need to engage the potential subject populations in the decision making process regarding research in their community.

Paul McNeill commented, "The assumption that society (or the community) should have a voice on ethics committees is based on a notion about the role of the lay member." The regulations do not privilege scientific expertise over community participation on the IRB. Instead, the regulations reserve an adequate number of chairs at the IRB table for both scientific expertise and community representation and note that the IRB should be "sufficiently qualified through the experience and expertise of its members, including consideration of race, gender, and cultural backgrounds and sensitivity to such issues as community attitudes, to promote respect for its advice and counsel in safeguarding the rights and welfare of human subjects." The National Commission endorsed a balance of scientific, individual, and community concerns on IRBs in order to guard against scientific self-interest and to demonstrate an "awareness and appreciation for the various qualities, values and needs of the diverse elements of the community served by the institution or in which it is located. A diverse membership will enhance the local IRB's credibility as well as the likelihood that its determinations will be sensitive to the concerns of those who conduct or participate in the research and other interested parties."

Community, however, consists of several distinct and sometimes intersecting groups, such as the community of potential research subjects, people located in a specific geographical area, people with similar interests, work, culture, or religious, racial, or ethnic background. The letter and the spirit of the National Commission IRB report and the federal regulations require sufficient scientific, cultural, and community expertise, and therefore, appear to support representative or democratic IRB membership, one that includes the participation of representatives of potential subject populations on the IRB. The federal regulations recognize that research is a social act involving particular social relationships. Such awareness underscores an important aspect of the spirit of the regulations and the intent behind local review, that is, the democratic constitution of a local IRB in order to balance the interests of science, society, and the individual. Though a nonscientific community member serves an important purpose on the local IRB, it is important to distinguish between such independent members and community members who are representative of or who directly advocate for subject populations. . . .

The role of community members on local IRBs evolved out of concern that a committee comprised exclusively of institutional representatives would be biased toward research and the interests of the institution.

NOTES AND QUESTIONS

1. With regard to the requirement that IRBs have a non-scientific member, the FDA provides the following guidance:

[N]urses, pharmacists and other biomedical health professionals should not be regarded to have "primary concerns in the non-scientific area." In the past, lawyers, clergy and ethicists have been cited as examples of persons whose primary concerns would be in non-scientific areas. Some members have training in both scientific and non-scientific disciplines, such as a J.D./R.N. While such members are of great value to an IRB, other members who are unambiguously non-scientific should be appointed to satisfy the non-scientist requirement.

FOOD AND DRUG ADMINISTRATION, INFORMATION SHEETS: GUIDANCE FOR INSTITUTIONAL REVIEW BOARDS AND CLINICAL INVESTIGATORS 8 (1998 Update).

2. Peckman notes that the regulations provide for an "adequate" number of community representatives on IRBs. In fact, the regulations only require that there be one unaffiliated member and one member who is a non-scientist. Is that an adequate number? How should adequacy be determined? Both the National Bioethics Advisory Commission (NBAC) and the Institute of Medicine have recommended that twenty-five percent of an IRB's members should be either unaffiliated, non-scientists, or chosen to represent the views of research subjects. See NATIONAL BIOETHICS ADVISORY COMMISSION, 1 ETHICAL AND POLICY ISSUES IN RESEARCH INVOLVING HUMAN PARTICIPANTS 63 (2001); INSTITUTE OF MEDICINE, RESPONSIBLE RESEARCH: A SYSTEMS APPROACH TO PROTECTING RESEARCH PARTICIPANTS 96 (2002) [hereinafter INSTITUTE OF MEDICINE, RESPONSIBLE RESEARCH]. Would that be a helpful change, and if so, why? Might there be any drawbacks to such a requirement? Note that Danish law requires that a majority of the members of its Research Ethics Committees be comprised of laypersons. See Jesse A. Goldner, An Overview of Legal Controls on Human Experimentation and the Regulatory Implications of Taking Professor Katz Seriously, 38 SAINT LOUIS U. L.J. 63, 107 (1993).

3. Richard Saver has compared IRBs to the boards of directors of corporations, which are also required to have "outside" (unaffiliated) members. Saver notes that outside directors on corporate boards typically become co-opted by the insiders, and thus have relatively little impact in altering a corporation's behavior. Thus, he suggests, the proposals for adding more unaffiliated members to IRBs might similarly have little impact. See Richard Saver, Medical Research Oversight from the Corporate Governance Perspective: Comparing Institutional Review Boards and Corporate Boards, 46 WM. & MARY L. REV. 619 (2004). In

evaluating this comparison, might it be relevant that service on a corporation's board of directors is considered to be a prestigious thing to do within the business community, and thus such positions are often actively sought after?

4. How should IRBs resolve the tension between having adequate scientific expertise to understand the scientific issues posed by complex protocols, and also having adequate non-scientific representation? Will increasing the non-scientific representation, as suggested by the NBAC, make it harder for IRBs to maintain adequate scientific representation? Should IRBs increase their number of members as a possible solution, or will the size of many IRBs become so large as to be unwieldy? Another route would be to use more scientific consultants: people who are not formally members of the IRB, but on whom the IRB can call for scientific expertise. *See* 45 C.F.R. § 46.107(f).

§ 4.03 PROCESS OF IRB REVIEW

There are two different ways in which an IRB can evaluate a new study to determine whether it is approvable. The first, which is often called "full" review, involves having the study evaluated at a meeting of the committee where enough members attend to constitute a quorum. This is the usual way in which studies involving the possibility of significant risks to subjects are reviewed. Some relatively low-risk studies can be reviewed in a more streamlined manner known as expedited review. The federal regulations provide guidance on how both of these types of review should take place.

[A] Full Review

45 C.F.R. § 46.108: IRB FUNCTIONS AND OPERATIONS; § 46.109: IRB REVIEW OF RESEARCH; AND § 46.111: CRITERIA FOR IRB APPROVAL OF RESEARCH

These provisions are reproduced in Appendix A, at pages A-8 and A-11. Please review them before proceeding.

GUIDANCE ON WRITTEN IRB PROCEDURES OFFICE FOR HUMAN RESEARCH PROTECTIONS JULY 11, 2002
http://www.hhs.gov/ohrp/humansubjects/guidance/irbgd702.htm.

(2) Research Review Materials

    (a) Initial Review Materials. HHS regulations at 45 CFR 46.111 set forth the criteria that must be satisfied in order for the IRB to approve research. These criteria include, among other things, determinations by the IRB regarding risks, potential benefits, informed consent, and safeguards for human subjects. In conducting the initial review of proposed research, IRBs must obtain information in sufficient detail to make the determinations required under HHS regulations at 45 CFR 46.111. Materials should include the full protocol, a proposed informed consent document, any relevant grant application(s), the investigator's brochure (if one exists), and any recruitment materials, including advertisements intended to be seen or heard by potential subjects. Furthermore, for HHS-supported multicenter clinical trials, the IRB should receive and review a copy of the HHS-approved sample informed consent document and the complete HHS-approved protocol, if they exist. Unless a primary reviewer system is used, all members should receive a copy of the complete documentation. These materials should be received by members sufficiently in advance of the meeting date to allow review of this material.

If the IRB uses a primary reviewer system, the primary reviewer(s) should do an in-depth review of all pertinent documentation (see previous paragraph). All other IRB members should at least receive and review a protocol summary (of sufficient detail to make the determinations required under HHS regulations at 45 CFR 46.111), the proposed informed consent document, and any recruitment materials, including advertisements intended to be seen or heard by potential subjects. In addition, the complete documentation should be available to all members for review.

NOTES AND QUESTIONS

1. As noted by OHRP, the criteria that an IRB must evaluate in reviewing a study are spelled out in 45 C.F.R. § 46.111. Most of these criteria are discussed in detail elsewhere in this book. Are the criteria specified in § 46.111 adequate for protecting human subjects, or are there other criteria that you would add? For a general discussion of this issue, not specifically referring to the regulations, see Ezekiel J. Emanuel et al., *What Makes Clinical Research Ethical?* 283 JAMA 2701 (2000).

2. For an attempt at providing a comprehensive list of the questions that an IRB should think about in reviewing a protocol, see Ernest D. Prentice & Dean L. Antonson, *A Protocol Review Guide to Reduce IRB Inconsistency*, 9 IRB, Jan.-Feb. 1987, at 9.

3. The OHRP guidance document excerpted above provides detailed information on what issues need to be covered in an IRB's written procedures, expanding on what is spelled out in 45 C.F.R. § 103(b)(4). It also discusses various issues relating to the documentation of IRB actions, such as what information must be in the minutes of IRB meetings, the requirement to document

the appropriate determinations before allowing waiver of the usual criteria for informed consent, and the requirement to document determinations relating to the risk level of a particular study and the period for which it has been approved. In general, an IRB is required to keep records of its action for a period of at least three years. *See* 45 C.F.R. § 115(b).

MAJORITY incl. 1 non-scientist

4. An IRB has 14 members. How many must be present for there to be a quorum? What if it had 15 members? If you had to make a guess, do you think IRBs would more commonly have an odd number of members or an even number of members?

108

5. The membership of an IRB at a university medical center consists of three doctors on the medical staff, two nurses who work there, a priest who works at the center, and a research scientist who works at a not-for-profit research center in that town. During a particular meeting, all of the members are in attendance, but the research scientist gets an important message and has to leave. Can they continue the meeting without her? Assume that she then returns to the meeting, but the priest has to go assist a dying patient. Can they continue the meeting then?

.Y   N

6. For an IRB with 14 members, imagine that eight members show up at a particular meeting. On one study, five members vote in favor of approval, and three vote against. According to the federal regulations, has the study been approved? What if, for another study, there are four members voting for approval, three opposed, and one who abstains? *Y   N*

7. As the OHRP document notes, IRBs are permitted to review a study by using a "primary reviewer" system. Under such a system, the IRB adopts a policy under which each study to be reviewed at a meeting is assigned ahead of time to one or two reviewers who will be given primary responsibility to present the study to the other members at the meeting. In fact, it is very common for IRBs to use such a system. Based on the information provided in the OHRP document, why might an IRB have a substantial incentive to adopt such a policy?

8. Sometimes it is not possible to get enough members in one room to have a quorum, due to people being out of town. In such circumstances, a meeting can be conducted via a conference call. *See* OPRR, IRB MEETINGS CONVENED VIA TELEPHONE CONFERENCE CALL, March 28, 2000, available at http://www.hhs.gov/ohrp/references/irbtel.pdf.

What Does It Mean to "Review" a Protocol? Johns Hopkins & OHRP
Bette-Jane Crigger
23 IRB, July-Aug. 2001, at 13.

Ellen Roche was a healthy, 24-year-old technician at the Johns Hopkins Asthma and Allergy Center when she volunteered to participate in a protocol designed to study the mechanism by which deep inspiration can protect a person's airways from stimuli that might cause them to spasm (bronchoprotection). On 4 May Ms. Roche received a dose of nebulized hexamethonium, a ganglionic blocker not approved for clinical use, to test the hypothesized neural mechanisms of bronchoprotection. The following day she developed a dry cough and shortness of breath on exertion. Over the next several days she reported flu-like symptoms and was seen by a member of the research team on 7 May. When she was contacted at home the following day she reported that she was going to see her primary care provider. When she was contacted again on the 9th she was still unwell and Dr. Togias [the principal investigator for the study] asked her to return to the laboratory for evaluation. Ms. Roche was running a fever, had decreased blood oxygen saturation after mild exertion, and a chest x-ray showed abnormalities. She was evaluated by the Johns Hopkins Bay Medical Center (UHBMC) emergency department and admitted to the hospital on the 9th.

Dr. Togias sent a letter to the IRB that day advising them of the serious adverse event and that the protocol would be "placed on hold at this point." At that time he also advised the IRB for the first time that a previous participant in the study had developed an adverse reaction to hexamethonium that had resolved without treatment.

Ms. Roche's condition continued to deteriorate and she was transferred to the intensive care unit on 14 May. She was intubated, but required increasing ventilatory support and dialysis for renal failure. Extensive diagnostic testing identified no infectious agent that could account for her steadily worsening condition. After considering possible further therapies, her family decided to withdraw life supports and Ms. Roche died on 2 June 2001.

John Hopkins' Investigation

An internal investigative committee reviewed the study records and other documents related to the protocol, including communication between the IRB and Dr. Togias, as well as Ms. Roche's medical records and autopsy report, and interviewed Dr. Togias, members of the research team, and the chair and a member of the Johns Hopkins Bay Medical Center IRB. The investigation sought to answer whether the study addressed an important scientific question and had been appropriately reviewed by the JHBMC IRB; whether the consent form signed by Ms. Roche and other subjects was appropriate; whether any coercion had been involved in recruiting Ms. Roche; whether the study was carried out appropriately; whether Ms. Roche had received prompt, appropriate medical care; and what had caused her death.

The investigation concluded that the study was designed to address an important scientific question but that the investigator and the IRB relied on inadequate data as to the pulmonary toxicity of hexamethonium. The committee further found that the consent form as approved by the IRB failed to disclose that the study agent was not approved by the FDA and was no longer used clinically, that the safety of inhaled hexamethonium was not known with certainty, and that there was a possibility of serious adverse consequences or death as a result of study participation. The committee noted as well that the IRB had not been notified of changes in the protocol after its approval, but also noted these were minor changes that would almost certainly have been approved and were unlikely to have had significant bearing on the outcome.

The report of the investigation concluded that the study had not involved coercion — although Ms. Roche was a technician in the Asthma and Allergy Center where it was conducted, she did not work in Dr. Togias's laboratory and there was no evidence that her employment was in any way conditioned by her participation. Ms. Roche received excellent medical care from the time she arrived at the emergency department, from staff members not affiliated with the research. Although autopsy revealed damage to her lungs, no specific etiology could be identified. The conclusion that she died as a result of the study agent was based on the timing of the dose of inhaled hexamethonium and development of symptoms, the absence of any identifiable infectious agent that might have caused her symptoms, the development of similar but less severe symptoms by another participant in the protocol, and previously reported pulmonary toxicity associated with hexamethonium administered intravenously.

OHRP's Findings

In its letter of 19 July suspending Hopkins' MPA, OHRP stressed the failure to identify pulmonary toxicity associated with hexamethonium and flaws in the approved consent form — including misleading description of the study agent as a "medication," failure to disclose that hexamethonium is not currently FDA approved for human use and has never been approved as an inhalant. OHRP reviewed not only the records related to the protocol in which Ms. Roche died, but also IRB files for more than 60 protocols and minutes of IRB meetings since 1998, and interviewed a total of 24 IRB members and all IRB staff of both the Johns Hopkins University School of Medicine (JHUSOM) and Johns Hopkins Bay Medical Center (JHBMC). Their findings revealed weaknesses in the IRB process overall.

With regard to the study itself, OHRP found that the investigators failed to advise the IRB that hexamethonium was labeled "for laboratory use only" by the manufacturer and did not provide — nor did the IRB request — information about the pharmacology, toxicity, or safety in humans of inhaled hexamethonium. The consent form did not identify hexamethonium as experimental, did not describe the protocol's escalating dose strategy, and did not describe the circumstances under which a subject's participation would be terminated by the investigator as required by 45 CFR 46.116. OHRP also cited the failure to notify the IRB of changes in the protocol or of the first subject's adverse reaction to the study agent, and the continuation of the study before the subject's symptoms had resolved.

Among weaknesses in the IRB process, OHRP found the practice of using "boilerplate" consent forms problematic, noting that such forms too readily lead to the omission of information important to disclose for particular studies and are frequently difficult to read. Further, continuing review practices did not meet guidelines set out by the agency in a letter to Hopkins of October 2000; the investigators concluded that as conducted such review was "not substantive [or] meaningful." Nor were IRB actions appropriately documented separately for individual protocols, they found, and minutes of IRB meetings often did not document the grounds on which changes in protocols were required. OHRP also noted that the IRBs failed to adhere to restrictions on the use of procedures for expedited review of changes to previously approved protocols set out at 45 CFR 46.110(b)(2).

Finally, although OHRP praised the culture of respect for the IRB process that it found among investigators at Hopkins, and the "sincere commitment" and dedication of IRB members and staff to protecting participants, the agency expressed concern that IRB members and chairs did not have a sufficiently detailed understanding of federal regulations to implement them appropriately in all cases.

What Counts as "Review"?

Among the many concerns OHRP identified, one particularly stands out, however: The agency's on-site investigation found that in initial review of protocols, IRBs at JHUSOM and JHBMC did not review this and most other protocols that did not meet criteria for expedited review at "convened meetings" of the full IRB, which OHRP judged to violate 45 CFR 46.108(b). The IRB minutes reviewed by the federal investigators suggested that for the most part, protocols under consideration were neither presented individually nor discussed in detail by the IRB with a majority of members present (Finding 8).

Prior to the suspension, Hopkins employed a multi-stage review process built around a system of executive subcommittees at each of its IRBs. As described in internal IRB guidelines, protocols were circulated to all members of the relevant IRB for comment. When a majority of members' comments had been returned, comments were reviewed by an executive subcommittee comprised of the chair and several other members of the IRB, which determined whether and which comments or questions to convey in writing to the investigator for response. Written responses from investigators were again considered by the executive subcommittee and further communication with the investigator undertaken as deemed necessary by the subcommittee. Protocols, with their correspondence, were then recirculated to IRB members before final approval at convened meetings. When significant concerns or questions remained, the investigator might be invited to attend a convened meeting to discuss the protocol.

The system, Hopkins argued in its 21 July response to OHRP's findings, "assures that all issues relevant to the review process are identified and documented prior to the convened meetings." Convened meetings of the full IRB then provide opportunity for further review and discussion before a protocol is approved. The matter, in Hopkins' view, is one of how 45 CFR 46.108(b) is to be interpreted. The university interpreted the regulation not to require individual presentation of protocols at IRB meetings. In light of OHRPs clear interpretation otherwise, Hopkins will now require protocols to be presented and discussed individually at convened meetings, and will document such discussions separately in IRB minutes.

The Outcome

On 22 July OHRP reinstated Hopkins' multiple project assurance, with some notable restrictions. All federally funded protocols that, being eligible for expedited review, had been so reviewed and approved may resume. Those protocols not eligible for expedited review that were reviewed at a convened meeting of one of the IRBs covered by the MPA will also be permitted to resume. All other protocols covered by the MPA that are not eligible for expedited review, whether federally funded or not, remain suspended until they are reviewed and approved by the appropriate IRB at a convened meeting.

Arguably, what lies at the heart of OHRP's concerns about the IRB process at Johns Hopkins, and indeed led to the "triage" review structure employed by the university, is the volume of work required of IRBs. Hopkins receives more federal funding for biomedical research than any other institution in the country, for which two institutional review boards have oversight responsibility. OHRP itself expressed concern that its findings "may be indicative of IRBs overburdened by the large volume of research for which it [sic] has oversight responsibility" and noted that more than two IRBs seem warranted. Similarly, it was concerned that the existing IRBs were not adequately staffed, both professionally and clerically, to carry out their mandate—minutes have not been recorded for over nine months.

Surely, Hopkins does not face these dilemmas alone.

NOTES AND QUESTIONS

1. Imagine that instead of using the subcommittee system described in Crigger's article, Hopkins had constituted each of the subcommittees as a separate IRB, and had made sure that each of the subcommittees met all of the regulatory requirements for being an IRB (i.e., there was an unaffiliated member, a non-scientific member, and so forth). For example, if there were initially four subcommittees, each with five members, and the full IRB initially had twenty

members, the new arrangement would involve four separate IRBs each with five members. Under those circumstances, would Hopkins have been in violation of the regulations?

2. Crigger says that at the heart of OHRP's concerns about the review process used at Hopkins was the volume of work required of IRBs. Assuming that this is indeed a problem, what are appropriate ways to eliminate that problem? Is changing from one large IRB to several smaller IRBs a good change? What does this do in terms of the workload of individual IRB members? What does this do in terms of the actual outcome, namely the adequacy of review given to each study?

3. At least some of the mistakes leading to Ellen Roche's death appear primarily related to scientific issues, such as lack of adequate information. In its review of what happened at Hopkins, OHRP noted, among other things, that the investigator and the IRB "failed to obtain published literature about the known association between hexamethonium and lung toxicity." (One of the reasons they did not find everything reported in the literature was that hexamethonium was no longer being used as a drug, and therefore some of the reports about toxicity were not contained in the online data banks, such as Medline, that are generally reviewed. To find all of the toxicity reports, someone would have also needed to do a separate search in the older literature that had not been transferred to online services, a search that one would rarely think about doing.) Assuming that the investigator had listed the risks of hexamethonium in the consent form, was the IRB under a duty to evaluate whether the list of risks was complete? As a general matter, what should IRBs do to ensure that scientific information submitted by an investigator is accurate and complete?

4. In a recent evaluation of the U.S. system for protecting research subjects, the Institute of Medicine (IOM) concluded that IRBs should not be expected to review studies for their scientific merit. As the IOM put it, "it is unrealistic to expect a single group of individuals to possess the requisite skills to competently carry out the many tasks needed to protect the rights and welfare of research participants." INSTITUTE OF MEDICINE, RESPONSIBLE RESEARCH, *supra*, at 72. The IOM accordingly recommended that there should be a separate mechanism for reviewing the scientific merit of a study, and that the results of that review should be given to the IRB, which would then concentrate on purely ethical issues. There would be a variety of ways in which the scientific review could take place, including the use of outside experts, such as panels in the National Institutes of Health or the FDA. In accord with this change, the IOM recommended that IRBs be renamed "research ethics review boards." Do you agree with the suggestion to split off scientific review to a separate mechanism? How would such a research ethics review board interact with the scientific review group? Would it be necessary to amend the regulations that give IRBs the ultimate authority to pass on risk/benefit ratios? Which of these two review groups would be charged with answering what is arguably the major eth-

ical question, namely whether the risks of a particular study are "worth it" given the potential scientific benefits?

While the following excerpt focuses on the process of risk-benefit assessment, its observations have implications for the process of IRB review more generally.

Rationalizing Risk Assessment
in Human Subject Research
Carl H. Coleman
46 ARIZ. L. REV. 1 (2004)

IRBs' current approach to evaluating protocols has several distinctive characteristics. First, decisions are made by a relatively small group of people who tend to come from similar professional and institutional backgrounds. In addition, deliberations are conducted behind closed doors, and minutes of meetings are made available to outsiders only under limited circumstances. In general, therefore, the process is both insular and secretive.

Second, the risk assessment process is highly unstructured; essentially, the members are simply given a set of protocols and asked for their reactions. The only specific guidance the members receive for this exercise is the general regulatory standard for approving research — i.e., whether the risks are "reasonable" in relation to the study's anticipated benefits. Each member is free to interpret this reasonableness standard as he or she sees fit. Because the members are not required to state reasons for their decisions, the process encourages reliance on impressionistic judgments, or "gut reactions."

Third, IRBs are rarely required to explain or justify their decisions. IRBs do not issue written opinions, and while they are required to keep minutes of meetings, these minutes often contain little substantive information about the basis of decisions, particularly when the IRB decides to approve a protocol. In addition, while federal agencies conduct audits of IRBs, these audits are infrequent and tend to focus on matters like documentation and record-keeping, not the substance of decisions about particular protocols. The prospect of a federal audit, therefore, creates little incentive for IRBs to develop articulable rationales for their decisions. The only time most IRB decisions receive serious scrutiny is in the rare event that an investigation or lawsuit is initiated following a significant injury, at which point any damage caused by an inappropriate decision has already been done.

Fourth, the system does not encourage IRBs to look beyond the specifics of particular protocols, or to develop general principles with applicability to more than one set of facts. In IRBs with longstanding memberships, customary ways of dealing with particular issues may develop informally, but no formal mechanisms exist to standardize risk-benefit assessments by incorporating prior decisions into current evaluations. There also is no mechanism for IRBs to learn about deliberations that have taken place at other institutions, except when issues happen to be publicized at conferences or in professional journals, both of which are relatively uncommon occurrences. As a result, IRBs are regularly challenged by issues of first impression — not necessarily issues that are new to the world of research, but issues that have never previously come before the particular IRB.

Finally, IRBs' independence, combined with the fact that IRB decisions are not appealable to any higher authority, leads to widely varying approaches to similar issues at different institutions. For example, commentators have noted widespread differences in how IRBs interpret the riskiness of common procedures like venipuncture, arterial puncture, gastric and intestinal intubation, and lumbar puncture. This variation is one of the reasons some investigators engage in the practice of "IRB shopping."

NOTES AND QUESTIONS

1. Coleman goes on to argue that the characteristics of IRB decision making described above are similar to those of common law juries, and that, given these similarities, "many of the problems with the jury deliberation process are also likely to apply to IRBs' review of research protocols." For example, he argues that the current decision-making process "leaves enormous discretion to the individuals entrusted with making the decisions," which both increases the likelihood of "arbitrariness and inconsistency" and risks "overemphasizing the values and attitudes of" the particular IRB members. "Indeed," he suggests, "a jury-like process of risk-benefit assessment may not even accurately reflect the values and attitudes of the individuals participating in the deliberative process. This apparent anomaly may arise because perceptions of risk are frequently distorted by a variety of cognitive biases, which are likely to be fueled by a decision-making system that relies on general impressions and case-by-case determinations." For example, "the manner in which risk information is presented, or 'framed,' can significantly influence individuals' perceptions of the magnitude of a risk." Similarly, people tend to "pay greater attention to risk information they have learned recently than information they learned a long time ago, and to trust 'detailed, concrete reports' about risk more than 'abstract though arguably more relevant ones.'" Coleman, *supra*, at 21.

2. What implications do these observations have for the efficacy of IRB review? If you believe that relatively unstructured, case-by-case decision making is problematic, what alternatives might work better? Would it help if IRBs, like appellate courts, were required to issue written opinions? Should an IRB be required to explain when it departs from reasoning it has embraced in the past,

or from approaches used by other IRBs confronting similar situations? Even if these mechanisms might be helpful, are they worth the added expense?

The Role of Institutional Review Boards in Protecting Human Subjects: Are We Really Ready to Fix a Broken System?
Hazel Glenn Beh
26 L. & PSYCHOL. REV. 1 (2002)

Why IRBs Fail To Protect Human Subjects

As many commentators have acknowledged, IRBs are often too weak, over-burdened, ignorant, or conflicted to adequately perform the important duties assigned to them by the federal system. The weaknesses in the IRB system are pervasive, and the resulting widely publicized gaffes should come as no surprise. Importantly, these deficiencies jeopardize the effectiveness of the federal system that relies heavily on IRBs to safeguard human subject research. Under federal regulations, the 3,000-5,000 local IRBs act as the gatekeepers standing between the researcher and her research. Remarkably, in spite of all the elaborate rules it promulgated, the federal government barely oversees the IRB system in order to ensure that it complies with its regulations. Expenditures on human subject protection are woefully inadequate. For example, "the National Institutes of Health spent less than 0.5 percent of its human research budget last year on activities aimed at protecting patients."

In 1998, the Office of Inspector General issued a comprehensive report warning that "the effectiveness of IRBs is in jeopardy." In particular, it found that changes in the nature and number of research proposals have strained the IRB system, and thus, they review "too much, too quickly, with too little expertise." Moreover, the Inspector General criticized that continuing review of projects is scant, IRB independence is threatened by conflicts, and members have too little training to perform their duties. Finally, the Inspector General complained that the effectiveness of the IRB system has not been subjected to critical evaluation, and "too much . . . attention now focuses on perfunctory review responsibilities yielding little protective value."

Without a doubt, IRBs are overworked. Scientists conduct thousands of studies across the United States at any given time, and researchers estimate that as many as 19 million individuals participate in human subject research each year. According to the Inspector General, "IRBs across the country are inundated with protocols," and the workload of the average IRB has increased to the point that they are unable to provide meaningful review. As a result, some IRBs provide "only one to two minutes of review per study." The rule requiring each institution to review study protocols conducted in its institution, even when the research is being conducted at many research sites, constitutes one source of overload. This process slows research, frustrates researchers, and unnecessarily taxes an already overburdened IRB system. IRBs expend "scarce resources on reviewing the same protocol that, in some cases, is being reviewed by hundreds of other IRBs, even when overall design and methods can only be changed with great difficulty."

In addition to being overburdened, IRB members are neither sufficiently trained in the substantive topic of ethical research conducted on human subjects, including issues of research design and informed consent, nor in the morass of federal requirements that guide the review process. Both the Inspector General and the National Bioethics Advisory Commission (NBAC) cited increased need for education of IRB members and recognized a shared obligation at the federal and at the institutional level. In its 2001 final report, NBAC explained that "despite this enduring recognition of the important role of education, the educational function of the oversight system has been only minimally implemented through federal programs." This failure to emphasize education "at the federal level was repeated at the local level, with institutions often failing to provide educational programs to their investigators, research staff, and IRB members." According to a 1995 survey, one-quarter of IRBs at universities "offered no training at all to their members" and a "vast majority" offered fewer than four hours of training to IRB members. This lack of training constitutes a fundamental flaw and is problematic because it "impedes [independent IRB members'] ability to serve as an effective counterbalance to institutional and scientific interests."

IRB education in ethics is particularly essential because there is no assurance that principal investigators and scientists have necessarily received training on ethical human subject research. In October 2000, for the first time, the National Institutes of Health (NIH) instituted a rule requiring all investigators submitting NIH applications to receive education in human subject protection. Although institutions may develop their own training programs, the NIH facilitates education by offering an online tutorial, initially developed for the NIH staff. Aside from that development, one cannot assume that the thousands of researchers in a variety of academic fields have received any training in the ethics of human subject research in the course of their education or otherwise.

The federal system is complex and this complexity presents its own obstacles to meaningful review. In addition to the actual regulations, there are dozens of Dear Colleague letters and Guidance Letters covering topics ranging from the circumstances under which an IRB can convene a meeting by telephone, to how an IRB can ensure informed consent to the non-English speaking subjects. IRBs are also required to understand the significant differences between provisions mandated by the Food and Drug Administration, NIH, and the Department of Human Services. As a result of the extensive list of rules, it is not uncommon for IRBs to miscalculate the complexities of the federal regulations.

Overwork has also resulted in IRB failure to adequately fulfill the continuing review obligations. As a result of the increased workload, IRBs have become preoccupied with form over substantively meaningful review of initial protocols, adverse events, and continuing reviews. As one critic stated, "IRBs are spending too much time editing informed-consent forms and too little time analyzing the risks and potential benefits posed by research." In fact, it is widely known that IRBs have long neglected continuing review obligations. Federal regulations require IRBs to undertake continuing review of ongoing research projects at least annually. As the Inspector General noted, however, "many IRBs find that with significant increases in the quantity of new research protocols, they have little time left for annual reviews," and they have focused "much more on complying with procedural requirements than on conducting substantive continuing review."

One facet of continuing review that is often neglected concerns adverse events. Researchers conducting studies with federal support must report adverse events to their own IRB and to the federal government. In spite of this reporting requirement, it is impossible to obtain an accurate count of the number of human subjects that suffer from adverse events each year as a result of their participation in research. One reason the extent of adverse events is unknown is that some research is not subject to federal reporting requirements at all. Underreporting is also a problem. Studies indicate that tens of thousands of adverse events as well as thousands of deaths are unreported in violation of federal law. For example, discussing gene therapy, one commentator wryly noted that:

> In the past year, researchers in the United States have been "catching up" on their reporting to regulators, and it now appears that at least 691 serious side effects — ranging from high fevers to serious infections and even seizures — have been experienced by experimental subjects in U.S. gene therapy trials using modified adenovirus vectors. Researchers claim that most of these side effects were caused by the subjects' underlying medical conditions, and undoubtedly this is so. Still, of the 691 serious side effects, only thirty-nine were reported — as regulations require — when they happened. The others were reported in the wake of Pennsylvania's program shutting down, no doubt because of fear of the same fate. More than 500 serious side effects were reported just this year, of which 130 occurred in the year 2000. This represents . . . a rate of failure to comply of almost ninety-five percent.

Significantly, the adverse effects of hexamethonium on Ellen Roche were not promptly reported. . . .

As NBAC dolefully noted, even when adverse events are reported, IRB review is a woefully ineffective mechanism for monitoring adverse events. Upon receiving an adverse event report, local IRBs are unable to "determine whether the event is frequent or rare, whether it is caused by their research as opposed to the underlying illness or standard treatment, or whether the adverse event is more common in the intervention group than in the control groups." It is nearly impossible for a committee to discern the significance of adverse events reported to the IRBs across the nation. In essence, it is like "looking for a needle in a haystack." Because they lack access to the necessary information needed to evaluate these reports, local IRBs are "not only wasting time attempting to analyze them but are also unable to make use of the data."

According to the Inspector General, similar to "the continuing review requirement, the Federal intent [underlying the reporting of adverse events requirement] was to foster substantive review. But here, too, the reality has been quite different." Fearing exposure to liability, sponsors have been increasingly likely to report. As a result, IRBs have become inundated with adverse event reports. In response to these and other gaps in safety monitoring, in 1998 NIH began to require its grantees to design and establish "Data Safety Monitoring Boards" for their clinical trials and to submit a data safety monitoring plan with each grant. These boards have duties distinct from the IRB and involve oversight and monitoring activities as they were intended to supplement, rather than supplant, the IRB system. [Data Safety Monitoring Boards are discussed in chapter 11 of this book, at page 475.]

The IRB system also suffers from more basic, systemic flaws that cannot be cured by simply easing workloads, fostering more diligence, and educating IRB members. These flaws spring from the interests, biases, and conflicts board members bring with them. Many critics have noted conflicts of interest among researchers, the institution, and IRB members. Those related to the IRB may be the most pernicious because they are more subtle and less easy to cure by regulation and disclosure than the more obvious financial conflicts that taint the institution and its researchers. In suggesting that the IRB may not be the appropriate body to perform continuing reviews, the Inspector General astutely noted that "the IRB process is rooted in trust," and as a result, it reviews protocols "in a collegial manner assuming the best of intentions on the part of researchers and sponsors." In fact, IRBs eschew the "watch-dog" role in favor of mutual trust, which "inhibits effective continuing review."

An additional problem plaguing the IRB system results from the fact that typically the membership is dominated by scientists, and therefore, the IRB has an inherent "systematic bias which favors the conduct of research." Current regulations require these bodies to consist of only one member who is unaffiliated with the institution, and one who is not involved in the sciences. No doubt there are competing values at stake in human subject research. The federal government invests in research because of society's core belief in the value of scientific research and discovery. On the other hand, the federal government established the IRB system because it recognized a paramount need to protect human subjects from scientific research abuses. By staffing the IRBs primarily with scientists, the government has failed to mitigate the natural bias of scientists and to accomplish the goals underlying the system.

Because an IRB is charged under federal law with protecting human subjects, and yet established to facilitate research at its institution, the board can succumb to conflicts and bias inherent from the outset. In order to obtain federal research money, institutions convene IRBs, and while the board's purpose is to protect human subjects, it is inescapable that the institution's objective is to comply with federal regulations so to obtain funding.

Collegiality and institutional loyalty may inhibit IRBs from conducting thorough and independent reviews of protocols. Most IRB members are employed as faculty or researchers at the institutions to which the investigators belong. These members realize "when sitting in judgment of a research protocol, that their proposals may soon be subjected to similar scrutiny." As a result, "it is unlikely that members of IRBs will hold investigators to a standard of disclosure and consent that would protect the subjects of research if doing so would place impediments on the conduct of research and, in turn, affect the well-being of their colleagues in decisive ways."

NOTES AND QUESTIONS

1. In 2000, the Office of Inspector General issued a follow-up to the 1998 report discussed by Beh. It noted that, since its initial report, there had been some progress in reforming the system, but "overall, few of our recommended reforms have been enacted." In particular, it found the following:

> *Flexibility and Accountability* — Minimal progress had been made in recasting Federal IRB requirements so that they grant IRBs greater flexibility and hold them more accountable for results. Too much IRB attention now focuses on review responsibilities of questionable protective value.

> *Oversight and Protections* — Minimal progress had been made in strengthening continuing protections for human subjects participating in research. Continuing IRB review of research after it has been initially reviewed is a low priority at many IRBs. IRBs know little of what actually occurs during the consent and research processes.

> *Education* — No educational requirements had been enacted for investigators or IRB members. The most important continuing protection for human subjects is the presence of well-trained and sensitized investigators and IRB members.

> *Conflicts of Interest* — There had been no progress in insulating IRBs from conflicts that can compromise their mission of protecting human subjects. The increased commercialization of research and the growing importance of research revenues for institutions heightens the potential for conflicts of interest in clinical research.

> *Workload* — Minimal progress had been made in moderating workload pressures of IRBs. IRBs are inundated with protocols and adverse event reports. With limited personnel and few resources, many IRBs are hard-pressed to give each review sufficient attention.

Federal Oversight — Minimal progress had been made in reengineering the Federal oversight process. Federal oversight of IRBs is not equipped to respond effectively to the changing pressures and needs of the current system of protections.

DEPARTMENT OF HEALTH AND HUMAN SERVICES, OFFICE OF INSPECTOR GENERAL, PROTECTING HUMAN RESEARCH SUBJECTS, STATUS OF RECOMMENDATIONS (2000). The report also concluded that the Common Rule was a major barrier to the adoption of many of the IOM's proposed changes, because many of the changes would require the Common Rule to be altered, and would thus need the approval of each of the seventeen federal agencies that had separately adopted the Common Rule for the studies that agency funds. OIG thus concluded that Congress would probably need to pass new legislation to alter this state of affairs in order for substantial reform to take place.

2. If you were able to implement some of the changes suggested by the OIG, which of them would you implement first? Why? What specific measures would you propose, either through legislation, regulation, or other mechanisms, to implement these changes?

3. In the discussion of the Hopkins hexamethonium study earlier in this chapter, it was noted that the IRB was criticized for not doing an adequate review to see if the investigator had listed all the possible risks of using the hexamethonium. If IRBs are indeed to have such a duty, how would it affect the issues raised in Beh's article? Who would perform this duty? Note that the IRB staff generally consists of administrators with no training in medical research.

4. The current system of review by local IRBs was formulated at a time when there were relatively few multicenter studies. For multicenter studies, local IRB review may be particularly problematic. A recent study of 31 IRBs reviewing the same nationwide cystic fibrosis genetic epidemiology protocol indicated that there were wide disparities in assessments of the level of risk of the study, the number of consent forms required, and the age ranges for which the "assent" of pediatric subjects would be necessary. The authors argued that centralized IRB review — review by one central board instead of many local ones — would both solve the variability problem and help "ensure that proper expertise is applied to each study, decrease the time required for review, and lessen the burden on local review boards." Noting the likely growth in multicenter epidemiology studies as a result of the Human Genome Project, the authors concluded, "The multicenter approval process is onerous because of inexperience with new technologies and science, outdated regulations, and a lack of unified comprehensive national standards." Rita McWilliams et al., *Problematic Variation in Local Institutional Review of a Multicenter Genetic Epidemiology Study*, 290 JAMA 366 (2003).

5. The idea of using a more centralized review process has had the greatest impact with regard to federally funded cancer studies, in which there already is a centralized IRB for certain types of adult and pediatric studies. In each

instance, an institution's "usual" IRB is asked to delegate much of the review authority to the central IRB, with the local IRB being responsible primarily for local issues. *See, e.g.*, NATIONAL CANCER INSTITUTE, THE CENTRAL INSTITUTIONAL REVIEW BOARD INITIATIVE, available at http://www.ncicirb.org; M.C. Christian et al., *A Central Institutional Review Board for Multi-Institutional Trials*, 346 NEW ENG. J. MED. 1405 (2002). What do you think of this approach? Is it possible to centralize IRB review without sacrificing the system's emphasis on local values and attitudes?

6. Taken one step further, the idea of centralized IRB review might suggest the creation of several "national IRBs" that would review all studies (or at least some major portion of them, such as all multi-center studies, or all federally funded studies). Consider the variety of issues that might arise with national IRBs: Who might be appointed to these bodies, by whom, and for what term of office? Would the deliberations of the national IRBs be subject to the Federal Advisory Committee Act (FACA) and thus be open to visitors? Would protesters have equal access to meetings? How would such committees balance the private interests of the researchers with the public pressures to act openly? Would the benefits of such national IRBs outweigh the costs?

7. There has been no shortage of other comprehensive reports suggesting ways to reform the system. At the end of her article (not included in the above excerpt), Beh took comfort in the recommendations of NBAC, which proposed a number of reforms, including better education, accreditation of human subject protection programs, more federal inspections of institutions, and clearer guidance regarding what conflicts of interest are not permitted. *See* NATIONAL BIOETHICS ADVISORY COMMISSION, 1 ETHICAL AND POLICY ISSUES IN RESEARCH INVOLVING HUMAN PARTICIPANTS (2001). Of those suggested reforms, the only one that appears to have had substantial progress is the effort to accredit human protection programs, discussed below, at page 202.

8. A third major report on how the system should be reformed is the Institute of Medicine's RESPONSIBLE RESEARCH, *supra*. For other discussions of problems with the current IRB system see, e.g., Harold Edgar & David J. Rothman, *The Institutional Review Board and Beyond: Future Challenges to the Ethics of Human Experimentation*, 73 MILBANK QUARTERLY 489 (1995); Sharona Hoffman, *Regulating Clinical Research: Informed Consent, Privacy, and IRBs*, 31 CAP. U. L. REV. 71 (2003); Ezekiel J. Emanuel et al., *Oversight of Human Participants Research: Identifying Problems to Evaluate Reform Proposals*, 141 ANNALS INTERNAL MED. 282 (2004).

[B] Expedited Review

Certain types of research can be reviewed by an IRB under a somewhat less rigorous process than is required of the average study. This less rigorous type of review is known as *expedited review*.

For a study to qualify for expedited review, it must: (1) involve no more than minimal risk to the subjects, and (2) fall within at least one of the specific categories of research that the Secretary of Health and Human Services has determined to be eligible for expedited review. A list of those specific categories has been established, and it is revised somewhat from time to time.

45 C.F.R. § 46.110: EXPEDITED REVIEW PROCEDURES

This provision is reproduced in Appendix A, at page A-9. Please review it before proceeding.

Categories of Research That May Be Reviewed by the Institutional Review Board (IRB) Through an Expedited Review Procedure
DEPARTMENT OF HEALTH AND HUMAN SERVICES
63 FED. REG. 60,364 (1998)

This document is reproduced in Appendix B. Please review it before proceeding.

NOTES AND QUESTIONS

1. Although expedited review is sometimes viewed by researchers as a way to get a protocol approved sooner than might otherwise be the case, the primary purpose of expedited review is to reduce the workload of the IRB. Unlike protocols that undergo full review, which have to be evaluated at a meeting of the entire IRB, protocols reviewed under the expedited review process need only be reviewed by the Chair of the IRB or a member designated by the Chair. The IRB, in its procedures and policies, must determine whether it permits expedited review of protocols and, if so, who is permitted to conduct that review. Expedited review may or may not lead to a researcher getting a protocol approved sooner than would take place under full review, depending on the IRB's procedures and policies.

2. OHRP has provided a decision chart on the topic of expedited review. *See* OFFICE FOR HUMAN RESEARCH PROTECTIONS, CHART 8: MAY THE IRB REVIEW BE DONE BY EXPEDITED PROCEDURES? available at http://www.hhs.gov/ohrp/human subjects/guidance/decisioncharts.htm.

3. Unlike the studies that meet the criteria for being "exempt," expedited studies remain fully subject to all of the requirements imposed on researchers by the regulations (such as the need for written consent forms, the requirements for obtaining a subject's consent, and so forth). In addition, they are also subject to the requirements imposed on IRBs regarding all other non-exempt

studies (such as the need for continuing annual review, although such review may also be conducted through an expedited process).

4. Categories (5) and (7) note that they may overlap with certain types of research that might be exempt. Can you give an example of a study for each of these categories that would *not* be exempt, but would be expeditable?

5. A researcher proposes to study whether otherwise healthy young adults (ages 21-24) who are less than five percent over their ideal body weight can lose weight by cutting out desserts from their diets. The subjects will be asked to record their food intake during a 30-day period, and will be weighed once a week. No other research procedures will be required. Does this study qualify for expedited review?

6. Review the discussion, at page 48 of Chapter 1, of the 1960s experiment in which Stanley Milgram put subjects in control of a machine that was supposed to be giving electrical shocks to someone in another room. Does this study meet the criteria for expedited review?

§ 4.04 PROPRIETARY AND INDEPENDENT IRBS

In recent years, there has been growth of a new type of institutional review board, one that does not serve and is not part of a single institution, but rather is freestanding and can be hired to do reviews for anyone who wishes to hire it. This is very different from the type of review boards envisioned when IRBs were first created. To some extent, the growth of this type of entity has been encouraged by the federal government. Dr. Greg Koski, the first head of OHRP, spoke of removing the "I" from IRBs, and allowing these independent entities to compete for the business of institutions conducting research with human subjects. Doing so would presumably lessen the possibility that IRBs would be too beholden to the institutions that they were part of. However, these independent IRBs raise questions of their own.

INSTITUTIONAL REVIEW BOARDS: THE EMERGENCE OF INDEPENDENT BOARDS
OFFICE OF INSPECTOR GENERAL, DEPARTMENT OF HEALTH AND HUMAN SERVICES
(1998)

Independent IRBs

These boards are not part of any organization in which research is conducted.

They are hired by research sponsors (most often pharmaceutical and device manufacturers) and investigators to review research plans.

Most are for-profit entities.

Some are owned by other organizations (such as contract research organizations that place clinical studies for research sponsors).

Some offer consultation, training, and other services in addition to traditional IRB services.

Board members are paid for their work, either on a per-meeting basis, an hourly basis, a per-protocol-reviewed basis, or some combination thereof. . . .

Independent IRBs are Playing an Increasingly Prominent Role in the Research Community.

While There are Relatively Few of Them, their Number Has Been Growing. The exact number of independent IRBs is not known, but the Consortium of Independent IRBs estimates that there are at least 15, and perhaps quite a few more. While 1 of these independent IRBs dates to 1968, at least 10 were established after 1980, and 4 of these were established after 1990. The increasing number of independent IRBs parallels an increasing number of research protocols being put forward by commercial sponsors.

They Oversee an Increasing Number of Research Plans. The number of research plans that the independent IRBs review is considerable and growing. In the last 2 years, independent IRBs we contacted reported an average increase in initial reviews of approximately 36 percent. In 1997, the independent IRBs we surveyed conducted an average of 256 initial reviews. The largest and oldest of them reviewed over 1,000 initial protocols and conducted over 4,000 continuing reviews in 1997, a caseload comparable with many IRBs in academic health centers.

The great preponderance of the research that independent IRBs oversee is sponsored by either pharmaceutical or device manufacturers and is conducted in physician offices outside of hospitals, medical clinics, or commercial-research facilities. A growth of research in such independent-investigator sites has contributed to the increase in the number of protocols that these IRBs review.

They are Now Reviewing HHS-Sponsored Research. Independent IRBs are increasingly being used for HHS-funded clinical studies. . . .

They Are Becoming More Involved with Hospital-Based Research. Independent IRBs become increasingly attractive to some hospitals as the quantity and complexity of their own IRBs' workloads increase. Four of the 11 independent IRBs with which we spoke already act as IRBs of record for one or more hospitals. One, in fact, had established a contract with a major academic health center IRB to review all commercially sponsored research plans for that IRB. A few other large research institutions have separated their commercially sponsored research from the Federal assurance requirements that apply to all HHS-funded research, thereby giving the institution greater flexibility in contracting with independent IRBs if it so chooses. Many of the experienced IRB officials with whom we spoke noted that such separations are becoming increasingly likely and present good market opportunities for independent IRBs.

Independent IRBs Offer Advantages That Institutional IRBs Find Difficult to Match.

They Are Geared to Making Quick Decisions on Research Plans. To commercial sponsors, time is money. Sponsors expect IRBs to do their work properly, but to do it quickly as well. Independent IRBs are organized to meet this expectation. It is widely recognized, by research sponsors and in the IRB community more generally, that they provide research sponsors with timely responses to their submissions. Thus, for instance, the independent IRBs we contacted reported that, on average, they were able to provide research sponsors with an approval or disapproval decision for initial, non-expedited research protocols in an average of about 11 days. By contrast, the IRBs in academic medical centers that we visited reported decisions in an average of about 37 days.

Independent IRBs have an inherent advantage in meeting timeliness expectations because they hire their board members with the understanding that the members will be regularly available to conduct reviews. Hospital IRB members, in contrast, are almost always volunteers with many competing demands for their time. Not surprisingly, independent IRBs tend to meet more frequently and can meet with minimal notice. The independent IRBs we contacted reported holding multiple board meetings each month. One independent IRB reported that it holds four meetings a week. Academic health centers and hospitals generally are hard-pressed to match that.

They Provide a Detached Source of Expertise. Independent IRBs are staffed by people who have no affiliation with the institutions whose research plans they review and who are unlikely to have collegial relationships with the investigators whose work they review. Thus, the independent IRBs can operate without being influenced by concerns about the financial well-being or prestige of the institution that employs them or the career interests of colleagues. One hospital official, who has worked with independent and hospital-based IRBs, underscored the importance of such detachment, pointing out that it leads to greater objectivity. IRB officials in other settings, however, are wary of such a conclusion.

They Provide Unified Reviews for Multi-site Trials. Some multi-site trials involve research sites that do not have their own IRBs or do not require that all local research be overseen by the site's own IRB. In such cases, independent IRBs can serve as a single entity reviewing the applicability of a specific research plan to various sites. This unified review eliminates the complications that result from multiple, local IRB reviews of a sponsor's research plan. It also facilitates analysis of adverse-event reports submitted from individual sites and, in so doing, can enhance protections for human subjects.

Yet, the Use of Independent IRBs Raises Concerns.

They Are Not Local Review Bodies. In the 1970s, when the current infrastructure of Federal protections for human research subjects was established and when relatively few national multi-site trials were underway, local review was regarded as essential. . . .

The OPRR's recent decision to grant assurances involving independent IRBs is based largely on the IRBs' commitments to stay well-informed about local sites. In response to OPRR and other concerned parties, the independent IRBs point to a variety of ways in which they keep abreast of the site circumstances. These include site visits, local contacts, relationships with local IRBs, newspaper clipping services, and other means. Many in the IRB field remain unconvinced that such compensatory efforts allow for adequate local representation.

They May Be Subject to Conflicts of Interest. Some IRB officials are concerned that an independent, for-profit IRB might compromise its review process to advance the financial well-being of the firm. Such concerns are heightened to the extent that corporate-equity owners or employees serve on the IRB review boards and are sustained to some extent by the fact that reviewers are paid for their services. The NIH policy for HHS-funded research reviews by for-profit IRBs is to prohibit equity owners from participating in the review process. There is no such policy for industry-sponsored studies submitted to FDA. As we noted earlier, the great preponderance of research overseen by independent IRBs is sponsored by either pharmaceutical or device manufacturers.

A contrast is often made with the academic health center, where, some IRB officials say, a long established research culture allows for greater IRB independence. In an increasingly competitive research environment, however, in which those centers are seeking to maximize clinical research revenues, the IRBs in these centers can also experience conflicting pressures.

They Heighten Concerns about IRB Shopping. For research that is not federally funded, sponsors have considerable discretion in their choice of an IRB. A problem here is that if one IRB finds fault with the sponsor's research plan, the sponsor might then contract with another IRB without informing it of the prior board's determinations. While applicable to all IRBs, this vulnerability is particularly germane to independent IRBs since nearly all the proposals they review are not federally funded. Some representatives of these boards emphasized this point to us and felt there was a good case for a Federal requirement that when submitting a research plan for review, sponsors must inform the IRB of any prior IRB reviews of that plan.

Conclusion

This report does not afford us a basis for assessing how well independent IRBs are performing. But, it does lead us to two concluding observations that have broader significance for the Federal system of human-subject protections.

First, independent IRBs have become a noteworthy part of the IRB landscape. They give research sponsors an alternative to the traditional, well-established IRBs. Particularly for non-federally funded research, they allow for these sponsors to engage in some shopping to determine what IRBs best meet their needs.

In that sense, they serve as competition to the longer established IRBs, especially those in academic health centers, and contribute to a marketplace ethic — one that is quite different from the ethic of 20 or even 10 years ago when IRB activity was carried out within a more clearly defined research culture. This development presents both opportunities as well as dangers. On the one hand, it encourages IRBs to undertake more timely and innovative approaches to their review processes. On the other hand, the competitive pressures to satisfy research sponsors can lead some IRBs to be less vigilant in protecting human subjects.

Second, independent IRBs raise important questions for Federal oversight. How can the Federal government best ensure that independent IRBs afford necessary protections? That the emerging competition does not compromise safeguards? That the advantages and efficiencies offered by independent IRBs are not undercut by unnecessary Federal prescriptions? Such questions underscore the importance of having a good understanding of the actual effectiveness of IRBs, whether they are independent or part of an organization that conducts research.

NOTES AND QUESTIONS

1. The use of independent IRBs appears to clash with one of the bedrock principles of the current system, namely that of local review. What steps are these independent IRBs taking to demonstrate that they, too, can meet the requirement for "local" review? Do these steps seem sufficient? The predecessor agency to OHRP provided detailed guidance about what measures these entities should take to apprise themselves of local circumstances. *See* OFFICE FOR PROTECTION FROM RESEARCH RISKS, KNOWLEDGE OF LOCAL RESEARCH CONTEXT (1998, updated in 2000), available at http://www.hhs.gov/ohrp/humansubjects/guidance/local.htm.

2. One of the possible problems with independent IRBs mentioned in the OIG report is that they may be willing to bend to the wishes of the institutions that hire them, perhaps too readily approving research so that institutions remain eager to use them. But somewhat paradoxically, increased independence has also been raised as a possible benefit of using these new entities: they would be immune from the pressure to approve studies that the members of an institution's own IRB might feel, given that such persons are mostly full-time employees of the institution. Which of the two types of IRBs do you think is likely to be more independent, and why? How might we collect information that might help in resolving this policy question?

3. In 2002, the FDA asked for public comment on mechanisms to combat sponsors' efforts to "IRB shop" until they find an IRB that will approve a particular study. Among the proposed mechanisms was a rule that would require researchers and sponsors of studies to inform any IRB reviewing a study of certain prior actions by other IRBs, such as a disapproval of the study. *See* FOOD

AND DRUG ADMINISTRATION, INSTITUTIONAL REVIEW BOARDS: REQUIRING SPONSORS AND INVESTIGATORS TO INFORM IRBS OF ANY PRIOR IRB REVIEWS, 67 FED. REG. 10,115 (2002). A similar rule already exists for studies that are conducted under the emergency research regulations (discussed in Chapter 7 at page 318). *See* 50 C.F.R. § 50.24(e). Apart from reducing forum shopping, are there other advantages to ensuring that IRBs are told about the thinking of other IRBs that have decided not to approve a study? What are the potential drawbacks to such an approach?

4. In an effort to further legitimize themselves, several independent IRBs have been among the first to participate in the voluntary process of IRB accreditation, as described in the next section of this chapter.

5. For additional discussions about independent IRBs, see, e.g., Evangeline D. Loh & Roger E. Meyer, *Medical Schools' Attitudes and Perceptions Regarding the Use of Central Institutional Review Boards*, 79 ACAD. MED. 644 (2004); Erica Heath, *The History, Function, and Future of Independent Institutional Review Boards*, in NATIONAL BIOETHICS ADVISORY COMMISSION, 2 ETHICAL AND POLICY ISSUES IN RESEARCH INVOLVING HUMAN PARTICIPANTS E-1 (2001); Trudo Lemmens & Benjamin Freedman, *Ethics for Sale? Conflict of Interest and Commercial Research Review Boards*, 78 MILBANK Q. 547 (2000).

§ 4.05 ACCREDITATION

As policymakers have searched for new ways to protect human subjects, they have sometimes borrowed from methods used to regulate health care institutions. One of the most recent such ideas is that of accrediting human research protection programs. Accreditation is different from the concept of licensing:

> Licensure is the mandatory governmental process whereby a health care facility receives the right to operate. In the United States, licensure operates on a state-by-state basis. A health care facility [such as a hospital or nursing home] cannot open its doors without a license from the appropriate state agency. . . . Accreditation is a private voluntary approval process through which a health care organization is evaluated and can receive a designation of competence and quality. Most private accreditation for health care organizations today is done under the auspices of the Joint Commission for the Accreditation of Healthcare Organizations (called "JCAHO).

MARK A. HALL ET AL., HEALTH CARE LAW AND ETHICS 1073 (6th ed. 2003).

Accrediting Programs to Protect Participants in Human Research: The IOM Report
Larry D. Scott
23 IRB, Sept.-Oct. 2001, at 13

Last year, the Department of Health and Human Services commissioned the Institute of Medicine (IOM) to study protection issues associated with human subjects' participation in clinical research. The initial phase of an anticipated two-phase study has now been completed and published in *Preserving Public Trust*. The report focuses on accreditation of what the IOM refers to as "human research participant protection programs" (HRPPPs). The use of this more global term recognizes that the institutional review board (IRB) is but one of several elements intrinsic to effective participant protection, the others being the institution itself, investigators, and even participants.

One outcome of this report, and perhaps the one of most value, is its illumination of the issues associated with protecting research participants. In acknowledging ongoing needs in this area *Preserving Public Trust* advocates, among other things, defining standards against which the performance of HRPPPs can be measured, having an accrediting body that is nongovernmental, and including all organizations involved in clinical research — not just the academic health centers. Another useful recommendation is to begin collecting data to define and quantify research involving human participation and existing systems for protection. This should be a priority goal not only in structuring an accreditation process but also in charting its impact.

The other major outcome of the IOM study is endorsement of the pilot accreditation program now in progress at the Department of Veterans Affairs (VA) as a general model for accreditation. This program was developed for VA by the National Committee on Quality Assurance (NCQA), an organization that accredits managed health care plans. The IOM examined both the NCQA program and a pilot project developed by Public Responsibility in Medicine and Research (PRIM&R) to be administered through the newly created, independent organization, Association for the Accreditation of Human Research Protection Programs (AAHRPP).

The IOM deemed the AAHRPP accreditation program to be less helpful as a model. AAHRPP focuses on research conducted in the academic health center setting and IRBs in particular; as such, the IOM felt it could not easily adapt to other research settings, including private industry, even though AAHRPP goals are appropriately broad. This criticism seems odd since the NCQA program endorsed was designed specifically for the VA, hardly a paradigm for the rest of the research world. Moreover, the NCQA program seeks primarily to insure implementation of current regulations, a limited goal at best and not one consistent with the HRPPP concept that is fundamental to this report. In contrast, AAHRPP uses existing regulations as a starting point rather than a framework. The report notes, however, that NCQA drew on its experience in managed care to incorporate continuous quality improvement mechanisms into its accreditation program. Such strategies explicitly look to achievement of core goals beyond regulatory compliance.

Although, the IOM endorsed the NCQA program, it qualified its support by suggesting six areas in which the program needed strengthening if it were to be more generally applied. That is, the program should specify:

- how investigators themselves will be reviewed

- whether and how research sponsors will be assessed

- how research participants will be involved in setting standards and accrediting protection programs

- how oversight mechanisms can assure safety in ongoing research

- how institutions can cultivate a culture that prioritizes protecting research participants, and

- mechanisms to hold institutions, and sponsors, accountable for funding, supporting, and rewarding human participant protection programs.

In the final analysis, the real danger of increasing federal oversight of research is alienation of investigators, while removing participant safety from the investigator's obligations. Hence the importance of a carefully applied accreditation system. By involving all parties in the research organization, participant welfare remains the top priority of investigators, the need for outside regulation can be minimized, and accreditation can indeed be viewed as a "mark of excellence" that is not only a measure of success but self-sustaining.

NOTES AND QUESTIONS

1. The two competing organizations that currently accredit human research protection programs each has its own web page promoting the advantages of its accreditation system. The Association for the Accreditation of Human Research Protections Programs (AAHRPP) is located at www.aahrpp.org. The Partnership for Human Research Protection, Inc. (PHRP, which is the successor to the NCQA program mentioned by Scott) has its Web site at www.phrp.org. For additional discussion about the goals of these two accreditation programs, see, e.g., Mary Faith Marshall & Mark Barnes, *The Partnership for Human Research Protection: Setting the Standard for Safety*, 2 MED. RESEARCH L. & POL'Y REP. (BNA) 862 (2003); Marjorie A. Speers, *AAHRPP's Peer-Reviewed Approach to Protecting Research Participants*, 3 MED. RESEARCH L.& POL'Y REP. (BNA) 55 (2004).

2. A later report from the IOM provided further discussion and analysis of the status of accreditation. It noted that AAHRPP had been responsive to the

concerns expressed by the earlier IOM report about the need for "broader utility" within the standards, by revising them so as to include more specific
requirements regarding participants and sponsors as well as attention to quality improvement efforts. INSTITUTE OF MEDICINE, RESPONSIBLE RESEARCH, *supra*,
at 171-77. For a review of what occurs during a site visit, see Alexander Otto,
*Richmond First Fully Accredited VA Center; AAHRPP OKs Site Despite Rival's
VA Contract*, 2 MED. RESEARCH L. & POL'Y REP. (BNA) 628 (2003).

3. Accreditation programs are usually voluntary; no one forces an institution
to become accredited. However, there are often interconnections between accreditation programs and government regulations. For example, a state may accept
JCAHO accreditation of a health care facility as sufficient proof that the facility qualifies for licensure. (And without that accreditation, the facility would
have to undergo an examination by state licensing personnel to verify that it
meets the appropriate standards.) Currently, there are no such interconnections
between accreditation of human subject protection programs and the federal
regulation of this field. Would it be a good thing for there to be such interconnections? For example, should human subject protection programs be required
to be licensed by the government, with accreditation from one (or perhaps
either) of the accreditation organizations as sufficient proof that a program
deserves a license? Given the limited resources of the regulatory agencies
(OHRP and the FDA), if an institution is accredited, should that minimize the
likelihood that the facility would be subject to random (as opposed to "for cause")
agency audits?

4. All sides of the debate about accreditation seem to agree that what is
needed is a method to encourage institutions to move from a culture of compliance to a culture of "conscience and compliance." The disagreement centers on
whether accreditation is a better way to achieve this goal than having the federal government play a stronger role in directly policing compliance with the regulations. In what ways might accreditation be a less effective way of protecting
human subjects? A skeptic might suggest that accreditation may merely lead
institutions to do the minimum necessary to keep their programs off the radar
screen. Would they be right?

5. Imagine that you are an administrative official at a university medical center, and that the president of the university has asked you to determine whether
or not the medical center should retain one of the two organizations to accredit
your institution's human research protections program. Identify the factors
that argue for and against obtaining accreditation. In general, do you think most
institutions will try to have their programs accredited? Why or why not?

Chapter 5

CONFLICTS OF INTEREST

As discussed in Chapter 2, changes in how research is conducted over the past several decades have led to substantial financial entanglements between researchers and the for-profit companies that sponsor much of their work. This circumstance, together with the deaths of some subjects in studies in which the investigators had ownership interests in the products being studied, has led to increasing concerns about the impact of conflicts of interest on the way that research is conducted.

§ 5.01 INVESTIGATOR CONFLICTS

Dealing with Conflicts of Interest in Biomedical Research: IRB Oversight as the Next Best Solution to the Abolitionist Approach
Jesse A. Goldner
28 J. L. Med. & Ethics 379 (2000)

In what has become one of the better known and more tragic stories involving problematic research, in 1999 an eighteen-year-old study subject, Jesse Gelsinger, died as a result of his participation in a gene therapy study at the University of Pennsylvania. Though suffering from a rare liver disorder, Gelsinger had been managing his illness on a combination of special drugs and diet. After his death, Food and Drug Administration (FDA) investigators concluded that he was placed on the protocol and given an infusion of genetic material despite the fact that his liver was not functioning at the minimal level required under study criteria. Moreover, researchers had not notified the agency of severe side effects experienced by prior subjects that should have resulted in halting the study, nor was the agency told of the death of four monkeys who had undergone similar treatment. The consent form signed by Gelsinger did not inform him of those events. Federal investigators determined that the University's Institute for Human Gene Therapy was unable to document that all patients had been informed of the risks and benefits of the procedures and that some patients should have been considered ineligible for the study because their illnesses were more serious than the protocols allowed.

Ultimately, the FDA suspended all active or pending gene therapy studies at the Institute after finding numerous deficiencies in the way the trial was run, and the University announced that the Institute would no longer experiment on people. The director of the Institute that conducted the research, James M.

Wilson, was identified as having a conflict of interest because he owned stock in Genovo, the company that financed research at the Institute. Both Wilson and the former dean of Pennsylvania's medical school had patents on some aspects of the procedure. Subsequently, Wilson admitted "he would gain stock worth $13.5-million from a biotechnology company in exchange for his shares of Genovo stock." In addition, the University's contract with Genovo gave the company rights to gene research discoveries at the Institute in exchange for substantial financial support. The University's equity interest in Genovo has been valued at $1.4 million dollars.

The Gelsinger family filed a lawsuit alleging negligence and fraud in recruiting their son for the research study. The defendants in this lawsuit were the University of Pennsylvania, the research team, three other doctors, and two hospitals. Part of the lawsuit claimed that the defendants intentionally failed to disclose their conflicts of interest. The suit was recently settled but the terms of the settlement were undisclosed.

Medical research on human subjects allows medical science to advance by the development of new medications, equipment, and procedures. Furthermore, it is a lucrative business. It is estimated that the average cost to develop a new medication can range from $300 million to $600 million. More than half of the 6 billion dollars spent annually for clinical trials worldwide is paid by pharmaceutical companies to investigators in the United States. Despite the fact that there has been a recent shift away from conducting research at academic centers, many research investigators are university faculty. Researcher-physicians and others involved in the research enterprise, therefore, in the broadest sense have a financial interest in conducting research trials. Thus, a potential conflict of interest exists when a physician is conducting an objective research protocol while still receiving compensation or other forms of support for the research conducted. The issue at hand is how best to protect research subjects from potentially unfortunate consequences of such conflicts of interest.

Given the government's recent flurry of activity in the area of human subject protections — largely focusing on the activities of institutional review boards (IRBs) whose charge is to protect subjects' rights — it is ironic that, until very recently, relatively little official attention has been directed toward the conflicts of interest of individual investigators that might adversely impact subjects' rights. The *New York Times* and the *Chronicle of Higher Education* have published numerous articles identifying and discussing the financial conflicts of interest arising from investigators' ties with the pharmaceutical industry. In addition, there has been increased recognition in the scientific community that financial conflicts of interest, of all types, can potentially bias the outcome of clinical trials, affect a subject's welfare, and diminish a subject's ability to provide fully informed consent.

Primary, secondary, and non-financial conflicts

Conflicts of interest in research can arise in two very different spheres: conflicts between different primary interests and those between primary and sec-

ondary interests. In their most general form, the primary interests of a physician-researcher are the health of his or her patients and the integrity of the
research. These primary interests should be the most important consideration
in any professional decision. In therapeutic encounters, for example, physicians are expected to attend solely to the welfare of the individual patient.
More realistically, however, perhaps one ought to say they are expected to
attend almost entirely to the patient's welfare. In research encounters, on the
other hand, patient-subjects are being used for scientific ends. Investigators,
therefore, are committed both to their present patient-subjects and to abstract,
future patients, thereby causing a conflict between competing primary interests.
In such a situation, the investigator must educate the potential subject on the
critical distinctions between clinical practice and research. In addition, the
investigator must correct the patient-subject's perception that an invitation to
participate in research is a professional recommendation solely intended to
serve the individual's treatment needs.

The focus of this paper, however, is not so much on these competing primary
interests, although in the ultimate analysis they may well come into play.
Rather, it is on the conflicts that exist between the physician's primary or ethical interests and his or her secondary or personal interests. The conflict of
interest here can be defined as a circumstance in which interests, such as career
advancement or financial gain, have an influence on the researcher's judgment
of a primary interest, such as a patient's welfare. Such circumstances present
the specter of altering physician-researcher judgments so that the risks to subjects participating in the research are increased.

A secondary interest is usually not illegitimate in itself — and may even be
a necessary part of professional practice. But, it is the relative weight of this secondary interest in professional decision-making that may be problematic and,
consequently, serve as the source of both financial and non-financial conflicts of
interest.

The desire to eliminate conflicts of interest arises from the natural belief that
physicians and other researchers should not engage in endeavors that could
endanger their ability to protect the interests of their patients. Regardless of the
treatment outcome, the determinative factors are the circumstances surrounding the physician's outside interests and the physician-patient relationship.

Conflicts of interest, of course, are by no means merely financial — at least
in the narrowest sense of that word. The true issue may not necessarily be one
of a physician's honesty or integrity but, rather, one of his or her unconscious
biases and influences, which may be subtle and difficult to detect. Some such
conflicts, however, can be equally insidious. Motivation to conduct research is an
enormously complex matter that no doubt differs among individuals. At one end
of the spectrum may be the altruistic, unselfish incentive to improve the lives
of others. At the other is the arguably crass, but surely comprehensible, human
desire to improve one's financial situation and level of creature comforts by
amassing and spending capital. Between these lies a range of potential sources

of motivation: the simple joy that comes from successful efforts and progress, the satisfaction felt when work is finally developed and completed, the desire to produce insights, and the quest for recognition through publications and professional advancement. Finally, institutional work environments themselves can generate immense pressures. . . .

I. INDIVIDUAL CONFLICTS OF INTEREST

The issue of individual conflicts of interest ordinarily arises when an investigator conducts a clinical study in which he or she has a financial interest. The investigator's financial interest in the research may manifest itself in a variety of ways. . . .

A. Per capita payments and finder's fees

The first situation in which an investigator's conflict of interest may arise involves clinical trials sponsored by pharmaceutical manufacturers. It is a common practice in the pharmaceutical industry to pay investigators for their recruiting of subjects on a per capita basis. To obtain a sufficient number of patient-subjects in an acceptable period of time, manufacturers offer investigators financial incentives to enter patients into studies. One commentator estimates that remuneration levels are as high as $3,000 per subject. Another indicates that such levels typically range from $2,000 to $5,000 per subject. These payments purportedly are intended to offset medical expenses incurred by the subject's participation, as well as the data management costs incurred by the investigator, but the amounts involved typically exceed these costs. In an academic setting, the researcher commonly uses money in excess of that required for conducting the study to purchase supplies and equipment or to support travel to scientific meetings. In addition, this money is often used to fund research efforts that may not have been judged sufficiently important or scientifically rigorous to warrant funding by government agencies via the standard peer review process. But particularly outside of academic environments, the money left over after study-related expenses have been met will remain in the researcher-physician's pocket.

In addition to the per capita payments, pharmaceutical sponsors frequently offer investigators, or their staff, incentives to boost subject enrollment. These incentives may be financial, often in the form of bonus payments per subject enrolled; or they may be non-financial, such as granting the investigator authorship on a corresponding study paper, providing the research site with office or medical equipment, or offering gifts such as books. There are several reasons, inherent in how the pharmaceutical industry operates, why sponsors offer these types of incentives. First, sponsors are pushing tight enrollment deadlines. These shorter deadlines reflect the pharmaceutical companies' desire to be as profitable as possible. The time for a drug patent starts running when the patent application is filed, which is prior to the clinical testing of the drug. Sponsors seek to shorten the testing phase so that they may recoup research and development costs before similar drugs appear on the market. Second, there is an intensified search for subjects. Sponsors need increasing numbers of subjects who meet particular eligibility criteria to fill more and larger clinical trials. As a result of these pressures, pharmaceutical sponsors must offer researchers incentives to meet the sponsors' needs.

There is a concern that comes with the pressure to enroll large numbers of subjects quickly. The fear is that investigators will encourage inappropriate or marginally appropriate subjects who do not meet the inclusion criteria to participate in the research. For example, it has been reported that patients have received drugs to treat conditions that they did not have, sometimes without being told that the drug was experimental. In such an instance, the investigator is compromising patient care in exchange for monetary gain, in addition to compromising the results of the study. A subject can also be considered inappropriate when other treatments or research protocols may be more beneficial for his or her particular condition. When an investigator enters a patient into a study when alternative treatments are known to be effective or thought to be superior, or when an investigator enrolls a patient who does not meet the study's inclusion or exclusion criteria, again he or she may be compromising patient care in exchange for monetary gain.

Aside from per capita payments, physicians may also receive "finder's fees" for referring patients to participate in clinical trials. The category of finder's fees includes the practice of "paying bonuses to physician-investigators, research nurses, and others involved in a pharmaceutical industry-sponsored research study in order to speed up subject recruitment to meet industry-imposed study completion deadlines." The practice of paying finder's fees has been pursued where there may not be an adequate patient population in a particular area where their research is being conducted.

Cynthia M. Dunn, a former drug industry executive who now directs the Clinical Research Institute at the University of Rochester, stated: "On one hand, many companies recognize it's [paying finder's fees] part of what we have to do to be competitive. On the other hand, they recognize they are setting up potential conflicts of interest for doctors." Some commentators have noted that the payment of finder's fees may encourage the enrollment of patients who do not properly meet inclusion criteria. Furthermore, finder's fees increase the total cost of clinical research, which is ultimately paid for by consumers. Other scholars have noted that, in practice, offering finder's fees is similar to paying fees for the referral of patients, which is prohibited. The underlying trust between the patient and the referring physician, researcher, and clinical research may be damaged when physicians are paid to refer the patient to a clinical study.

B. Gifts from industry sponsors

Another conflict of interest stemming from links with the pharmaceutical industry is the research-related gift. Gifts from companies to academic and other investigators can be in the form of biomaterials, discretionary funds, and support for students, research equipment or trips to professional meetings. A study in the *Journal of the American Medical Association* found that 43 percent of researchers who responded to a survey had received a research-related gift in the last three years. Of those researchers who had received a gift, 66 percent reported that the gift was important to their research. The survey results also suggest that corporate gifts may have been associated with a variety of donor restrictions and expectations. For example, some donors expected pre-publication review of any articles or reports stemming from the use of the gift, while others expected ownership of all patentable results from research in which the gift was used. In addition to difficulties stemming from the donor's expectations, research-related gifts are problematic in that they may cause an investigator to choose to develop or pursue one protocol over another out of a desire for future gifts. Alternatively, if an investigator is dependent on the gifts — similar to 13 percent of surveyed investigators who indicated that the gift was "essential" to their research — he or she may be inclined to publish or emphasize favorable results or minimize unfavorable aspects of a study, irrespective of the data, in order to help assure future gifts and support from a particular company.

Research indicates that, despite physician claims to the contrary, gifts have an effect on physicians. For example, a study published in the medical journal *Chest* examined the impact of an all-expense-paid trip to a resort hosting a seminar sponsored by a pharmaceutical company on physician prescribing patterns. The majority of the physicians interviewed insisted that this elaborate gift would not influence their prescribing decisions. The study demonstrated, however, that this promotional technique, used by some pharmaceutical companies, was associated with a significant increase in the prescribing of the promoted drugs at the institution studied. Thus, such enticements clearly influenced the behavior of the physicians in clinical practice. If minor gifts influence the prescribing conduct of physicians, then more major gift incentives are likely to have a pernicious effect on the projects physician-researchers pursue and the way in which researchers report outcomes. This is why it is important for universities and other research institutions to control the existence of this type of conflict of interest by maintaining an appropriate policy regarding gifts from industry.

C. Stock ownership and similar financial interests

A financial conflict of interest in the research setting may also occur when an investigator holds stock in, or serves as a paid consultant to, the manufacturer whose drugs or devices are under investigation. As noted earlier, a concern with these types of arrangements stems from the fear that the potential for profit may subtly affect an investigator's interpretation of his or her research or that the promise of large profits could affect the way the investigator presents his or her findings publicly. The potential for monetary gain could also influence the investigator's view of ethical issues. For example, if an investigator perceives the possible risk involved in the study to be great, he or she may attempt to offer the subjects higher levels of compensation as an inducement to enter the study. If the investigator is still unsuccessful in enrolling subjects, he or she may target institutions with populations such as the mentally ill or mentally retarded as a source of subjects. Even in situations where the potential for profit does not affect the investigator's work product, the perception of bias may linger in the minds of other investigators and lay observers.

In 1998, a comprehensive study of bias resulting from financial conflicts of interest was reported in an article published in the *New England Journal of Medicine*. This study surveyed eighty-nine investigators who had published research on calcium channel antagonists and found that 96 percent of the supportive authors had financial ties to the manufacturers. Only 60 percent of the authors of neutral papers and 37 percent of the authors of critical papers were found to have such ties. In addition, only two of the seventy papers analyzed in the study included disclosures of the investigator's financial relationship with the manufacturer. In part, as a result of this demonstration of the potential for bias, a relatively recent study indicated that some 15 percent of journals now require disclosure of stock ownership of companies the author is evaluating.

Recently, the *New England Journal of Medicine* reviewed its own conflict-of-interest policy and procedures. This review was initiated by a finding that the *Journal* had published an analysis favorable to two popular hair-loss treatments written by an investigator who had been a paid consultant to the companies producing the products. This investigator was also receiving research support from the companies. The *Journal* editor who was overseeing the article, Alastair Wood, was aware of the investigator's ties to the companies when the investigator was invited to do the comparison of the hair-loss treatments. The investigator was still a consultant at that time, but she assured Wood that she would cease those duties. The editor was satisfied with this arrangement. Moreover, the editor determined that the companies' continuing support of the investigator's research should not preclude her from writing the article since the grant money was being paid directly to the university where the investigator worked and not to the investigator personally.

When reports of the author's conflicts of interest were made public, the editor-in-chief of the *Journal* stated that the situation revealed inconsistencies between the *Journal's* policy and practice, which needed to be assessed. Sheldon Krimsky, a professor of urban and environmental policy, who studies the conflicts-of-interest policies of journals, stated that by publishing the review without the disclosure of the investigator's conflicts, readers may have been given a false sense of security about the reliability of the review. In Krimsky's own study, he found that few scientific journals required the disclosure of financial interests, but even those that do rarely publish such disclosures. The *New England Journal of Medicine* incident seems to confirm the results of Krimsky's study.

D. *Conflicts of interest related to the academic research environment*

All financial conflicts of interest facing individual investigators are not as overt as stock ownership, per capita payments, and gifts from pharmaceutical companies. There are, for example, conflicts of interest embedded in the highly competitive nature of academic research. Investigators often pursue clinical research in order to build their reputations and academic standing. In addition, investigators at different institutions may pursue the same clinical research simultaneously. Since recognition, future research grants, and job prospects generally go to those who publish first, and since criteria used to appoint, evaluate, and promote faculty emphasize publication output, investigators experience tremendous pressure to conduct and conclude research quickly. This pressure to produce continues unremittingly throughout an investigator's career. Therefore, an investigator's research may eventually fall prey to his or her desire for recognition. Although the investigator's motivations may not necessarily be directly or even largely financial in these situations, conflicts may stem as much from the desire for recognition or advancement as from corresponding increases in compensation.

University researchers also face financial conflicts of interest as a result of the passage of the Bayh-Dole Act in 1980, which "encourages academic institutions supported by federal grants to patent and license new products developed by their faculty members and to share royalties with the researchers." The National Institutes of Health (NIH) has a standard process for determining who can take title to an invention and file a patent application. After notifying the NIH of an invention, the awardee institution has two years to determine if it will do so, and the researcher himself will share in any profits. If the institution does not elect to take title, then the NIH can choose to do so, in which case the individual inventor also is guaranteed a portion of any royalties received. However, if the NIH does not take title, then the researcher-inventor himself may file for a patent.

After the researcher files for a patent, he or she may form a biotechnology company or enter into a joint venture with these types of companies. The stock options and directors' fees from these corporations may far exceed the salaries that the researchers receive from their universities. The potential for commercialization may create incentives for academic researchers to pursue areas of research that are likely to result in patentable inventions. At the least, it is encouraging researchers to think from a business perspective instead of a purely scientific one. Although this is an acceptable purpose, inadequate attention may have been given to conflicts of interest issues, which will always be a concern in an entrepreneurial environment.

Distribution of faculty practice plan revenues and the role of research in such distribution may also create a financial conflict of interest for academic investigators. Faculty practice plans typically are organized along departmental or divisional lines and operate autonomously. Traditionally, each department has broad latitude regarding its priorities, the research grants that it solicits, and its business practices. At many institutions, a portion of faculty practice plan revenues, ranging from 5 to 20 percent, is allocated to support general academic endeavors; this amount is commonly referred to as the "dean's tax." Another portion of faculty practice plan revenues finances the central administration, and the balance accrues to the individual medical department or division. After the departments or divisions cover administrative costs and invest appropriately in their practice, the remaining revenues typically are distributed to the clinical faculty.

Distribution of faculty practice plan revenues to clinical faculty occurs through a variety of means. The method currently employed by many medical schools, however, is a tripartite "base, supplemental, incentive" salary formula. The base salary is the guaranteed or "tenured" salary. The supplemental salary normally reflects the market value of the faculty member. This is negotiated on an annual basis and is usually contingent upon the availability of funds from faculty practice plan and other revenue sources. The incentive or bonus, which is also generally contingent upon the availability of funds from these sources, usually is reflective of "productivity," either individually or departmentally or both. In determining the amount of incentive salary, individual productivity may be measured on a point system in which the faculty member receives a designated number of points for contributions in areas including research, teaching, patient care, administration, and extracurricular activities.

Incentives, and even supplemental salary, can be linked to productivity. Research endeavors provide an opportunity to increase a physician-researcher's overall compensation. As a result, an investigator could feel pressure to complete as much research as possible in an effort to increase his level of compensation. Of course, under some other institutional incentive systems, such efforts may have a minimal effect on the investigators' overall compensation, particularly if the system places a heavy emphasis on production of clinical revenue through treating patients rather than through research projects. The changing world of institutional support, however, may radically alter this balance in the near future.

Curing Conflicts of Interest in Clinical Research:
Impossible Dreams and Harsh Realities
Patricia C. Kuszler
8 WID. L. SYMP. J. 115 (2001)

Although conflicts of interest have been a lurking danger for many years, they have only been addressed by law and institutional policy relatively recently. Now, there are a variety of federal regulations and guidelines, institutional policies, and professional association recommendations regarding conflicts of interest. Most recently, the Office for Human Research Protections (OHRP) has issued draft interim guidance on "Financial Relationships in Clinical Research." In issuing the draft guidance, the OHRP noted there is no recognized "best practice" with respect to handling conflict of interest questions. These draft guidelines were designed to stimulate consensus on a greater level of protection for human subjects. Unfortunately, there is little consensus among the many entities that have weighed in on the issue to date.

A. *Laws and Regulations Addressing Conflict of Interest*

At present there are no federal laws or regulations that are prescriptive regarding the types of financial interests that may be held by clinical researchers. Both the FDA and the Public Health Service (PHS) have issued regulations addressing conflicts of interest, but they are vague and inconsistent.

The FDA has had regulations in place since 1998 requiring investigators to have no financial interests in the product and technologies they are testing, with the exception of those disclosed and deemed allowable under the federal regulations. Any such allowable compensation cannot be tied to the outcome or results of the study. Payment by the sponsor to the investigator or the institution cannot exceed $25,000 in excess of the documented costs of conducting the research or clinical trial. Under the FDA regulations, this disclosure must be made during the time the study is being conducted and within one year after it has been completed. This disclosure is the responsibility of the investigator and must be made directly to the FDA.

Under the PHS regulations, institutions receiving federal grant funds must maintain a written, enforced policy on conflict of interest. This policy must provide for institutional review of significant financial interests of investigators before the research is commenced.

"Significant financial interests" means anything of monetary value, including but not limited to, salary or other payments for services (e.g., consulting fees or honoraria); equity interests (e.g., stocks, stock options or other ownership interests); and intellectual property rights (e.g., patents, copyrights and royalties from such rights). . . .

The PHS regulations are unclear in terms of specific guidance to the institution, containing only an undefined requirement that the institution take "reasonable steps" to manage conflicts.

Both the FDA and the PHS regulations focus heavily on disclosure. However, differences in government regulations addressing conflicts produce a baseline level of confusion. The PHS regulations require disclosure of the conflict to the research institution. In contrast, the FDA regulations require disclosure to the FDA. The reporting threshold for financial conflict of interest under the FDA regulations is $25,000, while under the Public Health Service, which applies to all NIH grants, the threshold is $10,000. Further complicating this issue is the fact that the royalty payments authorized under the Federal Technology Transfer Act, which are also a form of equity, have only a 15% dollar cap.

It is unclear in both sets of regulations how wide the scope of the disclosure should be; is it sufficient to disclose the conflict to the university and/or government agency, and is there a duty to disclose the conflict to subjects and patients in the formal consenting process? The federal regulations applying to research consent do not require such disclosure. There is an entirely different ethic and flavor to informed consent in the context of research. In research, informed consent focuses on emphasizing the unknowns of the experiment and on the fact the subject cannot necessarily expect benefit. In addition, a rigorous disclosure of risks is required. In traditional informed consent transactions, the goal is to disclose all of the known material information to the patient to aid them in making the most beneficial choice they can. The common law standard requiring disclosure of all facts that would be deemed "material" to the patient's or subject's decision-making would likely require disclosure of a financial conflict.

In the aftermath of the Gelsinger case, Donna Shalala, then Secretary of the Department of Health and Human Services, called for increased oversight of conflicts of interest. To that end, she appointed a twelve member National Human Research Protections Advisory Committee, designed to serve as the principal advisory body to the department on issues pertaining to human subjects protection and responsible conduct of human research. The Secretary also reconstituted the Office for the Protection from Research Risks (OPRR) as the new Office for Human Research Protections (OHRP), empowering it to lead efforts for protecting human subjects in biomedical and behavioral research.

In January 2001, OHRP issued Draft Interim Guidelines designed to "help IRBs [Institutional Review Boards], Clinical Investigators, and Institutions in carrying out their responsibilities to protect human subjects." These guidelines addressed the respective roles of institutions, clinical investigators, IRBs, and IRB members and staff. While not modifying existing law and regulation, the guidance does provide clues as to likely future trends. The guidance advocates strongly for communication of conflict of interest information to Human Subjects Committees so that they can consider how much of the information should be disclosed to subjects in the informed consent document. OHRP stressed the importance of Human Subjects Committees in management of conflicts of interest and noted that it is imperative that IRB members and staff are carefully vetted for any conflicts they may have as well. The guidance specifically states that research institutions are increasingly corporate partners with private sponsors and "should not lose sight of . . . their own conflicts." The guidance stops short of advocating a "prohibition" approach, but argues for enhanced disclosure and assiduous management of conflicts.

In addition, the OHRP draft guidelines stress the need for disclosure beyond the institution to the patient/subject and advocate inclusion of this information in the informed consent process. The FDA has expressed disagreement with this view, arguing that appropriate management of the conflict would eliminate the need for disclosure to the subject. Patients' rights activists argue that the patient or subject should be fully apprised of financial conflicts of interest during the consent process and that regulations should be revamped to reflect this requirement. They advocate mandatory, enforced disclosure of both investigator and institutional conflicts before the patient or subject begins the treatment.

Clinical investigators counter that providing complete information may be detrimental to the overall goals of informed consent. Patients may be unable to understand and assimilate the information sufficiently to draw their own conclusions as to the propriety of the conflict. Moreover, the complex informed consent document might chill participation in trials and lead to a perception that the conflict is more central than it actually is.

Moreover, there may be occasions when the patient/subject would be disadvantaged by having a conflicted investigator excluded from involvement in the trial. It may be that the conflicted scientist is the most qualified and knowledgeable person to conduct the trial. Indeed some argue that such concrete exclusion rules have already produced such anomalies. For example, the IOM does not allow anyone who has ever served on an advisory committee to author an IOM report on vaccine safety. This policy seeks to ensure that the IOM reports are unbiased and impartial. However, it may also mean that most of the experts and renowned specialists are excluded in favor of others who are less knowledgeable, less equipped, and less passionate about the subject matter.

There are also questions and concerns as to the optimal time for collection of information about conflicts of interest. For example, the recently issued draft guidance from the Office of Human Research Protections calls for collection and documentation of conflict information early in the trial, while the FDA requires a less stringent time frame.

Given the confusion and unanswered questions produced by the conflicting regulations and guidance, it is no wonder institutions that generally bear the burden for managing financial conflicts of interest exhibit similar disarray with respect to conflict of interest policies. Moreover, like the federal regulation, most institutions are silent with respect to nonfinancial conflicts of interest. Less quantifiable, this important class of conflicts is in an abyss with respect to recognition, much less management.

B. Institutional Policies on Conflict: Disclosure vs. Prohibition

Under the PHS regulations and the recently issued OHRP Draft Interim Guidance, the onus for "managing" conflicts falls upon the research institution. Once a conflict is disclosed, the institution must manage the conflict, determine what actions should be taken to reduce or eliminate the conflict, and impose any restrictions or modifications deemed necessary to ensure that the conflict does not bias the design, conduct, or reporting of the research project. Accordingly, research institutions have promulgated institutional policies that attempt to satisfy the limited federal regulations while simultaneously conforming to their institutional cultures. The result is a patchwork of policies with little consensus.

Several studies have recently reviewed institutional conflict of interest policies. The most notable of these reviewed 89 conflict of interest policies from leading research universities. There was little commonality among the policies. Fifty-five percent of the 89 conflict of interest policies reviewed required disclosures from all faculty, while 45% required disclosure only on the part of the principal investigator. The majority (88%) required disclosure about the financial interests of family members of the pertinent faculty member.

The dollar thresholds for disclosure were frequently more stringent than the existing PHS federal threshold of $10,000. However, the authors noted that this variable dollar threshold could be interpreted differently based on the institutional culture and values as well as the nature of the conflict. All of the policies dealt with financial conflicts of interest, but only a subset addressed other types of conflicts. Most of the policies described prohibited activities in a general sense rather than homing in on clinical research related taboos. The most common prohibition applied to researchers having financial interests in companies sponsoring their research. Only 19% of the reviewed policies had provisions specifically addressing clinical research. These provisions addressed limits on equity holdings in sponsors, disclosure of financial interests in published work, required disclosure of conflicts to the human subjects committee, and more stringent provisions for clinical versus non-clinical research.

Another study, in which the ten top medical schools were surveyed in terms of research funding, also found variability among conflict of interest policies. Although all ten universities required that faculty members disclose financial interests to university officials, they varied in terms of the dollar threshold for disclosure. Only four of the ten universities extended the disclosure rule to the entire research team, rather than just a cohort of the team.

There are increasing questions as to whether or not disclosure, even an expanded level of disclosure, is sufficient to adequately protect human subjects. Disclosure is but one of the models for managing conflicts of interest. It is criticized for being susceptible to loopholes and inconsistency. Increasingly, it is being viewed as "too cheap and easy" a method for addressing conflicts.

The other model is that of prohibition — a zero tolerance of financial conflict of interest. The prohibition model is criticized as having a chilling effect on research and development of new therapies and treatment. A few institutions, notably Harvard Medical School, have embraced a more prohibition-oriented model with respect to clinical research. These institutions argue that, in the case of clinical research, financial conflicts of interest may undermine clinical judgment. Equally concerning to Harvard and other proponents of more stringent conflict policies is the public perception that research which is biased has led to erosion of patient trust in medicine and the research enterprise.

Several leaders in medicine support a prohibition policy. They argue that disclosure merely "passes the buck" to the hapless subject/patient who is ill-equipped to assess its importance in the equation of impending care. At the most extreme, prohibition would be extended to all financial ties with sponsors, including speaking fees, consulting fees, sponsor-paid travel, and require that industry support be placed in general research support funds. Under the prohibition model, investigators with financial interests would be foreclosed from having authority over study design, data collection, and results interpretation, and sponsors would be forbidden from editorial involvement or pre-publication review of studies. Less draconian versions of prohibition would allow clinical investigators to be supported by a private sponsor, so long as the investigator had no stock, stock options, or decision-making position in the sponsoring company.

In justifying prohibition, adherents note that university-based investigators should be held to a higher standard than researchers working in commercial venues, because of their role in training and mentoring the next generation of scientists. This movement toward prohibition appears to be gaining favor. Advocates argue that the only way to solve conflict is to remove it completely by refusing to allow researchers to have a financial stake in the therapies they are researching.

IV. Redressing Conflicts: Palliating an Unresolvable Problem

In the wake of renewed attention to conflicts and the publication of the OHRP draft guidance, it is becoming increasingly clear that there is no easy solution to the complex issues of conflicts of interest. Researchers and reformers alike are essentially boxed into a corner by virtue of incentives of the Bayh-Dole and other technology transfer acts. Moreover, after two decades, technology transfer has forever changed the culture of biomedical research. At best, policymakers and regulators will be able to palliate conflict of interest problems, not eradicate them.

Testimony at National Institutes of Health, Conference on Human Subject Protection and Financial Conflicts of Interest
Marcia Angell
August 16, 2000

As we know, this conference was a response to Secretary Shalala's charge to "Identify new or improved means to manage financial conflicts of interest that could threaten the safety of research subjects or the objectivity of the research itself."

That language is important and I will come back to it later. I am going to begin this morning by defining a financial conflict of interest because there is often controversy on that score. A financial conflict of interest, I believe, is any financial association that would cause an investigator to prefer one outcome of his research to another.

Let me give you an example. If an investigator is comparing Drug A with Drug B and also owns a large amount of stock in the company that makes Drug A, he will prefer to find that Drug A is better than Drug B. That is the conflict of interest. Note that it is a function of the situation, not the investigator's response to that situation.

If the investigator then finds that Drug B is better, he may swallow his disappointment and report the facts objectively or, as Tom Bodenheimer pointed out, he may in many ways not report his findings objectively. According to this definition then, there is no such thing as a potential conflict of interest. The only thing potential about it is whether the conflict leads to bad research.

Note also that financial conflicts of interest are not inherent to the research enterprise. They are entirely optional, unlike the intellectual or personal conflicts of interest to which they are often compared, such as the desire for Nobel worthy results.

At one time financial associations with private industry were largely confined to drug companies awarding grants to academic institutions for research in areas of interest to both of them. In the best institutions, this was done at arm's length. The companies had no part in designing or analyzing the studies. They did not own the data and they certainly did not write the papers and control publication. The academic institutions, the best of them, insisted on this, and they were the watchdogs.

Things have changed dramatically in the past few years. Arm's length relationships are a thing of the past and financial arrangements are hardly limited to grant support. Companies now design studies to be carried out by investigators and academic medical centers who are little more than hired hands supplying the patients and collecting data.

The companies own the data. They analyze it and control publications. Such a study is not even necessarily of any real scientific importance or interest to the investigators. It may — particularly Phase 4 studies, it may instead be almost entirely of marketing importance to the sponsor.

For their part, academic institutions are increasingly involved in deals with the same companies, whose products their faculty members are studying. Some institutions are for a price allowing companies to set up research outposts in their hospitals and giving them access to students and house officers, as well as large numbers of patients. They are aligning then their interest with those of industry and allowing the boundaries between them to become ever more blurred.

Consider the story in last Thursday's *Wall Street Journal*. It reported that Targeted Genetics Corporation will acquire Genovo, Incorporated. As part of the deal, James Wilson will receive $13.5 million worth of stock in Targeted in exchange for his 30 percent equity interest in Genovo.

Recall that the University of Pennsylvania permitted Wilson to own a piece of Genovo, even while he was doing research on its products. Now, that is hardly surprising, given that Penn itself, according to the story, will receive $1.4 million worth of stock for its 3.2 percent stake in Genovo. Some watchdog.

This story is news because of the death of Jesse Gelsinger, but it is hardly unique in its outline. Incidentally, I sometimes think that there has been no piece of legislation quite like Bayh-Dole with respect to the enthusiasm and the expansiveness with which it is embraced. It believe it is often used as an excuse for making as much money as possible in as many possible ways.

Now, what about the integrity of the scientific literature. As Tom Bodenheimer summarized yesterday beautifully for us, there is plenty of strong evidence that investigators with financial ties to companies whose products they are studying are, indeed, more likely to publish studies favorable to those products. In my two decades at *The New England Journal of Medicine*, it was my clear impression that papers submitted by authors with financial conflicts of interest were far more likely to be biased in both design and interpretation.

In my view, the pervasive and manifold financial conflicts of interest that now exist have a number of bad effects, in addition to the threat to the integrity of the scientific literature and the risk to human subjects that primarily concern us here.

I don't have time to discuss those other negative effects. Suffice it to say, though, that we need to remember that the mission of investor-owned companies is quite different from the mission of academic medical centers. The primary purpose of the former, of the companies, is to increase the value of the shareholders' stock, which they do by securing patents and marketing their products.

Their purpose is not to educate nor even to carry out research, except secondarily as a means to their primary end. I believe that academics often forget this and they allow themselves to believe that marketing is really education. They allow themselves to believe that. With all this as background, what I would like to do in the time remaining to me here is to say a few words about the remedies that have been proposed at this conference and why I find most of them unsatisfactory.

The emphasis here has been on managing conflicts of interest. Managing is, in fact, the word used in Secretary Shalala's charge. In particular, the focus has been on disclosure to human subjects and on institutional oversight. In my view, disclosure simply passes the buck to the patient subject, who is left to wonder how the investigator will balance his competing interest. That is neither fair nor helpful to the subject who may be both sick and desperate and it certainly does nothing to remove the conflict of interest.

Caveat emptor is simply inappropriate in this setting. On the other hand, not disclosing a conflict of interest is even worse because it is fundamentally deceptive.

Patients naturally assume investigators are primarily interested in patient welfare and they have a right to know of anything that may shake that assumption.

To disclose or not to disclose then is a Hobson's Choice and the very difficulty of making that choice points to the underlying problem, the very existence of financial conflicts of interest.

Institutional oversight usually boils down to defining conflicts of interest that must be disclosed and documenting them on various pieces of paper. Some of the guidelines are truly mind boggling in their complexity and detail. For example, Harvard Medical School's guidelines widely acknowledged to be among the most stringent and the best, fill eight, closely-worded and nearly impenetrable pages. They deal with such matters as the dollar amount of equity interest investigators and specified family members may own in companies sponsoring their research. The answer seems to be $20,000 for spouse and dependent children.

In short all of this is about management, not about the wisdom of permitting the conflicts of interest in the first place. It is as though financial conflicts of interest were inherent to the enterprise, were a given of nature or a constitutional right, neither of which they are. I believe we need to stop dancing on the margins of this issue and deal with it head on.

The important question is whether financial conflicts of interest should exist, not how to work around them. Mind you, I am not opposed to cooperation with industry. Academic industrial collaborations have led to some important events, but the conflicts of interest that now abound in academic medicine go way beyond cooperation and many of them have no conceivably useful social purpose.

I would like to suggest the following guidelines. One, investigators who receive grant support from industry should have no other financial ties to those companies. Consider an analogy. Suppose a judge had before him a case of two contending companies and he had equity interests in one of those companies and he said not to worry. I am a good judge. This won't bother me. I will hear the case.

He would not be permitted to do that. Why should we?

Two, institutions should not accept grants with strings attached. Investigators should design and analyze their own studies, write their own papers and decide about publication.

Three, consultancy arrangements need to be carefully limited. I believe the argument that they bring new technologies to the bedside is greatly overblown, particularly in clinical research where the technology is usually developed.

Consultancies in academic medicine are virtually ubiquitous and they are more often about income supplementation and the good will thereby generated, than about technology transfer. Incidentally, the issue of good will, I think, is considerably underestimated.

Furthermore, technology transfer does not require that fees be paid directly to investigators. Income from limited consulting might instead go to a pool earmarked to support the missions of the institution. After all, investigators at academic medical centers have reasonably well-paying jobs. They do not need to jeopardize their objectivity, the very core and essence of what they do to increase their income.

Four, institutions should not become outposts for industry by allowing investor-owned companies to set up teaching or research centers in their hospitals and giving them access to the students, house officers and patients. I am aware that academic medical centers are now in difficult times financially and I sympathize with their plight. I really do. But the answer cannot be to sell themselves and their patients to industry.

Five, institutions and the senior officials should not have investments in any health care industry. The editors of *The New England Journal of Medicine* have long had such a rule and it has not been a hardship to us. Rubies, race horses, real estate, yes, we can invest in all of those, but not biotechnology or managed care companies.

Finally, and perhaps most important at this stage, institutions need to get together on this issue and develop a common policy. As it now stands, investigators may threaten to leave institutions with stringent policies and go to more lenient ones. That race to the bottom can be stopped only by the major academic medical centers joining together to do the right thing. I am well aware that my proposals might seem radical. That is because our society is now so drenched in market ideology that any resistance to it is considered quixotic.

But medicine and clinical research are special and I believe we have to protect their timeless values of service and disinterestedness. Patients should not have to wonder whether an investigator is motivated by financial gain and the public should not have to wonder whether medical research can be believed.

The only way to deal with the problem is to eliminate it as much as possible.

NOTES AND QUESTIONS

1. Goldner describes a wide variety of practices that create conflicts of interest. Which of them are the most troublesome? Which of them seem relatively minor?

2. Note the differences between the conflicts created by the "per capita" or "finder's fee practices," which often involve relatively small amounts of money (though, for a researcher who is enrolling many patients in a variety of studies, the total amounts can quickly become large) and affect many investigators who often have a minor role in a much larger study, and the "ownership interest" conflicts, which often involve millions of dollars, and affect only the few researchers

who played a major role in creating the new product. In terms of the overall research system, is one of these conflicts more troublesome than the other?

3. As part of its efforts to police payments to researchers, the federal government has begun to rely on the "fraud and abuse" laws, which are designed to ensure that federal Medicare and Medicaid funds are spent properly. In particular, the anti-kickback law makes it a federal crime for anyone to make or receive a payment for the purpose of encouraging the provision of medical services that will be paid for with federal funds. Federal prosecutors are now investigating the possible application of these rules to a variety of payment practices in the research area, such as payments by drug manufacturers to doctors for participation in "company-sponsored clinical trials that were little more than thinly disguised marketing efforts that required little effort on the doctors' part." Gardiner Harris, *As Doctor Writes Prescription, Drug Company Writes a Check*, N.Y. TIMES, June 27, 2004, sec. 1, at 1; *see also* Mark Barnes & Sara Krauss, *Conflicts of Interest in Human Research: Risks and Pitfalls of "Easy Money" in Research Funding*, 9 HEALTH L. REP. (BNA) 1378 (2000).

4. In March 2001, the Seattle Times ran a multi-part series about cancer studies conducted at Seattle's Fred Hutchinson Cancer Research Center. Although the main focus of the series related to whether adequate informed consent was obtained from subjects, the articles also noted that some researchers owned hundreds of thousands of dollars of stock in a company called Genetic Systems. That company, founded by three of the researchers who also had other continuing involvements in company operations, would own certain rights to some of the antibodies that were being investigated in the research. *See* Duff Wilson & David Heath, *The Blood-Cancer Experiment*, SEATTLE TIMES, March 11, 2001 at A1; Robert M. Nelson, *Protocol 126 and "The Hutch,"* 23 IRB, May-June 2001, at 14. In one of the lawsuits filed on behalf of subjects in these studies, a judge dismissed the financial conflict of interest claims, ruling that there was insufficient evidence. *See* David Heath & Luke Timmerman, *Jury Finds Hutch Not Negligent in 4 Deaths*, SEATTLE TIMES, Apr. 9, 2004, at A1.

5. A health law teacher, who served as provost of a university that conducts biomedical research, recently observed:

> We have all been there, walking away from a talk or a meeting and thinking: "They just don't get it." Sometimes, it is the lawyers shaking their heads about the doctors; and at other times, it is the doctors stunned speechless by the ignorance of the lawyers. For example, tell doctors that they have a "conflict of interest" in relation to a proposed protocol for research with human subjects, and they believe that you have accused them of unethical behavior. In my experience, doctors tend to assume that a conflict of interest exists only when they actually have made a "bad" decision motivated by their financial interest in the sponsor of the research. Lawyers (and, therefore, federal agencies regulating research) view conflicts as objective, structural, and rule-based. You could be a paragon of virtue, and you would be conflicted out of rep-

resenting a client if a prohibited conflict of interest exists. Doctors, in contrast, view conflicts of interest as relating to the individual's character and ability to resist temptation. We lawyers might say that doctors just don't get it when they get angry at us for telling them that they have a conflict of interest. And, perhaps, we just don't get it when we get defensive at their response and fail to understand their starting point.

Sandra H. Johnson, *Five Easy Pieces: Motifs of Health Law*, 14 HEALTH MATRIX 131 (2004).

6. Researchers at Stanford University and the University of California at San Francisco (UCSF) were recently surveyed to see how well they understood conflict-of-interest policies at those institutions. *See* Elizabeth A. Boyd et al., *Financial Conflict-of-Interest Policies in Clinical Research: Issues for Clinical Investigators*, 78 ACADEMIC MED. 769 (2003). At UCSF, more than half (58%) of the investigators could not correctly describe that institution's policies, which prohibited an investigator from "receiving compensation from the sponsor of a trial or holding a decision-making position within the company." (What things do you think are meant by "receiving compensation"?) "The most common misunderstanding was that the policy does not *prohibit* personal compensation, but only requires its disclosure. . . . In general, investigators felt that their own relationships with industry posed little risk either to them personally or to the profession." Is investigators' lack of knowledge about their institution's policies a problem? As long as investigators comply with reporting rules (such as an annual reporting requirement, with additional information required when a new study is begun) does it matter if they understand what type of conflicts are considered impermissible? Should we be troubled by investigators' perceptions that their relationships with industry are not a problem?

7. There continues to be a debate about whether the best approach for dealing with conflicts of interest is to prohibit them or to disclose them. What are the advantages and disadvantages of each of these strategies? For views on these issues, see, e.g., Sharmon Sollitto et al., *Intrinsic Conflicts of Interest in Clinical Research: A Need for Disclosure*, 13 KENNEDY INST. ETHICS J. 83 (2003); Mark Barnes & Patrik S. Florencio, *Investigator, IRB and Institutional Financial Conflicts of Interest in Human-Subjects Research: Past, Present and Future*, 32 SETON HALL L. REV. 525 (2002); Frances Miller, *Trusting Doctors: Tricky Business When It Comes to Clinical Research*, 81 B.U. L. REV. 423 (2001); Timothy Caulfield & Glenn Greiner, *Conflicts of Interest in Clinical Research: Addressing the Issue of Physician Reimbursement*, 30 J. L. MED. & ETHICS 305 (2002); Pilar Osorio, *Pills, Bills and Shills: Physician-Researcher's Conflicts of Interest*, 8 WID. L. SYMP. J. 75 (2001); Katherine S. Mangan, *Medical-Research Ethics Under the Microscope*, CHRONICLE HIGHER EDUC., July 25, 2003, at A22; OFFICE OF INSPECTOR GENERAL, DEPARTMENT OF HEALTH AND HUMAN SERVICES, RECRUITING HUMAN SUBJECTS: PRESSURES IN INDUSTRY SPONSORED CLINICAL RESEARCH (June 2000).

8. A variety of research organizations have issued reports about how to deal with conflicts of interest — perhaps hoping that if they create their own rules,

they will reduce the likelihood of government action. *See, e.g.,* ASSOCIATION OF AMERICAN UNIVERSITIES, TASK FORCE ON RESEARCH ACCOUNTABILITY, REPORT ON INDIVIDUAL AND INSTITUTIONAL FINANCIAL CONFLICT OF INTEREST (2001); ASSOCIATION OF AMERICAN MEDICAL COLLEGES, TASK FORCE ON FINANCIAL CONFLICTS OF INTEREST IN CLINICAL RESEARCH, PROTECTING SUBJECTS, PRESERVING TRUST, PROMOTING PROGRESS — POLICY AND GUIDELINES FOR THE OVERSIGHT OF INDIVIDUAL FINANCIAL INTERESTS IN HUMAN SUBJECTS RESEARCH (2001); Karine Morin et al., *Managing Conflicts of Interest in the Conduct of Clinical Trials,* 287 JAMA 78 (2002) (reporting new ethical opinion adopted by American Medical Association); Susan L. Coyle for the Ethics and Human Rights Committee, American College of Physicians, *Physician-Industry Relations, Part 1: Individual Physicians,* 136 ANNALS INTERNAL MED. 396 (2002); American Society of Clinical Oncology, *Background for Update of Conflict of Interest Policy,* 21 J. CLINICAL ONCOLOGY 2387 (2003).

Financial Relationships and Interests in Research Involving Human Subjects: Guidance for Human Subject Protection
Office of Public Health and Science, Department of Health and Human Services
69 FED. REG. 26,393 (2004)

D. Basis for This Document

. . . Concerns have grown that financial conflicts of interest in research, derived from financial relationships and the financial interests they create, may affect the rights and welfare of human research subjects. Financial interests are not prohibited, and not all financial interests cause conflicts of interest or affect the rights and welfare of human subjects. HHS recognizes the complexity of the relationships between government, academia, industry and others, and recognizes that these relationships often legitimately include financial relationships. However, to the extent financial interests may affect the rights and welfare of human subjects in research, IRBs, institutions, and investigators need to consider what actions regarding financial interests may be necessary to protect those subjects. . . .

II. Guidance for Institutions, IRBs and Investigators

A. *General Approaches to Address Financial Relationships and Interests in Research Involving Human Subjects*

The Department recommends that in particular, IRBs, institutions, and investigators consider whether specific financial relationships create financial interests in research studies that may adversely affect the rights and welfare of subjects. These entities may find it useful to include the following questions in their deliberations:

- What financial relationships and resulting financial interests cause potential or actual conflicts?

- At what levels should those potential or actual financial conflicts of interest be managed or eliminated?

- What procedures would be helpful, including those to

  - collect and evaluate information regarding financial relationships related to research,

  - determine whether those relationships potentially cause a conflict of interest, and

  - determine what actions are necessary to protect human subjects and ensure that those actions are taken?

- Who should be educated regarding financial conflict of interest issues and policies?

- What entity or entities would examine individual and/or institutional financial relationships and interests?

B. *Points for Consideration*

Financial interests determined to create a conflict of interest may be managed by eliminating them or mitigating their impact. A variety of methods or combinations of methods may be effective. Some methods may be implemented by institutions engaged in the conduct of research, and some methods may be implemented by IRBs or investigators. Some of those may apply before research begins, and some may apply during the conduct of the research.

In establishing and implementing methods to protect the rights and welfare of human subjects from conflicts of interest created by financial relationships of parties involved in research, the Department recommends that IRBs, institutions engaged in research, and investigators consider the questions below. Additional questions may be appropriate. The Department's intent is not to be exhaustive, but to suggest ways to examine the issues so that appropriate actions can be taken to protect the rights and welfare of human research subjects. The Department recognizes that a number of institutions currently address such issues in their consideration of financial interests of parties involved in human subject research.

- Does the research involve financial relationships that could create potential or actual conflicts of interest?

  - How is the research supported or financed?

  - Where and by whom was the study designed?

  - Where and by whom will the resulting data be analyzed?

- What interests are created by the financial relationships involved in the situation?
  - ◆ Do individuals or institutions receive any compensation that may be affected by the study outcome?
  - ◆ Do individuals or institutions involved in the research:
    - have any proprietary interests in the product including patents, trademarks, copyrights, and licensing agreements?
    - have an equity interest in the research sponsor and, if so, is the sponsor a publicly held company or non-publicly held company?
    - receive significant payments of other sorts? (e.g. grants, compensation in the form of equipment, retainers for ongoing consultation, or honoraria)
    - receive payment per participant or incentive payments, and are those payments reasonable?
- Given the financial relationships involved, is the institution an appropriate site for the research?
- How should financial relationships that potentially create a conflict of interest be managed?
- Would the rights and welfare of human subjects be better protected by any or a combination of the following:
  - ◆ reduction of the financial interest?
  - ◆ disclosure of the financial interest to prospective subjects?
  - ◆ separation of responsibilities for financial decisions and research decisions?
  - ◆ additional oversight or monitoring of the research?
  - ◆ an independent data and safety monitoring committee or similar monitoring body?
  - ◆ modification of role(s) of particular research staff or changes in location for certain research activities, e.g., a change of the person who seeks consent, or a change of investigator?
  - ◆ elimination of the financial interest?

C. *Specific Issues for Consideration*

1. Institutions

The Department recommends that institutions engaged in HHS conducted or supported human subjects research consider whether the following actions or other actions would help ensure that financial interests do not compromise the rights and welfare of human research subjects.

Actions to consider:

- Establishing the independence of institutional responsibility for research activities from the management of the institution's financial interests.

- Establish conflict of interest committees (COICs) or identifying other bodies or persons and procedures to

  - deal with individuals' or institutional financial interests in research or verify the absence of such interests and

  - address institutional financial interests in research.

- Establish criteria to determine what constitutes an institutional conflict of interest, including identifying leadership positions for which the individual's financial interests are such that they may need to be treated as institutional financial interests.

- Establish clear channels of communication between COICs and IRBs.

- Establish policies on providing information, recommendations, or findings from COIC deliberations to IRBs.

- Establish measures to foster the independence of IRBs and COICs.

- Determining whether particular individuals should report financial interests to the COIC. These individuals could include IRB members and staff and appropriate officials of the institution, along with investigators, among those who report financial interests to COICs.

- Establish procedures for disclosure of institutional financial relationships to COICs.

- Provide training to appropriate individuals regarding financial interest requirements.

- Using independent organizations to hold or administer the institution's financial interest.

- Include individuals from outside the institution in the review and oversight of financial interests in research.

- Establishing policies regarding the types of financial relationships that may be held by parties involved in the research and circumstances under which those financial relationships and interests may or may not be held.

[2. IRB Operations — *reprinted below at page 237.*]

3. IRB Review

The Department recommends that IRBs reviewing HHS conducted or supported human subjects research or FDA regulated human subjects research consider whether the following actions, or other actions related to conduct or oversight of research, would help ensure that financial interests do not compromise the rights and welfare of human research subjects.

Actions to consider:

- Determining whether methods used for management of financial interests of parties involved in the research adequately protect the rights and welfare of human subjects.

- Determining whether other actions are necessary to minimize risks to subjects.

- Determining the kind, amount, and level of detail of information to be provided to research subjects regarding the source of funding, funding arrangements, financial interests of parties involved in the research, and any financial interest management techniques applied.

4. Investigators

The Department recommends that investigators conducting human subjects research consider the potential effects that a financial relationship of any kind might have on the research or on interactions with research subjects, and what actions to take.

Actions to consider:

- Including information in the informed consent document, such as

  - the source of funding and funding arrangements for the conduct and review of research, or

  - information about a financial arrangement of an institution or an investigator and how it is being managed.

- Using special measures to modify the informed consent process when a potential or actual financial conflict exists, such as

  - having another individual who does not have a potential or actual conflict of interest involved in the consent process, especially when a potential or actual conflict of interest could influence the tone, presentation, or type of information presented during the consent process.

  - Using independent monitoring of the research.

NOTES AND QUESTIONS

1. This DHHS guidance is the final version of the interim guidance described in Kuszler's article. It was released approximately three years after the version that she described and reflected changes made as a result of public comments on the interim guidance. Based on her description of the earlier version, how substantially has this document changed during this three-year period?

2. In terms of the basic two approaches to conflicts of interest — prohibition versus disclosure — does one or another approach appear to predominate in the DHHS document?

3. How specific is the DHHS guidance? Is the level of specificity appropriate? Are there reasons some institutions might not be willing, on their own, to pass strict rules (for example, not allowing researchers to own stock in companies whose technology they are studying), but would welcome such rules if they were adopted by the government? If you were involved in compliance activities at an institution that was not yet one of the major players in receiving federal grants, what concerns might you have about enacting a strict conflict-of-interest policy?

§ 5.02 INSTITUTIONAL CONFLICTS

Financial Conflicts of Interest in Human Subjects Research: The Problem of Institutional Conflicts
Mark Barnes & Patrik S. Florencio
30 J. L. Med. & Ethics 390 (2002)

The Association of American Universities (AAU) has defined institutional financial conflicts of interest as situations in which:

> [T]he institution, any of its senior management or trustees, or a department, school, or other sub-unit, or an affiliated foundation or organization, has an external relationship or financial interest in a company that itself has a financial interest in a faculty research project. Senior managers or trustees may also have conflicts when they serve on the boards of (or otherwise have an official relationship with) organizations that have significant commercial transactions with the university. The existence (or appearance) of such conflicts can lead to actual bias, or suspicion about possible bias, in the review or conduct of research at the university. If they are not evaluated or managed, they may result in choices or actions that are incongruent with the missions, obligations, or the values of the university.

What is central to the AAU's definition of institutional financial conflicts of interest is that: (1) the conflict can arise from corporate (i.e., the institution or a subdivision of the institution) or individual (i.e., senior management, trustees, department chairs) relationships with, or financial holdings in, industry; (2) there is no *de minimis* threshold below which the conflict will be considered insignificant (i.e., all relationships or financial interests are viewed as potential conflicts); (3) the appearance of bias is as important as actual bias; and (4) if conflicts are not managed, they can lead to improper decision-making. . . .

[I]nstitutional conflicts of interest, like investigator conflicts of interest, may be financial or nonfinancial. Examples of nonfinancial institutional interests are the desire to enhance institutional reputation, originate innovative new technologies, develop safe and effective treatments for illnesses, and win prestigious research awards in order to be able to attract and maintain "star" faculty members and researchers to the institution, as well as to be able to compete successfully for sponsored research funding. These nonfinancial interests may generate conflicts through institutional pressure to achieve positive research results. Although nonfinancial interests have been widely acknowledged in the literature dealing with investigator conflicts of interest, nonfinancial conflicts of interest are generally thought to be effectively controlled through research oversight processes at institutions (e.g., IRB approval of only scientifically meritorious research protocols) and through the scientific method itself. Moreover, nonfinancial interests are much less easily identified than are financial interests and are therefore harder to regulate. . . .

How then might institutional financial conflicts of interest affect research outcomes or the health and safety of human research subjects participating in a trial at the institution? The issue of institutional financial conflicts of interest is premised on the assumption that institutional conflicts can influence researchers and institutional decision makers, including IRB members, IRB staff, and others employed by the institution. . . . The risk is that their professional judgment may be affected by institutional pressure to achieve a research end point that is favorable to the institution's reputation or financial interests. The institutional pressure may be indirect (e.g., researcher or institutional decision maker obliquely learns that the institution is heavily invested in the trial being conducted) or direct (e.g., he or she is notified by an institutional administrator or department chair of the institution's interest in the outcome of the trial). This institutional pressure may lead researchers and/or administrators to compromise their primary responsibilities toward assuring human subject welfare, scientific integrity, and institutional integrity. Examples of compromised primary responsibilities may include, among others: (1) the inadequate disclosure of study risks and exaggeration of potential study benefits in order to enhance subject enrollment; (2) enrollment of subjects not meeting eligibility criteria; (3) failure to exclude subjects meeting exclusion criteria; (4) failure to report adverse events to the IRB charged with overseeing the trial; (5) improper data manipulation; (6) failure to conduct rigorous initial and continuing review; and (7) failure to suspend or terminate trials when indicated. . . .

Management of institutional financial conflicts of interests

. . . While the close partnership between academia and for-profit industry has led to a surge in the rapidity with which scientific innovations are brought to market, this partnership has also led to a number of practices that are incompatible with academic values. For instance, clinical trial agreements between investigators and sponsors have sometimes contained "gag clauses" permitting the sponsor to delay publication of research findings for significant periods of time, or to outrightly prohibit publication when research results are unfavorable to the sponsor's product. In some cases, industry sponsors have taken legal action to enforce such clauses, even where the withholding of data could lead to research injuries. While "gag clauses" are simple to regulate in that they are usually easy to identify, and can then be modified or altogether negotiated out of clinical trial agreements, the nature and extent of the steps that should be taken to manage other problems associated with the growing nexus between academia and industry, such as the problem of institutional financial conflicts of interest, are less clear.

It is recommended that the primary methods for controlling institutional financial conflicts of interest should focus on assuring adequate separation of research activities from institutional investment activities, and instituting independent monitoring of clinical trials. While the erection of "firewalls" to assure adequate separation between researchers and those institutional officials responsible for the institution's corporate investments and relationships should be feasible to implement, isolating researchers from, for example, conflicted department chairs will be more difficult to achieve. For instance, in an academic medical center where the head of the department of cardiology has financially invested in a sponsor whose cardiac device is being tested by a faculty member of the department of cardiology, it may not be feasible, or even desirable, to largely restrict communication between the head of a cardiology department and the faculty member for the duration of the trial. First, regular interaction between department chairs and faculty members, for example, during faculty meetings, is necessary to the efficient operation of academic medical centers. Second, most clinical trials continue at least for months, and many carry on for years. Thus, while "firewalls" are an appropriate mechanism for managing institutional conflicts that arise from the institution's corporate investments and relationships, this mechanism may be less reasonable or practical in the case of certain institutional conflicts that arise from the personal investments and relationships of senior managers. In these cases, management of institutional conflicts ought to occur at various stages of the research process — for example, during trial enrollment, eligibility determinations, informed consent, physical examinations, data interpretation, and analysis — by outside, independent professionals.

PROTECTING SUBJECTS, PRESERVING TRUST, PROMOTING PROGRESS II: PRINCIPLES AND RECOMMENDATIONS FOR OVERSIGHT OF AN INSTITUTION'S FINANCIAL INTERESTS IN HUMAN SUBJECTS RESEARCH
ASSOCIATION OF AMERICAN MEDICAL COLLEGES, TASK FORCE ON FINANCIAL CONFLICTS OF INTEREST IN CLINICAL RESEARCH
13 (2002)

Academic institutions are privileged to serve as a public trust for the advancement, preservation, and dissemination of knowledge. These institutions have diverse obligations to students, faculty and staff; to legislators and regulators; to donors and benefactors; and to society at large. When meeting these obligations in the ordinary course of business, institutions must and do reconcile competing interests. In so doing, institutions recognize widely that policies must be made and decisions taken in a manner that is free of the taint of improper bias or conflict of interest.

Increasingly, academic institutions that conduct research also invest in — and accept the philanthropy of — commercial research sponsors. Regulators, legislators, journalists, and patient advocates have now begun to question whether such financial relationships may give rise to "institutional" conflicts of interest that could threaten research integrity and, especially troubling, potentially pose risks to human research subjects. Concern has arisen that existing institutional processes for resolving competing interests may be insufficient when the institution has a financial stake in the outcome of research and the safety and welfare of human subjects are at stake.

Although perceived risks to human subjects have received the greatest attention thus far, the growing perception that research institutions may have financial conflicts of interest also threatens to weaken public support for research. In an era of tremendous public investment in academic research, legislators and policymakers and others justifiably expect heightened public accountability from research institutions. . . .

CIRCUMSTANCES THAT IPSO FACTO MAY CREATE — OR APPEAR TO CREATE — INSTITUTIONAL CONFLICT OF INTEREST (ICOI) IN HUMAN SUBJECTS RESEARCH AND MUST THEREFORE RECEIVE CLOSE SCRUTINY

It is the view of the Task Force that certain financial relationships between institutions and commercial sponsors of human subjects research may present — or appear to present — a conflict of interest, even though an institution has fully separated all of its research and investment functions. Such circumstances warrant the highest degree of scrutiny in every instance in which they occur.

Accordingly, when one or more of the following circumstances exist, the institution should conduct a specific, fact-driven inquiry into whether the particular financial relationship may affect or reasonably appear to affect human subjects research conducted at or under the auspices of the institution:

A. When the institution is entitled to receive royalties from the sale of the investigational product that is the subject of the research;

B. When, though its technological licensing activities of investments related to such activities, the institution has obtained an equity interest or an entitlement to equity of any value (including options or warrants) in a *non-publicly traded* sponsor of human subjects research at the institution;

C. When, through technology licensing activities or investments related to such activities, the institution has obtained an ownership interest or an entitlement to equity (including options or warrants) of greater than $100,000 in value . . . in a *publicly-traded* sponsor of human subjects research at the institution; or

D. When, with regard to a specific research project to be conducted at or under the auspices of the institution, institutional officials with direct responsibility for human subjects research hold a significant financial interest in the commercial research sponsor or the investigational product. . . .

Institutional Conflict of Interest (ICOI) Committee

The Task Force recommends that an institution form a standing ICOI committee for the purpose of reviewing the circumstances of [institutional conflicts of interest]. The Task Force recommends that the ICOI committee members be individuals who have sufficient seniority, expertise, and independence to evaluate the competing interests at stake and make credible and effective recommendations. . . . One or more external ("public") members are strongly urged, as the inclusion of public members will increase the transparency of the committee's deliberations and enhance the credibility of its determinations.

NOTES AND QUESTIONS

1. Assume that a conflict of interest committee had been in existence at the University of Pennsylvania in 1999, when Jesse Gelsinger was participating in the gene modification study described at the beginning of this chapter. What should that committee have done with regard to the $1.4 million in stock that the University of Pennsylvania owned in the company that had rights to the patents? Should the committee have insisted that Penn sell the stock, on the ground that the conflict was impossible to manage? Do the readings tell you how such questions should be resolved?

2. Assume that a long-standing chairperson of a department of cardiology has developed a new type of pacemaker. The device has received FDA approval, but post-marketing surveillance studies are still underway. As a result of the chairman's prior work, he receives royalties on each pacemaker implanted by any physician. During a routine internal audit, it is noted that ninety percent

of the pacemakers implanted by department cardiologists since FDA approval was granted are of this type. Evidence indicates that, nationally, only fifteen percent of pacemakers implanted during the same period are of this type. When the departmental chair is questioned about this situation, his reply is that he believes that this pacemaker is better than competing devices in the vast majority of situations, that practically all of the junior cardiologists in the department were involved in earlier trials of the device, and that to his knowledge the other doctors in his department use it because they both share his views of its superiority and feel most comfortable using it because of their familiarity with it. If you were a member of the institution's conflict of interest committee, how would you handle this situation? What other information might you want to know?

§ 5.03 IRB CONFLICTS

In some circumstances, a member of an IRB may have a conflict of interest in connection with a particular protocol that the IRB is being asked to vote on. The federal regulations prohibit such members from participating in a vote.

45 C.F.R. § 46.107(e): IRB MEMBER CONFLICTS OF INTEREST

This provision is reproduced in Appendix A, at page A-8. Please review it before proceeding.

Financial Relationships and Interests
in Research Involving Human Subjects: Guidance
for Human Subject Protection
Office of Public Health and Science, Department
of Health and Human Services
69 FED. REG. 26,393 (2004)

The Department recommends that institutions engaged in human subjects research and IRBs that review HHS conducted or supported human subjects research or FDA regulated human subjects research consider whether establishing policies and procedures addressing IRB member potential and actual conflicts of interest as part of overall IRB policies and procedures would help ensure that financial interests do not compromise the rights and welfare of human research subjects. As noted, 45 CFR 46.107(e) and 21 CFR 56.107(e) prohibit an IRB member with a conflicting interest in a project from participating in the IRB's initial or continuing review, except to provide information as requested by the IRB.

Policies and procedures to consider:

- Reminding members of conflict of interest policies at each meeting and documenting any actions taken regarding IRB member conflicts of interest related to particular protocols.

- Developing educational materials for IRB members to ensure their awareness of federal regulations and institutional policies regarding financial relationships and interests in human subjects research.

PROTECTING SUBJECTS, PRESERVING TRUST, PROMOTING PROGRESS II: PRINCIPLES AND RECOMMENDATIONS FOR OVERSIGHT OF AN INSTITUTION'S FINANCIAL INTERESTS IN HUMAN SUBJECTS RESEARCH
ASSOCIATION OF AMERICAN MEDICAL COLLEGES, TASK FORCE ON FINANCIAL CONFLICTS OF INTEREST IN CLINICAL RESEARCH
13 (2002)

[T]he institution should require that IRB members report annually any personal and significant financial interests that might reasonably appear to be affected by the scope of their responsibilities. These reports should include significant financial interests in sponsors of human subjects research when the IRB member is aware that the company in question is or may become a sponsor of human subjects research at the institution. The reports of IRB members should be reviewed by the institution's [conflict of interest] committee, which should apply a presumption against significant individual financial interests in an investigational product or a commercial sponsor of the institution's human subject research, and stipulate that any member should recuse himself or herself in any such circumstance.

IRB members are required by federal regulations to recuse themselves from voting upon or participating in any deliberations concerning protocols in which they have conflicting interests. Institutional policies should reiterate that disclosure and recusal are required on a protocol-by-protocol basis for all IRB members. Institutions should require the IRB administrator to poll the IRB about potentially conflicting financial interests prior to the start of each meeting and to document the members' responses in the meeting minutes. Institutions should consider providing the IRB administrator with a list of the research sponsors in which one or more members hold a significant financial interest, to ensure that recusal occurs when necessary.

NOTES AND QUESTIONS

1. A group of researchers at Harvard Medical School sent questionnaires to medical school faculty members during 2001-2002 to find out if there are any special characteristics of those who serve as IRB members. One of their findings

was that about half (47%) of the faculty members who served on IRBs had served as consultants "to industry" within the past three years. This percentage was somewhat higher than the percentage (37%) for the faculty members who did not serve on IRBs, although the difference was not statistically significant. Regarding that finding, the study authors noted:

> Our previous research among life science faculty members has shown that associations with industry are related to scientific behavior, including delays in publishing research and trade secrecy. It is possible that relationships with companies could affect members' IRB-related activities and attitudes as well. This finding may be a cause for some concern given that faculty members serve as leaders on the IRB. The fact that almost half serve as consultants to industry (most of whom are likely compensated for their services) certainly raises the issue of financial conflicts of interest.

Eric G. Campbell et al., *Characteristics of Medical School Faculty Members Serving on Institutional Review Boards: Results of a National Survey*, 78 ACADEMIC MED. 831 (2003). What, if anything, should be done about this situation? Should faculty members who serve as consultants to industry be banned from sitting on IRBs? Should they be prevented from voting on all studies that are industry-sponsored, even if they are not serving as a consultant to the particular company sponsoring the study? Should nothing be done?

2. As noted above, federal regulations prohibit IRB members from participating in discussions or voting on protocols in which they have a conflict of interest, except to provide information requested by the IRB. However, the regulations do not specifically prohibit these members from being present when an IRB discusses or votes on the protocol. Should there be such a prohibition?

§ 5.04 DISCLOSING CONFLICTS OF INTEREST TO SUBJECTS

RECOMMENDATIONS ON
DEPARTMENT OF HEALTH AND HUMAN SERVICES' DRAFT INTERIM GUIDANCE ON FINANCIAL RELATIONSHIPS IN CLINICAL RESEARCH NATIONAL HUMAN RESEARCH PROTECTIONS ADVISORY COMMITTEE (NHRPAC)
AUGUST 23, 2001

One of the most difficult issues in establishing a conflicts of interest process is the extent to which troubling financial relationships or possible conflicts, once identified, must be disclosed to research subjects, or potential subjects, in the informed consent process. . . . NHRPAC's general sense has been that research subjects should be informed of "real" problems relating to financial relationships and conflicts of interest, but should not be burdened with information about problems that are arcane or speculative. . . .

How to tell patients in a meaningful and understandable way about these relevant financial relationships and conflicts, and about potential risks flowing from them, is a largely undefined process with no clear precedents. A very real risk here is that if presented with confusing, chaotic, and detailed but undigested information about investments and compensation and money flows, patients could be utterly confused, and their ability to make reasoned choices impaired rather than assisted. Another real risk is that patients may defer from participating in research if troubling financial relationships are exaggerated or ways of managing them are unclear. . . .

NHRPAC would advise that in a research protocol in which an actual conflict of interest has been identified in the financial disclosure process, subjects could be advised in the informed consent process (and/or in the form itself) of the possible conflict and the nature of that conflict, with the terms, conditions and extent of disclosure calibrated by the conflict of interest committee and the IRB to correspond to the level of the risk that the possible conflict poses. Conflict management strategies should also be disclosed, so that research subjects have general knowledge of the conflict of interest identification and management processes, and how these apply to the study in which the subject is considering her enrollment. Conflicts management strategies may include, for example, mandating independent monitoring of informed consent, outside evaluation of subjects' eligibility for a trial, independent review of adverse events reports and research records, and peer review of data analysis and interpretation. The method of disclosure of specific financial interests and any specific conflict management strategies may be referred to as "specific" disclosure of conflict of interest.

Alternatively, in cases in which the possible conflict of interest may be less tangible and more speculative, the IRB and the conflict of interest committee may choose to advise the potential research subjects in a more generic way. . . . This initial disclosure, however, would not contain, in this scenario, specific mention of where the possible conflict resides or of actual financial interests held. This method of disclosure may be referred to as "generic" disclosure.

A form of disclosure could include the following:

> Every research scientist and physician at Mercy Hospital, and Mercy Hospital itself, must disclose significant financial interests in private companies or entities that may be related to this research study. Our Hospital committees have reviewed this information and have concluded that there are some financial relationships between the researchers or Mercy itself on the one hand, and the company that is funding this research, on the other. [Insert some degree of specific disclosure here, if warranted, as to the interests and the conflicts management strategies.] However, after considering this information, our

Hospital committees believe that there are no conflicts of interest that [or no conflicts of interest that, when taken with the conflicts management strategies discussed above] will influence the way you will be treated in this study or the way in which this research study will be conducted. If you would like to have more information about Mercy Hospital's review process in general, or in regard to this study, please ask the researchers or the research coordinator, and they will assist you.

A minority of NHRPAC preferred that all actual relevant financial relationships (whether for the investigator or the institution) be disclosed in writing as part of the informed consent process, in order to provide complete transparency to research subjects. A majority, however, decline that approach, for several reasons. First, such an approach could well result in informed consent forms being made even more complicated than they are already. . . . Second, under the scheme proposed by NHRPAC, institutions and researchers would be required to actively disclose and evaluate financial relationships in all research activities, regardless of source of funding, and to manage all possible conflicts or troubling financial relationships identified; and, in fact, research should not, in NHRPAC's proposed and preferred approach, be allowed to proceed *unless the actual risks from troubling financial relationships have already been reduced to a level below "significant" through conflicts management strategies*. Therefore, under NHRPAC's approach, disclosure of troubling financial relationships or actual conflicts to research subjects is not the preferred methodology for protecting subjects . . . . Finally, a NHRPAC majority felt that an unvarying requirement that researchers' personal and private financial information be published in widely circulated and easily available informed consent forms is not respectful of researchers' own privacy interests, and should be employed only when the IRB and the conflict of interest committee think that such disclosure is indicated.

NOTES AND QUESTIONS

1. An early case regarding the duty of a physician to disclose research-related conflicts of interest is *Moore v. Regents of the University of California*, 793 P.2d 479 (Cal. 1990). In that case, a physician had used tissue removed from a patient to create a marketable product that was worth millions, and never told the patient that the research was taking place. The California Supreme Court concluded that this situation created a conflict of interest, and that the physician had a duty to disclose the conflict. The case is discussed in greater detail in Chapter 17, at page 729.

2. Following the approach recommended by NHRPAC, what should have been disclosed in the consent form for the gene study in which Jesse Gelsinger died? Write the text of such a disclosure paragraph.

3. The NHRPAC document gives a suggested paragraph for use when the conflict of interest is "less tangible" and "more speculative." What situations

does it have in mind where that suggested paragraph would be appropriate, as opposed to a more explicit disclosure? What do you think of this approach?

4. Suppose the consent form in the gene study in which Jesse Gelsinger died had fully disclosed that Dr. Wilson and the University of Pennsylvania owned millions of dollars of stock in the company that owned rights to the treatment being studied. How should a prospective subject use that information in deciding whether or not to enroll in the study? Might the fact that a company has been founded, with stock worth millions of dollars, indicate that the treatments being studied are considered very promising? Should a subject be troubled when offered enrollment in a study where there are no conflicts of interest because no one thinks it is worth investing money in the investigator's idea?

5. In a survey of 5,500 individuals who indicated a willingness to participate in clinical trials, sixty-four percent said that knowing about individual and institutional financial conflicts of interest was "extremely" or "very" important, and eighty-seven percent said that such information should be disclosed as part of the informed consent process. The respondents were given seven hypothetical studies involving conflicts of interest and asked whether knowledge of the conflicts would lead them to decline participation. A majority of respondents said that they would be willing to participate in all of the studies, but in some of the situations a large minority said that they would be reluctant to enroll. *See* S.Y.H. Kim et. al., *Potential Research Participants' Views Regarding Researcher and Institutional Financial Conflicts of Interest*, 30 J. MED. ETHICS 73 (2004).

6. How do the NHRPAC recommendations apply to the "per capita payments" discussed earlier in this chapter? Should the existence of such payments always be disclosed to subjects in the consent form? Or should they be disclosed only if the amount of the payment is large enough — and if that is the case, what should the cut-off amount be? If there is disclosure, should the consent form specifically mention what amount the researcher is getting for enrolling the subject? If you decide to disclose specific amounts, how do you deal with the complication that portions of these payments may reimburse the researcher for expenses they may incur in conducting the study? *See, e.g.*, Jammi N. Rao & J.J. Sant Cassia, *Ethics of Undisclosed Payments to Doctors Recruiting Patients in Clinical Trials*, 325 BRITISH MED. J. 36 (2002).

PART II
REVIEWING RESEARCH PROPOSALS: GENERAL CONSIDERATIONS

Chapter 6

RISK-BENEFIT ASSESSMENT

Virtually all research involves some degree of risk. The goal for IRBs is not to eliminate the risks of research, but to ensure that the risks have been minimized to the extent reasonably possible and that any remaining risks are justified by the benefits the study is likely to achieve. Identifying and weighing the risks and benefits of research are among the most important, and most challenging, components of IRB review. As you read this chapter, consider whether existing laws and policies provide appropriate standards and procedures for IRBs as they engage in the process of risk-benefit assessment. If they do not, consider how those laws and policies might be improved.

§ 6.01 THE ROLE OF RISK-BENEFIT ASSESSMENT IN RESEARCH OVERSIGHT

45 C.F.R. § 46.111(a)(1)-(2): CRITERIA FOR IRB APPROVAL OF RESEARCH

These provisions are reproduced in Appendix A, at page A-10. Please review them before proceeding.

THE NUREMBERG CODE

6. The degree of risk to be taken should never exceed that determined by the humanitarian importance of the problem to be solved by the experiment.

DECLARATION OF HELSINKI: ETHICAL PRINCIPLE FOR RESEARCH INVOLVING HUMAN SUBJECTS WORLD MEDICAL ASSOCIATION

16. Every medical research project involving human subjects should be preceded by careful assessment of predictable risks and burdens in comparison with foreseeable benefits to the subject or to others. This does not preclude the participation of healthy volunteers in medical research. The design of all studies should be publicly available.

17. Physicians should abstain from engaging in research projects involving human subjects unless they are confident that the risks involved have been adequately assessed and can be satisfactorily managed. Physicians should cease any

investigation if the risks are found to outweigh the potential benefits or if there is conclusive proof of positive and beneficial results.

18. Medical research involving human subjects should only be conducted if the importance of the objective outweighs the inherent risks and burdens to the subject. This is especially important when the human subjects are healthy volunteers.

NOTES AND QUESTIONS

1. Is risk-benefit assessment purely a utilitarian exercise, or are some risks so objectionable that they should never be authorized, regardless of the benefits a study is likely to achieve? In this regard, consider the Nuremberg Code's fifth principle: "No experiment should be conducted when there is an *a priori* reason to believe that death or disabling injury will occur; except perhaps in those experiments where the experimental physicians also serve as subjects." What types of studies might this provision preclude? Without this provision, might such studies be permissible under the sixth principle of the Code, quoted above?

2. How risky is biomedical research? Robert Levine argues that "it is not particularly hazardous to be a research subject," despite the common assumption to the contrary. In one study of participants in "nontherapeutic research," for example, "the risk of being disabled either temporarily or permanently was substantially less than that of being similarly harmed in an accident." ROBERT J. LEVINE, ETHICS AND REGULATION OF CLINICAL RESEARCH 2D ED. 39-40 (1988). Nonetheless, some studies can be quite risky. A 2001 review of three clinical trials involving critically ill patients found that 150 more deaths occurred among subjects receiving the experimental interventions than among subjects in the control groups, and that "[a]s many as one-half of these deaths were in excess of those needed to show that the treatment was ineffective or harmful at accepted thresholds for significance." Bradley D. Freeman et al., *Safeguarding Patients in Clinical Trials with High Mortality Rates*, 164 AM. J. RESPIRATORY CRITICAL CARE MED. 190 (2001).

3. What is the relationship between risk assessment and informed consent? Is it appropriate for IRBs to disapprove protocols because of their own determination that the risks are excessive, or should their role be limited to ensuring that the risks have been minimized to the extent reasonably possible and that prospective subjects are adequately informed about the risks — leaving the ultimate determination of whether the risks are acceptable to the subjects themselves? For competing views on this question, compare ROBERT M. VEATCH, THE PATIENT AS PARTNER: A THEORY OF HUMAN-EXPERIMENTATION ETHICS 56 (1987) ("If the right of self-determination for the competent, non-institutionalized adult is taken seriously, the instances when that right should be compromised on paternalistic grounds will be extremely limited if not non-existent.")

with Richard W. Garnett, *Why Informed Consent? Human Experimentation and the Ethics of Autonomy*, 36 CATHOLIC LAW. 455, 488 (1996) ("Dignity may require respecting autonomy-as-free-choice in some circumstances, but at the same time it may also require objective limits on practices, behaviors, procedures, and institutions which are in themselves inconsistent with the dignity of persons."). Do the federal regulations resolve this question?

§ 6.02 IDENTIFYING RISKS

[A] The Concept of Risk

The word "risk" is used to convey two interrelated concepts. First, it refers to the harmful outcomes that might result from a particular activity, as in the statement, "Death is an inherent risk of the procedure." Second, it refers to the likelihood that such an outcome will occur, as in the statement, "The procedure carries a 5 percent risk of death." A risk may be considered significant either because the nature of the feared outcome is especially serious, because the likelihood of that outcome is particularly high, or both. Thus, a relatively low likelihood of dying might be considered a significant risk, as might a much higher chance of experiencing a less severe outcome, such as short-term pain.

As the following excerpt suggests, the concept of risk is inherently imprecise, a fact that significantly complicates the process of IRB review.

Trust, Emotion, Sex, Politics, and Science: Surveying the Risk Assessment Battlefield
Paul Slovic
1997 U. CHI. LEGAL F. 59

Attempts to manage risk must confront the question: "What is risk?" The dominant conception views risk as "the chance of injury, damage, or loss." The probabilities and consequences of adverse events are assumed to be produced by physical and natural processes in ways that can be objectively quantified by risk assessment. Much social science analysis rejects this notion, arguing instead that risk is inherently subjective. In this view, risk does not exist "out there," independent of our minds and cultures, waiting to be measured. Instead, human beings have invented the concept [of] risk to help them understand and cope with the dangers and uncertainties of life. Although these dangers are real, there is no such thing as "real risk" or "objective risk." The nuclear engineer's probabilistic risk estimate for a nuclear accident or the toxicologist's quantitative estimate of a chemical's carcinogenic risk are both based on theoretical models, whose structure is subjective and assumption-laden, and whose inputs are dependent on judgment. As we shall see, nonscientists have their own models, assumptions, and subjective assessment techniques (intuitive risk assessments), which are sometimes very different from the scientists' models.

One way in which subjectivity permeates risk assessments is in the dependence of such assessments on judgments at every stage of the process, from the initial structuring of a risk problem to deciding which endpoints or consequences to include in the analysis, identifying and estimating exposures, choosing dose response relationships, and so on. For example, even the apparently simple task of choosing a risk measure for a well-defined endpoint such as human fatalities is surprisingly complex and judgmental. . . . Each way of summarizing deaths embodies its own set of values. For example, "reduction in life expectancy" treats deaths of young people as more important than deaths of older people, who have less life expectancy to lose. Simply counting fatalities treats deaths of the old and young as equivalent; it also treats as equivalent deaths that come immediately after mishaps and deaths that follow painful and debilitating disease. . . . One can easily imagine a range of arguments to justify different kinds of unequal weightings for different kinds of deaths, but to arrive at any selection requires a value judgment concerning which deaths one considers most undesirable. To treat the deaths as equal also involves a value judgment. . . .

Numerous research studies have demonstrated that different (but logically equivalent) ways of presenting the same risk information can lead to different evaluations and decisions. One dramatic example of this comes from a study by McNeil, Pauker, Sox, and Tversky, who asked people to imagine that they had lung cancer and had to choose between two therapies, surgery or radiation. The two therapies were described in some detail. Then, one group of subjects was presented with the cumulative probabilities of surviving for varying lengths of time after the treatment. A second group of subjects received the same cumulative probabilities framed in terms of dying rather than surviving (for instance, instead of being told that 68 percent of those having surgery will have survived after one year, they were told that 32 percent will have died). Framing the statistics in terms of dying changed the percentage of subjects choosing radiation therapy over surgery from 18 percent to 44 percent. The effect was as strong for physicians as for laypersons. . . .

[R]esearch has also shown that the public has a broad conception of risk, qualitative and complex, that incorporates considerations such as uncertainty, dread, catastrophic potential, controllability, equity, risk to future generations, and so forth, into the risk equation. In contrast, experts' perceptions of risk are not closely related to these dimensions or the characteristics that underlie them. Instead, studies show that experts tend to see riskiness as synonymous with expected mortality, consistent with the definition given above and consistent with the ways that risks tend to be characterized in risk assessments. As a result of these different perspectives, many conflicts over "risk" may result from experts and laypeople having different definitions of the concept. In this light, it is not surprising that expert recitations of "risk statistics" often do little to change people's attitudes and perceptions. . . .

Given the complex and subjective nature of risk, it should not surprise us that many interesting and provocative things occur when people judge risks. Recent studies have shown that factors such as gender, race, political worldviews, affiliation, emotional affect, and trust are strongly correlated with risk judgments. Equally important is that these factors influence the judgments of experts as well as judgments of laypersons. . . .

Whoever controls the definition of risk controls the rational solution to the problem at hand. If you define risk one way, then one option will rise to the top as the most cost-effective, or the safest, or the best. If you define it another way, perhaps incorporating qualitative characteristics and other contextual factors, you will likely get a different ordering of your action solutions. Defining risk is thus an exercise in power.

NOTES AND QUESTIONS

1. Social science research suggests that numerous cognitive biases affect individuals' judgments about risk. The McNeil study summarized in the previous excerpt is an example of what is commonly described as the "framing bias," which states that the manner in which risk information is presented will affect individuals' assessment of the significance of those risks. Another common bias is the "availability heuristic," which leads people to evaluate the riskiness of activities based on information that is easily called to mind (or "available"), even if that information is not representative of the activity's true risk. For example, reading about a recent airplane crash tends to increase people's perception of the riskiness of air travel, even if they know that airplane crashes are extremely rare. For a thorough discussion of these and other cognitive biases, see JUDGMENT UNDER UNCERTAINTY: HEURISTICS AND BIASES (D. Kahneman et al., eds., 1982) and THE PERCEPTION OF RISK (Paul Slovic ed., 2000). What are the implications of these cognitive biases for IRB review?

2. You have been asked to identify members for a new IRB. Given Slovic's observations about the factors influencing individuals' risk perceptions, what type of people would you want to select? Does Slovic's analysis suggest that the membership requirements for IRBs set forth in 45 C.F.R. § 46.107 should be modified? If so, how?

[B] Risks to Research Subjects

[1] Introduction: A Typology of Research Risks

Institutional Review Board Assessment of Risks and Benefits Associated with Research
in 2 NATIONAL BIOETHICS ADVISORY COMMISSION, ETHICAL AND POLICY ISSUES IN RESEARCH INVOLVING HUMAN PARTICIPANTS
Ernest D. Prentice & Bruce G. Gordon
L-1 (2001)

In general, risks may be categorized as physical, psychological, social, or economic. Another type of risk, which is less commonly associated with research in general, is legal risk. Risks of any of these types may occur in the setting of various biomedical or behavioral research projects, but physical risks, and to a lesser extent psychological risks, are most common in biomedical studies, while social, economic, and legal risks are often limited to behavioral or social science research. IRBs should recognize that these categories of risk are somewhat fluid in that a given risk may fall into two or more of the categories or multiple types of risk may be present in a single study.

Physical Risks

Physical risks are usually thought of as the possibility of pain, suffering, or physical injury. Such harms may be easy to identify in certain biomedical studies, such as phase III clinical trials of antihypertensive drugs, or may be yet unknown, as in the case of phase I dose and toxicity finding studies. Nonetheless, the pharmacology of a drug, and its similarity to other drugs, often provides enough information to predict some potential harms with reasonable certainty. Similarly, physical harms associated with other research interventions are often clear, e.g., the risk of ecchymosis with venipuncture, pain associated with lumbar puncture, myocardial infarction related to a maximal exercise treadmill test, sore throat as a consequence of bronchoscopy.

Physical risks may arise from withholding or withdrawal of effective therapy. For example, subjects in a trial of a new oral hypoglycemic drug may suffer harm if the new drug is not as effective as their standard therapy. Similarly, evaluation of new drugs often requires discontinuation of standard therapy followed by a so-called "wash-out period" during which time the subject receives no treatment. Although these periods are usually short, they are not without risk. Physical risk also includes the possibility that a subject may experience discomfort or mere inconvenience which may not rise to the level of an actual harm, such as pain or injury. These risks can easily be overlooked during the process of risk assessment. For example, the requirement to lie still in an MRI machine for an extended period of time during an imaging study may have associated discomfort or boredom for some subjects. A cardiac device study may require the subject to wear a Holter monitor for 48 hours, which would more than likely represent inconvenience. These less obvious risks should be considered by IRBs during their review.

Psychological Risks

Psychological risks may be readily apparent, although they are often less quantifiable. For example, withdrawal of antidepressant therapy in a wash-out period, or administration of placebo to subjects in a trial of a new therapy for depression may precipitate an episode of depression. Research involving genetic testing may have psychological risks associated with disclosure of a subject's likelihood of developing a disease for which there is no treatment or cure such as Huntington's chorea. Administration of a sensitive survey to adult subjects regarding domestic violence may provoke feelings of guilt, distress, and anger. There may also be a concomitant risk of precipitating further incidents of spousal abuse.

In some studies, the generation of psychological distress is expected and may be an end point of the study itself. A classical case that illustrates this point would be the "Obedience to Authority" experiments conducted by Milgram. [For a description of these studies, see Chapter 1, at page 48.] The risks of such a study would not be acceptable today under contemporary ethical standards but deception is still a fairly common component of behavioral research and, accordingly, there may be risks which must be considered by the IRB.

Some psychological risks may be more nebulous or not even related to the research procedure *per se*. For example, a prospective subject may be asked to donate allogeneic bone marrow to be used in an experimental manner to treat a patient with AIDS. He or she, however, may feel guilty for not wanting to participate in the research, especially when such a refusal is associated with a risk of harm to another party. Although the individual being asked to donate bone marrow is not yet a research subject, the psychological harm, i.e., feelings of guilt, is certainly associated with the process of consent for the study. IRBs, therefore, should be cognizant of this kind of risk.

Social Risks

Participants in research may experience social risks, that is, risk of harm to a person in the context of his or her social interactions with others. Examples include the risk of stigmatization as a result of testing positive for HIV, or the risk that genetic studies will disclose nonpaternity. Social risks are particularly associated with studies of private aspects of human behavior. . . . Indeed, the possibility of a breach of confidentiality is often the most significant risk of social science research. The degree of risk, however, is related to the sensitivity of the research data from the subject's perspective and the likelihood that unauthorized individuals could gain access to the data. In other words, discovery or disclosure of meaningless albeit personal information about a subject is certainly a "wrong" but does not rise to the level of a "harm." While the IRB should be more concerned about the possibility that a subject could suffer a harm, nonetheless, the Board should not dismiss a potential wrong.

Economic Risks

Research may pose economic risks to subjects. Participants in "high tech" clinical research may incur financial obligations for treatment which are significantly higher than those associated with standard therapy and, ultimately, no health benefit is realized. In some studies, subjects may need to take time off from work, or pay costs of transportation to the study center, which could impose a significant economic hardship. Subjects may also be exposed to the possibility of loss of insurability, associated with diagnosis of a chronic or life-threatening disease. Economic risk may even extend to a research participant's livelihood. For example, sociologic studies of employer-employee relationships may carry the risk of loss of employment if confidentiality is breached.

Legal Risks

Participation in research may present legal risks to the subject. For example, one IRB was asked to approve a study of paroled felons, which assessed the effect of time since release from prison on the incidence of repeat offenses. Subjects were asked to complete a survey of crimes committed three months and one year after release. The surveys contained linked codes so the responses of each subject could be compared at the two time points. Had the investigator been compelled by judicial order to provide data with subject identifiers to the court, the study participants would have incurred significant legal risk. Similar risks can easily be incurred in studies of possession and use of illicit drugs, sexual or physical abuse, or workplace theft. As Wolf points out, assuring confidentiality of research records may require the investigator and the IRB to be aware of various legal protections, such as Certificates of Confidentiality, for sensitive research data. [For a discussion of certificates of confidentiality, see Chapter 10, at page 452.]

NOTES AND QUESTIONS

1. Do you agree that the risks associated with the Milgram study "would not be acceptable today under contemporary ethical standards"? What, exactly, were the risks involved in that study? How would you evaluate their significance?

2. Risks to subjects should not be considered in isolation from one another. In some cases, "the interaction between . . . two risks is likely to be greater than the sum of their parts." NEW YORK STATE DEPARTMENT OF HEALTH WORKGROUP ON IRB GUIDELINES, SAFEGUARDING HEALTHY RESEARCH SUBJECTS: PROTECTING VOLUNTEERS FROM HARM (1999) (offering the example of "a Phase One trial of two new drugs expected to potentiate each other in preventing replication of a

dangerous virus," in which "there is a possibility that both drugs together could aggravate their known side effect of reducing the subject's white blood cells, thereby reducing immunity"). IRBs also should be aware that some subjects may be participating in multiple studies simultaneously or sequentially, which can increase the risk of otherwise routine interventions, such as X rays. *See id.* (urging IRBs to "ensure that researchers ensure the cumulative risks involved in utilizing subjects whose occupation is, in part or whole, being a research subject").

3. In addition to the specific risks described above, there is a more general risk that exists in all human studies – the risk of the unknown. *See* Robert J. Levine, *Uncertainty in Clinical Research*, 16 L. MED. & HEALTH CARE 174 (1988). For example, any time a relatively new drug is given to someone, there is a risk that some never-before-seen side effect might occur. Risks to future generations are especially difficult to predict, even when preclinical animal studies have been performed. Consider the case of DES, discussed in Chapter 1, at page 36. The full risks of this drug did not became apparent until the daughters of the women who took the drug entered reproductive age, when they began to experience higher-than-usual rates of cancer and reproductive problems.

4. In addition to risks that are unknown because they have not yet been discovered, sometimes even known risk information may be unavailable because it has been deliberately withheld. For example, in 2004, a controversy erupted when it was discovered that drug manufacturers had chosen not to publish studies suggesting that antidepressants increase the risk of suicidal ideation in children. In response, a group of leading medical journals agreed that it would no longer publish the results of any clinical trial unless the trial was registered at its inception in a public database. Such a database would make it more difficult for researchers and sponsors to hide the results of studies that produce negative results. *See* Catherine De Angelis et al., *Clinical Trial Registration: A Statement from the International Committee of Medical Journal Editors*, 351 NEW ENG. J. MED. 1250 (2004).

5. The IRB on which you serve is considering whether to approve a study sponsored by a large pharmaceutical company. All of the investigators affiliated with the study have agreed that they will not publish any information about the study without first obtaining the sponsor's approval. Should the IRB approve the study with this restriction in place? See Frank Davidoff et al., *Sponsorship, Authorship, and Accountability*, 345 NEW ENG. J. MED. 825 (2001) (joint statement by editors of medical journals indicating that they "will not review or publish articles based on studies that are conducted under conditions that allow the sponsor to have sole control of the data or to withold publication").

6. In his article, *The Ethical Analysis of Risk*, Charles Weijer presents the following two hypothetical cases:

    1. Several hypnotically suggestible, but otherwise healthy college students are randomly selected to receive one of three hypnotic sug-

gestions: partial deafness without awareness of the cause; partial deafness with awareness of the cause; and no deafness but an ear itch. The hypothesis is that people in the first group, as compared with those in the other two groups, will demonstrate more symptoms of paranoia. Subjects are assessed with a variety of measures, including psychometric scales and a scoring of observed behavior. After being evaluated, the subjects are hypnotized again, debriefed at the end of the study, and reassessed after one month.

2. The study involves the administration of a pencil-and-paper questionnaire to 400 Minneapolis high school students during regularly scheduled health classes. The survey seeks to document attitudes and behaviors related to HIV prevention. Accordingly, the adolescent participants are asked whether they are sexually active, what types of sexual activity they have experienced (e.g., oral, vaginal, or anal intercourse), and the sex(es) of their partners.

Charles Weijer, *The Ethical Analysis of Risk*, 28 J. L. MED. & ETHICS 344 (2000). For each of these cases, identify the risks to subjects who agree to participate in the research.

[2] Distinguishing the Risks of Research from the Risks of Interventions That Would Otherwise Be Performed

Subjects in clinical research are exposed to a variety of interventions. Some will receive investigational drugs or undergo innovative medical procedures, while others may receive a placebo or interventions that reflect the existing standard of care. All subjects are likely to undergo interventions for purposes of diagnosis, monitoring, or data collection, only some of which would be performed on patients receiving ordinary medical treatment. While all of these interventions are likely to have risks, only the risks *of the research* are relevant to the IRB's evaluation of the protocol.

IRB GUIDEBOOK Chapter 3A
U.S. DEPARTMENT OF HEALTH AND HUMAN SERVICES,
OFFICE FOR PROTECTION FROM RESEARCH RISKS
(1993)

In the process of determining what constitutes a risk, only the risks that may result from the research, as distinguished from those associated with therapies subjects would undergo even if not participating in research, should be considered. For example, if the research is designed to measure the behavioral results of physical interventions performed for therapeutic reasons (e.g., effects on memory of brain surgery performed for the relief of epilepsy), then only the risks presented by the memory tests should be considered when the IRB performs its risk/benefit analysis. It is possible for the risks of the research to be minimal even when the therapeutic procedure presents more than minimal risk. IRBs should recognize, however, that distinguishing therapeutic from research activities can sometimes require very fine line drawing. Before eliminating an activity from consideration in its risk/benefit analysis, the IRB should be certain that the activity truly constitutes therapy and not research.

It is important to recognize that the potential risks faced by research subjects may be posed by design features employed to assure valid results as well as by the particular interventions or maneuvers that may be performed in the course of the research. Subjects participating in a study whose research design involves random assignment to treatment groups face the chance that they may not receive the treatment that turns out to be more efficacious. Subjects participating in a double-masked study take the risk that the information necessary for individual treatment might not be available to the proper persons when needed. In behavioral, social, and some biomedical research, the methods for gathering information may pose the added risk of invasion of privacy and possible violations of confidentiality. Many risks of research are the risks inherent in the methodologies of gathering and analyzing data, although the more obvious risks may be those posed by particular interventions and procedures performed during the course of research.

NOTES AND QUESTIONS

1. How will the IRB know when one or more of the treatment groups include "therapies subjects would undergo even if not participating in research"? Should the IRB simply take the word of the principal investigator? Is it required to conduct its own independent review of the literature to determine what constitutes the current standard of care, or to solicit the opinion of an outside expert, assuming none of the members qualifies as an expert in the area? (In answering these questions, recall the FDA's criticisms of the Johns Hopkins' IRB regarding the study in which Ellen Roche died. *See* Chapter 4, at page 182.)

2. Even when a study is comparing two standard interventions, each of which is routinely offered to patients outside of research, the risks to subjects are likely to be greater than those faced by patients receiving the identical interventions outside of research.

Ordinarily, treatments are determined by patients' physicians based on individualized considerations of what would be most likely to help a particular patient. This process is short-circuited in controlled clinical trials by randomization. . . . Subjects in randomized trials also lose the right to select among treatments that, even if their main effects are identical, may have significantly different side effects. Or they may lose the ability to trade off potential efficacy in main effect against the severity of side effects. . . . The constraints of a scientific protocol – the document that sets down what therapeutic interventions are and are not permissible in the conduct of a particular study — may also compromise individual decision making. In ordinary practice physicians might decide to raise or lower the dose of a medication, discharge a patient from the hospital, or add or delete adjunctive treatments. The rigidities of a protocol may limit a physician's ability to take these steps, regardless of patients' desires — short of dropping patients from the study, which neither physician-researchers nor patients may want to do. . . . Finally, double-blind procedures, in which both patient-subjects and clinicians are kept in the dark about which group patients have been assigned to and what treatment they are receiving, are often considered essential to preventing bias in treatment or evaluation. In these situations subjects are at risk when information is unavailable to help physicians monitor a clinical course or diagnose adverse reactions.

JESSICA W. BERG ET AL., INFORMED CONSENT: LEGAL THEORY AND CLINICAL PRACTICE 2D ED. 281-83 (2001). How significant are these sorts of risks? Are they likely to be greater in some types of studies than in others?

[3] The Concept of Clinical Equipoise

As the previous section suggests, the process of randomization can itself be seen as a risk of clinical research, because it requires subjects to accept treatments according to random chance rather than an individualized assessment of their particular needs. In a seminal essay on research ethics, Charles Fried (who later became United States Solicitor General under President Ronald Reagan) argued that, even when both arms of a study involve standard medical treatment, the process of randomization sacrifices subjects' best interests:

Consider, for instance, the choice between medical and surgical intervention for acute unstable angina pectoris. I would suppose that a group of patients could be so defined that the risks and benefits of the two available courses of action were quite evenly balanced. But, when a particular patient is involved, with a particular set of symptoms, a particular diagnostic picture and a particular set of values and preferences . . . then one may doubt how often a physician carefully going into all of these particularities would conclude that the risks and benefits are truly equal. . . .

Perhaps, after all, this may happen, and may happen often enough to justify a significant number of RCT's [randomized controlled trials]. But before one concludes that the dilemma has really been dissolved in these cases, one must be quite careful to determine whether the condition of equipoise obtains just because it has been previously decided not to inquire too closely into the particular circumstances of the particular patient, proceeding rather on the balance of risks and benefits as they pertain to a larger group. One must be careful of this, because if the equipoise appears as a result of this failure of inquiry, then the sacrifice has indeed taken place, but only at another level, in a different way. One might say that the individual patient has perhaps not been sacrificed in the crude sense that the best available treatment has been withheld from him, but he has been sacrificed in that for the sake of the experimental design his interest in having his particular circumstances investigated has been sacrificed. But this amounts to the same thing.

CHARLES FRIED, MEDICAL EXPERIMENTATION: PERSONAL INTEGRITY AND SOCIAL POLICY 52-53 (1974).

In a now-classic essay, Dr. Benjamin Freedman argued that the randomized clinical trial need not conflict with the therapeutic interests of individual subjects. In the following excerpt from that essay, Dr. Freedman responds to the claim that randomization is unethical whenever there is some evidence supporting the use of one intervention over another.

Equipoise and the Ethics of Clinical Research
Benjamin Freedman
317 NEW ENG. J. MED. 141 (1987)

[W]e need to recall the basic reason for conducting clinical trials: there is a current or imminent conflict in the clinical community over what treatment is preferred for patients in a defined population P. The standard treatment is A, but some evidence suggests that B will be superior (because of its effectiveness or its reduction of undesirable side effects, or for some other reason). . . . Or there is a split in the clinical community, with some clinicians favoring A and others favoring B. Each side recognizes that the opposing side has evidence to support its position, yet each still thinks that overall its own view is correct. There exists (or, in the case of a novel therapy, there may soon exist) an honest, professional disagreement among expert clinicians about the preferred treatment. A clinical trial is instituted with the aim of resolving this dispute.

At this point, a state of "clinical equipoise" exists. There is no consensus within the expert clinical community about the comparative merits of the alternatives to be tested. We may state the formal conditions under which such a trial would be ethical as follows: at the start of the trial, there must be a state of clinical equipoise regarding the merits of the regimens to be tested, and the trial must be designed in such a way as to make it reasonable to expect that, if it is successfully concluded, clinical equipoise will be disturbed. In other words, the results of a successful clinical trial should be convincing enough to resolve the dispute among clinicians.

A state of clinical equipoise is consistent with a decided treatment preference on the part of the investigators. They must simply recognize that their less-favored treatment is preferred by colleagues whom they consider to be responsible and competent. Even if the interim results favor the preference of the investigators, treatment B, clinical equipoise persists as long as those results are too weak to influence the judgment of the community of clinicians, because of limited sample size, unresolved possibilities of side effects, or other factors. (This judgment can necessarily be made only by those who know the interim results — whether a data-monitoring committee or the investigators.) [Data monitoring committees are discussed in Chapter 11, at page 475.]

At the point when the accumulated evidence in favor of B is so strong that the committee or investigators believe no open-minded clinician informed of the results would still favor A, clinical equipoise has been disturbed. This may occur well short of the original schedule for the termination of the trial, for unexpected reasons. (Therapeutic effects or side effects may be much stronger than anticipated, for example, or a definable subgroup within population P may be recognized for which the results demonstrably disturb clinical equipoise.) Because of the arbitrary character of human judgment and persuasion, some ethical problems regarding the termination of a trial will remain. Clinical equipoise will confine these problems to unusual or extreme cases, however, and will allow us to cast persistent problems in the proper terms. For example, in the face of a strong established trend, must we continue the trial because of others' blind fealty to an arbitrary statistical bench mark?

Clearly, clinical equipoise is a far weaker — and more common — condition than theoretical equipoise. ["Theoretical equipoise," as defined by Freedman earlier in the article, refers to a "fragile" state of affairs when "overall, the evidence on behalf of two alternative treatment regimens is exactly balanced."] Is it ethical to conduct a trial on the basis of clinical equipoise, when theoretical equipoise is disturbed? Or, as Schafer and others have argued, is doing so a violation of the physician's obligation to provide patients with the best medical treatment?[4,5,14] Let us assume that the investigators have a decided preference for B but wish to conduct a trial on the grounds that clinical (not theoretical) equipoise exists. The ethics committee asks the investigators whether, if they or members of their families were within population P, they would not want to be treated with their preference, B? An affirmative answer is often thought to be fatal to the prospects for such a trial, yet the investigators answer in the affirmative. Would a trial satisfying this weaker form of equipoise be ethical?

I believe that it clearly is ethical. As Fried has emphasized,[3] competent (hence, ethical) medicine is social rather than individual in nature. Progress in medicine relies on progressive consensus within the medical and research communities. The ethics of medical practice grants no ethical or normative mean-

---

4 Marquis D. Leaving therapy to chance. Hastings Cent Rep 1983; 13(4): 40-7.

5 Schafer A. The ethics of the randomized clinical trial. N Eng J Med 1982; 307: 719-24.

14 Schafer A. The randomized clinical trial: for whose benefit? IRB: Rev. Hum Subj Res 1985; 7(2): 4-6.

3 Fried C. Medical experimentation: personal integrity and social policy. Amsterdam: North-Holland Publishing, 1974.

ing to a treatment preference, however powerful, that is based on a hunch or on anything less than evidence publicly presented and convincing to the clinical community. Persons are licensed as physicians after they demonstrate the acquisition of this professionally validated knowledge, not after they reveal a superior capacity for guessing. Normative judgments of their behavior — e.g., malpractice actions — rely on a comparison with what is done by the community of medical practitioners. Failure to follow a "treatment preference" not shared by this community and not based on information that would convince it could not be the basis for an allegation of legal or ethical malpractice. As Fried states: "[T]he conception of what is good medicine is the product of a professional consensus." By definition, in a state of clinical equipoise, "good medicine" finds the choice between A and B indifferent. . . .

The Implications of Clinical Equipoise

The theory of clinical equipoise has been formulated as an alternative to some current views on the ethics of human research. At the same time, it corresponds closely to a preanalytic concept held by many in the research and regulatory communities. Clinical equipoise serves, then, as a rational formulation of the approach of many toward research ethics; it does not so much change things as explain why they are the way they are.

Nevertheless, the precision afforded by the theory of clinical equipoise does help to clarify or reformulate some aspects of research ethics; I will mention only two.

First, there is a recurrent debate about the ethical propriety of conducting clinical trials of discredited treatments, such as Laetrile.[17] Often, substantial political pressure to conduct such tests is brought to bear by adherents of quack therapies. The theory of clinical equipoise suggests that when there is no support for a treatment regimen within the expert clinical community, the first ethical requirement of a trial — clinical equipoise — is lacking; it would therefore be unethical to conduct such a trial.

Second, Feinstein has criticized the tendency of clinical investigators to narrow excessively the conditions and hypotheses of a trial in order to ensure the validity of its results.[18] This "fastidious" approach purchases scientific manageability at the expense of an inability to apply the results to the "messy" conditions of clinical practice. The theory of clinical equipoise adds some strength to this criticism. Overly "fastidious" trials, designed to resolve some theoretical question, fail to satisfy the second ethical requirement of clinical research, since the special conditions of the trial will render it useless for influencing clinical decisions, even if it is successfully completed.

---

[17] Cowan DH. The ethics of clinical trials of ineffective therapy. IRB: Rev. Hum Subj Res 1981; 3(5): 10-1.

[18] Feinstein AR. An additional basic science for clinical medicine 4. II. The limitations of randomized trials.

The most important result of the concept of clinical equipoise, however, might be to relieve the current crisis of confidence in the ethics of clinical trials. Equipoise, properly understood, remains an ethical condition for clinical trials. It is consistent with much current practice. Clinicians and philosophers alike have been premature in calling for desperate measures to resolve problems of equipoise.

NOTES AND QUESTIONS

1. Under the federal regulations, are IRBs required to determine whether the interventions being offered in the different arms of a clinical trial are in a state of clinical equipoise? Might such an obligation be inferred from particular regulatory provisions? If such an obligation exists, what procedures should IRBs use to carry it out?

2. Deborah Hellman argues that the concept of clinical equipoise does not resolve the ethical dilemmas associated with randomization. Even when two interventions are in a state of clinical equipoise, she suggests, subjects may rationally prefer one of the interventions over the other. For example, individuals confronting a serious illness may prefer an unproven intervention that, if successful, has a chance of providing more extensive benefits than the existing standard of care, even if the new intervention may turn out not to work at all. Because individuals are unlikely to be indifferent between investigational interventions and standard treatments, she concludes, "we must recognize that the tension inherent in the use of the randomized clinical trial is real and fairly intractable. We ought not to try to evade it by offering false assurances that the interests of the individual patient in treatment are not being compromised." Deborah Hellman, *Evidence, Belief, and Action: The Failure of Equipoise to Resolve the Ethical Tension in the Randomized Clinical Trial*, 30 J. L. MED. & ETHICS 375, 378 (2002); *see also* Samuel Hellman & Deborah S. Hellman, *Of Mice But Not Men: Problems of the Randomized Clinical Trial*, 324 NEW ENG. J. MED. 1585 (1991).

3. The concept of clinical equipoise, as well as the critique of that concept offered by Hellman, rest on the assumption that "each patient must receive treatment that is best for her." Hellman, *supra* at 375. Does this assumption inappropriately conflate the ethics of research with the ethics of ordinary medical treatment? Why should we be concerned that a subject might be randomly assigned a less-than-optimal intervention, as long as the subject was informed about the risks and benefits of each arm of the study and provided informed consent to the process of randomization? Put another way, why should the risks of randomization not be treated like any other risk of a study — minimized to the extent possible, and then balanced against the expected benefits the study is expected to achieve? Consider this analysis by Robert Veatch:

Clinicians in normal clinical practice are sometimes not merely permitted but actually required to refrain from doing what they think is best for their patients. They must do so in those cases when the patient refuses to consent to the clinician's recommendations. So, similarly, clinicians are permitted to depart from the best therapeutic option in research when patients, based on their understanding and evaluation of the options, choose to be randomized. While traditional defenders of equipoise would see those departures are morally acceptable only when there is equipoise in the clinical community, a better rationale for RCTs is based on the reasonable consent of the subject. This occurs when patients are at or near what I have referred to as their personal *indifference points*. What is critical for the present discussion is that for patients to become subjects they need only be "approximately indifferent" to which treatment they get. They must be willing to intentionally forgo the treatment (if any) that they consider to be in their best interest. One good reason why they might be willing to forgo what they consider to be best is to make a contribution to science.

Robert M. Veatch, *Subject Indifference and the Justification of Placebo-Controlled Trials*, 2 AM. J. BIOETHICS, June 2002, at 12. By contrast, Kathleen Cranley Glass and Duff Waring argue, "Consent alone is an insufficient defense when a physician fails to act according to the established standard. Prospective research subjects should not be invited to consent to what by law would constitute negligence in the practice of medicine." Kathleen Cranley Glass & Duff Waring, *Effective Trial Design Need Not Conflict with Good Patient Care*, 2 AM. J. BIOETHICS, June 2002, at 25. Do you agree that offering a patient a less-than-optimal intervention outside of research would "constitute negligence in the practice of medicine," assuming the patient provides informed consent? *Cf.* Schneider v. Rivici, 817 F.2d 987 (2d Cir. 1987) (finding sufficient evidence to allow the jury to consider assumption of risk as a defense to a malpractice claim against a physician who treated a cancer patient with an approach described by some doctors as "snake oil").

4. When data accumulated during a study disturb the position of clinical equipoise that justified the study's initiation, it may be necessary to end the study early. In July 2002, for example, a large study of hormone replacement therapy in postmenopausal women was terminated early when preliminary data revealed that the drugs increased the risk of invasive breast cancer. *See* Gina Kolata, *Study Is Halted over Rise Seen in Cancer Risk*, N.Y. TIMES, July 9, 2002, at A1, col. 2. Whether preliminary results disturb the position of clinical equipoise depends on how the end points of the study have been defined. For example, in the United States, early studies of the effectiveness of zidovudine (AZT) as a treatment for early HIV infection were halted when preliminary results showed that subjects receiving AZT did not develop full-blown AIDS as quickly as subjects in the placebo control arm. However, European studies of the same medication continued because the European researchers had defined the relevant end point as death, not as the length of time of progression to AIDS.

Ultimately, the European studies found that the subjects who received AZT did not live any longer than those in the placebo-control arm. *See* Susan S. Ellenberg & Robert Temple, *Placebo-Controlled Trials and Active-Control Trials in the Evaluation of New Treatments – Part 2: Practical Issues and Specific Cases*, 133 ANNALS INTERNAL MED. 464 (2000).

[4] Clinical Equipoise and the Use of Placebo Controls

The concept of clinical equipoise is generally understood to mean that the various arms of a study not only must be in a position of equipoise vis-à-vis one another, but that they also be in a position of equipoise with respect to other interventions the subjects could receive outside of the study. Thus, the 2000 revision of the Declaration of Helsinki states, "The benefits, risks, burdens and effectiveness of a new method should be tested against those of the best current prophylactic, diagnostic, and therapeutic methods." WORLD MEDICAL ASSOCIATION, DECLARATION OF HELSINKI, ¶ 29. Taken literally, this principle suggests that placebo-controlled trials are appropriate only when no effective treatment exists for a particular condition, or when the treatments that exist are inadequate for a particular subset of patients. As the following excerpts indicate, however, such a restrictive position on the use of placebos does not enjoy universal support.

What Makes Placebo-Controlled Trials Unethical?
Franklin G. Miller & Howard Brody
2 AM. J. BIOETHICS, June 2002, at 3

Argument from Therapeutic Obligation

It is claimed that the use of placebo controls in clinical trials when proven effective treatments exist violates the duty of physicians to offer optimal medical care. Because patients who enroll in RCTs are seeking treatment, they should not be randomized to treatment known to be inferior. When existing treatments have been proven effective in previous RCTs, it is unethical to test an experimental or novel treatment against placebo, which is known to be inferior to standard treatment. Instead, new, promising treatments should be tested against standard, proven effective treatment. What makes it ethical to conduct an RCT comparing a new treatment with a standard treatment, but not with a placebo, is that experts in the clinical community are uncertain or in a state of disagreement about whether the new treatment is as good as or better than standard therapy. This state of uncertainty in the clinical community is known as "clinical equipoise." Use of placebo controls in the face of proven effective treatment violates clinical equipoise because it is already known that the placebo is inferior to standard treatment.

Underlying both clinical equipoise and the therapeutic obligation of physicians is the principle of therapeutic beneficence, central to medical ethics.

Physicians should promote the medical best interests of patients by offering optimal medical care, and the risks of prescribed treatments are justified by the potential therapeutic benefits to patients. Placebo-controlled trials of new treatments in conditions for which proven effective treatments exist contravene the principle of therapeutic beneficence. Placebo controls in this situation are contrary to the medical best interests of patients. Patients randomized to placebo forgo proven effective treatment or treatment with a novel intervention considered to be as good as or better than standard treatment. Accordingly, they are exposed to risks associated with lack of treatment that are not justified by potential medical benefits.

Critique of Argument from Therapeutic Obligation

The argument from therapeutic obligation and the principle of clinical equipoise as applied to placebo-controlled trials confuse the ethics of clinical medicine with the ethics of clinical research. Physicians in clinical practice have a duty to promote the medical best interests of patients by offering optimal medical care. In RCTs, however, physician-investigators are not offering personalized medical therapy for individual patients. Rather, they seek to answer clinically relevant scientific questions by conducting experiments that test the safety and efficacy of treatments in *groups* of patients. The process of treatment in RCTs differs radically from routine clinical practice. Treatment is selected randomly, not by an individualized assessment of what is best for a particular patient. Patient volunteers and physician-investigators often do not know who has been assigned to the experimental treatment and who to the control treatment, which may be a placebo. Protocols governing RCTs frequently restrict flexibility in dosing and use of concomitant medications. These features of research design are implemented to promote scientific validity, not to promote therapeutic benefit.

Owing to these fundamental differences in purpose and process, the ethics of clinical trials is not identical to the ethics of clinical medicine. Specifically, the obligations of physician-investigators are not the same as the obligations of physicians in routine clinical practice. Investigators have a duty to avoid exploiting research participants, not a therapeutic duty to provide optimal medical care. Accordingly, enrolling patient volunteers in placebo-controlled trials that withhold proven effective treatment is not fundamentally unethical as long as patients are not being exploited. Patients may be seeking medical benefits by enrolling in clinical trials; however, they are not being exploited if

1. they are not being exposed to excessive risks for the sake of scientific investigation; and

2. they understand that they are volunteering to participate in an experiment rather than receiving personalized medical care directed at their best interests

. . . The ethical irrelevance of the therapeutic obligation and the principle of clinical equipoise are concretely illustrated in the case of placebo-controlled trials that carry little or no risk from placebo assignment, despite withholding proven effective treatment. Consider a placebo-controlled trial of a new treatment for allergic rhinitis. There exist proven effective treatments for this condition. Nonetheless, it is difficult to see what could be morally wrong about a short-term trial comparing a novel treatment for allergic rhinitis with a placebo. Trial participants randomized to placebo may be more likely to suffer from mild to moderate discomfort associated with untreated allergic rhinitis. But individuals with this condition often forgo treatment, and short periods without treatment pose no risks to health. Many would probably consider this example to be a valid exception to an absolute prohibition of placebo-controlled trials in the face of proven effective treatments. Notice, however, the significance of recognizing an exception in this case and in comparable clinical trials. If it is ethically justifiable to conduct a placebo-controlled trial of a new treatment for allergic rhinitis, then *what counts ethically is not denial of treatment but lack of substantial risk to participants*. Furthermore, if placebo-controlled trials can be ethical when they pose low risk to research participants, then it is an open question whether they are justifiable in conditions such as depression and anxiety disorders, migraine or tension headaches, stable angina, and asthma. In patients with these conditions, randomization to placebo poses more serious risks of discomfort or temporary functional disability from lack of standard treatment but low risk of irreversible harm, provided that clinical trials implement appropriate safeguards for screening eligible participants, monitoring their condition, and withdrawing them from the trial and initiating standard treatment. . . .

The implications of adopting clinical equipoise for the ethics of clinical research in general, especially research without any prospect of medical benefit, deserve attention. If physician-investigators are subject to a therapeutic obligation in the case of clinical trials, which makes RCTs ethical only when they conform to clinical equipoise, it is puzzling that physician-investigators can ethically perform any research procedures that pose risks but no compensating therapeutic benefits to patient volunteers; for example, studies of pathophysiology that administer biopsies or lumbar punctures, or imaging procedures that use ionizing radiation. In other words, why should therapeutic beneficence govern clinical trials but not the whole of clinical research? . . .

The Argument from Scientific and Clinical Merit

It is also argued that placebo-controlled trials in the face of proven effective treatment lack scientific and clinical merit. The purpose of RCTs is to answer clinically relevant scientific questions about the safety and efficacy of treatments, with the ultimate aim of improving treatment. When proven effective treatments exist, there is no scientific or clinical value in testing a novel treatment against placebo. Instead, we want to know whether the new treatment is as good as or better than standard therapy, not whether it is better than "nothing" or no treatment.

This argument fails to come to grips with the methodological limitations of active-controlled trials, especially when they are designed to test the equivalence or "noninferiority" of an experimental and a standard treatment. There are powerful methodological considerations in favor of placebo-controlled trials both in the initial efficacy testing of experimental treatments and in the comparative evaluation of new and standard treatments. No new treatment should be introduced into clinical practice unless the expert community can be confident that it is effective. Superiority to placebo in a double-blind RCT is generally considered to be the most rigorous test of treatment efficacy. Accordingly, new treatments should be tested initially against placebo before being approved or validated, unless the use of placebo controls poses substantial risks of serious harm from withholding proven effective treatment.

In addition to their superior rigor, two-arm placebo-controlled trials generally require fewer research participants than active-controlled trials, making them more efficient. The reason for this is that the anticipated difference between the new treatment and placebo typically is greater than that between the new and standard treatments. The efficiency of placebo-controlled trials is ethically relevant because they permit rigorous testing with less cost than active-controlled trials, and they expose fewer research participants to potentially toxic or ineffective experimental treatments. How many initial placebo-controlled trials should be conducted, given the need to replicate scientific findings, and how many subjects should be included are matters of debatable judgment. From an ethical perspective, initial placebo-controlled trials of new treatments for conditions with already existing proven effective treatments should not enroll any more patient volunteers than is necessary to achieve a convincing demonstration of efficacy.

As the argument from scientific and clinical merit correctly asserts, once a new treatment has been shown to be better than placebo, it is important to evaluate its comparative efficacy by testing it against an existing standard treatment in an RCT. Nevertheless, there remain strong methodological reasons for including placebo controls in many trials comparing new and standard treatments in disorders with high rates of placebo response where standard treatments are only partially effective and not consistently found to be superior to placebos in clinical trials. Under these conditions, if a two-arm active-controlled trial between the new and the standard treatment shows no statistically significant difference between them, two inferences are possible. Either both the new and the standard treatments were effective in the study sample; or neither the new treatment nor the standard treatment were effective. Without a placebo control to validate the efficacy of the two treatments being compared, it may be difficult, if not impossible, to determine which inference is correct. Such active-controlled trials lack "internal validity." It follows that there are sound methodological reasons for including placebo controls in three-arm trials comparing new and standard treatments in conditions with high rates of placebo response where standard treatments are only partially effective, such as depression and anxiety disorders. . . .

The argument from scientific and clinical merit also adopts the false premise that placebo-controlled trials test whether new treatments are better than nothing or no treatment. Despite the recently published meta-analysis of clinical trials with placebo and "no treatment" arms, which cast doubt on the power and pervasiveness of the placebo effect, the jury remains out on whether the use of placebo controls is associated with therapeutic benefit. But even if placebo interventions in themselves are entirely lacking in therapeutic benefit, placebo controls are typically combined with interventions that have therapeutic potential. These include clinical attention from investigators and members of the research team, the therapeutic milieu of research hospitals, especially in the case of inpatient clinical trials, and ancillary treatments or rescue medications that are often provided to research participants randomized to placebo. Though participants randomized to placebo may receive treatment that is less than optimal, this is not the same as no treatment.

Avoiding a Jekyll-and-Hyde Approach to the Ethics of Clinical Research and Practice
Trudo Lemmens & Paul B. Miller
2 AM. J. BIOETHICS, June 2002, at 14

Where Freedman sought to provide a moral compass to physicians-researchers caught in the tension between the ends of research and practice, Miller and Brody suggest the adoption of split personalities in recognition of correspondingly split moral worlds and constitutive moral obligations. Researchers and clinicians inhabit different moral worlds, they argue, and are thus not bound by the same moral commitments. The researcher is morally committed to research; the clinician morally bound by a duty of care. This Jekyll-and-Hyde approach to ethics clearly offers an easy solution to the moral discomfort of a research community that is increasingly under pressure to perform placebo-controlled trials. However, physician-researchers who seek to adhere to a coherent moral code should find only false comfort in their solution. The realization of the tension between clinical research and practice in the debate surrounding the use of placebo controls is not genuinely solved through a sheer re-definition of the ethics of clinical research and practice which, without argument, finds in the differences between the activities grounds for their moral divorce.

In any other walk of life we tend to believe that people ought not to conduct themselves as professionals in a way that they would normally deem to be morally problematic. We tend to value moral integrity in all spheres of human activity. If anything, our expectations of moral integrity are only heightened with respect to professionals with whom we have relationships of care and trust. When meeting physicians in a medical context, patients expect that their best medical interests will be protected and promoted. They do not expect that physician-researchers will hold their therapeutic obligations in suspense at their discretion, whenever they believe they are involved in "research activities."

Yet Miller and Brody invite physician-researchers to do precisely that—to hang their fiduciary duty on the hook when they approach patients as researchers.

Miller and Brody might object to this characterization by stressing that it is their view that placebo controls are acceptable only when people are fully informed and not exposed to excessive levels of risk. The first part of this argument reflects an inordinate reliance on individual autonomy and ignores the real-life circumstances of research participation. The entire research review process is clearly an explicit, sustained, and systematic recognition of the insufficiency of informed consent. Many have pointed out how informed consent is an ideal that is hardly realized. And Freedman himself argued that we must be careful not to conflate the ethics of research with the ethics of consent. Any defensible ethic of research must account for the fact that many patients will be in a vulnerable and dependent position vis-à-vis their caregivers. Particularly when institutionalized, patients assume that those who show medical interest in their case are professional caregivers in whom trust is rightfully placed. Many patients may be under pressure to enter clinical trials as an alternative means by which to obtain access to needed care. One of us has received personal accounts of patients being offered participation in placebo-controlled trials as an alternative to waiting several months for standard treatment of a psychiatric condition. Even when recruited through advertisements, research subjects are often lured with alarming descriptions of the serious problems they have. Those who respond to well-designed publicity campaigns often do so because they long for medical attention and care. Still others participate in research because they lack health insurance and want to have at least a chance of receiving treatment. Although these circumstances may not necessarily be coercive and thus invalidate consent, they nevertheless call into question the appropriateness of relying on informed consent as the primary condition for the conduct of research. As Robin West eloquently stated,

> [c]onsensual acts of commerce, labor, or sexual intercourse are not morally good simply because they are not coerced: a bad trade is still bad, even if it is not theft; a bad job is still bad, even if it is not slavery; and bad sex is still bad sex, even if it is not rape.

Despite their positing of a clear distinction between the ethics of clinical research and practice, Miller and Brody recognize that clear lines are drawn with much difficulty in practice. In attempting to mollify the implications of their earlier insistence that placebos be considered nontherapeutic procedures, Miller and Brody point out that "placebo controls are typically combined with interventions that have therapeutic potential. These include clinical attention from investigators and members of the research team {and} the therapeutic milieu of research hospitals." Even if Jekyll could feel morally comfortable clothed in Hyde's hide, can one really expect the research subjects to be aware of such subtle and continuous transformations? Jekyll and Hyde wear the same white coat, speak the same language, and handle the same instruments. They seem the mirror image of one another to the unsuspecting patient.

As to the second part of their argument, we agree with Miller and Brody that some notion of significant/nonsignificant risk may play a role in determining the ethical acceptability of certain placebo-controlled trials, but only exceptionally. The relevance of the degree of risk exists not in isolation, however, but rather in sorting out the implications of clinical equipoise in marginal situations, as, for instance, where there might be some doubt as to the nature and extent of the superiority of "effective standard treatment." There are numerous minor conditions in society for which standard treatment is available but often avoided. Hay fever is often left untreated or is sometimes treated with alternative treatments that have not been scientifically validated. The risk of not taking any medication for these conditions is small, and this often influences peoples' decisions about whether to seek treatment or not. They may feel indifferent about the available treatments and feel happy to participate in a trial that could offer something better. The issue of the significance of the risk is in such cases not an independent condition but is rather intimately bound up with the questions surrounding what is to count as standard treatment and when the availability of standard treatments is to have normative force on the conduct of physician-researchers. In these conditions it is generally fine for physician-researchers to leave the decision of whether or not to participate solely in the hands of their patients, who often vote with their feet when determining what are acceptable treatments. Where the risks posed by the use of placebo controls are slight in light of available treatments, the therapeutic obligation must be felt with correspondingly decreased force, and the clinical equipoise condition may thus be applied with some latitude.

NOTES AND QUESTIONS

1. Why do Lemmens and Miller reject Miller and Brody's position? Are they suggesting that the risks of receiving a placebo are qualitatively different from the other risks of research? Do you think their position would be different if clinical research were not typically performed by physicians?

2. If it is inappropriate to give subjects placebos when standard treatment exists, why is it not also wrong to perform risky interventions on healthy volunteers? In both cases, subjects are being exposed to risks without any possibility of receiving a direct benefit.

3. In some situations, the FDA will refuse to approve a new drug unless the manufacturer can demonstrate that the drug performed better than a placebo in a controlled clinical trial. *See* Kenneth J. Rothman & Karin B. Michels, *The Continuing Unethical Use of Placebo Controls*, 331 NEW ENG. J. MED. 394 (1994) (noting the FDA's refusal to approve a new beta blocker because it had not been compared to a placebo, even though the new drug had been shown to be as effective as an already-approved drug). However, the FDA emphasizes that the use of placebos is "obviously not ethically acceptable where existing treatment is life-prolonging" or in studies "that expose subjects to a documented risk." FOOD

AND DRUG ADMINISTRATION, IRB INFORMATION SHEETS — DRUGS AND BIOLOGICS (1998), available at www.fda.gov/oc/ohrt/irbs/drugsbiologics.html#study.

4. The 2000 revision to the Declaration of Helsinki, quoted at the beginning of this section, states that the importance of offering subjects the "best current prophylactic, diagnostic, and therapeutic methods" does not preclude the use of placebos "in studies where no proven prophylactic, diagnostic or therapeutic method exists." Two years later, in response to concerns that this language placed undue restrictions on the use of placebos, the drafters of the Declaration inserted the following "note of clarification":

> The [World Medical Association] hereby reaffirms its position that extreme care must be taken in making use of a placebo-controlled trial and that in general this methodology should only be used in the absence of existing proven therapy. However, a placebo-controlled trial may be ethically acceptable, even if proven therapy is available, under the following circumstances:
>
> —Where for compelling and scientifically sound methodological reasons its use is necessary to determine the efficacy or safety of a prophylactic, diagnostic or therapeutic method; or
>
> —Where a prophylactic, diagnostic or therapeutic method is being investigated for a minor condition and the patients who receive placebo will not be subject to any additional risk of serious or irreversible harm.

WORLD MEDICAL ASSOCIATION, NOTE OF CLARIFICATION ON PARAGRAPH 29 OF THE WORLD MEDICAL ASSOCIATION DECLARATION OF HELSINKI (2002). Does this note of clarification adopt the position advocated by Miller and Brody?

5. In assessing the acceptability of a placebo-controlled trial, is it appropriate to consider the "best current prophylactic, diagnostic, and therapeutic methods" that exist anywhere in the world, or should the focus be on those methods that are actually available to the population from which prospective subjects will be drawn? This question has arisen in studies conducted in developing countries, where, as a practical matter, the "standard care" for many conditions is no treatment at all. Does the fact that individuals enrolled in research in such conditions would not receive any treatment whatsoever if they were not in a study justify giving those individuals placebo controls? Consider, for example, studies evaluating treatments to reduce the risk that HIV-positive pregnant women will transmit the virus to their offspring during pregnancy or childbirth. While some such treatments already exist, they are unavailable in third world countries because of their cost. Is it appropriate for researchers to test less expensive treatments in third world countries against placebo controls, or must they compare them to the expensive treatments that are used in the United States and other wealthy countries? *Compare* Peter Lurie & Sidney M. Wolfe, *Unethical Trials of Interventions to Reduce Perinatal Transmission of the Human Immunodeficiency Virus in Developing Countries*, 337 NEW ENG. J. MED. 853 (1997) (criticizing the use of placebo controls in such circumstances); *with*

Harold Varmus & David Satcher, *Ethical Complexities of Conducting Research in Developing Countries*, 337 NEW ENG. J. MED. 1003 (1997) (suggesting that it would be unethical *not* to conduct the studies with placebo controls, as the relevant question for third world women is whether the less expensive treatment is better than nothing, not whether it is better than treatments that are practically unavailable).

6. One of Miller and Brody's arguments is that placebo-controlled trials may create less overall risk than equivalence trials, because the use of a placebo may make it possible to enroll a smaller number of subjects and still produce statistically valid results. Responding to this point, Kathleen Cranley Glass and Duff Waring argue that "[n]o ethical theory or principle of law recognizes a duty to nontrial participants (those 'spared' exposure by using a PCT), or even to future patients, that trumps the physician-investigator's duty to patients recruited to the current trial." Kathleen Cranley Glass and Duff Waring, *Effective Trial Design Need Not Conflict with Good Patient Care*, 2 AM. J. BIOETHICS, June 2002, at 25. Should IRBs be concerned only with the *level* of risks imposed on the subjects in a study, or should they also consider whether the researchers are exposing *too many* people to risks by designing the study so that it requires too many subjects?

7. While placebos are most often used in drug studies, they are also sometimes used in surgical research. For example, in a study of individuals with osteoarthritis of the knee, subjects were randomly assigned to receive arthroscopic debridement, arthroscopic lavage, or "sham surgery." For subjects undergoing the sham procedure, surgeons made incisions in the knee and went through the motions of surgery, but no surgical procedures were actually performed. The researchers found that the subjects receiving the sham surgery did just as well as those in the two intervention groups. *See* J. Bruce Mosley et al., *A Controlled Trial of Arthroscopic Surgery for Osteoarthritis of the Knee*, 347 NEW ENG. J. MED. 81 (2002). Similarly, researchers used sham surgery to evaluate the efficacy of transplanting fetal tissue cells into the brains of Parkinson's disease patients. Subjects who received the sham surgery had holes drilled into their head, but nothing was inserted into their brains. As it turned out, the subjects who received the sham surgery generally did much better than those in the active treatment group; many of those who received the fetal tissue transplants not only failed to show any overall improvement, but also exhibited debilitating side effects. *See* Gina Kolata, *Parkinson's Research Is Set Back by Failure of Fetal Cell Implants*, N.Y. TIMES, March 8, 2001, at A1. Should IRBs evaluate the appropriateness of using placebo controls in surgical studies according to the same standards they would apply to the use of placebos in drug trials, or does sham surgery raise additional ethical issues? *See* Ruth Macklin, *The Ethical Problems with Sham Surgery in Clinical Research*, 341 NEW ENG. J. MED. 992 (1999).

[5] **Washouts and Challenge Studies**

Two aspects of research design may trigger the manifestation of symptoms in individuals with underlying medical conditions. First, subjects may become symptomatic during a "placebo washout," a period in which subjects are taken off their existing medications, either to investigate the impact on subjects of foregoing their usual medications or to provide a clean slate prior to beginning a new investigational drug. Second, subjects may develop symptoms of their underlying condition during "challenge studies," a type of trial that is expressly designed to provoke the manifestation of symptoms in otherwise stable subjects. Both of these techniques are used in many types of biomedical research, but they have become particularly controversial in psychiatric studies. The following excerpts describe the fatal consequences of a washout period in a study of schizophrenia patients at UCLA.

For the Sake of Science
Joy Horowitz
Los Angeles Times Magazine, Sept. 11, 1994

At 8:43 A.M. March 28, 1991, two UCLA campus police officers responding to an emergency call found a burly young man lying face down outside of Boelter Hall. He had jumped from the roof of the nine-story classroom building; at 9:23 he was pronounced dead at UCLA Medical Center. His name was Tony Lamadrid.

A coroner's report included this notation: "This 23-year-old male with a history of depression and schizophrenia was being treated for same at UCLA Medical Center Psychiatric Department . . . (his) social worker was . . . trying to place him into a new psychiatric program and was trying to convince decedent on 3-22-91 to commit himself to UCLA because she felt he was suicidal. Decedent contacted his brother, Enrique Lamadrid, and advised him he wanted to take poison to end it all. . . ."

In the days that followed, police discovered an answering machine tape that included a message from Debbie Gioia-Hasick, his social worker at UCLA's Aftercare Clinic. "Hi, Tony. It's Debbie," she began, "Even later today, (if) you're just feeling really bad, go over to UCLA and just check yourself into the hospital. Tell them you're suicidal and that you think you're really going to hurt yourself. Check yourself in, and then we'll go from there."

But the institution that was supposed to help Tony Lamadrid had another interest in him as well. From 1985 to 1989, according to government records, he had been both a patient at the UCLA Medical Center and an active participant in a sweeping psychiatric study approved by the university. In the spring of 1991, even though he was no longer directly involved in experiments, Lamadrid continued to be monitored by the research staff, including Gioia-Hasick. The study, "Developmental Processes in Schizophrenic Disorders," was directed by psychologist Keith H. Nuechterlein, with psychiatrist Michael Gitlin, and its aim was to gather data on the how and why of schizophrenic relapse. . . .

The research included two protocols, approved by the university's Human Subjects Protection Committee and by the government. The first involved putting the patient-subjects on a standardized dose of the antipsychotic drug Prolixin while the researchers tracked their symptoms and tested for factors associated with relapses, defined as a "return to a state of active and severe psychotic symptoms." The variables to be studied included environmental stresses thought to trigger symptoms — "high expressed emotion" within families, for example, things like emotional over-involvement, criticism and hostility — and physiological components such as "smooth pursuit eye movements," breathing rate, blood pressure and the like.

Every two weeks, a van would pick up the participants at home and bring them to the Aftercare Clinic, where they received a shot of Prolixin, attended group therapy sessions and saw their social worker and a psychiatrist. From time to time, the subjects and their families filled out questionnaires and were interviewed; they were given MRI scans and hooked to electrodes.

In the controversial second protocol of the experiment, the researchers continued to track symptoms and test for relapse variables, but now the patient-subjects were withdrawn from the stabilizing Prolixin in a "Double Blind Drug Crossover and Removal." The subjects were randomly divided into two groups, with 12 weeks on medication, then 12 weeks on a placebo, or vice versa. After that, "all clinically appropriate" subjects — those who had remained relatively stable on a placebo —received no medication at all for as long as 18 months.

The goal of "Developmental Processes" was to identify predictors of schizophrenic psychosis. Such research, the doctors said, would not only further basic understanding of the disease, it would be of immense practical value in treatment, especially the results of the drug-withdrawal protocol. That information could help establish when and if recent-onset patients could do without medication, and thereby escape such horrific side effects as tardive dyskinesia, a sometimes irreversible neuromuscular disorder marked by facial grimaces, tics, trembling hands and tongue thrusts.

And the risks? "The potential risk in the study," one of Nuechterlein's grant applications said of the second protocol, "is that clinical exacerbation or relapse can be expected to occur in some of our patient subjects, probably in most. . . ." By comparison, the application indicated, if the patient-subjects stayed on antipsychotics, most would also be expected to backslide, but "the exacerbation or relapse would be later in many cases. . . ." If the symptoms were deemed serious according to certain criteria, a "decompensating" participant would be withdrawn from the study and treated "as per the clinical needs" of the situation. In any case, the researchers expected some of their patient-subjects to regress to the point of experiencing "hallucinations, unusual thought content, bizarreness, self-neglect, hostility, depressive mood and suicidality." They just didn't know who, or when. . . .

By the time Tony Lamadrid joined the second protocol in 1987, however, Nuechterlein and Gitlin's risk hypothesis was being backed up by their preliminary data. Most of their patient-subjects were relapsing. According to a document obtained through the Freedom of Information Act, on Feb. 10, 1986, a government peer review team, conducting a site visit of the project, expressed concern over the ethical implications of these preliminary results. In its summary report, the team noted that "a comment was made about the risk/benefit ratio for the withdrawal protocol, since, to date, 11 of 14 patients have relapsed during the 18 months of neuroleptic (drug) withdrawal."

Nuechterlein responded with a list of benefits, saying, "that most study patients are eager to discontinue neuroleptics, that many clinicians would consider drug discontinuation to be clinically indicated by this time, and that the study will yield clinically important information about predictors of early relapse." Ultimately, the NIMH [National Institutes of Mental Health] reviewers were satisfied: "In light of project staff's ability to reinstate neuroleptics very rapidly if clinical decompensation begins, the site visitors judged that subjects are adequately protected." . . .

The 1986 grant application omitted specific references to exactly how relapsing patient-subjects like Tony Lamadrid would be handled. In a 1988 application, the methodology was more specific: Participants would be removed from the study (and presumably remedicated) when their symptoms were rated at specific levels. But rating symptoms is something of a judgment call, the doctors would later admit, and the protocol description also said that the participants' clinical interests would be deferred, at least temporarily, until the researchers could conduct their tests and make their measurements: "Information-processing, psychological, and blood testing will be done, and the patient will then be treated. . . ."

As troubling is a 1988 article Nuechterlein and one of his graduate students published in the Journal of Abnormal Psychology. They analyzed relapses in the UCLA study that reached the "severe or extremely severe level," noting that the research had not been restricted "by the necessity to increase medication to avoid a possible relapse." However rapidly decompensation was treated during the protocols, this sub-analysis found 17 instances of severe psychotic symptoms in 23 patient-subjects. Later, Nuechterlein would say that the choice of words in the article had been bad, and that it didn't accurately reflect the criteria for relapse and remediation in the main study.

Some families I spoke to said their relatives were put back on medication as soon as they noticed minor symptoms, like acting bizarrely or not sleeping or pacing. One parent, whom the researchers asked to speak to me and who requested anonymity, told me how much she respected Gitlin, explaining he would "break the blind" (intervene during the double-blind phase) at any time.

The problem was she lacked authority over her adult son, who was relapsing on the placebo but "fooling everyone" — hearing voices yet denying it because he wanted to stay off the medication. She began crying. "I'll tell you the truth," she said of the study during which her son was hospitalized. "I don't resent the fact that my son went through it. But I wish he hadn't. It caused him a lot of pain. And a lot of months of recuperation." At one point during the recuperation, she said, he tried to jump out of his car on the freeway.

Other families say their efforts to reinstate medication were rebuffed, and whatever the study called for, they allege that the doctors' response to relapse was inadequate. . . . Gregory Aller, now 30 and attending UCLA part-time, recently told a congressional panel what happened during the months in 1990 that his parents said they were begging the research leaders to reinstate his medication but were told that their insistence on becoming involved was part of their son's problem:

> This time my symptoms were much more severe than the symptoms at the onset of my schizophrenia. What ensued was a nightmare. My ability to concentrate fell apart. I was unable to do schoolwork. I became manic and hyperactive. Some days I would hardly sleep at all. One night I woke up screaming, actually believing that I was sprouting another leg. I started to have paranoid delusions about government agents chasing me. I became violent with my father and threatened to kill him. I believed there were hidden cameras on the wall of my parents' living room. Much later, still in a delusional state, I started hitch-hiking to Washington to assassinate President Bush. Though I had slipped back into paranoid symptoms, my doctor asked me if I felt I needed medication. Since I was paranoid by that time, I said I was fine, I didn't need medication. Dr. Gitlin never delved into what was really going on in my life.

Elizabeth de Balogh, 34, another UCLA subject-patient, now lives in an Artesia board and care home. She blames herself for her predicament. At UCLA, she says, she was stabilized for a year — able to drive and go to the beach and hold a job. But then, as she participated in the drug withdrawal protocol, her life began slipping away. She thought musical notes were chasing her and her "eyes rolled up," meaning she would hallucinate. "But I wanted to get off the medications," she says. "So, it's not really their fault, I guess." Her long blond hair is washed, her purple dress and scarf offset by sneakers, no socks. Her vivid blue eyes grow sad, her little-girlish voice plaintive. "Why didn't they give me medications when I got sick?" Looking agitated, she says, "I'm starting to get bad thoughts. I'm scared the devil is trying to take my soul away from me." . . .

Ask anyone closely involved in the UCLA schizophrenia research project and he will tell you that the study has absolutely nothing to do with purposefully relapsing schizophrenic patients. "In no way," says Michael Gitlin, "were we trying to create or produce relapse in any way, shape or form." Says Keith Nuechterlein: "The simple idea that someone would accuse us of things like being unethical, and gee, trying to induce relapses and making all our patients do poorly — it just blew my mind."

Statement of Don A. Rockwell, M.D., Director, Neuropsychiatric Hospital, University of California, Los Angeles, before the House Subcommittee on Regulation, Business Opportunities, and Technology of the Committee on Small Business, U.S. House of Representatives
May 23, 1994

Over the past three years, a UCLA schizophrenia study has been under review by the federal Office for Protection from Research Risks (OPRR), which was investigating allegations regarding informed consent made by some family members of patients in the study. UCLA fully cooperated with the review. As a result of the OPRR review, UCLA is making several significant changes in documenting its informed consent and review process, including establishing an independent Data and Safety Monitoring Board to oversee those studies in which the clinical researchers are also responsible for the clinical care of psychiatric study subjects, and augmenting the three non-UCLA members of the campus's medical IRB with one or more subject representatives, who would represent the research subject's perspective on studies involving subjects with severe psychiatric disorders. . . .

In order to fully understand the UCLA study, it is absolutely essential to understand three important facts about schizophrenia and its treatment:

1. Although there are many medications that are commonly prescribed to minimize the symptoms of schizophrenia, each of them has significant drawbacks that limit their effectiveness. All of the typical, commonly prescribed medications for schizophrenia have serious side effects (including a potentially irreversible movement disorder called tardive dyskinesia) and common uncomfortable side-effects (muscular stiffness, dry mouth, sleepiness, etc.). As a result, many people in the early stages of schizophrenia refuse to take their medication or take themselves off medication against their doctors' advice.

2. There is a wide variation among patients in their degree of recovery during the years after initial onset of schizophrenia. For patients who are doing well, it is not clear to physicians how long to continue ongoing outpatient medication, which involves further risk of serious side-effects. Some patients do well during periods off medication, while others do not. Similarly, some patients do well on medication and others relapse despite being on medication.

3. Because of the above-mentioned problems with medication and because of the variability among patients, it is common clinical practice worldwide for doctors to give patients periods without medication during the initial years after the onset of schizophrenia. These periods need to be closely monitored, since some patients do well without medication, while others do not. Little is known about the factors that determine which patients will do well off medication and which will not. One of the specific goals of the UCLA study was to identify factors that predict the need for short-term outpatient medication versus long-term, continuous medication. This is a key issue in the treatment of the early stages of schizophrenia, as noted above.

The treatment protocol in the UCLA study was similar to what is done in everyday clinical practice with patients in the initial years after the onset of schizophrenia. The study was not designed to cause relapse, but to observe patients for periods on medication and off medication, since this is what typically occurs in community practice.

None of the patients who participated in the study was deliberately allowed to experience a relapse. As in common clinical practice, the UCLA doctors would intervene by recommending medication and/or additional therapy if the patient showed signs of a psychotic exacerbation, which involves less intense symptom changes than a relapse.

How Was the UCLA Study Conducted?

The UCLA study consisted of three phases. Before entering each phase, the potential study subjects were presented with both written and oral information about the study. . . . For Phase One, potential subjects signed written consent forms that explained the initial screening interview procedure, that allowed the researchers to contact the patients' significant others, and that explained the testing procedures of this phase, and the fact that medication and other treatment would be provided at an outpatient research program at UCLA. Additional details were described orally and any questions were answered. The nature of the study and associated treatment were also described to close family members, who signed a form consenting to their own participation in some study measures. Over the course of the study, even before the OPRR review, the written consent information was refined at several points, as we gained more information on ways to enhance the informed consent process. For example, more details regarding the starting medication dosage were added.

In the first phase, patients with recent-onset schizophrenia (that is, with an initial schizophrenic episode within the past two years) were started on a dose of 12.5 mg Prolixin Decanoate every two weeks. As in community practice, the dosage was a starting point, not an unchangeable dosage. It was later adjusted upward or downward if needed, depending on the patient's symptoms and the drug's side-effects. The 12.5 mg starting dosage was determined by a comprehensive review of the scientific literature regarding Prolixin Decanoate and recent-onset schizophrenia.

In Phase One, the patients were seen at least every two weeks in the UCLA Aftercare Program. Medication and symptoms were monitored by a psychiatrist. A case manager provided training in everyday living and coping skills, and also monitored symptoms. Close family members were invited to a family education program. Family members were also encouraged to contact the staff if they had any questions or concerns. The staff also worked to keep family members informed about treatment, unless patients exercised their right to restrict such information. Adult patients have the right to exclude family members from being involved in their care, if they wish, and some patients in the study exercised this right.

Following Phase One, those patients whose medications had been monitored for at least one year and who were clinically stable for at least three months were offered the opportunity to participate in Phase Two. Phase Two was designed to mimic the common medical practice in the community, which is to give recent-onset schizophrenia patients trial periods off medication to determine if they can continue to do well without the medication. In Phase Two, study participants continued to be monitored in the UCLA Aftercare Program at least every two weeks, but had a 12-week period on medication followed by a 12-week period on a placebo, or vice versa. In addition, close family members were encouraged to call the staff if they noticed any change in the patient's symptoms. More frequent visits to the Aftercare Program were recommended as clinically indicated. If patients did not show significant symptoms during this period, they were offered the opportunity to try a longer period without medication, to determine whether they would continue to do well without continuous medication.

During Phase Two, the researchers monitored the patients for any signs of exacerbation or relapse. In fact, in Phase Two the researchers used more sensitive procedures than standard medical practice to determine at the earliest possible point if someone was experiencing a psychotic exacerbation. Following Phase Two, patients could continue to receive treatment at the UCLA Aftercare Program, where they can be monitored and their medication is given as needed.

Did the Study Intentionally Cause Subjects to Relapse?

Unfortunately, relapse among patients with schizophrenia is common, even with medication. None of the patients who participated in the UCLA study was deliberately allowed to relapse. As occurs in community practice, some of the study subjects did experience a relapse. The rate of relapse in Phase One of the UCLA study was 18 percent for a one year period, which is in the low end of the national average yearly relapse rate of 15 - 35 percent for schizophrenic patients on medication. Thus, in the UCLA study, patients off medication relapsed, and patients on medication relapsed. In its review of the study, the OPRR report found "no demonstrable basis for rejecting the UCLA IRB's determination that the methodological design of the Schizophrenic Disorders research is scientifically and ethically justifiable." (OPRR Report, p. 17 (May 11, 1994)) . . .

A crucial point that has often been overlooked is the "clinical override" aspect of the study. At any point in the study, the researchers could (and in fact did) override the study criteria to provide medication or other treatment if needed by the patient. The patient's best interest always came first. Some patients in the UCLA study refused to go back on medication. When that happened, UCLA staff worked with the patient, and, as appropriate, close family members and others to urge the patient to resume medication. However, a physician cannot force adult patients to take or resume medication against their will, without a court proceeding.

NOTES AND QUESTIONS

1. An investigation by the federal Office of Protection from Research Risks (OPRR; the predecessor of OHRP) concluded that the UCLA researchers had violated informed consent requirements, but that the study design and care given the subjects was otherwise appropriate. *See* Horowitz, *supra*.

2. What does the debate about the use of placebo controls suggest about the use of placebo washouts? If you believe that placebos should not be used when effective treatment for a condition exists, must you also object to the use of placebo washouts for patients whose current treatment is working?

3. If a study similar to the UCLA experiment were presented to your IRB, would you approve it? What conditions might you impose to minimize the risks? Would it be appropriate to limit washout studies to inpatient settings?

4. In 1999, OPRR faulted researchers at Mt. Sinai School of Medicine in New York for a 1987 study in which stabilized schizophrenic patients were taken off their medications and given L-dopa, a substance known to induce psychotic symptoms. All of the patients experienced a relapse of their symptoms, and some became violent or suicidal. *See* Dolores Kong, *Study Harmed Mentally Ill, Agency Reports*, BOSTON GLOBE, Feb. 9, 1999, at A8. If you had been on the IRB reviewing this study, do you think the use of L-dopa in this manner would have struck you as problematic? Now that you are aware of this incident, will it affect your balancing of the risks and benefits of challenge studies in psychiatric subjects? Should IRBs set limits on the nature, duration, or setting of challenge studies?

5. For further discussion of the ethical issues raised by challenge studies, see Franklin G. Miller & Donald L. Rosenstein, *Psychiatric Symptom-Provoking Studies: An Ethical Analysis*, 42 BIOLOGICAL PSYCHIATRY 403 (1997).

[C]   Risks to Others

National Bioethics Advisory Commission,
1 ETHICAL AND POLICY ISSUES IN RESEARCH INVOLVING HUMAN PARTICIPANTS
72-73 (2001)

Risks may accrue not only to research participants, but also to persons not directly involved in research, such as to the participants' family, loved ones, other contacts, social groups, and to society in general. . . .

For example, in a study of a new live virus vaccine, there may be risks to participants' family members or other contacts who could contract the attenuated disease. In some states, there may be legal risk to parents whose minor children participate in a study of illegal activity. Genetic research may result in certain groups being associated with certain diseases, thus exposing members of those groups to the possibility of stigmatization or discrimination in insurance or employment. Society in general may incur harm related to research involving procedures, such as xenotransplantation or studies of viruses in which there may be some potential of releasing pathogenic organisms.

Current regulations focus only on individual participants. However, other individuals and communities not directly involved in research can also bear risks that are associated with a research study, but that are not acknowledged or mentioned in the regulations. If IRBs focus only on risks to individual research participants, they fail to apply fully the principle of beneficence, because the scope of this principle can extend beyond the individual participants in the research.

NOTES AND QUESTIONS

1. Washout periods may pose risks to nonsubjects as well as to the subjects themselves. As noted above, one of the subjects who was taken off his medications in the UCLA schizophrenia study threatened to kill his father before leaving for Washington, D.C. in an attempt to assassinate the President. *See* Horowitz, *supra.*

2. Breaches of confidentiality can pose risks to nonsubjects, particularly when research data involves information that has relevance for the subject's family members. For further discussion of this issue, see Chapter 10, at page 450.

3. Genetics research poses special risks to the interests of nonsubjects, including members of the subject's family and individuals with a similar racial or ethnic heritage. These issues are discussed in Chapter 17, at page 709.

[D] "Minimal Risk" Research Under the Federal Regulations

The determination that a study involves "minimal risk" is relevant to several areas of the federal regulations:

- *Expedited review* — Certain categories of minimal risk research may be approved through expedited procedures, without the involvement of the full IRB. *See* 45 C.F.R. § 46.110; *see also* Chapter 4, at page 196.

- *Waiver of informed consent* — IRBs may approve consent procedures that differ from those usually required, or waive the requirement of informed consent entirely, in certain types of minimal risk studies. *See* 45 C.F.R. § 46.116; *see also* Chapter 7, at page 313.

- *Waiver of written consent* — IRBs may waive the requirement for written documentation of informed consent in certain types of minimal risk studies. *See* 45 C.F.R. § 46.117; *see also* Chapter 7, at page 317.

- *Protected classes* — For research with pregnant women, fetuses, prisoners, and children, studies involving more than minimal risks are subject to stringent limitations. *See* Chapters 9 and 16 (pregnant women and fetuses), 15 (prisoners), and 13 (children).

Except for the Subpart of the regulations that governs prison research, which contains its own definition of "minimal risk," the term "minimal risk" under the federal regulations "means that the probability and magnitude of harm or discomfort anticipated in the research are not greater in and of themselves than those ordinarily encountered in daily life or during the performance of routine physical or psychological examinations or tests." 45 C.F.R. § 46.102(i). As the following excerpt explains, the meaning of this definition has engendered considerable debate.

1 ETHICAL AND POLICY ISSUES IN RESEARCH INVOLVING HUMAN PARTICIPANTS
NATIONAL BIOETHICS ADVISORY COMMISSION
83 (2001)

The definition of minimal risk in federal regulations does not specify an unambiguous standard. That is, risks involved in the research study are compared to those encountered in daily life, but it is unclear whether daily life applies to healthy individuals or the target group of the research. Existing sources of guidance offer conflicting interpretations of the standard to be used in determining level of risk. In the context of its discussion of research involving children, the National Commission defined a so-called absolute standard when it defined minimal risk as "the probability and magnitude of physical or psychological harm that is normally encountered in the daily lives, or in the routine medical or psychological examination, of healthy children." This standard was not adopted in the regulations pertaining to research involving children. However, DHHS regulations concerning research involving prisoners limit minimal risk to the experience of healthy individuals. In 1993, OPRR endorsed such an absolute standard interpretation for Subpart A. OPRR's interpretation is inconsistent with DHHS' intention as expressed in the preamble of the 1981 version of 45 C.F.R. 46 which stated that "the risks of harm ordinarily encountered in daily life means those risks encountered in the daily lives of the subjects of the research." If minimal risk is not characterized in terms of the daily life and experiences of healthy individuals, then it might be taken to refer to the daily life and experiences of research participants. If this is the case, then the same intervention could be classified as minimal risk or greater than minimal risk, depending on the health status of the research participants and their particular experiences. For example, a bone marrow aspiration would not be considered minimal risk in relation to the daily life of a healthy individual, but it might well be determined to fall within this category in relation to the experience of a person with acute leukemia. Such an understanding entails a relative standard for minimal risk.

A relative standard for minimal risk would allow ill participants to be exposed to greater risks than healthy participants. Such a standard would impose disproportionate burdens of research on the ill and provide weaker protections for them than for healthy individuals. This would violate the ethical principle of justice.

NOTES AND QUESTIONS

1. In place of the existing definition, NBAC recommended that the definition of "minimal risk" be tied to the daily lives of the "general population," a standard that falls between the "relative" standard described in the excerpt and the "healthy individuals" standard used in the regulations governing prisoners. Which of these three standards do you find preferable?

2. Several studies have found widespread variation in IRBs' interpretation of the minimal risk standard. *See, e.g.,* M. Alexander Otto, *Advance Directive, Minimal Risk Mandate Could Hamper Vulnerable Subject Research*, 1 MED. RESEARCH L. & POL'Y REP. (BNA) 352 (2002) (reporting survey of 200 IRB chairs, which found significant disagreement about whether procedures like magnetic resonance imaging and allergy skin testing constituted more than a minimal risk); Loretta M. Kopelman, *Pediatric Research Regulations Under Legal Scrutiny: Grimes Narrows Their Interpretation*, 30 J. L. MED. & ETHICS 38, 45 (2002) (discussing studies showing widespread differences in how IRBs interpret the riskiness of common procedures like venipuncture, arterial puncture, gastric and intestinal intubation, and lumbar puncture). Is this inconsistency problematic? Would a different definition of minimal risk yield more consistent interpretations?

§ 6.03 IDENTIFYING BENEFITS

Federal regulations direct IRBs to balance risks to subjects against "antici-pated benefits, if any, to subjects, and the importance of the knowledge that may reasonably be expected to result." 45 C.F.R. § 111(a)(2). In carrying out this task, what potential benefits may IRBs appropriately take into account?

[A] Potential Benefits to Research Subjects

ETHICS AND REGULATION OF CLINICAL RESEARCH
ROBERT J. LEVINE
(2d ed. 1988)

With regard to benefits to subjects, I shall assume that it is always appro-priate to weigh and to offer direct health-related benefits if their probability and magnitude are stated correctly. Let us instead focus on some sorts of direct benefits to subjects about which there are controversies as to whether they ought to be weighed or offered. These are economic, psychosocial, and kinship benefits. . . .

Psychosocial Benefits. Patients who know they have terminal illnesses and patients who are depressed will often respond favorably to the notion that investigators are not only interested in them but also are attempting to devise something that might offer relief or, perhaps, cure. Some patients with cancer in whom all validated modes of therapy have been tried without success become optimistic when the prospect of trying an investigational drug is offered. The patient may be relieved to learn that he or she need not give up hope because there is yet another possibility for relief and that he or she is not about to be abandoned by health professionals. Many individuals who are depressed or anxious or both will experience relief as they assume the role of subject; in the relatively sheltered research environment, they are largely divested of the bur-dens of some sorts of decision-making.

Individuals who are concerned about their sense of worth may welcome the opportunity to appear valuable to themselves as well as to others; doing some-thing that they consider altruistic enhances their sense of personal worth. Among examples of such individuals are some elderly persons and some pris-oners (who might, incidentally, hope that their altruistic tendencies will be appreciated by those who make parole decisions).

In some social groups, playing the role of subject may bring an individual con-siderable prestige. Some may be flattered to be the subject or object of attention of so many important people. This is particularly true of individuals who become eligible for the role by virtue of having a rare disease. Others gain what they consider substantial prestige or satisfy their tendency to exhibitionism through participation in research that attracts great publicity, e.g., Walter Reed's studies on yellow fever.

Many bored persons find that participation in research is a welcome diversion. Although this is discussed most commonly in relation to prisoners and those institutionalized as mentally infirm, patients hospitalized in acute general medical services, after the busy first day or two, commonly state that they prefer being used as research subjects or teaching material to the ennui of daytime television.

Kinship Benefits. Some persons experience as a personal benefit the belief that their actions will produce direct benefits to others. Thus they may be willing to assume the burdens of the role of research subject in order to better the lives of theirs. In general their motivation to do this is higher when they either are related to or have a sense of kinship with the prospective beneficiaries. To the extent that the individual is motivated by a sense of kinship with increasingly large groups of humans, the largest group being the entire human species, the motivation increasingly approximates altruism or charity.

Perhaps the closest sense of kinship one can feel is with one's self. Some persons may become subjects of basic research on diseases with which they are afflicted hoping that they will contribute to the development of knowledge about their disease. This knowledge, in turn, might lead to the development of improved therapy for their disease; thus, they may hope for a direct health-related benefit in the future, particularly if they have a chronic disease. Alternatively, they might feel a sense of kinship with others with the same disease, hoping that in the future some direct benefit might accrue to them.

Within families, persons are often motivated by the prospect of kinship benefits; this is particularly relevant to research in the fields of genetics and transplantation. Persons are generally more likely to offer bone marrow to a relative than to a stranger. The father or mother of a child with phenylketonuria might be willing to participate in research designed to perfect techniques for detecting heterozygous carriers although it will bring no direct benefit to them or their child; they already know they are carriers. However, if a better method for carrier detection is discovered, it would be likely to provide direct health benefit to another relative who is phenotypically normal but who might be a carrier.

A sense of kinship might be based on racial or ethnic factors. Thus, some Jews might be motivated to serve as normal controls for research designed to explore the pathogenesis or therapy of Tay-Sachs disease; blacks might volunteer for similar roles in research related to sickle cell anemia.

Women who are about to have abortions may feel a sense of kinship with other pregnant women who expect to continue their pregnancies to term; among such women in the future might be the woman who is now planning an abortion. Thus, she might be motivated to participate in research made possible by virtue of the fact that she has planned to have an abortion, research designed to develop knowledge that might be of benefit to pregnant women who expect to carry their pregnancies to term.

It is customary to appeal to kinship interests and altruism when prospective subjects are capable of consenting for themselves. Kinship interests are commonly weighed by those who are considering whether one can justify research involving vulnerable subjects or those incapable of consent. For example, arguments for justification of research on the dying person or dying fetus have been grounded in presumptions of their "interest" in the welfare of others like them. Some arguments supporting the involvement of children in research have even gone so far as to construe a limited moral obligation to such acts of charity.

Defining and Describing Benefit Appropriately in Clinical Trials
Nancy M.P. King
28 J. L. MED. & ETHICS 332 (2000)

There are three distinguishable types of benefit possible from research:

- Direct benefit to subjects, which is properly defined as benefit arising from receiving the intervention being studied;

- Collateral benefit to subjects . . ., which is benefit arising from being a subject, even if one does not receive the experimental intervention (for example, a free physical exam and testing, free medical care and other extras, or the personal gratification of altruism);

- Aspirational benefit, or benefit to society and to future patients, which arises from the results of the study.

Payment to subjects, though technically a collateral benefit, is classified and treated separately in research ethics and policy. . . .

When investigators argue that "patients do better on-study," so that enrolling in research is their best treatment option, they are making a collateral benefit claim. The provision of collateral benefit in a research project raises issues of justice in two ways. First, providing a potentially higher standard of care to those enrolled in research than those receiving standard treatment potentially discourages the improvement of standard treatment. Second, because collateral benefits are entirely under the control of research investigators and sponsors, their provision poses the risk of manipulating or possibly even coercing participation from subjects who are disadvantaged or otherwise vulnerable. At the very least, questions are raised about the standard of care and about the best ways to provide and finance health care for those in need.

Yet the problem of collateral benefit may be more complicated still. Remember that what distinguishes collateral benefit from direct benefit is that direct benefit is linked to the intervention under study and collateral benefit is available to all subjects simply by virtue of being in the study. There are several new research design trends that seek to make it difficult to distinguish between these two types of benefit. Conflation of direct and collateral benefit serves the argument that research is the best treatment, which in turn makes it difficult to remember that patients may also be subjects.

Some thoughtful investigators and policy makers have begun to broaden their definitions of the intervention being studied as well as to design studies that include several stages in order to maximize the potential for direct benefit to subjects. This is most readily seen in psychiatric research, especially drug trials and comparisons of drug and non-drug interventions, and is largely a response to public concern about placebo designs, challenge studies, and washout periods. Proponents of this viewpoint do not consider the potential benefit from the study drug in isolation from the rest of the study. They do not regard study design features that minimize risk or provide collateral benefit (e.g., monitoring and testing, rescue medications, non-study physician available to monitor subjects — all means of minimizing risks to subjects; crossover designs and post-study open label extensions — two means of ensuring that all subjects gain at least limited access to the drug being studied) in isolation, either. Instead, they take it all together, rolling risk-minimization features and collateral benefit features into one package, and view the whole study as providing direct benefit. According to this view, the whole study has been designed to maximize the potential for direct benefit to all subjects.

Robert Levine has called this view, which takes all the components of the study as a whole, "the fallacy of the package deal." He has condemned it when it is used to label an entire study "nontherapeutic," as has been done in the past, because it contains some unproven and/or purely research components. But its use as described here turns the "fallacy of the package deal" to the opposite effect — to label an entire study "therapeutic" despite the clearly experimental character and unproven benefit of its central component, i.e., the drug being studied.

This view rightly recognizes that a treatment program has many interconnected features and components and that maximizing potential benefit for patients requires a grasp of this dynamic complexity. Analogizing from the treatment setting, this view considers a research protocol to be a plan for cutting-edge treatment — but the analogy goes too far. A research protocol is not treatment, no matter how much all parties wish it so. Treatment requires genuine attention to the best interests of the patient as an individual, including individual attention and individual tailoring or complete changing of any regimen for maximal efficacy. Even if the organization, scope, and duration of a clinical trial were compatible with these goals, the uncertainties and unknowns attendant upon use of an unproven intervention make individual tailoring almost meaningless, especially in early-phase trials. Moreover, the trialists' mandate to collect data systematically makes individual tailoring largely incompatible with the development of generalizable knowledge.

NOTES AND QUESTIONS

1. As King notes, payment to subjects is typically not considered a "benefit" of research for purposes of the IRB's risk-benefit assessment. That has not always been the case. *See* Ruth Macklin, *The Paradoxical Case of Payment as Benefit to Research Subjects*, 11 IRB, Nov.-Dec. 1989, at 1 (criticizing the FDA's characterization of payments to subjects as a "benefit" of research). The FDA's position has since been changed. *See* Chapter 8, at page 395. Why shouldn't payment to subjects be considered a benefit of research? Does it make sense to treat financial costs to subjects as a risk of research, *see supra* page 252, but to exclude payments to subjects from the IRB's assessment of benefit? If payments to subjects are not treated as benefits, should the psychosocial and kinship benefits described by Levine also be excluded from the IRB's consideration?

2. Why is King concerned about including so-called "collateral benefits" in the IRB's risk-benefit assessment? If individuals will receive better overall care in the context of a study, is it necessarily wrong for IRBs to consider those benefits in evaluating the acceptability of research-related risks?

[B] The Production of Knowledge as a Benefit of Research

The production of generalizable knowledge is the *raison d'être* of research. Unless a study holds out a reasonable prospect of producing generalizable knowledge, the risks of research cannot be justified, regardless of whether the subjects may receive a direct benefit from participating in the study. (Make sure you understand why this conclusion necessarily follows from the risk assessment standard set forth in 45 C.F.R. § 111(a)(2).) Of course, in studies in which there is no possibility of benefiting the subjects directly, the potential to generate knowledge is the only benefit the IRB can balance against risk.

Institutional Review Board Assessment of Risks and Benefits Associated with Research
in 2 National Bioethics Advisory Commission, Ethical and Policy Issues in Research Involving Human Participants
Ernest D. Prentice & Bruce G. Gordon
L-1 (2001)

Research is commonly divided into "therapeutic" and "nontherapeutic." Although the distinction between the two is not as clear as it would seem, nonetheless the division has some value, particularly in the IRB's assessment of study related benefits. Typically, therapeutic research or "research on therapy," as it has been more correctly described, is not performed solely to produce generalizable knowledge, but also has the intent of providing a direct medical benefit to the subject. . . .

Nontherapeutic research, in contrast, has no intent of producing a diagnostic, preventive, or therapeutic benefit to the subject. Although subjects of nontherapeutic research are usually healthy volunteers, this is not always the case. For example, a study of the salivary cortisol levels in patients hospitalized after severe trauma would be considered "nontherapeutic" research without any direct health benefit to the subject. In other cases, participation in nontherapeutic research may yield information that is of benefit to the subject. For example, a study that measures maximal oxygen consumption during sustained exercise may be of value to a long-distance runner in establishing training goals or a study that includes comprehensive educational and psychological testing may be of value to a subject planning his or her career path. . . .

In the setting of nontherapeutic research, benefits to society in terms of knowledge to be gained may be the only clearly identifiable benefit. Societal gain without direct benefit to the subject, however, may not be sufficient justification, especially when vulnerable populations are involved.

NOTES AND QUESTIONS

1. Whether research is likely to produce generalizable knowledge depends in part on the adequacy of the study design. Thus, methodological analysis is an important component of IRB review. The importance of sound research methodology means that studies with too few subjects to produce statistically valid information should generally not be conducted. However, with rare diseases, it may be impossible to recruit a sufficient number of subjects to produce a statistically valid study. In these circumstances, it has been suggested that researchers conduct "prospectively designed meta-analyses," i.e., a series of small-scale studies designed so that their results can be combined to draw statistically valid conclusions. *See* Scott D. Halpern et al., *The Continuing Unethical Conduct of Underpowered Clinical Trials*, 288 JAMA 358 (2002) ("[O]nly prospectively designed meta-analyses can justify the risks to participants in individually underpowered trials because they provide sufficient assurance that a study's results will eventually contribute to valuable or important knowledge.").

2. Generalizable knowledge, in and of itself, is not necessarily a "benefit" sufficient to justify risk. Instead, "[i]f one holds the view that the primary objective of a trial is to provide knowledge that is able to be directly translated into an improved treatment choice, a trial needs to be designed so that reasonable clinicians would allow its results to influence their choice of treatment." Benjamin Freedman & Stanley H. Shapiro, *Ethics and Statistics in Clinical Research: Towards a More Comprehensive Examination*, 42 J. STATISTICAL PLANNING & INFERENCE 233 (1994). This means that the study must be designed to show more than a statistically significant difference between the two arms of the

study. Rather, it should "provide sufficient evidence to conclude that the treatment difference exceeds a value . . . such that the treatment of choice would be altered." *Id.*

Producing clinically useful information may make it impossible to adhere to a scientifically "fastidious" study design:

> When a controlled trial imposes rigid criteria, the aim is to narrow the population to two groups similar in as many relevant respects as feasibly may be determined, differing only in the allocation of treatment of the two groups. Such a "fastidious" trial is intended to present the cleanest possible scientific comparison. That choice, though, loses in generalizability what it may have gained in validity. The trial is intended to teach us something about the treatment of patients, who do not have the luxury of checking a list of eligibility criteria before choosing to become ill. The clinical goal of a trial — to achieve results that rationally contribute to decisions about patient care — can be sacrificed in "fastidious" trials to an unyielding commitment to scientific validity.

> The choice of a point along the continuum between maximally "fastidious" trials (i.e., those with tightly-controlled eligibility criteria) and supremely "sloppy" ones has an important ethical component. This is made more clear by rephrasing the issue at stake: What is the *ethos* of a clinical trial? — To yield valid, reproducible knowledge; or, to improve patient care?

> As a practical matter, of course, these two often come in tandem: Patient care ought not be influenced by the results of experiments of poor design and necessarily equivocal interpretation. Does that imply that considerations of generalizability should always yield to validity? Such a decision-rule is often inherent in the stepwise progression of clinical trials, that may begin by testing a treatment in a very narrow population, and, upon achieving success, mounts trials in a progressively broader patient population. This strategy, under the best of circumstances, results in serious downstream costs: The bulk of the patient population needs to await the results of a series of trials, a process that can take ten years or more, before seeing an improvement in their condition. The strategy also raises the empirical likelihood that as the trials slowly and carefully progress, clinicians whose primary concern is with treating patients will begin to adopt the treatment under study for their sloppy, undifferentiated patient population. Accrual of patients in the later stages of trials will slip, as more patients have access to the new treatment off trial, thereby avoiding the risk of enrolling in the trial and being randomized to the old regimen. All of this, of course, implicates a further ethical question: Is it justified to carry this stepwise plan through to completion, as evidence accumulates that the treatment in question is likely to be effective on a broad population?

Id. How can IRBs reconcile this tension between scientific validity and clinical generalizability?

§ 6.04   BALANCING RISKS AND BENEFITS

ETHICAL PRINCIPLES AND GUIDELINES FOR THE PROTECTION OF HUMAN SUBJECTS OF RESEARCH (THE BELMONT REPORT) NATIONAL COMMISSION FOR THE PROTECTION OF HUMAN SUBJECTS OF BIOMEDICAL AND BEHAVIORAL RESEARCH
(1979)

It is commonly said that benefits and risks must be "balanced" and shown to be "in a favorable ratio." The metaphorical character of these terms draws attention to the difficulty of making precise judgments. Only on rare occasions will quantitative techniques be available for the scrutiny of research protocols. However, the idea of systematic, nonarbitrary analysis of risks and benefits should be emulated insofar as possible. This ideal requires those making decisions about the justifiability of research to be thorough in the accumulation and assessment of information about all aspects of the research, and to consider alternatives systematically. This procedure renders the assessment of research more rigorous and precise, while making communication between review board members and investigators less subject to misinterpretation, misinformation and conflicting judgments. Thus, there should first be a determination of the validity of the presuppositions of the research; then the nature, probability and magnitude of risk should be distinguished with as much clarity as possible. The method of ascertaining risks should be explicit, especially where there is no alternative to the use of such vague categories as small or slight risk. It should also be determined whether an investigator's estimates of the probability of harm or benefits are reasonable, as judged by known facts or other available studies.

Finally, assessment of the justifiability of research should reflect at least the following considerations: (i) Brutal or inhumane treatment of human subjects is never morally justified. (ii) Risks should be reduced to those necessary to achieve the research objective. It should be determined whether it is in fact necessary to use human subjects at all. Risk can perhaps never be entirely eliminated, but it can often be reduced by careful attention to alternative procedures. (iii) When research involves significant risk of serious impairment, review committees should be extraordinarily insistent on the justification of the risk (looking usually to the likelihood of benefit to the subject — or, in some rare cases, to the manifest voluntariness of the participation). (iv) When vulnerable populations are involved in research, the appropriateness of involving them should itself be demonstrated. A number of variables go into such judgments, including the nature and degree of risk, the condition of the particular population involved, and the nature and level of the anticipated benefits. (v) Relevant risks and benefits must be thoroughly arrayed in documents and procedures used in the informed consent process.

The Incommensurability of Research Risks and Benefits: Practical Help for Research Ethics Committees
Douglas K. Martin et al.
17 IRB, Mar.-Apr. 1995, at 8

There are two types of incommensurability regarding research risks and benefits. First, risks and benefits for subjects may affect different domains of health status. For example, a subject may incur a physical risk in expectation of a potential psychological benefit. Second, in some research, risks and benefits may affect different people. For example, in some cases the risks of research may be borne by the subject, but the direct benefits (possible therapeutic effects of the intervention) and the indirect benefits (the development or contribution to generalizable knowledge that is a defining feature of research) accrue to others — to future patients and science. The following three examples illustrate both of these types of incommensurability in medical research.

Live-Donor Lung Transplantation

Lung transplantation is a viable treatment option for patients with end-stage lung disease, but many potential recipients die before a donor lung becomes available. To help meet the demand for donor lungs, researchers have attempted experimental live-donor lung transplantation. What are the potential risks and benefits of this research? For the donor, the risk is that of lobectomy, which has a mortality rate of less than 1% and possible long-term effects on pulmonary function; the potential benefit is knowing that one has attempted to save the life of another, usually a loved one. For the recipient, the risks are those of receiving only a lobe of lung rather than a whole lung and that the transplanted lobe will not grow along with the recipient so that it may become insufficient to support adequate pulmonary function; the potential benefit is a reduced chance of dying while awaiting transplant. In live-donor lung transplantation, the principal risk is assumed by the donor but the principal benefit accrues to the recipient. Moreover, donors assume a physical risk but potentially gain a psychological benefit. The risks and benefits are of different types with no common measurement, and are distributed between different people.

Renal Biopsy for Diabetic Kidney Disease

Because renal biopsy is the only means of identifying structural changes early in the evolution of diabetic kidney disease, it has been proposed as a logical part of research into the pathogenesis of this disease. Research renal biopsy offers no direct benefit to the individual undergoing the procedure other than the satisfaction the subject might feel as a result of "furthering science." The physical risk of research renal biopsy to the subject is unknown, but is expected to be less than the risk of renal biopsy for clinical indications; the risk is short-term, finite, and experienced by the subject. The benefits of research renal biopsies are long-term, imprecise, and experienced by future patients, or communities who suffer from diabetic kidney disease (for example, Pima Indians, a community whose prevalence of diabetic kidney disease is very high). These risks and benefits affect different domains and they accrue to different people.

Phase I Drug Trials

Although substantial knowledge about investigational new drugs is obtained from extensive animal studies before exposure to humans, many of the undesirable effects of drug use are evident only in human trials. Phase I studies help to evaluate pharmacological activity, toxicity, absorption, metabolism and excretion, and involve measurements of blood and urinary levels. In most phase I studies the subjects are healthy volunteers, although phase I cancer trials restrict enrollment to subjects who have cancer since anti-cancer drugs are toxic. In phase I trials, subjects assume the direct risk of toxicity and side effects. While these subjects may benefit from the knowledge that they have helped society, it is unlikely that they will benefit directly from the study drug. The benefits of phase I drug studies accrue to society in general (or an unidentified subgroup of society who may one day require treatment using the drug under study). There are different types of risks and benefits in Phase I drug studies and they are distributed between different people. . . .

RECs [research ethics committees] cannot assess the balance of incommensurable risks and benefits. Nevertheless, RECs still have the responsibility for approving or rejecting research protocols according to the ethical merit of each proposal, and the risk-benefit analysis is part of this evaluation. RECs could benefit from the input of potential subjects and beneficiaries. First, only the individuals involved know how different incommensurable consequences will affect them personally. This is the common currency, or common scale, that allows potential subjects or beneficiaries to "weigh" risks and benefits, or determine the acceptability of the risk-benefit "ratio." Second, only the community of potential subjects and beneficiaries can assess the acceptability of potential risks when the harms and benefits that result from research will accrue to different people within the community. In particular, only those who might be harmed by research can judge whether the potential benefits to others within the community justify the risks.

In the case of research that involves incommensurable risks and benefits, we propose that RECs encourage investigators to consult the community of potential research subjects, specifically with regard to judgments about potential risks and benefits for subjects. Furthermore, RECs should request that investigators incorporate the information acquired from the consultation when developing the research protocol. RECs would then be better informed regarding the acceptability of risks and benefits in a research protocol, and better able to make their judgment about the protocol.

Consultation, before or during protocol development, could be done by sending out a "letter of intent" to members of the community of potential research subjects. In the examples we provided, investigators could survey parents of children with chronic lung disease, patients with diabetic kidney disease, or patients with the type of cancer being investigated in a proposed phase I drug trial. The letter of intent would outline the proposed procedures and describe the potential risks and benefits, then invite the potential subjects to provide their reaction with specific reference to the mix of potential harms and benefits. This information could then be submitted to the REC as part of the research proposal.

Note that our purpose is not to address whether RECs should accept or reject research protocols. RECs are making such decisions currently. However, we believe that the way in which they have been asked to appraise risks and benefits in the process of making these judgments is infeasible. We have proposed a feasible, principled method to accomplish this task.

The federal regulations direct IRBs to balance the risks to subjects against (1) potential benefits to subjects; and (2) the knowledge expected to result from the research. Does this mean that IRBs should *combine* the potential benefits to subjects and the potential contribution to knowledge, and then balance those combined benefits against the total level of risks? Or should the IRB attempt to disaggregate the potential benefits to subjects from the potential contribution to knowledge? In the following excerpt, the National Bioethics Advisory Commission urges IRBs to adopt the latter approach.

NATIONAL BIOETHICS ADVISORY COMMISSION
1 ETHICAL AND POLICY ISSUES IN RESEARCH INVOLVING HUMAN PARTICIPANTS
76-78 (2001)

Charles Weijer has proposed a framework based on a "component analysis" that he believes provides a better ethical analysis of research that contains a mixture of components — some that offer the prospect of direct benefit to research participants and others with the sole intent of answering the research question(s). In the context of a research study, *all* components are designed to answer the research question(s). Components may include one or more procedures. However, some components also offer the prospect of direct benefit to research participants, while others do not; the latter *solely* offer the potential societal benefit of knowledge. For example, a research study designed to test whether aspirin or acetaminophen reduces fever more effectively uses a number of procedures, including the administration of aspirin to one group; the administration of acetaminophen to another group; the randomization of participants to these two groups; and the measurement of fever. All of these procedures are included in the study design because they are needed to answer the research question(s). However, some of these procedures are also designed to offer the prospect of direct benefit to participants — for example, the administration of aspirin or of acetaminophen. Others, such as randomization, temperature taking, and chart comparisons, do not offer the prospect of such direct benefits; their *sole* intent is to answer the research question(s). Although a research study must be examined in its entirety, the two types of components should be judged differently.

The component-based approach to the analysis of risks and potential benefits requires IRBs to sort research study procedures into these two types of components to determine their ethical acceptability. The first type consists of those components containing particular procedures that may offer the prospect of direct benefit to participants. The second type includes procedures that do not. Most procedures in a research study are easily classified into one of these two types of components. However, in some studies, it might not be clear into which component the procedures best fit — for example, a survey involving a questionnaire and measurements of health in which clinically meaningful results (e.g., blood pressure) are reported back to participants, but no treatment is offered. Further, in any research study using diagnostic procedures that might provide useful health information to the participant in addition to the information provided for the study — such as the use of CAT scans to study brain activity that could also identify tumors—the classification of such procedures may be ambiguous and therefore requires careful consideration by the IRB.

IRBs should be able to identify whether a clear and direct benefit to society or the research participants might result from participating in the study. However, IRBs should be cautious in classifying procedures as offering the prospect of direct benefit. In fact, if it is not clear that a procedure also offers the prospect of direct benefit, IRBs should treat the procedure as one solely designed to answer the research question(s). A major advantage of this approach is that it avoids justifying the risks of procedures that are designed solely to answer the research questions based on the likelihood that another procedure in the protocol is likely to provide a benefit.

To the extent possible, IRBs should independently weigh the risks and potential benefits of each type of procedure. The risks associated with individual procedures offering the prospect of direct benefits are justified in relation to their potential to benefit the participant in addition to their potential to generate knowledge, and those procedures designed solely to answer the research question(s) are justified in relation to their potential to generate knowledge. . . .

Components Designed Solely to Answer the Research Question(s)

All research involves the administration of procedures and use of methods *solely* for the purpose of answering the research question(s). These procedures or methods can be questionnaires, interviews, chart reviews and use of existing data, observations, randomization, and clinical procedures such as blood draws. Many health services studies and most epidemiological, behavioral, and social science studies as well as historical research involve only such components.

By definition, risks associated with components containing procedures designed *solely* to answer the research question(s) can be justified only by the potential benefit associated with the knowledge gained, not by the potential direct benefits to individual participants. [Benjamin] Freedman argued that this judgment requires the opinion of both scientific experts and community representatives. Community representatives might come from geographic areas or from affected participant communities (e.g., persons with a particular disorder). Involving community representatives can be challenging, as it is sometimes difficult to define relevant groups or individuals who can represent the community. As risks increase, scrutiny from the communities that may be affected by the research findings will help to ensure public confidence and trust that participants are offered "reasonable choices."

Components That Also Offer the Prospect of Direct Benefits

Clinical and other types of research studies might include procedures that, in addition to answering the research question(s), also offer the prospect of direct benefit to participants, such as drug interventions, surgical and medical procedures, or educational, psychological, and behavioral interventions. They might also include diagnostic and other procedures that guide the administration of treatment, even if these procedures are not routinely administered. Studies with components containing procedures of this kind pose their own distinctive challenge in the ethical analysis of risks and potential benefits.

Here too, IRBs must determine whether the relation between risks and potential benefits is reasonable. To do so, IRBs should determine whether the procedures meet the criteria of research equipoise in addition to being justified in terms of the potential knowledge gain for society. Investigators and IRBs should understand that the term *research equipoise* applies to any type of research involving interventions or procedures that offer the prospect of direct benefit to participants, which would include, for example, health education interventions, clinical psychology interventions, and public health interventions.

NOTES AND QUESTIONS

1. What are the advantages and disadvantages of the component-based approach to risk-benefit assessment, as compared to an approach that lumps together potential benefits to subjects and potential contributions to knowledge? Which type of approach is likely to lead IRBs to request changes to more protocols?

2. How should IRBs deal with the incommensurability problem discussed in the article by Martin et al.? Is the type of community consultation suggested in

the excerpt the best way to deal with the problem?

3. Can the possibility of producing generalizable knowledge, in itself, ever justify significant risks to research subjects, or should high-risk research be limited to studies in which there is also a prospect of direct benefits to the subjects themselves? For differing views on this question, compare Royal College of Physicians, *Research on Healthy Volunteers: A Report of the Royal College of Physicians*, 20 J. ROYAL COLLEGE OF PHYSICIANS 245 (1986) (concluding that it is unacceptable to conduct greater-than-minimal-risk research with normal healthy volunteers) with NEW YORK STATE DEPARTMENT OF HEALTH WORKGROUP ON IRB GUIDELINES, SAFEGUARDING HEALTHY RESEARCH SUBJECTS: PROTECTING VOLUNTEERS FROM HARM (1999) (arguing that "personal autonomy should enable an individual to choose to participate in a scientifically valid more-than-minimal-risk study as long as the risks are disclosed to the individual, the individual understands the extent of those risks, any incentives offered are appropriate, and the individual provides informed consent").

4. Alex Rajczi argues that it will often be impossible for IRBs to determine whether a particular study "will do more good than harm," given the difficulty of estimating the likelihood of harms and benefits and the lack of objective measures for valuing good or bad outcomes. Moreover, Rajczi suggests, even if such calculations were possible, it would be inappropriate for IRBs to condition approval of research on a showing that the study will do more good than harm. Instead, the standard for risk-benefit assessment should be based on what Rajczi calls "the agreement principle":

> A protocol has an acceptable combination of risks and benefits if it would be entered into by *competent and informed decision-makers* — that is, people who (i) have a set of values that is at least minimally consistent, stable, and affirmed as their own, (ii) are informed about the nature of the protocol in question, and (iii) reason clearly about whether to enter the protocol using those values. Otherwise, it does not.

Alex Rajczi, *Making Risk-Benefit Assessment of Medical Research Protocols*, 32 J. L. MED. & ETHICS 338, 342 (2004). Do you agree? What objections might be raised to Rajczi's proposal?

§ 6.05 MINIMIZING RISKS

The federal regulations direct IRBs to ensure that risks to subjects are minimized "(i) by using procedures which are consistent with sound research design and which do not unnecessarily expose subjects to risk, and (ii) whenever appropriate, by using procedures already being performed on the subjects for diagnostic or treatment purposes." 45 C.F.R. § 46.111(a).

Safeguarding Healthy Research Subjects: Protecting Volunteers from Harm New York State Department of Health Workgroup on IRB Guidelines
(1999)

Unnecessary risks to subjects, no matter how small, can never be justified. Accordingly, IRBs should ensure that researchers minimize risks. To fulfill this obligation, IRBs should inquire about the following:

- Necessity of proposed procedures — Are the procedures proposed as part of the research design necessary to the question under investigation?

- Safety of proposed procedures — Is there a safer way to carry out the proposed procedure? Does the equipment that will be utilized meet safety standards? Will procedures be performed by competent and properly qualified individuals? Investigators are responsible for identifying the safest method of conducting their proposed research. If the investigators know or learn of a potentially safer method than the one proposed, even if it requires substantially more costly equipment or procedures, they should provide that information to the IRB along with a discussion of the advantages and disadvantages of the alternative methodology.

- Number of subjects exposed — Have the researchers ensured that the fewest people necessary will be exposed to any given risk? To answer this question, statistical tools such as power analysis should be considered by the IRB in the approval process.

NOTES AND QUESTIONS

1. How should IRBs go about determining whether a particular risk is "unnecessary"? In addition to considering the availability of methods to reduce or eliminate the risk, should IRBs also take into account the costs of those methods?

2. In what way might using placebo controls help researchers carry out some of the obligations suggested by the New York State workgroup?

Chapter 7

INFORMED CONSENT

Informed consent is the primary mechanism used to incorporate prospective subjects' preferences, values, fears, and expectations into decisions about enrolling and continuing in research. It is important to distinguish the doctrine of informed consent to research from that governing informed consent to medical care. The requirements for obtaining informed consent to medical care were honed by state courts around the time of the civil rights movement as patients struggled to establish the prominence of their decisions in the face of a long-standing tradition of medical paternalism. The principles governing informed consent to research, by contrast, emerged from the Nuremberg Code and the work of national and international ethics commissions. Those principles are now incorporated into the federal regulations governing human subject protection.

While our ultimate goal in this chapter is to explore the role of informed consent in the research setting, we begin by examining the principles governing informed consent to medical care. We do so because, as these two related notions of informed consent have developed, each has been informed by the other. Understanding the doctrine of informed consent to medical care is therefore an important foundation for exploring informed consent to research. In addition, the law governing informed consent to medical care is much better developed than the law governing informed consent to research. Legal principles developed in the context of medical treatment are a useful basis for thinking through some of the unresolved questions in the research setting.

As you read through these materials, think about the similarities and differences between the researcher-subject relationship and the ordinary physician-patient relationship. How might some of these distinctions be relevant to the doctrine of informed consent? In addition, consider why there appears to be such a significant gap between the legal and ethical ideals of informed consent and what actually happens in real-world settings. What measures might be undertaken to narrow that gap? Is it realistic to expect that the practice of informed consent will measure up to the doctrine's lofty goals in all situations?

§ 7.01 FROM CONSENT TO MEDICAL CARE TO CONSENT TO RESEARCH

[A] Informed Consent to Medical Care

[1] Case Law

The modern law of informed consent to medical care has contributed to a fundamental shift in the relationship between physicians and patients. As the Institute of Medicine has observed,

> The ethical ideal of informed consent, grounded in the philosophical concept of autonomy, represents a departure from the paternalistic traditions of medicine revealed in the Hippocratic text, in which physicians were told to direct their commitment to the health and well-being of their patients, but were not instructed to foster their independence of thought or individual choice. In the Hippocratic text, physicians are exhorted to keep patients from "harm and injustice" . . . not to give a "deadly drug" . . . and to "come for the benefit of the sick."
>
> In the late 1950s and the 1960s, however, judges began to propose in court opinions that one of the duties of the physician was to share sufficient information or "reasonable disclosure" with the patient so that the patient could choose among available medical options. In addition to the idea of professional duty was the developing legal concept of self-determination. In [the 1914 case] *Schloendorff* v. *Society of New York Hospital,* Judge Cardozo stated that "Every human being of adult years and sound mind shall have the right to determine what shall be done with his own body. . . ." This idea of liberty or self-determination evolved to include decisions about choices in medicine.
>
> Concurrent with the legal development of these concepts, the higher profile of medical ethical analysis and the various rights movements, including the patient rights discussions, led to an ongoing discussion in medicine about the doctor-patient relationship. The result of that discussion, in the context of the legal opinions and scholarship, was the general agreement that paternalism was no longer appropriate as the guiding philosophy of medicine and physician practice. The physician was exhorted to discuss, deliberate, and share with the patient so that this relationship could provide the basis for individually appropriate patient choice.

INSTITUTE OF MEDICINE, NATIONAL ACADEMY OF SCIENCES, RESPONSIBLE RESEARCH: A SYSTEMS APPROACH TO PROTECTING RESEARCH PARTICIPANTS 120-21 (2002).

While the *Schloendorff* case noted above was significant in its recognition of the patient's right to self-determination, that case merely recognized that it was wrong for doctors to operate on a woman when she had specifically told them she did not want an operation. From *Schloendorff* through the first half of the twentieth century, there was not yet any requirement that specific types of information be given to patients before they agreed to surgery or other medical treatment. The term "informed consent" does not appear until 1957 in a California case, *Salgo v. Leland Stanford Jr. University Board of Trustees,* 317 P.2d 170 (Cal. Ct. App. 1957).

As you read the following case, be aware that it was a ground-breaking departure from the usual manner of determining what disclosures a physician must make to a patient. This case was brought as a medical malpractice action, a type of negligence claim. As discussed in Chapter 12, malpractice actions typically require proof that the physician deviated from the "standard of care," and the standard of care has traditionally been determined by looking at the medical community's customary practices. *See* Chapter 12, at page 499. Until *Canterbury,* it was assumed that the standard of care for obtaining informed consent, like other medical standards of care, was set by medical custom.

CANTERBURY v. SPENCE
United States Court of Appeals for the District of Columbia Circuit
464 F.2d 772 (D.C. Cir. 1972)

It is well established that the physician must seek and secure his patient's consent before commencing an operation or other course of treatment. It is also clear that the consent, to be efficacious, must be free from imposition upon the patient. It is the settled rule that therapy not authorized by the patient may amount to a tort — a common law battery — by the physician. And it is evident that it is normally impossible to obtain a consent worthy of the name unless the physician first elucidates the options and the perils for the patient's edification. Thus the physician has long borne a duty, on pain of liability for unauthorized treatment, to make adequate disclosure to the patient. The evolution of the obligation to communicate for the patient's benefit as well as the physician's protection has hardly involved an extraordinary restructuring of the law.

Duty to disclose has gained recognition in a large number of American jurisdictions, but more largely on a different rationale. The majority of courts dealing with the problem have made the duty depend on whether it was the custom of physicians practicing in the community to make the particular disclosure to the patient. If so, the physician may be held liable for an unreasonable and injurious failure to divulge, but there can be no recovery unless the omission forsakes a practice prevalent in the profession. We agree that the physician's noncompliance with a professional custom to reveal, like any other departure from prevailing medical practice, may give rise to liability to the patient. We do not agree that the patient's cause of action is dependent upon the existence and nonperformance of a relevant professional tradition.

There are, in our view, formidable obstacles to acceptance of the notion that the physician's obligation to disclose is either germinated or limited by medical practice. To begin with, the reality of any discernible custom reflecting a professional consensus on communication of option and risk information to patients is open to serious doubt. We sense the danger that what in fact is no custom at all may be taken as an affirmative custom to maintain silence, and that physician-witnesses to the so-called custom may state merely their personal opinions as to what they or others would do under given conditions. . . . Respect for the patient's right of self-determination on particular therapy demands a standard set by law for physicians rather than one which physicians may or may not impose upon themselves. . . .

In our view, the patient's right of self-decision shapes the boundaries of the duty to reveal. That right can be effectively exercised only if the patient possesses enough information to enable an intelligent choice. The scope of the physician's communications to the patient, then, must be measured by the patient's need, and that need is the information material to the decision. Thus the test for determining whether a particular peril must be divulged is its materiality to the patient's decision: all risks potentially affecting the decision must be unmasked. And to safeguard the patient's interest in achieving his own determination on treatment, the law must itself set the standard for adequate disclosure.

Optimally for the patient, exposure of a risk would be mandatory whenever the patient would deem it significant to his decision, either singly or in combination with other risks. Such a requirement, however, would summon the physician to second-guess the patient, whose ideas on materiality could hardly be known to the physician. That would make an undue demand upon medical practitioners, whose conduct, like that of others, is to be measured in terms of reasonableness. Consonantly with orthodox negligence doctrine, the physician's liability for nondisclosure is to be determined on the basis of foresight, not hindsight; no less than any other aspect of negligence, the issue of nondisclosure must be approached from the viewpoint of the reasonableness of the physician's divulgence in terms of what he knows or should know to be the patient's informational needs. If, but only if, the fact-finder can say that the physician's communication was unreasonably inadequate is an imposition of liability legally or morally justified.

Of necessity, the content of the disclosure rests in the first instance with the physician. Ordinarily it is only he who is in a position to identify particular dangers; always he must make a judgment, in terms of materiality, as to whether and to what extent revelation to the patient is called for. He cannot know with complete exactitude what the patient would consider important to his decision, but on the basis of his medical training and experience he can sense how the average, reasonable patient expectably would react. Indeed, with knowledge of, or ability to learn, his patient's background and current condition, he is in a position superior to that of most others — attorneys, for example — who are called upon to make judgments on pain of liability in damages for unreasonable miscalculation.

From these considerations we derive the breadth of the disclosure of risks legally to be required. The scope of the standard is not subjective as to either the physician or the patient; it remains objective with due regard for the patient's informational needs and with suitable leeway for the physician's situation. In broad outline, we agree that "[a] risk is thus material when a reasonable person, in what the physician knows or should know to be the patient's position, would be likely to attach significance to the risk or cluster of risks in deciding whether or not to forego the proposed therapy." . . .

Two exceptions to the general rule of disclosure have been noted by the courts. Each is in the nature of a physician's privilege not to disclose, and the reasoning underlying them is appealing. Each, indeed, is but a recognition that, as important as is the patient's right to know, it is greatly outweighed by the magnitudinous circumstances giving rise to the privilege. The first comes into play when the patient is unconscious or otherwise incapable of consenting, and harm from a failure to treat is imminent and outweighs any harm threatened by the proposed treatment. When a genuine emergency of that sort arises, it is settled that the impracticality of conferring with the patient dispenses with need for it. Even in situations of that character the physician should, as current law requires, attempt to secure a relative's consent if possible. But if time is too short to accommodate discussion, obviously the physician should proceed with the treatment.

The second exception obtains when risk-disclosure poses such a threat of detriment to the patient as to become unfeasible or contraindicated from a medical point of view. It is recognized that patients occasionally become so ill or emotionally distraught on disclosure as to foreclose a rational decision, or complicate or hinder the treatment, or perhaps even pose psychological damage to the patient. Where that is so, the cases have generally held that the physician is armed with a privilege to keep the information from the patient, and we think it clear that portents of that type may justify the physician in action he deems medically warranted. The critical inquiry is whether the physician responded to a sound medical judgment that communication of the risk information would present a threat to the patient's well-being.

The physician's privilege to withhold information for therapeutic reasons must be carefully circumscribed, however, for otherwise it might devour the disclosure rule itself. The privilege does not accept the paternalistic notion that the physician may remain silent simply because divulgence might prompt the patient to forego therapy the physician feels the patient really needs. That attitude presumes instability or perversity for even the normal patient, and runs counter to the foundation principle that the patient should and ordinarily can make the choice for himself. Nor does the privilege contemplate operation save where the patient's reaction to risk information, as reasonably foreseen by the physician, is menacing. And even in a situation of that kind, disclosure to a close relative with a view to securing consent to the proposed treatment may be the only alternative open to the physician.

NOTES AND QUESTIONS

1. Can you speculate on the reaction of the physician community to this new process of determining patients' informational needs?

2. The *Canterbury* approach, which is sometimes referred to as the "reasonable patient" standard of disclosure, is the law in about half the states. Most other states limit physicians' disclosure obligations to the information that a reasonable practitioner would ordinarily disclose (the "professional standard"). *See* Ketchup v. Howard, 543 S.E.2d 371, 381 (Ga. Ct. App. 2000) (the appendix to the opinion describes the laws of every state). Given the arguments in support of the reasonable patient standard set forth in *Canterbury*, why do you think so many states have adopted the professional standard? Which of the two approaches do you think is preferable?

3. Note that both the reasonable patient standard and the professional standard are objective standards: the adequacy of the physician's disclosure is judged by either what a "reasonable patient" would want to know or what a "reasonable practitioner" would ordinarily disclose. What would a subjective approach to informed consent look like? Why do you think most states have not adopted a subjective approach?

4. Even under the objective reasonable patient standard, physicians may be required to modify their disclosures based on the informational needs of a particular patient. A patient may indicate, for example, that she is particularly concerned about a certain type of risk that most people would probably not consider material. If a doctor is put on notice in this way, she may be required to disclose information relevant to the patient's idiosyncratic needs. *See,* e.g., Hartke v. McKelway, 707 F.2d 1544 (D.D.C. 1983).

5. Note that *Canterbury* creates two exceptions to the rule requiring informed consent: one applies when the patient is unconscious or otherwise incapable of consenting; the second applies when there would be direct and immediate harm to the patient from the disclosure. Does the opinion make a persuasive case for these exceptions in the clinical context? Do you think that the same exceptions should apply in research?

6. Informed consent to clinical care may or may not involve having a patient read and sign a written document (a consent form). In a few situations, state legislation requires the use of such forms. Many states, for example, have laws requiring written informed consent to genetic testing. *See,* e.g., N.Y. CIV. RIGHTS LAW § 79-l(2)(a). In most instances, however, the decision whether to use a consent form is up to the health care provider. Typically, providers choose to use consent forms only when the treatment involves some type of invasive procedure, such as surgery. These forms are often "boilerplate," in the sense that patients undergoing very different procedures may end up reading and signing the same form. There will commonly be blank lines to be filled in with the names of the procedure and the doctor who will perform it. As will be discussed later in this

chapter, the use of consent forms in research is subject to much stricter regulation.

7. Based on what you know about the purpose of informed consent to medical care is the current approach to consent forms too lax? Should physicians be required to create written consent forms describing the major risks, benefits, and alternatives to a particular treatment, and allow patients to read the form (and perhaps even require them to sign it)? What would be the possible benefits of such an approach? What would be the downsides?

8. When patients sue for damages based on a physician's failure to disclose information about the risks, benefits, or alternatives of treatment, they must prove not only that the physician deviated from the applicable disclosure standard, but also that this deviation was the cause of the patient's injuries. Issues related to proving causation in informed consent cases are discussed in Chapter 12, at page 514, in the context of tort actions against researchers.

[2] Medical Practice Guidelines

STATEMENT OF THE AMERICAN MEDICAL ASSOCIATION COUNCIL ON ETHICAL AND JUDICIAL AFFAIRS
(adopted by the House of Delegates, March 1981)
http://www.ama-assn.org/ceja

The patient's right of self-decision can be effectively exercised only if the patient possesses enough information to enable an intelligent choice. The patient should make his or her own determination on treatment. The physician's obligation is to present the medical facts accurately to the patient or to the individual responsible for the patient's care and to make recommendations for management in accordance with good medical practice. The physician has an ethical obligation to help the patient make choices from among the therapeutic alternatives consistent with good medical practice. Informed consent is a basic social policy for which exceptions are permitted: (1) where the patient is unconscious or otherwise incapable of consenting and harm from failure to treat is imminent; or (2) when risk disclosure poses such a serious psychological threat of detriment to the patient as to be medically contraindicated. Social policy does not accept the paternalistic view that the physician may remain silent because divulgence might prompt the patient to forego needed therapy. Rational, informed patients should not be expected to act uniformly, even under similar circumstances, in agreeing to or refusing treatment.

NOTES AND QUESTIONS

1. Practice guidelines are neither statutes nor regulations. They are generally adopted by professional associations in an effort to foster good patterns of professional behavior. They do not, in and of themselves, establish the standard of care, but they are evidence of the profession's goals for itself. They are often referred to in litigation as one element in establishing the legal standard of care. *See* Michelle M. Mello, *Of Swords and Shields: The Role of Clinical Practice Guidelines in Medical Malpractice Litigation*, 149 U. Pa. L. Rev. 645 (2001).

2. You have all seen a physician at some time in your life. What were your expectations or hopes for that encounter? Were they fulfilled? Imagine that you are considering enrolling in a research protocol. What would you expect or want to discuss with the researcher? How might these expectations and desires contrast with those you would have in an ordinary clinical encounter?

[B] Informed Consent to Innovative Treatment

Doctors not infrequently offer patients new or unproven interventions as part of a patient's medical care. These situations are similar to research in that the patient is being asked to consent to something whose safety and efficacy have not yet been established. However, in the clinical context, the intervention is being offered because the doctor thinks it is the best choice for the patient; in research, by contrast, the goal is to develop generalizable knowledge. Because these situations differ from both ordinary medical treatment and formal research, they raise unique informed consent issues.

Waived Consent for Emergency Research
Norman Fost
24 Am. J. L. & Med. 163 (1998)

It has long been accepted that the standards for consent should be higher in the research setting than in ordinary care. Research is much more tightly regulated than standard treatment, with its succession of barriers from reviews of proposals for funding, approval of an IRB, detailed requirements for informed consent and review at the time of publication. There are several reasons for this, including the history of serious transgressions, particularly the horrific disclosures of the Nuremberg trials. Laws are not written until they are first broken. In addition, compared with standard care, experimentation is reasonably convenient to regulate due to its limited frequency and the existence of "tollgates," such as FDA approval and NIH funding.

This elaborate and generally effective regulatory infrastructure provides more protection to a patient in a clinical trial than a patient receiving routine care. In contrast, a physician providing routine care has considerable liberty to experiment on his patients. This experimentation is commonly termed "innovative therapy." The central differences between innovative therapy and research are that, in the former, there is relatively no regulatory oversight and a minimal likelihood that generally applicable knowledge will result. In the trenchant words of Paul Lietman, "As long as you promise not to learn anything from what you're doing, you don't have to go through an IRB."

For several reasons, the likelihood of patient exposure to innovative therapy — essentially unreviewed, uncontrolled experimentation — as compared with regulated research is arguably higher in the emergency and critical care settings than elsewhere. The pressure of clinical work leaves little time for physicians to design and implement research studies. Physicians attracted to emergency and critical care may be more inclined to action than scholarly activities. Moreover, the difficulties of obtaining IRB consent, coupled with complying with the federal regulation, have long been seen as barriers to conducting well-designed prospective studies in emergency settings.

Innovative therapy often had disastrous consequences. Many invasive, dangerous interventions were used for decades before physicians realized that such procedures were unacceptably toxic, ineffective or both. Thousands of children were killed or injured by these therapeutic misadventures. Although systematic comparisons are difficult, comparable examples of such widespread harm rarely result from well-designed, peer-reviewed clinical trials. Prospective review reduces the possibility for harm, filtering out many poorly thought out research designs through requiring researchers to satisfy particular requirements. Such requirements may include literature reviews and animal studies when appropriate; screening investigators for competence to conduct proposed studies; requiring justifications for sample size to reduce the number of potential subjects exposed to risk; interim review, by either an IRB or a data monitoring committee; and disseminating results through presentations at scientific meetings and publication. . . .

If this analysis is correct, then it follows that the standards for consent should be highest in those settings in which other mechanisms for protecting patients from harm are absent; namely, innovative therapy.

It might be said in response that the researcher has a conflict of interest in serving two masters: future patients versus the patient before him. It is this conflict that leads the physician/investigator to compromise the interests of his patient in the name of science, society and perhaps personal advancement. But the potential for these conflicts has been largely buffered in recent decades by the many layers of oversight in clinical research. The egregiously unethical practices that were common thirty years ago are now rare, presumably because of this extensive multi-layered oversight. For reasons such as undue confidence in technology, an impulse to action, and the absence of sufficient brakes on a physician's enthusiasm, an innovative therapist in the emergency setting has neither consent nor oversight to protect the patient from unwarranted experimenting.

NOTES AND QUESTIONS

1. To better understand these informed consent issues, review the discussion in Chapter 3 of the differences between research and clinical innovation. *See* Chapter 3, at page 109.

2. In what ways should the process of obtaining a patient's informed consent to innovative therapy differ from obtaining informed consent to standard care? How should the informed consent discussion be conducted by the physician? Should physicians always use a written consent form when they provide innovative treatment? If so, what should the form say?

3. Courts addressing the issue of consent to innovative therapy have generally agreed that a doctor must inform the patient about the innovative nature of the treatment. For example, in *Estrada v. Jaques*, 321 S.E. 2d 240 (N.C. Ct. App. 1984), a gunshot wound had caused damage to a blood vessel in a patient's leg. The surgeons treated this by using a new technique, one they had read about in a journal but had never before used, involving putting a steel coil into the vessel to block the blood flow. The treatment failed, and the patient had to have his leg amputated. The court found that there was a lack of informed consent: "If the health care provider has a duty to inform of *known* risks for *established* procedures, common sense and the purposes of the statute equally require that the health care provider inform the patient of any *uncertainty* regarding the risks associated with *experimental* procedures. This includes the experimental nature of the procedure and the known or projected most likely risks."

4. What type of oversight mechanisms are physicians subject to when they provide innovative care to their patients? How do these mechanisms differ from those applicable to research? Are physicians really free to "experiment" on their patients without any legal consequences?

5. What would the consequences be of categorizing all innovative therapy as research? Would this be an advance in the ethics of research or a barrier to developing new treatments? Would such a policy be enforceable?

6. Do you agree with Fost that receiving innovative care from a physician is riskier than being in a research study?

7. Fost states that it "has long been accepted that the standards for consent should be higher in the research setting than in ordinary care." This is certainly the accepted wisdom. What reasons support such a difference? Are they convincing to you? For a minority view, see Lars Noah, *Informed Consent and the Elusive Dichotomy between Standard and Experimental Therapy*, 28 AM. J. L. & MED. 361 (2002).

[C] Informed Consent to Research

Human Experimentation and Human Rights
Jay Katz
38 St. Louis L.J. 7, 12-18 (1993)

Physician-investigators have long maintained that clinical research and therapy, more often than not, are indistinguishable; that the drugs or therapies they subject to scientific study frequently are, or could be, proffered to patients in therapeutic settings; and that the only difference between their scientific endeavors and clinical practice resides in the objective evaluation of efficacy and risk-benefits to which they submit their interventions. Thus, since vast uncertainties and ignorance about effectiveness and risk-benefits are ubiquitous in the practice of medicine, every medical intervention, therapeutic or investigative in intent, constitutes an experiment. Moreover, investigators are apt to argue that in clinical practice patients are exposed to unnecessary, scientifically unproven, ineffective, and at times dangerous therapies about which patients learn little because their physicians believe in the therapies and their unwarranted beliefs are shared by many of their professional peers. In this view, clinical research differs from practice only in its endeavors not to perpetuate these uncertainties, but to resolve them once and for all for the benefit of future patients and perhaps even for the patient-subjects involved in clinical trials. Indeed, investigators maintain that clinical research is an enterprise more moral than clinical practice because ultimately it will safeguard patients and future patients from the slings and arrows of useless, if not dangerous, therapies. Therefore, it is grossly unfair not to extend the considerable discretion which doctors enjoy in making decisions on behalf of patients in therapeutic settings to investigators, and instead subject them to onerous review procedures regarding informed consent.

These contentions speak to the latitude physicians are given generally in making decisions on behalf of patients, despite the requirement for informed consent. For even in clinical practice the doctrine of informed consent continues to be an empty ritual not only because it does not require physicians to disclose the uncertainties inherent in their interventions, about which investigators are so correctly concerned, but also because the doctrine remains so inattentive to its underlying *idea* that patients and physicians must make decisions jointly, with ultimate decision-making authority residing in the patient and *not* in the physician. Yet, all these problems notwithstanding, the doctrine of informed consent, as currently articulated, imposes similar disclosure and consent obligations for therapy and research, with the only difference being that for research the informed consent process is subjected to review by IRBs. In application, however, disclosure and consent are taken all too lightly in both settings because physicians and physician-investigators do not consider patients and patient-subjects as equal partners in the decision-making process.

All the arguments about similarities between research and practice or complaints about inequitable burdens overlook an issue that speaks to the crucial importance of informed consent in research: In therapeutic encounters, unlike research encounters, physicians are expected to attend solely to the welfare of the individual patient before them. Throughout medical history this expectation has given physicians considerable discretion and authority to make decisions on behalf of patients. More recently, to be sure, such discretion and authority have been questioned on many grounds. I shall mention only two. First, since many of the diagnostic and therapeutic options now available allow patients to make choices that can have a decisive impact on the quality of future life, what a physician thinks is best may not necessarily comport with a patient's overall needs. Second, because the available options may have an impact on physicians' economic rewards, physicians' self-interests can readily influence their professional recommendations.

Indeed, the doctrine of informed consent was promulgated in 1957 in response to both of these new realities. Judges thought that the introduction of new powerful diagnostic and treatment modalities, which promised great benefits but could also inflict considerable harm, required that patients be given a greater voice in the medical decision-making process. Yet, informed consent notwithstanding, the physician-patient encounter continues to be shaped by the belief, shared by doctors and patients, that in therapeutic settings doctors at least try to do their level best for the individual patient who seeks their help and, therefore, the doctor's recommendations can be trusted.

In clinical research, on the other hand, patient-subjects are also being used for the ends of science. One cannot dismiss with impunity the implications of this difference. In these situations investigators are committed both to real, present patients and abstract, future patients. Individual patient-centered therapy gives way to a collective patient-centered endeavor in which the abstraction of the research question tends to objectify the person-patient. It does so to a significantly greater extent than in therapeutic interactions, even though similar problems of objectification arise in therapeutic settings when doctors attend too much to the disease of the body in the bed and not to the person before them.

The readiness with which clinical research continues to be viewed as an extension of clinical practice, both similarly grounded in the millennia-long Hippocratic commitment to the welfare of the individual patient, overlooks the transformation of medical practice since the age of medical science. Throughout most of medical history, research was limited to careful bedside observation of the effects of innovative treatments, with the interests of the individual patient as a polestar. In today's world, on the other hand, the interests of patient-subjects may yield to varying extents to the interests of science. This revolutionary development has not been accompanied by a thoroughgoing reexamination of physicians' ethical obligations in a post-Hippocratic age.

Examples in point are the many cooperative clinical trials, generally randomized clinical trials (RCTs), in which institutions throughout the United

States participate and which are designed to evaluate the effectiveness of various treatment modalities for breast cancer, coronary artery disease, prostate cancer and stroke. In the conduct of such clinical trials, conflicts between the interests of patients and science are ever-present and are all too readily swept aside by viewing patient-subjects less as subjects and more as patients who can only benefit from participation in such clinical trials. Convictions of therapeutic benefit thus shape decisively the informed consent dialogue in clinical research, aided and abetted by patients' belief that their doctors have their interest uppermost in mind.

This belief is at best only partially warranted. Investigators have other personal and professional interests which can only be kept in check if both physician-investigators and patient-subjects fully appreciate that both are engaged in an enterprise in which patient-subjects are also being asked to serve as means for science's ends and that other therapeutic alternatives are often available which do not involve a research dimension.

From all I have said so far, it follows that a major problem which compromises the protection afforded to subjects of research resides in the obfuscation of the boundaries between clinical research and clinical practice. It is therefore imperative to view clinical research as a distinct category, sharply delineated from clinical practice.

The need for such sharp distinctions may fade once physicians no longer exercise such sweeping authority over patients' medical fate. In *The Silent World of Doctor and Patient,* I not only questioned this authority but also argued that the doctrine of informed consent has insufficiently reduced this authority. Thus, patients have not been provided with meaningful opportunities to make their own choices. If the time ever comes when patients' rights to autonomy and self-determination are truly respected, the problem to which I now turn — the impact of the ideology of medical professionalism on clinical research — will be less pressing. It is this ideology which has given, and continues to give, physicians considerable latitude to decide for patients, in the belief that doctors can be trusted because their self-interest will yield to patients' interests. While I have already suggested that this is a questionable assumption for therapeutic settings, it surely is an untenable one for clinical research where physician-investigators have dual allegiances — to their patient-subjects and the research protocol.

NOTES AND QUESTIONS

1. According to Katz, what are the major differences between being a patient and being a research subject?

2. Katz is widely acknowledged as a leading critic of the methods by which doctors currently obtain patients' informed consent in the clinical care setting. His landmark work, *The Silent World of Doctor and Patient,* provides a history

of informed consent and suggests that the concept has provided far less protection to patients than it might appear. (The book, though written in 1984, is well worth reading by anyone with a serious interest in informed consent.) Given his attitude toward informed consent practices in clinical care, it is not surprising that he is even more troubled by what happens in the research setting.

3. Katz's primary concern appears to be that individuals asked to participate in research will not understand what it means to be a research subject: as he more artfully puts it, there is an "obfuscation of the boundaries between clinical research and clinical practice." What things should a researcher do to help a person understand what it means to be a research subject? Are there specific pieces of information that should be provided, either in a consent form or during a discussion?

4. Katz acknowledges a proposition to which all physicians would agree: too much of medicine is "seat-of-the-pants" rather than evidence based. Indeed, the recent movement for "evidence-based" medicine is an attempt to remedy this sloppiness in practice. *See, e.g.*, Evidence-Based Medicine Working Group, *Evidence-Based Medicine: A New Approach to Teaching the Practice of Medicine*, 268 JAMA 2420 (1992). But does this lack of rigor in practice undercut the longstanding distinction between practice and research? Does clinical practice need the same sort of rigor that applies in the research setting?

5. Thomas Percival's *Code of Medical Ethics*, published in 1803, had an interesting approach to the emerging notion of research:

> Whenever cases occur, attended with circumstances not heretofore observed, or in which the ordinary modes of practice have been attempted without success, it is for the public good and in especial degree advantageous to the poor (who, being the most numerous class of this society, are the greatest beneficiaries of the healing art) that new remedies and new methods of chirurgical treatment should be devised but, in the accomplishment of the new salutary purpose, the gentlemen of the faculty should be scrupulously and conscientiously governed by sound reason, just analogy, or well-authenticated facts. And no such trials should be instituted without a previous consultation of the physicians or surgeons according to the nature of the case.

GEORGE J. ANNAS & MICHAEL A. GRODIN, THE NAZI DOCTORS AND THE NUREMBERG CODE: HUMAN RIGHTS IN HUMAN EXPERIMENTATION 124 (1992). How would you characterize Percival's approach to prospective research subjects? With whom might he have consulted in preparing his experiments? Are the subjects to be consulted at all or merely to be happy at the attention accorded their situation?

6. There is an extensive literature about informed consent to research. *See, e.g.*, Jesse A. Goldner, *An Overview of Legal Controls on Human Experimentation and the Regulatory Implications of Taking Professor Katz Seriously*, 38 ST. LOUIS L.J. 63 (1993); George J. Annas, *Questing for Grails: Duplicity, Betrayal*

and Self-Deception in Postmodern Medical Research, 12 J. CONTEMP. HEALTH L. & POL'Y 297 (1996); Karine Morin, *The Standard of Disclosure in Human Subject Experimentation*, 19 J. LEG. MED. 157 (1998); Richard W. Garnett, *Why Informed Consent? Human Experimentation and the Ethics of Autonomy*, 36 CATH. LAW. 455 (1996); Richard Delgado & Helen Leskovac, *Informed Consent in Human Experimentation: Bridging the Gap Between Ethical Thought and Current Practice*, 34 UCLA L. REV. 67 (1986); GEORGE J. ANNAS ET AL., INFORMED CONSENT TO HUMAN EXPERIMENTATION: THE SUBJECT'S DILEMMA (1977); Alexander Morgan Capron, *Informed Consent in Catastrophic Disease Research and Treatment*, 123 U. PA. L. REV. 340 (1974).

THE NUREMBERG CODE

1. The voluntary consent of the human subject is absolutely essential.

This means that the person involved should have legal capacity to give consent; should be so situated as to be able to exercise free power of choice, without the intervention of any element of force, fraud, deceit, duress, over-reaching, or other ulterior form of constraint or coercion; and should have sufficient knowledge and comprehension of the elements of the subject matter involved as to enable him to make an understanding and enlightened decision. This latter element requires that before the acceptance of an affirmative decision by the experimental subject there should be made known to him the nature, duration, and purpose of the experiment; the method and means by which it is to be conducted; all inconveniences and hazards reasonably to be expected; and the effects upon his health or person which may possibly come from his participation in the experiment.

The duty and responsibility for ascertaining the quality of the consent rests upon each individual who initiates, directs or engages in the experiment. It is a personal duty and responsibility which may not be delegated to another with impunity.

NOTES AND QUESTIONS

1. The Nuremberg Code is to a large extent the source of the principles that underlie all modern codes of research ethics, including the far more detailed federal regulations. Notice how almost every phrase in section 1 of the Code has led to its own special category of issues in modern times. See if you can identify some of them. For example, for what types of subjects might we be concerned about "legal capacity to give consent"? Which subjects might be subjected to "duress"?

2. Earlier portions of this chapter highlighted the differences between consent to medical care and consent to research. To what extent does the Nuremberg Code's provision on informed consent reflect the special concerns about

participation in research? How well does the Code reflect the concerns expressed in Katz's article? In what way does this Code provision demand more than would be required to obtain a patient's consent to medical care?

3. Can you conceive of research that would be of such little risk and such great benefit to society that informed consent should not be required? Consider a protocol that is attempting to change the behavior of child-abusing parents. It would involve surveillance through a one-way mirror in a day care center, in order to gather data that could later be used to help other parents be more caring and less abusive. No negative consequences would flow to the parents who are the subjects of the research — their faces and voices would be scrambled so that they would not be recognizable to the researchers. If they knew that they were being watched it would change their behavior and then lessen the utility of the research. Could an IRB reasonably find that this research is so critical for children and so insignificant for the subjects that it should be permitted to proceed without the parents being aware of it and its methodology? How might you describe the boundary between research that is permissible without the informed consent of the subject and research that would require full informed consent? *See, e.g.*, Robert D. Truog et al., *Is Informed Consent Always Necessary for Randomized, Controlled Trials?* 340 NEW ENG. J. MED. 804 (1999); *see also infra*, at page 313 (discussing waivers of informed consent).

§ 7.02 FEDERAL REGULATIONS GOVERNING INFORMED CONSENT TO RESEARCH

[A] General Requirements

45 C.F.R. §§ 46.116(a)-(b) AND 117(a)-(b): GENERAL REQUIREMENTS FOR OBTAINING AND DOCUMENTING INFORMED CONSENT

These provisions are reproduced in Appendix A, at page A-12. Please review them before proceeding.

NOTES AND QUESTIONS

1. Consider the similarities and differences in goal, tone, diction, moral content, and directive language between the Nuremberg Code and the federal regulations. Which one is more likely to be of help to researchers who are designing protocols? Which would offer greater guidance to an IRB? Which proffers greater protections for human subjects and why? Imagine that you were a lawyer, claiming that your client had been inadequately informed of the risks of a research study. Might some of the broad language in the Nuremberg Code be

more helpful to you than the narrower requirements in the regulations? What phrases from the Code might you emphasize to a jury?

2. As in the Nuremberg Code, the federal regulations make the informed consent of the research subject a critical requirement for proceeding with research. In contrast to the Code, however, the regulations permit a "legally authorized representative" to consent on behalf of the subject under certain circumstances. Are you comfortable with allowing consent by a legally authorized representative? This issue is explored in detail in Chapter 14.

3. What is the goal of the first paragraph of section 46.116? How would you restate its intentions? Make a list of the elements of the paragraph that are most important. Do any of these statements — exhortations — seem at odds with one another? Can you speculate on why these requirements are collected in one paragraph rather than arrayed as specific subsections?

4. How, if at all, does section 46.117 advance the cause of protecting human subjects?

[B] Waivers and Alterations of the Usual Requirements

[1] General Waivers

45 C.F.R. §§ 46.116(c)-(d): WAIVERS AND ALTERATIONS OF THE CONSENT PROCEDURE

These provisions are reproduced in Appendix A, at page A-13. Please review them before proceeding.

Veterans Administration, Office of Research Oversight, Bi-Monthly Teleconference
September 10, 2003
http://www1.va.gov/oro/docs/09-10-03.rtf

The second waiver of consent or alteration of consent element(s) [i.e., 45 C.F.R. § 46.116(d)], used quite frequently, is when the research entails only minimal risk and there is a compelling reason to alter or waive consent. . . . There are many examples in which this waiver might be appropriate. One example would be large-scale epidemiological research using medical records where the research required maintaining identifiers, perhaps to link records. The presence of identifiers means that the research project would not be eligible for an exemption, but the scale and time periods covered might make it exceedingly difficult to carry out the research if consent from all participants were required. If the IRB determines the research is minimal risk, and if the threat to a subject's privacy and confidentiality has been minimized to the extent possible, then that research might be a candidate for invoking the waiver of consent. This waiver may also be applied when consent will be obtained but some required element of consent must be altered for the research to be feasible. An example would be a study of different ways of referring people for follow-up care after they come to an emergency room. In this situation, there is an opportunity to get the subject's consent to participate in the research, but the research is testing different ways to make the referrals and the major outcome variable is whether the subjects actually show up for the follow-up appointment. If you tell the subjects that the reason for doing the research is to see if they follow-up with a doctor's appointment, you're likely to bias the research, and produce data of questionable validity. In that case, the IRB may allow the investigator to withhold some information from the subjects, even though the regulations normally would require a full explanation of the purposes of the research as part of the informed consent procedure. If, as in this case, the research might not be practicably performed unless the IRB approved withholding the information, and if all the other criteria are met, then the information may be withheld.

THE GEORGE WASHINGTON UNIVERSITY

COMMITTEE ON HUMAN RESEARCH INSTITUTIONAL REVIEW BOARD

Section II. Waiver of or Alteration to the Informed Consent Process (written or otherwise):

In order to be eligible for waiver/alteration of the informed consent process, you must meet all of the criteria outlined below.

1. Does the proposed research, in its entirety, involve greater than minimal risk? (Minimal risk is defined as the probability and magnitude of harm or discomfort anticipated in the research which are not greater in and of themselves than those ordinarily encountered in daily life or during the performance of routine physical or psychological examinations or tests.)

   ☐ **Yes.** If yes, your study is ineligible for waiver of informed consent under 45 CFR 46.116(d). However, your study may be eligible for exception from Informed Consent requirements for emergency research under 21 CFR Part 50.24. *21 CFR 50.24 applies to FDA studies only*. [For a discussion of these FDA regulations, *see infra*, page 321.]

   ☐ **No.** If no, go to question 2 below.

2. Could the proposed research be practically carried out without the waiver?

   ☐ **Yes.** If yes, your study is ineligible for waiver of informed consent.

☐ **No.** If no, please explain in the space below and continue with question 3 below:

3. Will the requested waiver of informed consent affect the rights and welfare of the subjects?

☐ **Yes.** If yes, your study is ineligible for waiver of informed consent.

☐ **No.** If no, please explain in the space below and continue with question 4 below.

4. When appropriate, will pertinent information be provided to subjects later?

☐ **Yes.** If yes, your study is eligible for waiver of informed consent.

☐ **No.** If no, please explain in the space below.

NOTES AND QUESTIONS

1. Note that studies involving FDA-regulated products are not eligible for waivers of informed consent under these provisions, as such studies are also subject to the FDA regulations, which do not provide for such waivers. This is one of the few differences between the FDA regulations and the Common Rule. *See* Appendix C.

2. What is the likely rationale behind 45 C.F.R. § 46.116(c)? Can you conceive of research that might fit within the language of that section for which a waiver of informed consent would *not* be appropriate?

3. OHRP has provided a decision chart on the topic of waivers under § 46.116(d). *See* Office for Human Research Protections, *Chart 10: May Informed Consent Be Waived or Consent Elements Be Altered under 45 CFR 46.116(d)?* available at http://www.hhs.gov/ohrp/humansubjects/guidance/decision charts.htm.

4. In what types of situations might it be important to provide "additional pertinent information" to subjects pursuant to 45 C.F.R. § 46.116(d)(4)? How can IRBs ensure that researchers carry out their obligations under this provision?

5. Does § 46.116(d) effectively create an obligation for some individuals to participate in research? Reconsider the hypothetical protocol involving the one-way mirror observation of child abusing mothers (discussed at page 312). Could it be approved under § 46.116(d)?

6. Hospitalized patients, because they spend so much time in bed, are often at risk of developing blood clots in the veins of their legs. These blood clots can break off and travel to other organs (such as the lungs) and cause serious medical problems, including death. Some patients are at an especially high risk of developing these blood clots. There are certain drugs (which, like most drugs,

can produce serious unwanted side effects) that can be used to reduce the likelihood of developing blood clots. A group of researchers wrote a computer program that looked at patients' medical records to identify patients who are at a high risk for developing blood clots and thus should perhaps receive a clot-preventing drug. The researchers proposed to apply the computer program to all the patients admitted to a hospital over a three–year period. For patients determined to be at high risk, half would be randomized so that their doctors received an e-mail notifying them of the high-risk status; for the other half, no such e-mail would be sent. *See* Nils Kucher et al., *Electronic Alerts to Prevent Venous Thromboembolism among Hospitalized Patients*, 352 NEW ENG. J. MED. 969 (2005). Should this study qualify for a waiver of informed consent, so that none of the patients would be need to be told that they are in the study? How do you think a patient would feel if he developed a blood clot and later found out he was in the study and had been randomized to the group whose doctors did not receive the e-mail messages? Another issue raised by this set of facts is the dividing line between quality improvement initiatives and research studies, which was discussed in Chapter 3 at page 115. Should these events be considered a quality improvement initiative, in which case there would be no need for any review by an IRB?

7. What are the advantages and drawbacks of allowing exceptions to the informed consent requirement? What approach does the Nuremberg Code take on these issues?

8. One of the most common areas in which IRBs are asked to waive informed consent is psychological research. Psychologists often seek permission to "deceive" research subjects because, if the subjects know what is going to happen to them and why, that knowledge may alter the very behavior that is being studied. The study by Stanley Milgram, discussed in Chapter 1, at page 48, is an example of such a "deception" study. Take another look at that study. Under the current regulations, would it be appropriate for an IRB to approve that study under the waiver rules?

9. One proposed solution to the deception issue is so-called "authorized deception," in which the researcher would reveal to the subject that the study involves some element of deception and proceed only if the subject agrees to be deceived. What do you think about this approach? Would it have worked in the Milgram study? *See, e.g.*, David Wendler & Franklin G. Miller, *Deception in the Pursuit of Science*, 164 ARCH. INTERNAL MED. 597 (2004); Franklin G. Miller & David Wendler, *Assessing the Ethics of Ethics Research: A Case Study*, 26 IRB, Mar.-Apr. 2004, at 9; David Wendler, *Deception in Medical and Behavioral Research: Is It Ever Acceptable?* 74 MILBANK Q. 87 (1996).

10. Another area in which waivers of the informed consent requirement are often sought is research involving stored tissue samples. The appropriateness of waiving consent in this context is discussed in Chapter 17, at page 718.

45 C.F.R. § 46.117(c): WAIVER OF USUAL RULES
FOR DOCUMENTING INFORMED CONSENT

This provision is reproduced in Appendix A, at page A-15. Please review it before proceeding.

Unlike the waivers permitted under sections 46.116(c) and (d), which allow researchers to dispense with the consent requirement entirely, all that section 117(c) does is alter the paperwork requirements. Even if a section 117(c) waiver is granted, the researcher still must obtain the subject's informed consent. The difference between the two types of waivers

> is clear if you imagine the experience of a prospective research subject. If consent has been waived, the subject may never know that he or she was part of a research study. If documentation is waived, the subject is fully aware of the research, because there has been an oral consent procedure, even though there is no documentation of that procedure.

Veterans Administration Teleconference, *supra*. OHRP has provided a decision chart on this topic. *See* Office for Human Research Protections, *Chart 11: May Documentation of Informed Consent Be Waived Under 45 CFR 46.117(c)?* available at http://www.hhs.gov/ohrp/humansubjects/guidance/decisioncharts.htm.

NOTES AND QUESTIONS

1. A geriatric physician, working in a well-respected, academically connected nursing home, is interested in gathering some pilot data about "gait" and then designing a large study that will examine whether gait correlates with falls and with developing dementia. What she would like to do is have nursing home residents walk three times from her desk to the window in her office, some 20 feet and back. That is the extent of the research. The residents will use their usual supports, cane, walker or slider or walk unassisted. Whatever is the usual means of locomotion will be used in the study. No photographs or videos will be taken of the residents. Does the geriatrician need the signed informed consent of the individual residents? What if the residents refuse to sign but state that they are happy to have her watch them? What about family members who are concerned that research with their relatives is being conducted without their knowledge?

2. Assume that the IRB approved the following consent form:

> You have been asked to be part of a pilot study that is designed to see whether there might be a connection between how you walk and whether you fall, and whether you are having memory problems. You

will be asked to walk three times from Dr. Jones's desk to her window and back — that is all. She will watch you walk and then make some notes in her research book. She will note your name and the day you walked for her. She will then review your medical record.

This paragraph was followed by all of the "boilerplate" material about the research office in the facility, the compensation clause, the alternatives (non-participation), and the right to refuse at the outset and at any time during the study. The form was one and one-half single-spaced pages. Most residents refused to sign it. What should Dr. Jones do? Should she return to the IRB and request a waiver of documentation pursuant to section 117(c)? What argues for or against the IRB's approval of a "waivered" process?

[2] Waivers in Emergency Research

All jurisdictions, either by case law or by statute, permit persons to receive medical treatment in an emergency without the prior provision of informed consent. These statutes and cases reason that the person cannot provide the consent precisely because of the need for care and, if capable, would provide adequate permission. This clinical reasoning, however, did not carry over to the research arena.

Critical Care Research and Informed Consent
Richard S. Saver
75 N.C. L. Rev. 205 (1996)

Approximately 350,000 people suffer sudden heart attacks in the United States each year. Most die. Bystanders resuscitate only a small percentage of persons experiencing cardiac arrest. Of those who live long enough to be admitted to a hospital, less than twenty-five percent survive to leave. Among this group, many are often irreversibly impaired by brain damage, organ malfunctions, and other devastating complications.

Given these grim statistics, researchers have questioned whether standard cardiopulmonary resuscitation (CPR) techniques can be improved in terms of better survival rates or quality of life factors for post-cardiac arrest victims. Because current CPR practices were developed on a mostly theoretical basis, few controlled studies of CPR techniques or other cardiac arrest treatments have been conducted. Thus, much of what has become standard medical therapy for use in resuscitative clinical care has not been sufficiently evaluated by investigational trials that demonstrate safety or effectiveness. Research in this area has been impeded by the near impossibility of satisfying legal standards for informed consent. Until recent regulatory reforms, the applicable law, consisting primarily of federal regulations governing human subjects research, required that prospective informed consent be obtained from subjects before the administration of experimental therapies, with few available exceptions. For example, the Food and Drug Administration (FDA) recently halted clinical trials of the "Cardiopump" active compression-decompression cardiopulmonary resuscitation device, a plunger-like mechanism developed for the administration of new CPR techniques. FDA stopped the Cardiopump trials in part because subjects were unable to provide prospective consent to participate in the research.

Obtaining the prospective informed consent from a patient under circumstances such as cardiac arrest is impossible. The patient is unable to communicate and/or lacks decisional capacity, but the experimental therapy must be applied before the patient stabilizes and regains the capability of providing legally effective consent. This article refers to such situations as "critical care." In critical care settings, the patient's decisional or communicational incapacity may be temporary or permanent. Typical conditions that impair the critical care patient include stroke, coma, seizure, cardiac arrest, senility, depression of mental faculties, drug overdose, head trauma, poisoning, hemorrhagic shock, acute asthma attacks, and pulmonary embolism. The state of incapacity may be slowly progressive, as with the cognitive impairments arising from dementia or Alzheimer's disease or sudden and severe, such as can occur with head trauma or the onset of a coma. Satisfying the informed consent requirements proves problematic even with conscious critical care patients because they experience extreme duress and often cannot provide legally effective consent. Indeed, critical care patients able to respond to questions about research participation often later do not remember having consented to become subjects.

The legal difficulties and controversy surrounding the Cardiopump trials demonstrate a fundamental problem common to critical care research. Although researchers have developed investigational technologies and techniques that can be applied to patients in critical care situations, many such therapies require rapid application to be effective and satisfying the informed consent requirement presents a significant obstacle to clinical investigations. Apart from the Cardiopump trials, several other experimental investigations have grounded to a halt because of liability concerns related to waiving informed consent. This occurs at a time of renewed concern about the ethical conduct of medical experimentation generally and, as a result, increased sensitivity toward the need for obtaining subjects' fully informed consent.

Numerous commentators criticize the informed consent doctrine as elevating ritual and form over substance because it requires procedures which do not advance the patient's understanding, are easily subject to manipulation, and impose burdensome information exchange costs. Thus, there have been calls to change the informed consent standards and expressly require that investigators engage in frank and extended discussions with patients about the experimental nature of the proposed activity in order to ensure that subjects are not coerced or misled. But in critical care situations, there simply is no time for an extended dialogue between investigator and subject about the nature of the experiment. In such settings, it is impossible to comply even with the minimum legal standards already criticized as deficient and inadequate.

The legal requirement for informed consent, although historically rooted in the protections against bodily injury under the battery doctrine, derives continued support from the ethical and common-law principle that patients should be respected as persons capable and entitled to control their own medical care decisions. If patients are to be treated as autonomous agents, they must be provided material information relating to the risks and benefits of a proposed medical treatment and its alternatives in order to effectively decide whether to participate in the research. Validation of this broad underlying principle of the informed consent doctrine "requires that we deliberate before we decide."

Consequently, nowhere is the gap between legal theory and the realities of medical practice more evident than in application of the traditional informed consent doctrine to critical care research. The reasoned deliberation of the patient contemplated by the informed consent doctrine is simply not feasible when the patient suffers decisional or communicational incapacity and there is a limited time window for administering an experimental treatment. Thus, rigid application of informed consent requirements in critical care settings severely limits medical researchers' ability to test and study new therapies, preventing the efficient diffusion of beneficial medical technologies.

In a significant new regulatory development, the FDA has proposed amendments to its informed consent regulations that would relax the informed consent requirements in the critical care setting. In response to criticisms of the current obstacles to conducting critical care research, the FDA has proposed to revise its regulations to allow waiver of informed consent under limited circumstances. Relaxing the informed consent requirement for critical care research raises difficult issues regarding the physician-patient relationship and biomedical research. At one end of the spectrum are firmly held beliefs about individualism and patient autonomy as well as underlying concerns for patient safety in light of the egregious medical experiments of previous decades. Countervailing considerations include the societal benefits gained by systematic testing of medical technologies and the professional commitment, and at times paternalistic impulse, of physicians to act in their patients' best interests, especially where the patients cannot act for themselves. At bottom, it seems a terrible choice between forcing patients to become mere experimental objects or protecting these same patients to death.

As explained in further detail below, the FDA has proposed to strike the balance in favor of increased experimentation. FDA's proposed rules permit waiver of informed consent where: (i) the subject is in a life-threatening situation; (ii) available treatments are unproven or unsatisfactory; (iii) the subject cannot consent because of the medical condition; (iv) the intervention must be administered before consent from the patient or a representative is feasible; and (v) the risk of the intervention is reasonable in light of what is known about the medical condition, the current therapy, and the proposed intervention. Once the

FDA rules are issued in final form, the Department of Health and Human Services (HHS) is expected to harmonize its separate informed consent regulations through amendment and/or waiver so that both agencies will permit waiver of consent for critical care research under the same circumstances.

The proposed rules referred to in Saver's article were indeed adopted by both the FDA and the Department of Health and Human Services (DHHS) in late 1996. The FDA's version of the waiver was incorporated into the regulations, and can be found at 21 C.F.R. § 50.24. The DHHS version was not made a part of 45 C.F.R. Part 46, but instead was announced in the Federal Register pursuant to the Secretary's general authority to waive particular aspects of the regulations. *See* 45 C.F.R. § 46.101(i) ("Unless otherwise required by law, Department or Agency heads may waive the applicability of some or all of the provisions of this policy to specific research activities or classes or research activities otherwise covered by this policy."). The following excerpt sets forth the determinations that an IRB must make in order to comply with DHHS's criteria for waiving consent in emergency research.

REPORT: INFORMED CONSENT REQUIREMENTS IN EMERGENCY RESEARCH
OFFICE FOR PROTECTION FROM RESEARCH RISKS
October 31, 1996
http://www.hhs.gov/ohrp/humansubjects/guidance/hsdc97-01.htm\

(1) The human subjects are in a life-threatening situation, available treatments are unproven or unsatisfactory, and the collection of valid scientific evidence, which may include evidence obtained through randomized placebo-controlled investigations, is necessary to determine the safety and effectiveness of particular interventions.

(2) Obtaining informed consent is not feasible because:

   (i)   the subjects will not be able to give their informed consent as a result of their medical condition;

   (ii)   the intervention involved in the research must be administered before consent from the subjects' legally authorized representatives is feasible; and

   (iii)   there is no reasonable way to identify prospectively the individuals likely to become eligible for participation in the research.

(3) Participation in the research holds out the prospect of direct benefit to the subjects because:

(i) subjects are facing a life-threatening situation that necessitates intervention;

(ii) appropriate animal and other preclinical studies have been conducted, and the information derived from those studies and related evidence support the potential for the intervention to provide a direct benefit to the individual subjects; and

(iii) risks associated with the research are reasonable in relation to what is known about the medical condition of the potential class of subjects, the risks and benefits of standard therapy, if any, and what is known about the risks and benefits of the proposed intervention or activity.

(4) The research could not practicably be carried out without the waiver.

(5) The proposed research protocol defines the length of the potential therapeutic window based on scientific evidence, and the investigator has committed to attempting to contact a legally authorized representative for each subject within that window of time and, if feasible, to asking the legally authorized representative contacted for consent within that window rather than proceeding without consent. The investigator will summarize efforts made to contact representatives and make this information available to the IRB at the time of continuing review.

(6) The IRB has reviewed and approved informed consent procedures and an informed consent document in accord with Sections 46.116 and 46.117 of 45 CFR Part 46. These procedures and the informed consent document are to be used with subjects or their legally authorized representatives in situations where use of such procedures and documents is feasible. The IRB has reviewed and approved procedures and information to be used when providing an opportunity for a family member to object to a subject's participation in the research consistent with paragraph . . . (7)(v) of this waiver.

(7) Additional protections of the rights and welfare of the subjects will be provided, including, at least:

(i) consultation (including, where appropriate, consultation carried out by the IRB) with representatives of the communities in which the research will be conducted and from which the subjects will be drawn;

(ii) public disclosure to the communities in which the research will be conducted and from which the subjects will be drawn, prior to initiation of the research, of plans for the research and its risks and expected benefits;

(iii) public disclosure of sufficient information following completion of the research to apprise the community and researchers of the study, including the demographic characteristics of the research population, and its results;

(iv) establishment of an independent data monitoring committee to exercise oversight of the research; and

(v) if obtaining informed consent is not feasible and a legally authorized representative is not reasonably available, the investigator has committed, if feasible, to attempting to contact within the therapeutic window the subject's family member who is not a legally authorized representative, and asking whether he or she objects to the subject's participation in the research. The investigator will summarize efforts made to contact family members and make this information available to the IRB at the time of continuing review.

In addition, the IRB is responsible for ensuring that procedures are in place to inform, at the earliest feasible opportunity, each subject, or if the subject remains incapacitated, a legally authorized representative of the subject, or if such a representative is not reasonably available, a family member, of the subject's inclusion in the research, the details of the research and other information contained in the informed consent document. The IRB shall also ensure that there is a procedure to inform the subject, or if the subject remains incapacitated, a legally authorized representative of the subject, or if such a representative is not reasonably available, a family member, that he or she may discontinue the subject's participation at any time without penalty or loss of benefits to which the subject is otherwise entitled. If a legally authorized representative or family member is told about the research and the subject's condition improves, the subject is also to be informed as soon as feasible. If a subject is entered into research with waived consent and the subject dies before a legally authorized representative or family member can be contacted, information about the research is to be provided to the subject's legally authorized representative or family member, if feasible.

NOTES AND QUESTIONS

1. Here is how one institution has attempted to introduce these rules to its investigators:

Both FDA and OHRP permit [an IRB] to approve a research project designed to test new emergency therapies which — due to the critical condition of the patient and the need to administer the therapies within a short amount of time — may necessitate enrolling the subject in the research before a legally authorized representative is available to provide informed consent. . . . These federal waivers, however, require that this type of research be conducted in accordance with state law, as well as meet strict requirements. New Mexico law does not specifically address the propriety of enrolling subjects into research studies without informed consent. Typically, treating patients without obtaining consent may result in a claim of battery or lack of informed consent. However, because there is no New Mexico law that prohibits the conduct of this research, and the research is only permitted where there is no acceptable alternative treatment and the research holds out the prospect of direct benefit to the subject, we believe that these studies may be conducted at the UNMHSC, *provided* that all of the protections of the federal regulations are strictly followed. An HRRC [Human Research Review Committee, which is what the IRBs at the University of New Mexico are called] approval of a project under this waiver will permit investigators to enroll subjects who are unable to provide consent into their studies. Among other protections, this regulation/waiver uses a *"community consultation"* process to obtain the views of the community from which the likely subjects will be drawn, as well as the community in which the research will be conducted, prior to the initiation of research. . . . Community consultation (including consultation by the HRRC, as appropriate) must occur with the communities from which the subjects will be drawn *and* in which the research will be conducted *before* HRRC approval. The purpose of this consultation is to give these communities the opportunity to understand the proposed clinical investigation and its risks and benefits, and to discuss and raise objections to the investigation. The HRRCs must consider this community discussion when reviewing the investigation, and may decide, among other things, that it is appropriate to exclude certain groups from participation, or that wider community consultation is necessary. The HRRCs may consider:

- Having public meetings in the community to discuss the protocol (some institutions have used church meetings, club meetings, and special meetings, among other things);

- Establishing a separate panel of members of the community from which the subjects will be drawn;

- Including consultants to the HRRC from the community from which the subjects will be drawn (this alone would not be sufficient however); and

- Developing other mechanisms to ensure community involvement and input in the HRRC's decision making process (such as using the media, professional surveyors, etc.).

The HRRCs are responsible for listening to and considering the community's support, concerns, etc., and then ultimately deciding whether the investigation should be modified, approved, or disapproved. Thus, the community consultation will take place before the HRRC can approve the project. While a sponsor may provide the HRRCs information on community consultation, the HRRCs bear the responsibility for ensuring the adequacy of the community consultation requirements. In addition, the HRRCs have the responsibility for deciding what information should be disclosed to the community (information on risks/

benefits, relevant information from the investigational brochure, information on informed consent and on the protocol).

Human Research Review Committees [HRRC], *Manual for Conducting Human Subject Research*, University of New Mexico Health Sciences Center, http://hsc.unm.edu/som/research/hrrc/MANUAL.html#sevenfivefive.

2. University A meets with the "community board" in its area and discloses its plans. University B convenes a meeting of church, synagogue, and mosque groups. University C places advertisements in the local newspapers and asks for comments. University D has a slot on a local radio call-in program and answers questions from callers. Are any of these plans adequate?

3. The FDA has provided some tentative guidance about the community consultation requirement:

> Before a clinical study may be initiated, the IRB must find and document that consultation has occurred with representatives of the community(ies) in which the research will take place and from which research subjects may be drawn. . . . Community consultation means providing the opportunity for discussions with, and soliciting opinions from the community(ies) in which the study will take place and from which the study subjects will be drawn. These communities may not always be the same; when they are not the same, both communities should be consulted. The *community in which the research will take place* is the geographic area, e.g., city or region, where the hospital or clinical investigator study site is located. The *community from which subjects will be drawn* may be characterized by analyzing the demographics of previous hospital patients with the emergent condition under study. For example, the IRB or clinical investigator might review the hospital records of the last 50-100 patients admitted to the emergency room for the condition under study and tabulate characteristics (gender, age, ethnicity, geographic locale, etc.).

Food and Drug Administration, Draft Guidance, Guidance for Institutional Review Boards, Clinical Investigators, and Sponsors: Exception from Informed Consent Requirements for Emergency Research (2000), available at http://www.fda.gov/ora/compliance_ref/bimo/err_guide.htm#COMMUNITYA. How would you interpret the type and quality of the discussion that this rule requires? With whom should it be conducted?

4. In 2003, researchers examined data from four studies approved under the emergency regulations. They discovered "one-way" efforts to comply with the community consultation requirement, such as the distribution of announcements, and some "two-way" routes, such as focus groups and public meetings. The "one-way" methods predominated. A minority of participating hospitals announced mechanisms of advance refusal or collected quantitative data on public opinion. The researchers concluded that community consultation should be more carefully considered by the FDA in future applications. *See* A.N. Shah &

Jeremy Sugarman, *Protecting Research Subjects under the Waiver of Informed Consent for Emergency Research: Experiences with Efforts to Inform the Community*, 41 ANNALS EMERG. MED. 79 (2003). Given these findings, should the FDA and OHRP provide more specific guidance to institutions about the community consultation requirement? What specifically should these agencies say?

5. What is an IRB supposed to do with the information it gathers during its community consultation? The University of New Mexico manual says that the IRB should "listen to" and "consider" the views expressed by members of the community. Presumably, in many instances members of the community will have differing views. What if a large majority of the members support the research, but there is a vocal minority that believe it would be outrageous if they ended up participating in the study? Should the size of that minority matter? The strength of their convictions? Similar issues have been raised with respect to proposals for community consultation in the context of genetics research. *See* Chapter 17, at page 710.

6. Waivers of informed consent to emergency research are authorized only for patients in "life threatening" situations. Should the rules have been drawn more broadly to permit waivers of consent for research with patients in intractable pain, or patients with serious disabilities? Like patients in life-threatening situations, these patients have daunting problems that are insufficiently addressed by researchers in large part because of the difficulty of obtaining informed consent.

7. Or should the rules have been drawn even more narrowly? Consider one of the first studies approved under the rules permitting waivers of consent in emergency research. The study concerned HemAssist, a blood substitute. Artificial blood has a number of potential advantages: it would obviate the need for typing and match and, if effective, it would alleviate chronic shortages of blood. The research involved two groups of patients, trauma patients for whom consent was waived and elective surgery patients who were able to provide consent. Patients were randomly assigned to HemAssist or a saline placebo. When the blind was broken and the control group found to have a higher survival rate, the study was stopped for trauma patients. It continued for the surgical arm of the study. A number of concerns have been raised by critics, including possible exploitation of minority members, excessive leeway for researcher designs and egos, and the possibility that the use of ineffective experimental interventions will be a barrier to adequate insurance payments, which tend to exclude "experimental" treatments. *See* Mary Anderlik, *"You're Telling Me I Was Given Artificial Blood?": The Controversy over Emergency Research*, available at http://www.law.uh.edu/healthlawperspectives/Bioethics/981027Emergency.html.

8. The Belmont Report identified three governing principles of research ethics: respect for persons, beneficence and justice. *See* Chapter 2, at page 54. The relaxation of informed consent requirements in emergency research places less emphasis on the former and more on the latter two. Is that appropriate in this context? Should it be expanded to other circumstances in which the ability

of the patient/subject to make decisions is in question? For example, should it be the case for all incapacitated adults that autonomy takes second place to considerations of justice?

9. For additional discussion of the emergency research rules, *see, e.g.,* Sandra J. Carnahan, *Promoting Medical Research Without Sacrificing Patient Autonomy: Legal and Ethical Issues Raised by the Waiver of Informed Consent for Emergency Research,* 52 OKLA. L. REV. 565 (1999); Norman Fost, *Waived Consent for Emergency Research,* 24 AM. J. L. MED. 163 (1998); Symposium, *In Case of Emergency: No Need for Consent,* 27 HASTINGS CENTER REP., Jan.-Feb. 1997, at 7.

§ 7.03 IMPLEMENTING THE FEDERAL REGULATIONS

[A] The Consent Form

A Guide to Understanding Informed Consent
National Cancer Institute
http://www.cancer.gov/clinicaltrials/conducting/informed-consent-guide

If you and your physician have found a clinical trial that is of interest to you and for which you are eligible (that is, you meet requirements such as type and stage of cancer, age, treatment history, overall health, and others), you will need information in order to make a decision about whether to participate in the trial. Making a decision about participating in a research study involves understanding the potential risks and benefits as well as your rights and responsibilities. The presentation and discussion of these important issues are part of the process called informed consent. This guide will tell you what to expect during the informed consent process, explain its importance to clinical research participants, and describe how it fits into a larger system that protects the welfare of people who take part in clinical trials.

A Definition of Informed Consent

You may already have experience with signing consent forms for other kinds of medical procedures, such as surgery, or for cancer treatments such as radiation or chemotherapy. However, informed consent for a clinical trial involves much more than just reading and signing a piece of paper. Rather, it involves two essential parts: a document and a process.

The informed consent *document* provides a summary of the clinical trial (including its purpose, the treatment procedures and schedule, potential risks and benefits, alternatives to participation, etc.) and explains your rights as a participant. It is designed to begin the informed consent process, which consists of conversations between you and the research team. If you then decide to enter the trial, you give your official consent by signing the document. You can keep a copy and use it as an information resource throughout the course of the trial.

The informed consent *process* provides you with ongoing explanations that will help you make educated decisions about whether to begin or continue participating in a trial. Researchers and health professionals know that a written document alone may not ensure that you fully understand what participation means. Therefore, before you make your decision, the research team will discuss with you the trial's purpose, procedures, risks and potential benefits, and your rights as a participant. If you decide to participate, the team will continue to update you on any new information that may affect your situation. Before, during, and even after the trial, you will have the opportunity to ask questions and raise concerns. Thus, informed consent is an ongoing, interactive process, rather than a one-time information session.

SAMPLE CONSENT FORM ACCOMPANYING RECOMMENDATIONS FOR THE DEVELOPMENT OF INFORMED CONSENT DOCUMENTS FOR CANCER CLINICAL TRIALS
COMPREHENSIVE WORKING GROUP ON INFORMED CONSENT IN CANCER CLINICAL TRIALS FOR THE NATIONAL CANCER INSTITUTE
(August 1998)

A RANDOMIZED TRIAL EVALUATING THE WORTH OF TAXOL FOLLOWING DOXORUBICIN (ADRIAMYCIN)/CYCLOPHOSPHAMIDE (CYTOXAN) IN BREAST CANCER

This is a clinical trial (a type of research study). Clinical trials only include patients who choose to take part. Please take your time to make your decision. Discuss it with your friends and family.

You are being asked to take part in this research study because your breast cancer has spread to one or more of your underarm lymph nodes.

WHY IS THIS STUDY BEING DONE?

The purpose of this research study is to find out whether adding the drug Taxol (paclitaxel) to a commonly-used chemotherapy is better than the commonly-used chemotherapy by itself at preventing your cancer from coming back. The study also will see what side effects there are from adding Taxol to the commonly-used chemotherapy.

Taxol has been found to be effective in treating patients with advanced breast cancer. In this study, we want to see whether Taxol will be a useful addition to the treatment of patients with early-stage breast cancer and to see whether the side effects seem to be worth the possible benefit.

HOW MANY PEOPLE WILL TAKE PART IN THE STUDY?

About 2,450 people will take part in this study.

WHAT IS INVOLVED IN THE STUDY?

Please refer to the diagram at the end of this form.   (₁)

Medical tests:
The following tests must be done to make sure that you are eligible for this   (₁)
study. None of these tests are experimental. They are routine. Depending on
when you last had them, you may need to repeat some of these tests:

- Mammogram

- Blood tests

- Chest x-ray

- Gynecologic exam

- Electrocardiogram

- Bone scan

- A special x-ray to study the heart (MUGA scan)

Many of the tests will also be repeated during the study. If you participate
in this study, some of these tests may be done more frequently than if you
were not taking part in this research study.

Procedures (treatment):   (₁)
If you are eligible and agree to take part in this study, you will get two com-
monly-used chemotherapy drugs called Adriamycin (doxorubcin) and
Cytoxan (cyclophosphamide).

These drugs will be given into your vein while you are in the doctor's office
or clinic every 21 days for 4 visits. The procedure will take about 2 hours.
The doses of the drugs may be changed if you have side effects. You will not
need to be hospitalized unless you have serious side effects.

If you are older than 50, you will also take tamoxifen pills daily for 5 years.
If you are younger than 50, you will get tamoxifen if your tumor has a positive estrogen or progesterone (ER/PR) hormone receptor test.

The Adriamycin and Cytoxan plus tamoxifen are usual treatments that
would likely be given whether or not you are on this study.

Randomization (assignment to a group):   (₁)
   After completing the chemotherapy with Adriamycin and Cytoxan, you
will be randomized to one of the study groups. Randomization means that
you are put into a group by chance. It is like the flip of a coin, and assignment is done by a computer. Neither you nor the researcher choose what
group you will be in. You will have an equal chance to be placed in either
group.

Group 1: Does not get Taxol.

Group 2: Gets Taxol (by vein over 3 hours in the clinic or doctor's office every 21 days for 4 visits.)

How Long Will I Be in the Study?

(1) Your chemotherapy will last 4 to 8 months and the tamoxifen therapy will last for 5 years. Every 6 months you will come in for follow-up blood tests. We would like to keep track of your medical condition for the rest of your life to look at the long-term effects of the study. The researchers can take you off the study early for reasons such as:

• The treatment does not work in your cancer.

• Your health gets worse.

• You are unable to meet the requirements of the study (for example, you do not return for follow-up visits).

What Are the Risks of the Study?

(2) While on the study, you are at risk for these side effects. Most of them are listed in this form, but they will vary from person to person. There may be other side effects that we cannot predict. Other drugs will be given to make the side effects less serious and uncomfortable. (b)(1)

Many side effects go away shortly after the drugs are stopped, but in some cases, side effects may be serious and/or long-lasting or permanent. Some may be life-threatening. Talk with the researcher about this. You may also want to talk to your regular doctor and/or read more about the drugs on the sheets attached to this form.

Reproductive risks: You should not become pregnant while on this study. You should not nurse your baby while on this study. Also, some of the drugs may cause sterility (make you unable to have children in the future). Ask for more information if this applies to you.

Side effects of treatment:
Groups 1 and 2
Adriamycin and Cytoxan (commonly used chemotherapy)

Very likely:
• Lowered white blood count that may lead to an infection
  (If you get an infection or your white blood count becomes very low, you will get daily shots of G-CSF (Neupogen). G-CSF helps your white blood cells multiply to fight infections. Some patients get pain in their bones with the G-CSF.)

• Lowered platelets count which may lead to an increase in bruising or bleeding

• (If count gets too low, you may need platelet transfusions.)

- Lowered red blood cells count may cause anemia, tiredness, shortness of breath
  (If count gets too low, you may need blood transfusions.)

- Nausea, vomiting, or diarrhea

- Complete hair loss

- Skin and nail discoloration

- Irregular or permanent stoppage of menstrual cycles

- Mouth sores

- Time away from work

Less likely:
- Blood in the urine

- Heart damage (very rare at these doses)

- Irregular heart beat (may occur right after drug is given)

- Skin damage due to leakage of drug

- Acute leukemia (very rare at these doses)

Tamoxifen (part of commonly used anticancer drug regimen):
While on Tamoxifen you should have an annual pelvic exam. If you have abnormal vaginal bleeding, pelvic discomfort (pressure or pain), or other changes, report this to your regular doctor or the researcher as soon as possible. These might be related to changes in the uterus. Changes to the lining of the uterus can sometimes turn into a cancer of the uterus.

Very likely:
- Hot flashes

- Vaginal dryness or discharge

Less likely:
- Eye problems, increased risk of developing cataracts (clouding of eye)

- Uterine cancer

- Ovarian cysts or endometriosis (spillage of uterine cells outside the uterus)

- Blood clots (may be life-threatening)

- Inflammation of the liver

Side effects of the study drug (Taxol):

Group 2 only

Taxol

Many of these side effects occur with Adriamycin and Cytoxan that you will already have received as part of the commonly-used chemotherapy. This study will determine whether Taxol increases the severity of these side effects.

Also, three drugs will be given before the Taxol to control an allergic reaction that might occur. These are:
- A steroid similar to cortisone (dexamethasone [Decadron])

(A brief, vaginal tingling sensation is possible when this drug is given.)

- An antacid (metoclopramide [Reglan])

- An antihistamine (diphenhydramine [Benadryl])

Very likely:
- Lowered white blood count may lead to an infection

- Lowered platelets may lead to an increase in bruising or bleeding

- Lowered red blood cells may lead to anemia, tiredness, or shortness of breath

- Nausea, vomiting, or diarrhea

- Complete hair loss

- Irregular menstrual cycles or permanent menstrual stoppage

- Numbness or tingling in fingers or toes

- Pain in muscles and joints

Less likely:
- Allergic reactions (may happen during injection)

- Inflammation of pancreas and large bowel

- Irregular heart beat

- Inflammation of the liver

For more information about risks and side effects, ask the researcher or your regular doctor or contact _____.

ARE THERE BENEFITS TO TAKING PART IN THE STUDY?

There may or may not be direct medical benefits to you from taking part in this study. The expected benefit of taking part in the study is predicted to be similar to that of getting commonly-used chemotherapy without being in the study. Although Taxol has been shown to be effective in women with advanced breast cancer, it is unknown whether the addition of Taxol to commonly-used chemotherapy will improve the outcome for women with less advanced breast cancer.

The information learned from this study should help future patients with breast cancer.

WHAT OTHER OPTIONS ARE THERE?

(4)

Instead of being in this study, you have these options:

- Chemotherapy with Adriamycin and Cytoxan

- Chemotherapy with other drugs that are as effective as Adriamycin and Cytoxan

- Tamoxifen

- No chemotherapy

Discuss these options with your regular doctor.

WHAT ABOUT CONFIDENTIALITY?

(5)

Efforts will be made to keep your personal information confidential. We cannot guarantee absolute confidentiality. Your personal information may be disclosed if required by law.

Organizations that may inspect and/or copy your research records for quality assurance and data analysis include groups such as:

- The National Cancer Institute

- The Food and Drug Administration

- The National Surgical Adjuvant Project for Breast and Bowel Cancer

- Bristol-Myers Squibb Company, which is providing the study drug Taxol without charge

WHAT ARE THE COSTS?

(6)

Taking part in this study may lead to added costs to you or your insurance company. Please ask about any expected added costs or insurance problems.

In the case of injury or illness resulting from this study, emergency medical treatment is available but will be provided at the usual charge. No funds have been set aside to compensate you in the event of injury. You will be charged for continuing medical care and/or hospitalization at the usual rate.

(b)(3)

You will receive no payment for taking part in this study. You may be charged for the drugs other than Taxol that are used in this study. The researcher will explain the policy at this institution.

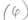

What Are My Rights as a Participant?

Taking part in this study is voluntary. Your decision about taking part in the study will not affect your medical care at this institution.

If you agree to take part and then decide against it, you can withdraw for any reason. If you decide to stop taking part in the study, you should talk to the researcher so it can be done safely. Leaving the study will not result in any penalty or lost benefits to which you are otherwise entitled.

A Data Safety and Monitoring Board, an independent group of experts, will be reviewing the data from this research throughout the study. We will tell you about new information from this board or other studies that may affect your health, welfare, or willingness to stay on this study.

Whom Do I Call If I Have Questions or Problems?

If you have questions about the study, or if you think you have had a study-related injury, you should call RESEARCHER at TELEPHONE NUMBER.

If you have questions about your rights as a research participant, call NAME OF CENTER Institutional Review Board or Patient Representative at TELEPHONE NUMBER.

Where Can I Get More Information?

You may call the NCI's **Cancer Information Service** at: **1-800-4-CANCER (1-800-422-6237)** or **TTY: 1-800-332-8615**

Or visit the **NCI Web site** at: **http://www.cancer.gov/**

A copy of the protocol (study plan) will be available at your request.

Please read the additional information provided with this form.

Signature

I agree to take part in this study.

Participant _____ Date _____

Attachment: Study Plan

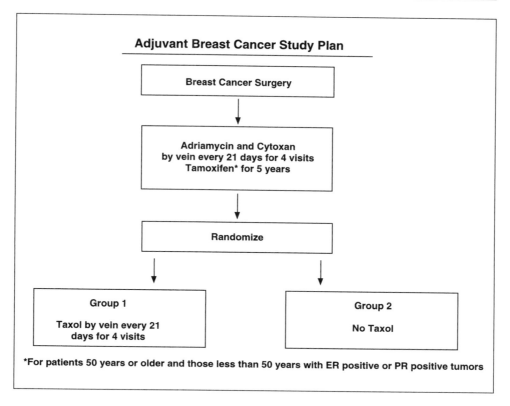

Adjuvant Breast Cancer Study Plan

Breast Cancer Surgery

Adriamycin and Cytoxan
by vein every 21 days for 4 visits
Tamoxifen* for 5 years

Randomize

Group 1

Taxol by vein every 21
days for 4 visits

Group 2

No Taxol

*For patients 50 years or older and those less than 50 years with ER positive or PR positive tumors

NOTES AND QUESTIONS

1. This consent form is based on several years of work by a distinguished group of experts gathered by officials from the National Cancer Institute. The experts were asked to come up with a solution for the problem that "many informed consent documents have become too long and complex, and do not provide a sound basis for informed decision-making." If you had breast cancer, do you think this document would give you all of the information you would want to know in deciding whether to be in the study? Is there any additional information you would want to have? Are there any parts of the form that you think are unclear?

2. The complete set of recommendations, together with templates for writing a consent form, is available on the web at http://www.cancer.gov/clinicaltrials/understanding/simplification-of-informed-consent-docs/page1.

3. Go through this form and find the sections that contain each of the required elements specified by items (1) through (8) of 45 C.F.R. § 46.116(a). Do you think that the form adequately meets each of these requirements?

4. Which of the six "additional elements" specified in section 116(b) are included in this form (and where are they)?   NO

(b)(2)
(b)(4)
(b)(5)

5. Notice that the description of the required and additional elements in sections 116(a) and (b) are very general. Apart from occasional consent form templates, such as the NCI template, there is very little guidance from the federal government about how much information needs to be in a consent form in order to comply with the regulations.

6. Review the discussion earlier in this chapter (at page 302) of the two types of standards — "professional" and "reasonable patient" — used to evaluate the adequacy of physicians' disclosure to patients in the clinical setting. Which of these standards appears more appropriate in determining the adequacy of disclosure in a research consent form? Who would you look to for purposes of applying a "professional" standard? A "reasonable patient" standard? These questions are explored further in Chapter 12, at page 511.

7. Compared to most consent forms currently being used in government-funded cancer studies, this form is unusually simple. It is not uncommon for cancer consent forms — particularly those used in pediatric cancer studies — to include several pages (sometimes eight or more) of lists or charts of side effects of drugs, because chemotherapy drugs are often very toxic. Is it appropriate for consent forms to be written in this way? Would it be acceptable, for a study in which the drugs cause numerous life-threatening side effects, to merely list a few of them, and state that there are many more similar side effects that are not listed in the form, and that a full list of those side effects is available upon request?

8. Does the model form adequately explain the differences between being a research subject and being a patient? Does it sufficiently distinguish between the risks "of the study" and the risks of interventions that subjects would undergo if they were receiving chemotherapy outside of research?

9. The regulations appear to contemplate that informed consent is obtained when a subject initially agrees to participate in a study. It is not uncommon that, over time, changes will be made in the protocol for a study, which will affect what happens to the subjects. Are there some changes that a subject can merely be told about orally, and others for which there should be another "consenting" process, with the signing of a revision or addendum to the initial consent form? If so, which types of changes should fall into each of these categories? *See* Dave Wendler & Jonathan Rackoff, *Consent for Continuing Research Participation: What Is It and When Should It Be Obtained?* 24 IRB, May-June 2002, at 1.

The Hidden Alternative: Getting Investigational Treatments Off-Study
Jerry Menikoff
361 LANCET 63 (2003)

[A] particular form of investigational treatment is [sometimes] available not only as one arm of a randomized research trial, but also as a treatment provided directly by a patient's doctor, independent of a research study. Hundreds if not thousands of research studies involve exactly this situation. In such a circumstance, disclosure of the off-study availability of the investigational treatment may lead prospective subjects to opt for the "sure thing" of getting the treatment outside of the study instead of being randomized in the study. Medical science may consequently be deprived of the important information that the study might produce. . . .

This article will highlight a related yet rarely mentioned phenomenon . . . : it appears that in many clinical trials, prospective subjects are *not* being advised about the availability of an experimental treatment outside of the study. Moreover, there is good reason to suspect that many of these subjects, had they been advised of that option, would not have participated in such studies. In effect, these subjects — those most likely to be poorly educated and thus vulnerable to manipulation — are being deceived, and their participation may not be fully voluntary. . . .

Confirmation of the fact that non-disclosure of experimental alternatives is common comes from what the U.S. government itself describes as "one of the largest breast cancer prevention studies ever": the NCI-sponsored Study of Tamoxifen and Raloxifene (STAR), comparing the efficacy of those two drugs in preventing breast cancer in women at high risk. Tamoxifen has already been demonstrated to reduce the risk of developing breast cancer, and is approved by the FDA for such use. There is some early evidence (from a study that was not specifically looking at breast cancer) to suggest that raloxifene, a marketed drug approved by the FDA for use in preventing osteoporosis, might also prevent such cancer, and perhaps might have fewer side effects (such as avoiding the increased risk of endometrial cancer associated with tamoxifen). In the double-blind STAR study being conducted in the U.S. and Canada, 22,000 women will be randomized between the two drugs. For five years each of these women will take one of the drugs, but will not know which they are taking.

With regard to the alternatives to participating in the STAR study, the sample consent form (approved by both the FDA and NCI) states that

> [i]nstead of being in this study, you can decide to do one or more of the following:
>
> • Perform self-breast exams, have breast exams done by a doctor or nurse, and get regular mammograms.
>
> • If you live in the U.S., ask your doctor to prescribe tamoxifen for you.
>
> • Request surgery to remove both breasts.

There is no mention of the fact that a subject could perhaps find a doctor who is willing, outside of this study, to prescribe raloxifene to prevent breast cancer. That this possibility is far from hypothetical is demonstrated by an interesting source: a lawsuit by the manufacturer of tamoxifen against the manufacturer of raloxifene, to prevent the latter company from inappropriately giving doctors information about the possible benefits of raloxifene in preventing breast cancer. Evidence in that case included market research demonstrating that more than one-third of the physicians surveyed acknowledged that at least some of their prescriptions for raloxifene had been written for the primary purpose of breast cancer prevention. . . .

Is obtaining, outside of a study, an investigational treatment that constitutes one arm of that study, an "appropriate alternative" to participating in the study? Some commentators appear to think that it is not. Consider the comments of Dr. D. Lawrence Wickerham, a co-leader of tamoxifen studies such as the STAR study, who has been quoted in the *New York Times* as stating that "[a]t the moment, it's too early to use raloxifene to prevent breast cancer outside of a clinical trial [such as the STAR study]. . . . We don't yet know raloxifene's long-term benefits or risks." Similar comments have been made with regard to the appropriateness of giving modified versions of HDC-ABMT, such as tandem transplantation or immune modulation, to women with breast cancer. As noted in a recent *New England Journal of Medicine* editorial, such investigational treatments "can neither be justified nor supported outside of clinical trials."

These conclusions merit further scrutiny. As Dr. Wickerham correctly notes, there would be a degree of uncertainty about some aspects of the benefits, or risks, or both, of such an investigational treatment. Does that fact in itself mean that getting that treatment outside of the study is not an "appropriate" alternative for a prospective study subject? With regard to the risks side of the analysis, a person who opts to get the treatment outside of the study will in many cases be exposed to *exactly the same risks* as a person who is randomized to that experimental treatment after enrolling in the study. Thus, the fact that the risks of the experimental treatment are still not fully known does not appear to be, in all cases, a reason for arguing against getting the treatment outside the study.

With regard to the benefits side of the equation, the very fact that the experimental treatment is being used as one arm in a study, with the other arm being standard care, would suggest the existence of "clinical equipoise": "an honest disagreement in the expert clinical community regarding the comparative merits of two or more forms of treatment for a given condition." Thus, there is a starting presumption that using the treatment for the stated purpose, although efficacy has not yet been fully proven, is not unreasonable. In addition, there may be definite benefits to some subjects from going outside the study. A subject may be trying to get into a study that randomizes between standard treatment X and unproven treatment Y precisely because *she wants to get a chance at treatment Y*. Indeed, this is likely to be the case for many, if not most, people who enroll in such a study. . . .

Given that there are in many instances no greater risks, and that there might be significantly greater benefits (at least as perceived by the patient), it would seem that the possibility of getting the investigational treatment outside of the study would be a very appropriate alternative for many subjects. . . .

Applying these concepts to the STAR study, we can imagine a hypothetical osteoporosis patient who is contemplating entering that study. She is particularly intrigued by the idea of taking raloxifene, a drug that might prevent breast cancer, improve her osteoporosis, and yet (unlike tamoxifen) not increase her risk of endometrial cancer. She knows that if she enters that study, she has only a 50% chance of ending up getting raloxifene, and she won't even know whether or not she is getting it. How is she any "worse off" if she instead goes to a doctor and that doctor gives her raloxifene for the next five years? The testing done in the STAR study consists of semi-annual breast exams and an annual routine blood test. Her private doctor can equally easily do all of this. The risk to her appears identical, whether she gets the raloxifene in the study or outside of it. On the other hand, given the fact of her osteoporosis, the benefits to her might well favor being certain of getting the raloxifene. If the study is stopped at any point due to compelling early results, her doctor will learn those results in exactly the same way that doctors participating in the study do. Under these circumstances, it is difficult *not* to conclude that getting raloxifene outside of the study is a perfectly appropriate alternative for her, and thus that option should be disclosed to her.

NOTES AND QUESTIONS

1. Does 45 C.F.R. § 46.116(a)(4) require the type of disclosure suggested in this excerpt?

2. If researchers were required to inform prospective subjects about the availability of unproven therapies, how would they decide which unproven therapies to include? For many medical problems, there are large numbers of alternative therapies, many of which are controversial (such as nutritional and vitamin treatments for cancer). Would all of these have to be listed? Does this create a problem for the approach suggested in the article? *See* Schiff v. Prados, 112 Cal. Rptr. 2d 171 (Cal. Ct. App. 2001) (concluding that parents of child with cancer did not have to be told about the availability of "anitneoplaston" treatment from an FDA-sanctioned and highly controversial Texas physician, Stanislaw Burzynski, but basing that conclusion on the fact that such treatment would have been illegal in California). Does the answer to this question depend on whether a "professional" or "reasonable patient" (or "reasonable subject") standard is applied?

3. Is Dr. Wickerham's argument sometimes correct? Could the new therapy being tested in some studies be so risky that it should be considered malpractice to provide it to a patient outside of a study, even if the patient consents? If that were the case, what should the consent form tell the subject about the risks and benefits of participating in such a study?

4. In 1990, Daniel Klais, newly diagnosed with head and neck cancer, was offered an opportunity at the prestigious Cleveland Clinic to be a subject in a study that randomized subjects between standard care alone (radiation and surgery), and standard care combined with chemotherapy. He allegedly told the doctors that he really wanted to get the chemotherapy. He was enrolled in the study and ended up being assigned to the standard care arm. While he was put into remission, five years after treatment, the cancer came back in an advanced and untreatable form. (The results of the study showed that the chemotherapy was very effective, and he likely would have been cured had he gotten it.) He sued the doctors and the Cleveland Clinic, claiming that they should have informed him, among other things, that the chemotherapy was directly available from doctors in Cleveland. While the trial court threw out the case, the appellate court reinstated it, saying that it should go to trial on the issue of whether informed consent had been properly obtained. *Stewart. v. Cleveland Clinic Foundation*, 736 N.E.2d 491 (Ohio Ct. App. 1999). Klais died in 1997, and the case was subsequently settled on undisclosed terms. In evaluating the legal issues in this case, what should be the significance of the fact that Daniel Klais made it clear that he wanted the chemotherapy?

5. Another claim made by Klais related to the fact that there had been previous phase 2 studies of chemotherapy that suggested that it was effective in treating his type of cancer; the trial he was being enrolled in was a phase 3 study. He claimed he should have been told about that tentative evidence of efficacy. The consent form did not disclose it. Do you think this is a valid point? What does section 46.116(a) require a consent form to say about the results of preliminary studies of a new treatment? Take another look at the sample consent form earlier in this chapter: what does it say about any earlier studies of the new treatment? (Note that because drugs are generally studied in stages — phase 2 taking place before phase 3 — it will often be the case in phase 3 studies that there will be results from some previous studies, and usually those results will at least be somewhat optimistic, or else the researchers probably would not have gone on to conduct the phase 3 study.)

Defining and Describing Benefit Appropriately in Clinical Trials
Nancy M.P. King
28 J. L. MED. & ETHICS 332 (2000)

Institutional review boards (IRBs) and investigators are used to talking about risks of harm. Both low risks of great harm and high risks of small harm must be disclosed to prospective subjects and should be explained and categorized in ways that help potential subjects to understand and weigh them appropriately. Everyone on an IRB has probably spent time at meetings arguing over whether a three-page bulleted list of risk description is helpful or overkill for prospective subjects. Yet only a small fraction of all the time and attention lavished on risk disclosure has been devoted to discussing whether and when potential benefit to subjects can reasonably be claimed and, if so, how it should be described in the consent form and process. . . .

Instead of detailed discussion designed to promote careful assessment and reasonable decision-making, prospective subjects are more likely to read "boilerplate" statements, such as the following, in the benefit section of the consent form:

- "It is not known whether your participation in this research study will have a beneficial effect."

- "You may not benefit from this research study."

- "Personal benefit cannot be guaranteed."

- Or the standard version used in much oncology research, "A potential benefit is control of your disease, if you should respond to these treatments. However, it is possible that your condition could worsen despite treatment."

Often, this is the only description of potential benefit in the entire document, aside from the aspirational benefit description in the purpose section. The vagueness of these statements is particularly troubling because they are so general that they could be applied to any standard treatment of proven effectiveness and, therefore, do nothing to distinguish research from treatment or to signal the uncertainty appropriate to most research settings. Surely we can do better than this.

Several examples of improved benefit boilerplate statements follow:

"This medical research project is not expected to benefit you" (scholars from the University of Pennsylvania's Bioethics Center have recommended that this statement be prominently placed near the beginning of all consent forms for Phase I studies).

"What you need to know before entering a clinical trial: You are not a patient" (the headline on a sidebar in a *U.S. News Online* story about the brief suspension of Duke University's federal authorization to perform human subjects research in April 1999).

Are these better? Yes. Are they good enough? No. The problem is that detail and evidence are required when direct benefit is being discussed. Boilerplate is simply inadequate; it is essential to particularize.

The following statement, compiled from three consent forms for early-stage research that had unusually detailed benefit sections, may serve as one example of particularization:

This research project is primarily testing the safety of an experimental intervention with which we have little experience. It is not likely that participation will benefit you. Results of earlier research have shown that a few subjects experienced reduction in symptoms, but most did not benefit in any way. We hope that the tumor may become smaller for a period of time, but we do not know if this will occur or for how long any benefit will last.

It is obvious how much more this attention to detail requires of both investigators and IRBs — namely, to craft and review descriptions of potential benefit whenever it can be reasonably claimed and to be sure that claims of potential benefit are adequately supported and not overstated. But because so little attention has been given to describing and discussing benefit in research, improvements here could greatly improve decision-making.

NOTES AND QUESTIONS

1. It is extremely common to see the benefits section of a consent form include language such as "No benefits are guaranteed." Defenders of this language say that it is very honest, and that it makes it clear to subjects that no one is promising them any benefits at all. Do you agree? How might a subject misinterpret this language? *sounds like some might still exist*

2. Take another look at the benefits section in the sample consent form provided earlier in this chapter. Does it adequately describe the potential benefits of participating in the study?

3. A study on patients with pneumonia involves treating them with the drug that would be given as standard care, but also giving them extra X rays and other tests so that the researchers can find out more about pneumonia treatment. The benefits section of the consent form says, "The direct benefit to you from participating in this study is that you will receive the accepted treatment for your pneumonia." Is this language acceptable? *treatment isn't a benefit*

4. A study is being conducted on people with a particular type of kidney infection. There is a standard antibiotic that is given to such patients. The study randomizes subjects 50-50 between that antibiotic and a new so-called "me too" antibiotic: it is not expected to be any more effective than standard care, although it may have somewhat different side effects. It is made by a company that competes with the company that makes the standard antibiotic. That company wants to get part of the share of the market for treating kidney infections. What should the benefits section of the consent form say?

5. As discussed in Chapter 3, Phase 1 studies are the first stage in evaluating a drug. The purpose of such studies is not to determine whether the drug works, but merely to determine the amount of the drug that subjects can tolerate before unacceptable side effects are seen. In Phase 1 cancer studies, the chance that the drug will positively affect the course of the patient's disease is less than five percent, and even if this occurs, it is usually only in the form of a shrinkage of the tumor as seen on X rays, with no increase in length of sur-

vival or quality of life. (For an evaluation of recent trends in such studies, *see* Thomas G. Roberts, Jr. et al., *Trends in the Risks and Benefits to Patients with Cancer Participating in Phase 1 Clinical Trials*, 292 JAMA 2130 (2004); Eric X. Chen & Ian F. Tannock, *Risks and Benefits of Phase 1 Clinical Trials Evaluating New Anticancer Agents: A Case for More Innovation*, 292 JAMA 2150 (2004).) In fact, usually the drugs being studied will *decrease* the subject's quality of life. Yet there is substantial evidence that participants in these studies often have wildly unrealistic views of possible benefits, such as thinking that participation will give them additional years of life.

In a prominent "Special Article" published in the *New England Journal of Medicine*, the ethics department of the NIH published the results of a study of consent forms, to see if the wording of the forms played a significant role in creating the common misunderstanding on the part of subjects. *See* Christine Grady et al., *Consent Forms for Oncology Trials*, 348 NEW ENG. J. MED. 1496, 1497 (2003). Their conclusion was that the wording of the consent forms was *not* a major factor in causing the misunderstanding. The reason for their conclusion was in part that the consent forms rarely promised a benefit. Most of the time, the forms merely said that benefits were uncertain (presumably by using language such as "benefits are not guaranteed" or "you may or may not benefit"). Is it possible to fault the consent forms even if they did not promise that subjects would benefit? Should IRBs require that consent forms in Phase 1 studies affirmatively state that it is highly unlikely that subjects will benefit? Should they include a statement like the one proposed by the Harvard oncologist who used to be in charge of Phase 1 cancer studies there? "Based on prior experience, the chance that you will feel better or live longer as a result of participating in this study is almost zero." Is this language better or worse than a sentence such as, "This medical research project is not expected to benefit you." Why? *See* Matthew Miller, *Phase I Cancer Trials: A Collusion of Misunderstanding*, 30 HASTINGS CENTER REP., July-Aug. 2000, at 34.

6. A recent analysis of adult cancer Phase 1 studies taking place between 1991 and 2002 demonstrated that different types of Phase 1 studies produced different results. "Classic" Phase 1 trials, in which only one chemotherapy drug was being given to subjects, were shown to have relatively low likelihood of benefit, consistent with previous thinking. Studies in which subjects were given at least one proven medication had a greater likelihood of benefiting subjects. *See* Elizabeth Horstmann et al., *Risks and Benefits of Phase I Oncology Trials, 1991 through 2002*, 352 NEW ENG. J. MED. 895 (2005); Razelle Kurzrock & Robert S. Benjamin, *Risks and Benefits of Phase I Oncology Trials, Revisited*, NEW ENG. J. MED. 930 (2005). Based on this information, should the language of the benefits section of consent forms differ based on the type of Phase 1 study being conducted?

[B] Informed Consent as a Process

RESPONSIBLE RESEARCH: A SYSTEMS APPROACH
TO PROTECTING RESEARCH PARTICIPANTS
INSTITUTE OF MEDICINE, NATIONAL ACADEMY OF SCIENCES
119-23 (2003)

Once a protocol has been developed, reviewed, and approved for scientific and ethical acceptability, the investigator must recruit individuals to participate in the research. The voluntary informed consent of the individual is a central element of participant protection. In addition, the informed consent process is a critical means by which investigators can establish the trust and confidence of participants. As such, informed consent can influence and shape long-term relationships with the study population and the general public.

Since the publication of *The Belmont Report: Ethical Principles and Guidelines for the Protection of Human Subjects of Research (Belmont Report)* and the report on IRBs by the National Commission for the Protection of Human Subjects of Biomedical and Behavioral Research in 1978, informed consent and IRB review have served as the primary procedural safeguards in human research in the United States. The centrality of informed consent to the research process was reiterated in a 1982 report by the subsequent President's Commission for the Study of Ethical Problems in Medicine and Biomedical and Behavioral Research, which identified informed consent as an "ethical imperative" to distinguish it from and raise it above the de minimis nature of law or regulation.

The continued importance of informed consent as a moral imperative is reflected in the attention it has received as a subject of research on the effectiveness of human research safeguards. A vast literature on informed consent has emerged in recent decades. Indeed, informed consent has been an ongoing subject of investigation by federal advisory committees, bioethics centers, and individual scholars.

However, the safeguards necessary to protect informed consent have been undermined in recent years by several factors, including the advancing complexity of science, threats to privacy, the conflation of institutional risk management with disclosure in consent forms, conflicts of interest, the inadequate time available for in-depth consideration of protocols by many IRBs, and the lack of investigators and reviewers sufficiently trained in biomedical, behavioral, and public health ethics. Other parts of this report discuss the role of the program in promoting informed consent by participants. This section addresses the *process* of assuring informed participation at the level of interactions between the investigator and the participant.

The Concept of Informed Consent

The meaning of the phrase "informed consent" has become distorted over the last two decades as concerns of institutional risk managers have overwhelmed the patient-centered spirit of the Common Rule. In the committee's view, the intent of this analysis is to recover the original concept of informed consent by disentangling the strands of meaning now woven together under that label, identify and preserve those parts of the current practice needed to empower participants, and rejuvenate and nurture a participant-centered process.

> *Recommendation 4.1*: The informed consent process should be an ongoing, interactive dialogue between research staff and research participants involving the disclosure and exchange of relevant information, discussion of that information, and assessment of the individual's understanding of the discussion.

. . . [I]n the specific context of research, the iterative set of federal regulations and the related multinational documents made clear that the informed and voluntary consent of the capable research participant was the norm for legally and ethically valid informed consent. Unfortunately, however, this ideal has been trampled by the research power structure and the realities of self-protective behavior often demonstrated by sponsors and research organizations.

The idea of the process of informed consent as one that provides for sharing information with and educating the research participant has fallen prey to the idea of informed consent as a document to be signed by the participant, constructed by the research sponsor or site to comply with the regulations. In medical treatment and clinical research, these documents typically include lengthy descriptions of diagnoses, prognoses, treatment alternatives, risks and benefits of the alternative treatments, the risk of no treatment, the right to refuse, the commitment to provide care even in the face of refusal, and the injury compensation policy of the sponsoring institution. The purpose of the document appears to be compliance with regulations, but the spirit of the document is clearly the articulation of every possible danger so that any subsequent participant complaint can be countered with the argument that the participant had been informed and had accepted this risk. The length, complexity, linguistic sophistication, and generally daunting nature of such documents are not conducive to increasing understanding, but rather serve to overwhelm the patient-participant.

Informed consent should never be focused merely on a written form, which constitutes only a fragment of the process. A structured conversation between the participant and a member of the research team should occur when it is required by the nature of the research, as it usually is in research involving significant risks. From a purely ethical standpoint, the purpose of the written form is to document and record that the ethically relevant information has been discussed. However, whatever role it may play in relation to potential legal liability, a signed form is not sufficient evidence of an ethically valid informed consent.

Informed Consent as an Ongoing Process

Emerging data show that informed consent is most effective as an evolving process, as opposed to a static, one-time disclosure event and/or signing of a consent form. Jeremy Sugarman, an expert on informed consent and the ethics of research involving humans, advised the committee during his testimony that informed consent should be considered an inherent component of the research process itself (not an adjunct exercise) in the form of an ongoing conversation that occurs at each research encounter or before each intervention. Ideally, the disclosure of information during the informed consent process takes place as a bilateral process involving an exchange of questions and answers between a research participant and a research investigator. This interplay is an important and potentially challenging process, as it requires the person obtaining consent to gauge the appropriate level of language and technical detail suitable for the participant's understanding.

Conceptually, informed consent should be construed as an evolving decision making process, rather than as simple "permission." This model of "ongoing conversation and decision making" allows for reinforcement of previously disclosed information, introduction of new information, and respect for autonomous participant decision making. The act of obtaining *written* consent is tangential to the *process* of informed consent and merely provides a mechanism to document and record that ethically relevant communication has taken place.

Particularly in instances of clinical research, investigators face many difficulties in communicating to potential participants the complex set of procedures, side effects, long-term risks, trade-offs relative to alternatives, and other information relevant to study participation. This task is not impossible, however. The challenge is to spend the necessary time and resources to prepare the appropriate language and ensure that communication truly occurs.

A Goodness-of-Fit Ethic for Informed Consent
Celia B. Fisher
30 Fordham Urb. L.J. 159, 161-62 (2002)

Informed consent to medical treatment and research represents a mutual agreement between a practitioner and patient, the validity of which requires that the consent be informed, rational, voluntary, and competent. The informed aspect of consent requires that practitioners provide information about the purpose, procedures, potential risks and benefits, and alternative options of treatment or research sufficient for an individual to make a reasoned decision. Such information, however, may not be sufficient for individuals with mental disorders who either lack general knowledge about health care treatments and patient rights, or who have not had the opportunity to make autonomous decisions. In these situations, a goodness-of-fit between the person and consent context might require modifying consent procedures to include "reasonable disclosure" of practical information about those general aspects of health care, or research essential for a knowledgeable decision to be made.

To meet the rational requirement of informed consent, an individual needs to be able to understand the information presented and appreciate the consequences to oneself of agreeing or declining treatment or research participation. Although impairments in abstract reasoning can limit this ability, matching the language level of consent information to that of a patient/participant with a mental disorder, and modifying those aspects of the consent setting that may be stress provoking for that particular individual, can reduce person-context consent vulnerability.

The voluntary requirement of consent is meant to insure that individuals are not coerced into participation, and are free to withdraw from treatment or biomedical research at any time. In some contexts people with mental disorders may be particularly vulnerable to coercion and exploitation. For example, they may fear disapproval from family caretakers or may feel that they must be compliant in deference to the authority of the requesting practitioner. Some may have had little experience in exercising their rights, or may fear the discontinuation of other services if they are living in a treatment residence. Modifying the consent setting to reduce the perception of power inequities, to provide opportunities to practice decision-making, and to construct concrete ways of demonstrating that other services will not be compromised, can strengthen the goodness-of-fit between person and consent setting.

NOTES AND QUESTIONS

1. This article mentions that ethically valid informed consent must be "informed, rational, voluntary and competent." Do people usually act "rationally" when they make important decisions? *See* Russell B. Korobkin & Thomas S. Ulen, *Law and Behavioral Science: Removing the Rationality Assumption from Law and Economics*, 88 CALIF. L. REV. 1051 (2000) (discussing social science research that calls into question the assumption that people act rationally). If medical decisions depend on factors such as a person's approach to authority, response to difficult medical data, assessment of varying probability estimates, historical experience with physicians, and complex relationships with family members, is it even possible to deem a particular decision "rational" or "irrational"?

2. The IOM report is committed to the idea of informed consent as an ongoing process. By contrast, many IRBs focus more on ensuring that the consent form discloses all the information required under the federal regulations. Which approach do you think best reflects the nature of the concept and the demands of the research setting? Which should be the model to which researchers aspire?

If there is a dissonance in the answers to the last two questions, how might a closer association be achieved?

Remaining Faithful to the Promises Given: Maintaining Standards in Changing Times
Nancy Dubler
32 SETON HALL L. REV. 563, 567-69 (2002)

II. ENSURING THE ADEQUACY OF THE INFORMED CONSENT PROCESS

. . . Informed consent forms regularly run from eight to sixteen pages of single-spaced recitation. They are barriers to, rather than supports for, critical individual thinking. What they do is calm the worries of the risk managers whose job it is to get all of the most contingent possible risks onto the paper trail of the research. Things are not as dire in the clinical care context, as fewer professionals are involved in the process, and the discussion is likely to be directed by the responsible clinician who has some relationship with and commitment to the patient. In the context of research, the potential subject and the researcher are likely to be strangers, and the conversation is thus totally in the hands of the planners and designers. When the suggestion was offered that these forms be accompanied by a "road map" to give the subject some idea of relative and most important risks, the liability attorney present at the discussion vetoed the idea. He offered the logic that the road map would substitute for the indigestible reality of the form and would not protect the sponsor and the investigator.

Creative alternatives are not beyond conception. Disclosure forms might contain layers of information — the most relevant in the body of the form, and the least important in an appendix. Potential research subjects could choose the level of risk of interest to them. The data could be placed in categories of risk described in the document with references for further research. Some patients and subjects have an almost inexhaustible thirst for information, seeking their own answers on the Internet, whereas others are content to accept the statement of the researcher that this is a good protocol to join. The former should be respected, and the latter — who need help evaluating research possibilities — are further deterred from undertaking such an evaluation by the current impenetrable process.

What should a better informed consent process look like? We know how an empowering discussion with a potential subject could be conducted. First of all, it would have to be a process that engages the subject on an escalating plane of complexity and abstraction. It would have to begin with the fact that this is research and that we do not know the answer to the question posed. In some cases, it means that we do not yet appreciate all of the risks and cannot predict what the consequences will be. In others — randomized clinical trials of approved interventions — it means that we do not know which is best. In placebo-controlled trials, it means that we do not know if the intervention proposed is better than no intervention at all. Evaluating the reading levels of the language of the informed consent documents has become the norm. But understanding the language may not provide real facility with the concepts. We can teach about these concepts as a precondition to engaging the potential subject. All it requires is time and money.

RESPONSIBLE RESEARCH: A SYSTEMS APPROACH TO PROTECTING RESEARCH PARTICIPANTS
INSTITUTE OF MEDICINE, NATIONAL ACADEMY OF SCIENCES
123-25 (2003)

[Note that in the IOM report an IRB is called a Research Ethics Review Board (ERB).]

Role of Consent Forms

In current practice, so-called informed consent forms are best characterized as consent forms. Additional documents (or appendixes to the basic consent form) that contain the boilerplate language directed at the legal protection of the institution rather than informing participants represent disclosure documents. These documents make little contribution to the process of communication and mutual understanding that is central to obtaining ethically valid informed consent. In contrast, the term "informed consent" should refer to the interactive process of education, discussion, and support that permits the potential participant to understand the options and apply a personal scale of values and preferences to those options in order to reach a decision about enrolling in a study.

The present convention, adhered to by investigators and followed by IRBs, is to review the consent form as the mechanism used to obtain informed consent, which is not sufficient as a process of involving and empowering the participant and promoting participant understanding. In the future, it should be up to the research organization's attorneys to decide whether the consent form and the disclosure documents are legally adequate; that is not the job of the Research ERB. Instead, the Research ERB should be expected to review the consent form to determine if it meets the federal standard and to decide whether a shorter, more accessible document might be used as a blueprint for the ensuing conversation with potential participants and as an aid to promoting understanding and choice. If a shorter form were offered, it might be useful to refer the participant to the sections in the full consent form that elaborate on the items in the short form. This would permit the participant to grasp the major procedures and their attendant risks, benefits, and alternatives and then explore them in greater depth. This process would facilitate understanding rather than impede comprehension, which, unfortunately, is often the result of the present use of lengthy consent forms.

Accomplishing the goal of real understanding as a precondition to a meaningful decision to participate will require a sea change in Research ERB and investigator perception and practice. Based on anecdotes and committee member experience, some investigator-participant exchanges are limited to answering questions such as, "What do you think I should do?" Such impoverished interactions utterly fail to link the skill and wisdom of the practitioner with the questions and concerns of the participant.

Disclosure of the nature of the study and its procedures, risks, benefits, and alternatives is a central pillar of the informed consent process. However, although it is necessary, it is not sufficient to support a process with real integrity. Disclosure information, presented comprehensively without overwhelming detail, is a pivotal aspect of the informed consent discussion, as without it potential participants will not have an adequate basis for decision making. Therefore, the committee encourages the development of innovative mechanisms (including written, electronic, or video instruments) to genuinely inform participants and promote understanding as well as record the interaction between the research staff and the potential participant.

In addition to this knowledge, the research professional's experience, perspectives, opinions, and recommendations are essential. Indeed, it might be more appropriate to label the process "advised consent" rather than "informed consent." This change would accommodate the interactive and supportive nature of the ideal process that assumes that information is the starting point of a discussion that alternates between participant questions and investigator responses and that helps participants understand the abstractions of benefit and risk in the context of a specific research situation and his or her personal needs and medical history.

An ideal informed consent process might use a brief document to present the basic material first and then offer the potential participant the opportunity to pose additional questions, as well as sufficient time to consider a more comprehensive document that may also be provided. It should always be stated in the case of nontherapeutic research that the project is research and not therapy. Appropriate help should be available to assist the participant in assuring that he or she understands the relevant issues and receives answers to all questions. In addition, special attention to the informed consent process should be provided for participants with language barriers, diminished capacity, and known vulnerabilities — both to facilitate informed consent and to avoid denying special groups access to human studies.

NOTES AND QUESTIONS

1. Review 45 C.F.R. § 46.116 and consider how you might address the objections raised in the excerpts above. What sort of conversation could you create

that would meet the objections and yet provide the information that the regulations require?

2. If you were to have a conversation with a prospective subject in the Taxol study (for which we provided a sample consent form earlier in this chapter), how would you introduce your discussion? What would be the major points that you would want to convey? What would be the setting for your discussion?

3. How might a researcher pilot-test an informed consent document? Should there be a requirement to field test the document and process with prospective subjects? Would it be useful to have a set of focus groups? Should researchers always be required to test-run the informed consent process before it is used?

4. For a review of the literature about the efficacy of interventions to improve the understanding of subjects, see James Flory & Ezekiel Emanuel, *Interventions to Improve Research Participants' Understanding in Informed Consent for Research: A Systematic Review*, 292 JAMA 1593 (2004).

[C] An Informed Consent Script

An Informed Consent Script for Adolescent Trials Network (ATN) 105
(National Institute of Child Health and Human Development)
(developed as a template by Nancy Dubler)

Title of Protocol:
Short-Cycle Therapy in Adolescents with Established Viral Suppression: Virologic and Immunologic Comparison to Adolescents on Non-interrupted Therapy

Model for a Script

Good morning:

I would like to talk to you this morning about the new research study that we have and that you might want to join.

You know that you are infected with the HIV virus and you have been taking medication for some time to try to control the infection. You have been doing very well and the HIV virus in your blood is very low as indicated by your viral load tests. We think that is because you are taking HAART (Highly Active Antiretroviral Therapy) that is keeping the virus from taking over. We think that you have been doing well with taking your medications. As part of our program here at _____ , we want to learn how to better take care of young people infected with HIV. We do this through research trials, which I will be discussing with you shortly.

First let me ask you: How has it been to take your medications when you are supposed to? Has it been difficult? Have you ever not taken them? Does it happen often or rarely that you don't take the medications?

Let me explain it to you. Right now, doctors tell everyone that they must take all their medicines, every day, at the right times. But we know that there are lots of patients, and maybe lots and lots of young people who don't take their medicines exactly on schedule. We don't know exactly what that will mean for them and for the development of the virus in their bodies. We suspect that some of these young people may do just as well with a skip every now and then but we do not know. On the other hand, we do know that stopping the medications may also make the body more resistant to the good things that the medicines do. The issue is that we really don't know what does or does not happen when someone stops taking the medicines for a while. So we would like to find out because if young people can take weekend breaks from their HIV medicines it might slow down some of the HIV medicine's bad effects and it might make it easier for young people to take the HIV medicines during the week, knowing the weekend would be free. We think that this may be possible for young people infected with HIV but only for those who have had a good response to the medicines with low viral load counts.

Tell me what sort of person you are — do you like to take risks? Are you a person who wants to be involved in something new?

Basically, if you agree to become a part of this research study, you will placed, by chance — like the flip of a coin — into one of two groups. One group will continue taking medicine on the usual schedule and one group will stop taking the medications on weekends. That is really all that the study will do — you will continue as usual or you will only take your drugs on the weekdays and skip taking them on the weekends. That is all that the study is; it is simple. But the really important point to remember is that WE DON'T KNOW IF STOPPING FOR A FEW DAYS EACH WEEK WILL BE A GOOD THING FOR YOUR HEALTH OR MIGHT MAKE YOUR HEALTH WORSE.

But there are other things that will be important to you if you come into the study.

If you come into the research study you will have to come to the clinic every other Monday for a month and then one Monday per month until the end of the six months of the project. Depending on which arm of the study you are in and how you are doing you might be asked to come to the clinic even more often. Whenever you do come to the clinic you will be asked to give some blood so that we can check how you are doing on your medications and how well they are controlling the growth of the virus.

Tell me in your own words what you think the study is about and how it might help or harm you. . . .

That really is all that this research study is about — seeing whether it is a good thing for young people with a low viral load from their HIV infection to stop medications on a regular basis.

But there are some things that you should think about.

First of all, as I said, this is research. That means that we really do not know if you will do better or maybe get sicker if you decide to come into this research.

If you are put in the group that continues to take your medicine 24/7, you have to be sure to do that. This group is called the control group. We use it to compare. We will not be able to tell if the weekends off group is dangerous or OK if we do not have a group that stays steady. So if you decide to join the study, you have to be willing to stay on your medicine like you have been doing if you get put in the group that continues.

If you are put in the group that stops for the weekends, it might happen that you will not do well and your virus will begin to grow. We will be watching your viral load very closely and if this started to happen we would tell you to go back and take your medications again on a daily basis. But it could happen that you would get worse and that you might not do as well afterwards on the same medications that had been working before . . . we just don't know. But it might be that you would do just as well with fewer days of medications and that would mean that you would get a break every week and might have an immune system that was stronger. We just don't know.

This conversation that we are having is called an "Informed Assent" conversation.[1] We call it that because we want you to think about this choice that you have. We are trying to be very honest with you and we want you to think with us, ask whatever questions that you want and try and think through whether you want to be a part of this research. We need to emphasize that you are really free to come into the research or not. It is totally your choice. If you decide not to you will be seen by your usual medical team and they will try and do what they think is best for your HIV care.

> *This is a really important point so I want to talk about it a bit. Do you usually talk about decisions with your parents? Do they know about your HIV infection? Does anybody know about your infection? Tell me how you make decisions about what to do with your medical care for HIV.*

> *So, let us talk for a bit about who you are and what sorts of things matter to you: Do you like to be first in the line or do you like to wait and see what happens to those in the front before you move too close? How do you feel about your own health? Do you think that you are doing well and don't want to rock the boat or do you feel that you would like to be part of the group that may help to learn more about this virus? Do you like to take risks or are you more of a conservative person who likes to take the advice of people who you think have the best advice to offer? How would*

---

[1] As discussed in Chapter 13, the regulations governing research with children require researchers to obtain the "permission" of the parents and, in some cases, the "assent" of the child. *See* Chapter 13, at page 538.

you think about this choice that I am presenting to you? Tell me your thoughts.

There is also another big issue for you to think about. If you decide to go into this study you will have to tell at least one of your parents. One of your parents will have to agree to your coming into this research. If you have not told your parents, this might be a real opportunity. On the other hand it might be really hard for you. If you are really not going to share your HIV with your parents then joining this study is not going to be possible for you.

Let us talk a bit more about your parents. Tell me what they are like and why you have told / not told them about your virus?

So, these are the things that are really important for you to understand:

1. *This is a research study and we really do not know if it will help you or make you worse. Remember you will know which study group you are in because if you are in the experimental group you will be told not to take your medicines on the weekend. It may be that if you are in the experimental group and you are not doing well on the weekends off plan that when you go back on medications you will not do as well. We just don't know.*

2. *If you come into the study it will mean that you will have to tell your parents, or at least one of them, and that you will have to come to the clinic on some Mondays, maybe in addition to your regular visits . . . that is really the only change in your life.*

3. *You really can say yes or no to me right now and you can say no later even if you say yes now. This is a choice for you and you should think about it carefully.*

Finally let me promise you that if we learn anything about this research we will let you know.

Thank you for coming to talk with me.

NOTES AND QUESTIONS

1. Might this sort of a script serve as a model for informed consent discussions in general? *No – too condescending!*

2. If informed consent is obtained through a "script" process, what sort of documentation should be required? Should the subject be required to initial the form after each section of the discussion? Do you think subjects would find that helpful? Might it interfere with the process?

3. Critics might charge that this discussion is "manipulative" and is designed to convince the subject to agree by engaging him or her in a dialogue meant to disarm his or her objections. Is this a reasonable objection? *Y*

§ 7.04 DEFICIENCIES IN THE INFORMED CONSENT PROCESS

[A] The Therapeutic Misconception

False Hopes and Best Data: Consent to Research and the Therapeutic Misconception
Paul S. Appelbaum, et al.
17 HASTINGS CENTER REP., April 1987, at 20

[A psychiatric patient, after several days of discussion with a psychiatrist and after reading a consent form, agrees to participate in a research study that randomizes him to receive either a placebo or a medication.] Yet when the patient is asked why he agreed to be in the study, he offers some disquieting information. The medication he will receive, he believes, will be the one most likely to help him out. He ruled out the possibility that he might receive a placebo, because that would not be likely to do him much good. In short, this man, now both a patient and a subject, has interpreted, even distorted, the information he received to maintain his view — obviously based on his wishes — that every aspect of the research project to which he had consented was designed to benefit him directly. This belief, which is far from uncommon, we call the "therapeutic misconception." To maintain a therapeutic misconception is to deny the possibility that there may be major disadvantages to participating in clinical research that stem from the nature of the research process itself. . . .

The unique aspects of clinical research include the goal of creating generalizable knowledge; the techniques of randomization; and the use of a study protocol, control groups, and double-blind procedures. Do these elements create a body of risks or disadvantages for research subjects? The answer lies in understanding how the scientific method is often incompatible with one of the first principles of clinical treatment — the value that the legal philosopher Charles Fried calls "personal care."

According to the principle of personal care, a physician's first obligation is solely to the patient's well-being. A corollary is that the physician will take whatever measures are available to maximize the chances of a successful outcome. A failure to adhere to this principle creates at least a potential disadvantage for the clinical research subject: there is always the chance that the subject's interests may become secondary to other demands on the physician-researcher's loyalties. And the methods of science inhibit the application of personal care. . . .

Studies on Consent

Our findings suggest that research subjects systematically misinterpret the risk/benefit ratio of participating in research because they fail to understand the underlying scientific methodology.

This conclusion is based on our observations of consent transactions in four research studies on the treatment of psychiatric illness, and our interviews with the subjects immediately after consent was obtained. The studies varied in the extent of the information they provided to subjects. Two of the studies compared the effects of two medications on a psychiatric disorder (one used, in addition, a placebo control group). A third study examined the relative efficacy of two dosage ranges of the same medication. And a fourth examined two different social interventions in chronic psychiatric illness, compared with a control group.

The populations in these studies ranged from actively psychotic schizophrenic patients to nonpsychotic, and in some cases, minimally symptomatic, borderline, and depressed patients. Our questions were based on information included on the consent form with regard to the understanding of randomized or chance assignment; and the use of control groups, formal protocols, and double-blind techniques. Eighty-eight patients comprised the final data pool, but since all of the issues addressed here were not relevant to each project the sample size varied for each question.

We found that fifty-five of eighty subjects (69 percent) had no comprehension of the actual basis for their random assignment to treatment groups, while only twenty-two of eighty (28 percent) had a complete understanding of the randomization process. Thirty-two subjects stated their explicit belief that assignment would be made on the basis of their therapeutic needs. Interestingly, many of these subjects constructed elaborate but entirely fictional means by which an assignment would be made that was in their best interests. This was particularly evident when information about group assignment was limited to the written consent forms and not covered in the oral disclosure; subjects filled vacuums of knowledge with assumptions that decisions would be made in their best interests.

Similar findings were evident concerning other aspects of scientific design. With regard to nontreatment control groups and placebos, fourteen of thirty-three (44 percent) subjects failed to recognize that some patients who desired treatment would not receive it. Concerning use of a double-blind, twenty-six of sixty-seven subjects (39 percent) did not understand that their physician would not know which medication they would receive; an additional sixteen of sixty-seven subjects (24 percent) had only partially understood this. Most striking of all, only six of sixty-eight subjects (9 percent) were able to recognize a single way in which joining a protocol would restrict the treatment they could receive. In the two drug studies in which adjustment of medication dosage was tightly restricted, twenty-two of forty-four subjects (50 percent) said explicitly that they thought their dosage would be adjusted according to their individual needs. . . .

Various theoretical explanations of our findings could support this view. Most people have been socialized to believe that physicians (at least ethical ones) always provide personal care. It may therefore be very difficult, perhaps nearly impossible, to persuade subjects that *this* encounter is different, particularly if the researcher is also the treating physician, who has previously satisfied the subject's expectations of personal care. Further, insofar as much clinical research involves persons who are acutely ill and in some distress, the well-known tendency of patients to regress and entrust their well-being to an authority figure would undercut any effort to dispel the therapeutic misconception.

In response, more of our data must be explored. In each of the studies we observed, one cell of subjects was the target of an augmented informational process, which supplemented the investigator's disclosures to subjects with a "preconsent discussion." This discussion was led by a member of our research team who was trained to teach potential subjects about such things as the key methodologic aspects of the research project, especially methods that might conflict with the principle of personal care.

By introducing a neutral discloser, distinct from the patient's treatment team, we shifted the emphasis of the disclosure to focus on the ways in which research differs from treatment. Of the subjects who received this special education, eight of sixteen (50 percent) recognized that randomization would be used, as opposed to thirteen of the fifty-one (25 percent) remaining subjects; five of five (100 percent) understood how placebos would be employed in the single study that used them, compared with eleven of the fifteen (73 percent) remaining subjects; nine of sixteen (56 percent) comprehended the use of a double blind while only fifteen of fifty-one (31 percent) remaining subjects did so; and five of seventeen (29 percent) initially recognized other limits on their treatment as a result of constraints in the protocol, compared with one of the fifty-one (2 percent) other subjects.

Our data suggest that many subjects can be taught that research *is* markedly different from ordinary treatment. Other efforts to educate subjects about the use of scientific methodology offer comparably encouraging results. There is no reason to believe that subjects will refuse to hear clear-cut efforts to dispel the therapeutic misconception. . . .

Who should have the task of explaining the therapeutic misconception to subjects? Clearly, investigators should be encouraged to discuss such issues with subjects and to include them on consent forms, but several problems arise here. First, it is decidedly *not* in investigators' self-interest for them to disabuse potential subjects of the therapeutic misconception. Experienced investigators, as we have reported elsewhere, view the recruitment of research subjects as an intricate and extended effort to win the potential subject's trust. One of our subjects in this study described the process in these words: "It was almost as if they were courting me. . . . everything was presented in the best possible light." One could argue that it is unrealistic to expect investigators to raise additional doubts about the benefits that subjects can expect; any effort in that regard will result in resistance by investigators, particularly those who have yet to internalize the justifications for informed consent in general.

In 1994, President Clinton created a committee to investigate government-sponsored human radiation experiments that took place between 1944 and 1974. (These experiments are discussed in more detail in Chapter 1, at page 44.) In addition to its main task, the Advisory Committee on Human Radiation Experiments also investigated how researchers obtained informed consent to radiation experiments during the period 1990-1993 (which they called the Research Proposal Review Project, or RPRP). The Committee also conducted the Subject Interview Study (SIS), which interviewed people to examine why they chose to participate or not participate in research studies.

Final Report
Advisory Committee on Human Radiation Experiments (ACHRE)
at 760-62 (1995)
http://www.eh.doe.gov/ohre/roadmap/achre/report.html

The findings of the SIS underscore what other, smaller studies also have identified — that patient-subjects generally decide to participate in medical research because they believe that being in research is the best way to improve their medical condition. In the SIS, we could not determine whether the patients had unrealistic expectations about how likely it was that they might benefit from being in research, or what form that benefit might take. Other empirical studies suggest that some subjects do have an inadequate, sometimes exaggerated understanding of the potential benefits of the research in which they are participating. In the RPRP, we reviewed consent forms that appeared to overpromise what research could likely offer the ill patient and underplay the effect of the research on the patient's quality of life. These were the kinds of disclosures that could easily be interpreted by a patient desperate for hope as offering much more than realistically could be expected. . . .

One of the most powerful themes to emerge from the SIS is the role of trust in patients' decisions to participate in research, a finding that has been observed in other studies as well. It was common for patients in the SIS to say that they had joined a research project at the suggestion of their physician and that they trusted that their physician would never endorse an option that was not in their best interest. This trust underscores the much-discussed tension in the role of physician-investigator, whose duties as a healer and as a scientist inherently conflict. This trust that patients place in their physicians often is generalized to the medical and research community as a whole. Some patients expressed faith not only in their doctors but also in the institutions where they were receiving medical care. These patients believed that hospitals would never permit research to be conducted that was not good for the patient-subjects. The trust that patients have in physicians and hospitals underscores the importance of . . . [our] concern, based on our review of the documents in the RPRP, that IRBs may not always be properly structured to ensure that the medical interests of ill patients are adequately protected. . . .

The theme of trust discerned in the SIS also has implications for how properly to view the role of informed consent in protecting the rights and interests of human subjects. For many of the patients who based their decision to be in research on their trust in their physicians, the informed consent process and the informed consent form were of little importance. . . .

The SIS and the RPRP also both speak to the current confusion between research and "standard care" in medical practice. The same therapy that is part of a research protocol, and therefore must receive IRB approval, can proceed outside of the research setting and not be subject to IRB oversight. This leads to understandable confusion on the part of subjects as to whether they are participating in research, receiving standard care, or some combination. It is thus perhaps not surprising that research subjects occasionally seem unaware of their participation in research, even when there is evidence they have signed consent forms. This finding was observed in the SIS, though the methodology of the study did not allow us to probe the reasons some subjects appeared unaware of their participation.

The confusion between research and alternative medical interventions is mirrored in the language used to communicate to patients in the informed consent process and in the language of patients themselves. In the SIS, the patients surveyed viewed *experiments* as involving unproven treatment of greater risk, while *clinical investigation* or *study* conveyed less uncertainty and were perceived as offering a greater chance of personal benefit. None of the consent forms we reviewed in the RPRP used the term *experiment*.

The Ubiquity and Utility of the Therapeutic Misconception
Rebecca Dresser
19 Soc. Phil. & Pol'y 271, 290-93 (2002)

Two general responses to the therapeutic misconception are possible. One is to accept it as an inevitable consequence of conducting research with patients. This has been the de facto response since Appelbaum, Roth and Lidz first described the therapeutic misconception. Despite periodic expressions of concern, the research system and the larger society continue to tolerate — and to promote — the conflation of research and therapy. Indeed, proposals by [some] explicitly endorse this response.

The alternative response is to take corrective action. Appelbaum and his colleagues showed that minor changes in the research setting increased patients' ability to understand the differences between research and therapy. Moreover, a host of additional possible changes have not yet been tried. Revisions in the conduct and presentation of research have a reasonable chance of changing how patients think about study participation. . . .

suggesting for correcting the therapeutic misconception.

Numerous other strategies have been offered for reducing the therapeutic misconception. Some focus on changes in consent forms. Simpler forms could communicate information to potential study participants more effectively. For instance, researchers could prepare a one-page form highlighting the most important information, including "the major benefits and risks of participation" as well as "the difference between the ways in which [patients] will be approached in the research context and the treatment they would expect to receive in the ordinary clinical setting." Furthermore, researchers conducting Phase I trials could create forms that emphasize study participants' low chance of receiving a health benefit by "includ[ing] the phrase, prominently displayed in bold type on the first page, 'This medical research project is not expected to benefit you.'"

Physicians could also act to discourage the therapeutic misconception. Physicians discussing the possibility of trial enrollment with their patients could be more "sensitive to the extraordinary power of their recommendations." They could present research not "simply as a new intervention with possibilities for beneficial effects, but as an intervention with little evidence suggesting whether effects will be beneficial or harmful." To separate their research and patient-care roles, physician-investigators could designate another person to discuss study information with patients.

All members of research teams could do more to reduce the therapeutic misconception. Researchers could explicitly state that their "primary loyalty is to future patients." They could also begin their discussion of randomization, placebo groups, and other research methods by announcing that study participants will be treated differently from patients and that study procedures are designed to promote valid data collection, not to promote what is best for participants. To counter their conversational tendencies to confuse research and therapy, researchers could prepare videotapes and interactive computer exercises that clearly delineate how study participation differs from clinical care. They could also administer questionnaires to evaluate how well prospective participants comprehend this information.

The therapeutic misconception could also be reduced through changes in the monetary reward system used in research. At minimum, IRBs and federal officials could require physicians who receive payments for trial referrals to tell patients about this arrangement. Such disclosure could raise patients' awareness that such referrals are not part of their ordinary treatment. Similarly, oversight bodies could require that patients be informed of any payment that physician-investigators conducting research will receive from research sponsors. If federal agencies prohibited referral fees and payment other than reasonable reimbursement for study costs, physicians would have fewer incentives to characterize studies as therapy.

Revisions in research advertisements and other recruitment publicity could promote patient understanding as well. Officials and IRBs could require sponsors and researchers to, when applicable, alert readers and listeners to major study risks and a study's use of placebo groups. Another idea is to offer payment to patients for research participation. The theory here is that payment could be an effective reminder that study participation is principally a service to others rather than a form of medical care.

These various measures could begin to erode the therapeutic misconception. In my view, however, more drastic change will be required. First, to counter the pervasive characterization of trials as treatment, researchers must give patients stark, bold and dramatic signs that research is different from clinical care. Simple environmental changes could have a strong impact on patient perceptions. For example, instead of the white coats associated with medical care, investigators could wear red ones. Instead of meeting with patients in a hospital or another health-care setting, investigators could be housed in separate buildings or areas clearly designated as research facilities.

Second, material progress in eliminating the therapeutic misconception will require change beyond the research setting. Federal officials, patient advocates, and journalists communicating with the public must provide better information about what trial participation offers patients. References to trials as being cutting-edge therapy must be replaced with realistic descriptions of the extra burdens and uncertainties that trial participants face. References to trials as being opportunities for patients to secure high-quality personal treatment must be replaced with messages stressing the altruistic nature of research participation. Finally, references to research "breakthroughs" and "medical miracles" must be replaced with language depicting the true course of science — slow and incremental advances combined with multiple setbacks and stumbling blocks. In sum, public discourse about research must convey a more sober and qualified picture of what patients can gain and lose from enrolling in research studies.

NOTES AND QUESTIONS

1. The therapeutic misconception is problematic because it can interfere with subjects' ability to provide genuine informed consent. Consider the discussion in the *Belmont Report* of the three essential elements of informed consent: information, comprehension, and voluntariness. How does the therapeutic misconception potentially undermine each of these elements?

2. A study published in *JAMA* looked at the ability of parents of children diagnosed with leukemia to understand the concept of randomization. They were invited to enroll their children in a study under which the participants would be placed in one of four active study arms. Randomization was explained by physicians in eighty-three percent of cases studied, and a consent document was presented during the conference in ninety-five percent of cases. Interviews after the conference demonstrated that sixty-eight (50%) of one hundred thirty-seven parents did not understand randomization. Although physicians described the trial as voluntary in ninety-seven percent of cases, eighteen percent of par-

ents did not understand that they were free to refuse study enrollment. Nineteen percent of parents reported feeling pressure to enroll in the randomized clinical trial. The right to withdraw was discussed in seventy-two percent of cases, but twenty percent of parents did not know that their child could withdraw from the trial at any time. The authors reached the following conclusion:

> Therapeutic misconception has been shown to be prevalent in clinical research, and our results suggest that it may be important in the context of childhood cancer. In these RCTs, parents may expect their child to be randomized to the best treatment based on the child's clinical characteristics. These findings highlight the need to improve the quality of informed consent.

Eric Kodish et al., *Communication of Randomization in Childhood Leukemia Trials*, 291 JAMA 470 (2004).

3. The therapeutic misconception is likely to be more significant in some situations than in others. Consider how the impact of the therapeutic misconception might differ in the following scenarios: (1) a physician recommends to her patient that the patient enroll in a clinical trial testing a new treatment for the patient's disease; (2) a physician conducting a clinical trial invites individuals she has never met before to enroll in the study; (3) a physician recruits "normal healthy volunteers" to participate in a study about the impact of pollutants on lung functioning; (4) a public health worker who is not a physician invites members of the community to participate in a study about the long-term benefits of regular exercise.

4. Dresser observes that the status quo appears to be an acceptance of the fact that subjects will frequently be unaware of the differences between being in a research study and being a patient. As she notes, prominent scholars seem to be willing to live with this situation. Why do you think that is the case?

5. Make a list of Dresser's suggested changes, and put them in order from those that are most likely to reduce the therapeutic misconception to those least likely to do so. If you were to decide which changes to make, which would you implement, and why? What level of resources would you be willing to devote to these efforts?

6. Instead of the language suggested by Dresser, should a researcher be required to state, in a *Miranda* warning fashion: "I am not here to serve your interest? What I might do may hurt you. Beware!"?

7. Some have suggested, similar to one of Dresser's recommendations, that the therapeutic misconception could be greatly minimized by precluding the patient's personal physician from being the person who obtains informed consent for participation in a study that the physician is conducting. *See, e.g.,* OFFICE OF INSPECTOR GENERAL, DEPARTMENT OF HEALTH AND HUMAN SERVICES, RECRUITING HUMAN SUBJECTS: PRESSURES IN INDUSTRY SPONSORED CLINICAL RESEARCH 54 (2000). Would you support such a rule? What might be the downside?

8. A further extension of that idea would be to create a separate class of research personnel who function only as researchers, not as providers of clinical care. When a person participated in research, they would go to a separate facility or wing of a hospital, clearly labeled as a "Research Center," and they would not be treated by anyone who functions as a clinician. What do you think of that idea?

9. For additional discussion of the therapeutic misconception, see, e.g., Paul S. Appelbaum et al., *Therapeutic Misconception in Clinical Research: Frequency and Risk Factors*, 26 IRB, Mar.-Apr. 2004, at 1; Charles W. Lidz & Paul S. Appelbaum, *The Therapeutic Misconception: Problems and Solutions*, 40(9) (Supp.) MED. CARE V-55 (2002); JESSICA BERG ET AL., INFORMED CONSENT: LEGAL THEORY AND CLINICAL PRACTICE 288-99 (2d ed. 2001).

[B] Failure to Convey Information

Family's Debate
Mirrored Scientists' on Gene Therapy Risk
Deborah Nelson & Rick Weiss
WASHINGTON POST, Sept. 30, 1999, at A7

Just before Paul Gelsinger sent his son off to Philadelphia to take part in a gene therapy experiment for the teenager's childhood disease, the Tucson man had a heated dining room debate with his mother-in-law over the wisdom of the trip.

He's healthy, she argued. He's doing well on his current treatment. Why take the gamble? It's a low-risk study, Gelsinger told her. He wants to do it. And it might lead to a cure for the rare genetic ailment he had, called ornithine transcarbamylase deficiency.

["Ornithine Transcarbamylase Deficiency is part of a urea cycle disorder. A urea cycle disorder is a genetic disorder caused by a deficiency of one of the enzymes in the urea cycle. The urea cycle involves a series of biochemical steps that takes place in the liver, in which nitrogen, a component of protein, is removed from the blood and converted into urea. There are five steps to the urea cycle, each of them requiring a specific enzyme. When one of these enzymes is missing, nitrogen accumulates and is converted into ammonia, a highly toxic substance, instead of urea. Ammonia reaches the brain through the blood, where it may cause irreversible brain damage and/or death. Ornithine transcarbamylase is one of these deficiencies. Urea cycle disorders are tragic illnesses that are characterized by excessive amounts of ammonia in the blood. Without treatment, these disorders can cause behavioral disorders, mental retardation, coma, or even death." Children's National Medical Center, *Human Ornithine Transcarbamylase*, available at http://www.cnmcresearch.org/glossary.asp.]

"Turns out she was right," the devastated father said yesterday.

Gelsinger's son died shortly after starting the pioneering treatment at the University of Pennsylvania in Philadelphia — the first apparent casualty since scientists began experimenting with ways to permanently alter disease-causing genes. The death is being investigated by the university and federal officials.

Although he didn't know it at the time, Gelsinger's argument with his mother-in-law was a dinner table replay of a similarly vigorous discussion over a meeting room table four years ago, when a federal advisory committee wrestled with whether to endorse the controversial study.

Of particular concern to committee members was the researchers' decision to experiment on patients who were doing well on conventional treatment or no treatment at all. The first round of human testing for new therapies is usually done on ill patients who haven't responded to standard treatments, and thus have less to lose by trying unproven approaches.

The Pennsylvania protocol was discussed at length at that December 1995 meeting of the Recombinant DNA Advisory Committee (RAC), an advisory group to the director of the National Institutes of Health that examines the scientific and ethical basis of all proposed gene therapy experiments involving federal funds.

Robert P. Erickson, an RAC member affiliated with the University of Arizona, opened the discussion with several criticisms of the proposed experiment. The study was not justified, he said, in part because the procedure was very "invasive" — a catheter would have to be threaded through critical blood vessels and the new genes would be delivered directly into the liver via millions of living viruses that had the potential to trigger organ damage — and because most of the patients to be studied were in good health and many in fact had never experienced symptoms.

At a minimum, he suggested, the viruses should be delivered through a less dangerous intravenous line. The Philadelphia researchers, in attendance at the meeting, accepted that advice. But ultimately they used the original approach anyway because of fears that the intravenous approach might create problems of its own by delivering the new genes to the wrong parts of the body.

That reversal was approved in private meetings with the Food and Drug Administration, but was never reviewed in public by the RAC — a fact that concerned some committee members, who did not learn about the change until they read it in newspapers yesterday.

"The public and the RAC didn't know," said LeRoy B. Walters, a Georgetown University ethicist who sat on the committee. "I think the early years of a promising area like gene therapy ought to be out in the light of day."

Researchers said on Tuesday that the method of delivery is one of several possible reasons that Jesse Gelsinger went into multiple organ failure soon after getting his first infusion of new genes — although none of the previous 17 patients had suffered any ill effects from the treatment.

NOTES AND QUESTIONS

1. The researcher in charge of the study in which Jesse Gelsinger participated had originally planned to use dying babies as research subjects. Arthur Caplan, a bioethicist at the University of Pennsylvania, advised against that approach. Caplan argued that "parents of dying infants are incapable of giving informed consent because 'they are coerced by the disease of their child.' " Instead, Caplan advised the researcher to study stable adults, female carriers, or men with partial enzyme deficiencies. Sheryl Gay Stolberg, *The Biotech Death of Jesse Gelsinger*, N.Y. TIMES, Nov. 28, 1999, Sec. 6, p. 137 (quoting Arthur Caplan). What do you think of Caplan's analysis?

2. What sorts of information should have been given to Jesse Gelsinger and his parents? Should they have been told about the RAC meeting? Should they have been given the minutes of the meetings? Should they have been told about the animal studies that preceded the research with human subjects in which four of the monkeys under treatment died? What about the fact that the researcher and the University of Pennsylvania had equity interests in the company that was sponsoring the research? *See* Chapter 5, at page 207. How should an IRB establish the standard for sharing information?

3. Would it be useful to test potential subjects after they have been engaged in a discussion and after they have read the form? What sort of questions would you want to ask? Should researchers test the prospective subjects on the specifics or just determine that they understand that it is research and that they might be harmed by it? Should they be required to explore the individual's personal objectives, values, and concerns and determine whether they have adequately assessed the research in light of those factors?

4. IRBs often establish readability standards for consent forms, requiring that they be written at a relatively easy-to-understand level (such as eighth grade or lower). In 2003, a study found that ninety-two percent of IRBs that posted readability standards for consent forms on the Internet also posted templates for writing consent forms that were written at a level that violated the IRB's own recommended readability standards. *See* Michael K. Paasche-Orlow et al., *Readability Standards for Informed-Consent Forms as Compared with Actual Readability*, 348 NEW ENG. J. MED. 721 (2003).

[C] Cultural and Gender-Based Barriers to Informed Consent

Ethnicity and Attitudes Toward Patient Autonomy
Leslie J. Blackhall et al.
274 JAMA 820, 823-24 (1995)

[Although this article discusses a study about informed consent in the clinical setting, its comments have equal relevance in the research setting.]

Korean-American and Mexican-American subjects were less likely than European-American and African-American subjects to believe that the patient should be told the truth about the diagnosis and prognosis of a serious illness and were less likely to believe that the patient should make decisions about the use of life support. . . .

The decision-making style exhibited by most of the Mexican-American and Korean-American subjects in our study might best be described as family centered. Although the patient autonomy model does not exclude family involvement, in this family-centered model, it is the sole responsibility of the family to hear bad news about the patient's diagnosis and prognosis and to make the difficult decisions about life support. Several prior studies of the issue of telling the diagnosis of cancer with different ethnic groups [such as Italians, Greeks, Chinese and others] have yielded similar results. . . .

Thus, belief in the ideal of patient autonomy is far from universal. . . .

Many questions remain to be answered about how this family-centered model functions in actual practice. Do patients who are not told the diagnosis usually know it anyway? . . . What is the perceived harm when the medical community violates cultural conventions and insists on telling the truth to the patient? . . .

[W]e believe it is vital to uncover the usually unspoken beliefs and assumptions that are common among patients of particular ethnicities to raise the sensitivity of physicians and others who work with these groups. Understanding that such attitudes exist will allow physicians to recognize and avoid potential difficulties in communication and to elicit and negotiate differences when they occur. In particular, we suggest that physicians ask patients if they wish to be informed about their illness and be involved in making decisions about their care or if they prefer that their family handles such matters. In either case, the patient's wishes should be respected. Allowing patients to choose a family-centered decision-making style does not mean abandoning our commitment to individual autonomy or its legal expression in the doctrine of informed consent. Rather, it means broadening our view of autonomy so that respect for persons includes respect for the cultural values they bring with them to the decision-making process.

NOTES AND QUESTIONS

1. If you were attempting to enroll somebody from one of the cultural groups described in this excerpt, would it be appropriate to assume that she shares the attitudes abut decision making identified in the excerpt? If you determined that she would prefer to have her family members make decisions on her behalf, how far would the federal regulations permit you to go in respecting those wishes? Would you insist on a discussion with the subject about the information contained in the consent form? Would you require that the subject read the consent form? Would you allow someone to consent to be in a research study even if that person has not yet been told that they have cancer if the study is investigating treatments for cancer?

2. If the researcher and prospective subjects come from different cultures, are most comfortable speaking in different languages, and have different attitudes and assumptions about physicians, research, and medical care, how can the researcher bridge the gap? Should she hire people from the community of subjects to act as advocates for the subjects? Should she hire interpreters? Should the consent form be translated into the subject's primary language? How should the researcher or the IRB determine the nature and extent of the efforts that should be undertaken? For the FDA's answers to some of these questions, see Question 51, in FDA Information Sheets (1998) at page 14, http://www.fda.gov/oc/ohrt/irbs/default.htm. How might 45 C.F.R. § 46.117(b)(2) be helpful in documenting that the subject's consent has been adequately obtained?

3. In *Diaz v. Hillsborough County Hospital Authority*, 2000 U.S. Dist. LEXIS 14,061 (M.D. Fla. 2000), a group of poor, non-English-speaking women alleged that, while they were pregnant, their physicians put them in a study designed to reduce the risk of respiratory problems in premature babies, without the women's knowledge or consent. As part of the study, the women were required to undergo as many as ten amniocentesis exams. According to the women's attorney, there were no bilingual staff; the women were simply told to come in and sign the consent forms, all of which were in English. *See* Peter Aronson, *A Medical Indignity*, NAT'L L.J., March 27, 2000, at A1. The *Diaz* case is discussed further in Chapter 12, at page 517.

4. For a moving account about how cultural differences between doctors and patients (in the clinical setting) can lead to a tragic outcome, see ANNE FADIMAN, THE SPIRIT CATCHES YOU AND YOU FALL DOWN: A HMONG CHILD, HER AMERICAN DOCTORS, AND THE COLLISION OF TWO CULTURES (1997).

Gender Matters: Implications for Clinical Research and Women's Health Care
Karen H. Rothenberg
32 HOUS. L. REV. 1201 (1996)

In her book, *You Just Don't Understand*, Deborah Tannen has described differences in the communication styles of men and women. Some of these differences may, in part, explain why gender matters in medical care. Because communication is the fundamental instrument by which physician and patient relate to each other and attempt to achieve therapeutic goals, the relationship between physician and patient is central to the process of health care delivery. Physicians must promote trust — they must hear the patient's story.

As one author has observed, "institutional authority of the physician and acquiescence to that authority by the patient, fostered frequently by gender expectations, can make it difficult for patients to assert their informational needs." For example, women who believe they have serious diseases may present their worries in a vague manner in an effort to avoid being labeled hypochondriacs.

The most difficult physician-patient relationships tend to be between male physicians and female patients. Some research has shown that male physicians may discourage information exchange with female patients. For example, compared to male physicians, female physicians engage in significantly more positive talk, partnership-building, question-asking, and information-giving. Similarly, when with female physicians, patients talk more during the medical visit and appear to participate more actively in the medical dialogue. The longest visits are between female physicians and female patients and the shortest between male physicians and female patients.

Both male and female patients are more willing to disclose symptoms to a physician of the same sex than to a physician of opposite sex. Research has shown that female-female interactions are characterized by fewer interruptions of patients by physicians. Fear and embarrassment may in fact be further barriers to health care, especially among special population groups, including low income blacks, Hispanics, and women over fifty.

A few recent studies have, in fact, surveyed women's attitudes about physician-patient communication. In the 1993 Commonwealth Fund study of over 2,500 women and 1,000 men, 1 out of 4 women (compared to 12% of men) said that they had been "'talked down to'" or treated like a child by their physician. Nearly 1 out of 5 women (compared to 7% of men) had been told that a reported medical condition was "'all in your head.'"

Communication barriers may be of particular concern to the older female population. In addition to sensory losses and concerns about the use of medical jargon, psychosocial factors were a major concern. Older women may fear being labeled as a nuisance, hypochondriac, or "'crabby old woman.'" Many older women report being intimidated by doctors and consider them as god-like entities who are busy with important matters and should not be bothered with their trivial aches and pains. Older women may feel particularly timid about private or embarrassing information and are likely to accept poorly communicated explanations, believing they are the ones who are at fault.

NOTES AND QUESTIONS

1. What are the implications of Rothenberg's observations for obtaining informed consent to research?

2. When the NIH awards grants for studies in which subjects will primarily be either men or women, should it favor applications from research teams made up of persons of the same gender as the prospective subjects?

3. Are there circumstances in which it might be appropriate to have separate male and female versions of a consent form? In what types of studies might this be considered? How might the two versions differ?

4. In addition to gender, subjects' sexual orientation or gender identity may affect their ability to communicate with researchers. Consider a researcher who informs a prospective subject that she should avoid becoming pregnant during the course of a study, and that she can do this by either using contraception or abstaining from sex. While that statement might seem innocuous to a heterosexual woman, it could come across as insensitive to a woman in a same-sex relationship. Is it possible that a lesbian's reaction to such a statement would affect her communications with the researcher about other issues? In what other circumstances might it be especially important for researchers to avoid making assumptions about subjects' sexual orientation or gender identity?

Chapter 8

RECRUITING AND PAYING SUBJECTS

As the material in Chapter 2 indicates, the clinical research environment has changed dramatically during the past decade and a half. Clinical trials have become more commercial and competitive, creating difficulties in finding enough subjects to bring new treatments to market within the desired time frame. The number and complexity of new treatments has led to a need for greater numbers of subjects, placing more pressure on investigators to expedite enrollment. Moreover, a site's ability to recruit subjects rapidly is a major factor in a sponsor's decision to contract with that site. The result has led to some disturbing recruitment practices. This chapter explores these practices, as well as related questions about offering payments to research subjects as either an inducement or a reward.

§ 8.01 RECRUITING SUBJECTS

[A] Overview of the Issues

RECRUITING HUMAN SUBJECTS: PRESSURES IN INDUSTRY
SPONSORED CLINICAL RESEARCH
OFFICE OF INSPECTOR GENERAL, DEPARTMENT OF HEALTH
AND HUMAN SERVICES
17-20 (2000)
oig.hhs.gov/oei/reports/oei-01-97-00195.pdf

Offering Incentives

> ". . . The order on the author list will be determined by the number of patients enrolled, so that the center which enrolls the highest number of patients will obtain first authorship . . ."
>
> **From a sponsor-investigator contract**

The use of certain recruitment methods illustrates the transformation of clinical research into a traditional business model. Sponsors provide incentives, both financial and nonfinancial (see box), to investigators to encourage speedy enrollment and/or reward those that recruit certain numbers of subjects.

Also, whereas before each site was allotted a certain number of subject slots, many trials now are conducted as "competitive enrollment." Because sponsors pay sites per subject enrolled, competitive enrollment penalizes those sites with a slow start-up period and encourages aggressive recruiting.

The use of financial enrollment bonuses appears to have increased somewhat in the past few years, despite evidence that such incentives are often ineffective. A coordinator we spoke with reinforced this notion when she told us her site "had gotten burned by enrollment bonuses in the past" because it enrolled all of its subjects before the bonus was offered. She told us, "we'll think about that the next time around," and possibly wait to enroll all of their subjects.

It is important to distinguish the financial incentives used to encourage timely recruitment from the sponsor payments to investigators for costs associated with conducting clinical research. Research costs vary significantly based on the requirements of the trial and can be very high when many expensive procedures are involved. When we refer to financial incentives for recruitment, we are referring to payments given to investigators purely to encourage speedy enrollment. Sponsors offer these incentives most often as an enrollment deadline nears or is passed.

The distinction between payment and enrollment incentives, however, can get blurred in practice. As sponsors continue to cut initial study budgets, many investigators that we spoke with reported that bonuses can help sites recoup the costs of conducting trials. These investigators often stated that they would rather have the initial study budgets accurately reflect the trials' costs. One investigator discussed a study in which he was initially paid $12,000 per subject enrolled. After other investigators in the trial complained to the sponsor of excessively tight budgets, the sponsor added a $30,000 bonus once a site enrolled its first six subjects and, after these first six subjects were enrolled, the site would receive an additional $6,000 per subject. The investigator, in describing this bonus scheme, emphasized that the sponsor had chosen to reimburse investigators by using bonuses to encourage recruitment rather than just revising the contract to reimburse investigators $18,000 per subject enrolled.

Targeting Own Patients

For many investigators, their own patients are a vital source of subjects. Nearly all of the investigators we spoke with told us that they first tried to enroll any of their patients that were eligible. As an investigator at an academic center told us, he saw a direct correlation between his clinic time and his ability to recruit. When he reduced his clinic time to one half-day per week, his recruitment declined significantly; when he increased his time, his recruitment resumed accordingly. Similarly, investigators who lack certain types of patients often experience difficulties enrolling for those trials. For example, an academic physician we spoke with told us he had a hard time recruiting for one of his clinical trials because the trial focused on a common ailment. At the tertiary care center where he practiced, he rarely saw such common diseases, which are easily treated by community physicians.

Patients are an important source of subjects in both academic and independent research settings. Even though many independent centers are freestanding entities, these sites contract with investigators who specialize in the condition under study, in large part because the investigators have potentially eligible subjects among their patients. The investigators will then refer their patients to the research site.

> ## Looking for Trials!
>
> We are a large family practice with 4 physicians and 3 Physician Assistants. We have two full time coordinators and a computerized patient data base of 40,000 patients. . . . We are looking for Phase2-Phase 4 trials as well as postmarketing studies. We can actively recruit patients for any study that can be conducted in the Family Practice setting.
>
> **An Internet advertisement directed to sponsors by a private practice seeking research opportunities.**

An advantage to using one's own patient base is the relative speed and ease with which investigators can reach these potential subjects. In fact, when asked what sponsors are looking for in placing a research study, both sponsor representatives and investigators told us that access to eligible patients is key. Sponsors seek out investigators and sites with large patient populations when looking to place trials. Investigators recognize this and, in turn, have begun to advertise their large patient bases. Such advertisements are numerous and prominent, particularly on the Internet, as investigators reach out to sponsors to place a trial with them (see box).

Seeking Additional Patient Bases

When sponsors and investigators need more subjects, they target their search efforts to reach large groups of potentially eligible subjects, such as other physicians' patient bases or disease advocacy groups. Occasionally, investigators offer fees to encourage referrals from other physicians or nurses. For example, one coordinator told us that a site she had formerly worked at offered $75 to physicians or nurses for each subject referred. Another investigator told us about a local site that offered referring physicians a reimbursement of 10 percent more than Medicare reimburses for services that this physician provided as part of the trial.

The researchers we spoke with said that they rarely hear referral fees offered. This may be due, in part, to the fact that many investigators find referrals to be an unsuccessful method of identifying additional subjects. The investigators who found referrals fruitless believed other physicians lack the time and the interest in research to approach their patients about participating. In addition, several academic physicians felt that community physicians were concerned that if they referred their patients to a trial, the academic investigators might take over all of the patients' care, thus "stealing" their patients.

Advocacy groups and student populations are another source of subjects. Advocacy groups often encourage researchers to develop new treatments for their disease. Many of these groups are eager to disseminate research information through their member networks and newsletters. Several investigators told us that they sometimes give presentations at advocacy meetings in which they try to mention their ongoing research protocols. For trials requiring healthy subjects, many sponsors and investigators reach out to student populations. Areas of high research activity are often located close to large universities.

Promotion and Advertising

Advertisements seeking human subjects are common. They can be found in newspapers, on the radio, the Internet, television, or as posters in, for example, public transportation or hospitals. Ads can be very expensive, especially in certain parts of the country. Because of this, many researchers are reluctant to use them unless absolutely necessary. Several researchers told us that ads are cost-effective only for studies in which the eligible population is large and widely dispersed (i.e., depression or heart disease) as opposed to rarer conditions such as cystic fibrosis.

Recently, sponsors and CROs [contract research organizations, described in Chapter 2, at page 78] have been helping sites recruit by initiating national recruitment campaigns for multi-site trials. The national efforts have spawned a new industry of patient recruitment firms and research marketing companies who are creating professional, elaborate marketing packages. Staff at the sites we spoke with report they are receiving more advertising from the sponsors at the start of the trial (including posters, fliers, and even prerecorded radio announcements for the local stations) than in years past. Many of these national advertisements include toll-free numbers. Call centers may provide operators who can screen respondents according to the trial's eligibility criteria and can schedule appointments at sites most convenient to callers. Or, the toll-free number may automatically transfer to a phone at the closest site.

The Internet is a fast-growing medium for advertising to potential subjects. As health care consumers make efforts to become more informed about their options, they are turning to the Internet as an important resource. Sponsors and/or investigators may post information about a trial on their website or on central listings of active research. There are several central listings and, in the past several months alone, there have been two announcements of alliances between healthcare websites and clinical trial organizations to post trial information on the Internet. Information on the Internet may prove particularly beneficial in recruiting for trials involving rare diseases where any one site may have only a small number of eligible subjects in its area.

Investigators told us that they have recently seen more press releases or television news segments describing their research and any promising progress the research may hold. Though not explicitly advertisements, the segments can generate numerous responses.

NOTES AND QUESTIONS

1. As part of the Office of Inspector General (OIG) study, IRB officials and others involved with clinical research were interviewed regarding their concerns about recruitment practices. The most fundamental concerns noted were that the consent process would be undermined as a result of investigators' misrepresenting the true nature of their research and that subjects would be unduly influenced to participate due to their trust in their physician. (This concern relates to the problem of the "therapeutic misconception," the tendency of subjects to confuse research with therapy. That issue is discussed at length in Chapter 7, at page 355.) In addition, however, those interviewed voiced fears about individuals other than the patient's physician searching medical records (such as a researcher given complete access to a medical center's computer files) and contacting patients about participation, and the possible misuse of other records, such as disease registries, school records, or mailing lists. (As discussed in Chapter 10, federal regulations governing patient privacy limit the circumstances under which researchers can access identifiable medical records. See Chapter 10, at page 459.) A final area of concern was the fear that some investigators would enroll ineligible subjects to meet quotas and satisfy sponsors.

2. The OIG study also concluded that oversight of subject recruitment was minimal and largely unresponsive to emerging concerns. The study determined that IRBs' limited review of recruitment was due in part to their perceived lack of authority to review these practices and to the minimal guidance provided by DHHS on acceptable recruitment practices. Similarly, it criticized DHHS for paying insufficient attention to recruitment practices in their site inspections of IRBs and investigators.

3. In 1996, the *Wall Street Journal* published a lengthy article detailing methods used by Eli Lilly to recruit healthy volunteers for its in-house Phase 1 drug studies, noting that Lilly offered $85 per day, below the industry average of $125-$250. The article claimed that, rather than advertising for Phase I subjects, Lilly relied on a "steady stream of homeless people, who come to Indianapolis seeking admittance to Lilly's research clinic," despite denials by Lilly executives. It quoted a veteran nurse at Lilly who claimed that the majority of its subjects were homeless alcoholics. It noted that many of these individuals utilized a variety of techniques to detoxify and mask their liver enzyme test results to be admitted to the studies. Often, they would lie and indicate that they had been sober for two months instead of a few days. The men were grateful for the "easy money" that could amount to more than $4,600 to $5,200 for a nine-week study. The article noted concerns about the lack of voluntary consent

from such subjects and the fact that over-utilization of homeless men violates federal policy regarding the equitable selection of research participants. An FDA official was quoted as saying that using homeless individuals circumvented FDA rules that were designed "to discourage disadvantaged people from participating in studies simply to escape 'the horrible situation of their lives.'"

Moreover, it was noted, there are reasons to be concerned about the use of alcoholics in these studies. For example, alcoholics might assume that adverse reactions to investigational drugs are the result of detoxification, or they might not report adverse reactions out of fears of being withdrawn from the study. The result would be that side effects would go unreported, skewing the safety profile of the drug and creating a dangerous situation for later subjects who might enter a Phase 2 study. In addition, heavy drinkers often metabolize drugs more slowly than others, leading to inaccurate data about a drug's half-life. *See* Laurie P. Cohen, *It's 'Quick Cash' to Habitues of Indianapolis Shelters; It Vanishes Quickly, Too*, WALL STREET JOURNAL, November 14, 1996.

4. You are a member of the IRB at your hospital. A protocol for researching a new cancer drug has been presented to the board. A small, new pharmaceutical company is sponsoring the research, and the drug involved is one of only two being pursued by the company. The principal investigator, a member of your medical staff who is not an employee of the hospital, will receive an eight percent equity or ownership interest in the company for conducting this research. In addition, the company will reimburse the hospital for 148 percent of its actual costs in conducting the study (e.g. laboratory tests, MRIs, etc.). Should the IRB approve this arrangement? What about the following alternative arrangements?

   a. The principal investigator will be paid $5,000 for each subject he or she enrolls in the study. The protocol calls for a total of 105 participants, and it is expected that 35 will be enrolled at each of three study sites.

   b. The principal investigator will be paid an hourly rate, to be established by reference to his or her annual income from clinical activities during the prior year, for whatever time he or she spends conducting the study. The hospital will be reimbursed in the manner described above. In addition, any physician on the hospital staff who refers a patient to the study staff will receive a bonus of $1,000 per subject if the patient ultimately enrolls and completes the protocol.

   c. Any physician on the medical staff who refers a patient who ultimately enrolls in the study will be reimbursed up to $3,500 for travel expenses, meals and lodging, and registration fees to attend a continuing medical education conference.

5. Several professional organizations, including the American Medical Association and the American College of Physicians, assert that financial incentives for referrals create an "unethical conflict of interest," and should be prohibited. Several other medical associations, though not prohibiting such

arrangements outright, advise that investigators at least disclose to potential subjects the existence and identity of a funding source for the study. Policies of academic medical centers and healthcare systems are similarly varied. Some of these institutions prohibit any payments to investigators intended to encourage subject recruitment, while others allow payments to cover expenses that investigators actually incur to hasten enrollment, such as additional advertising costs. *See* OFFICE OF INSPECTOR GENERAL, DEPARTMENT OF HEALTH AND HUMAN SERVICES, RECRUITING HUMAN SUBJECTS: SAMPLE GUIDELINES FOR PRACTICE 8-9 (2000), available at oig.hhs.gov/oei/reports/oei-01-97-00196.pdf.

6. In some situations, recruitment incentives could result in violations of a federal law designed to prevent the government from being cheated (known as the False Claims statute) if, for example, researchers and institutions hide the costs of finder's fees within other budgetary categories and then seek reimbursement for such amounts by government funding agencies. In addition, the federal Anti-Kickback Act criminalizes manufacturers and clinicians who make payments intended to induce the use of services covered by the various federal health programs such as Medicare and Medicaid. Presumably, this would include finders' fees for referrals of patients to trials funded by federal health programs, or even for privately sponsored studies if Medicare or Medicaid will be covering the costs of routine clinical care provided to the patient in the course of the study. *See* Paul E. Kalb and Kristin Graham Koehler, *Legal Issues in Scientific Research,* 287 JAMA 85 (2002); *see also* Chapter 5, at page 225.

7. Consider the following real advertisement:

New Treatment for Patients with Liver Cancer/Colon Cancer

████████ Medical Center Researchers Seek Participants in Gene Therapy & Radiofrequency (RF) Clinical Trials

If you are suffering from colon cancer which has spread to the liver, you may be eligible to participate in these clinical trials. In the gene therapy trial, patients will receive p53 gene therapy and liver-directed chemotherapy, administered by a totally implantable pump.

Source: OFFICE OF INSPECTOR GENERAL, DEPARTMENT OF HEALTH AND HUMAN SERVICES, RECRUITING HUMAN SUBJECTS: PRESSURES IN INDUSTRY-SPONSORED CLINICAL RESEARCH 21 (2000).

What about this advertisement might be potentially misleading? Are the implications of the ad sufficient to invalidate informed consent? Is the ad simply a necessity in today's difficult recruitment market?

[B] Agency and Institutional Guidance

Both the Food and Drug Administration (FDA) and the Office for Human Research Protections (OHRP) have developed guidance to assist IRBs in overseeing the recruitment of subjects.

[1] FDA

INFORMATION SHEETS: GUIDANCE FOR INSTITUTIONAL REVIEW BOARDS AND CLINICAL INVESTIGATORS, RECRUITING STUDY SUBJECTS
FOOD AND DRUG ADMINISTRATION
(1998)

The IRB should review the methods and material that investigators propose to use to recruit subjects. . . .

A. Media Advertising

Direct advertising for research subjects, i.e., advertising that is intended to be seen or heard by prospective subjects to solicit their participation in a study, is not, in and of itself, an objectionable practice. Direct advertising includes, but is not necessarily limited to: newspaper, radio, TV, bulletin boards, posters, and flyers that are intended for prospective subjects. *Not included* are: (1) communications intended to be seen or heard by health professionals, such as "dear doctor" letters and doctor-to-doctor letters (even when soliciting for study subjects), (2) news stories and (3) publicity intended for other audiences, such as financial page advertisements directed toward prospective investors.

IRB review and approval of listings of clinical trials on the internet would provide no additional safeguard and is not required when the system format limits the information provided to basic trial information, such as: the title; purpose of the study; protocol summary; basic eligibility criteria; study site location(s); and how to contact the site for further information. Examples of clinical trial listing services that do not require prospective IRB approval include the National Cancer Institute's cancer clinical trial listing (PDQ) and the government-sponsored AIDS Clinical Trials Information Service (ACTIS). However, when the opportunity to add additional descriptive information is not precluded by the data base system, IRB review and approval may assure that the additional information does not promise or imply a certainty of cure or other benefit beyond what is contained in the protocol and the informed consent document.

FDA considers direct advertising for study subjects to be the start of the informed consent and subject selection process. Advertisements should be reviewed and approved by the IRB as part of the package for initial review. However, when the clinical investigator decides at a later date to advertise for subjects, the advertising may be considered an amendment to the ongoing study. When such advertisements are easily compared to the approved consent document, the IRB chair, or other designated IRB member, may review and approve by expedited means, as provided by 21 CFR § 56.110(b)(2). When the IRB reviewer has doubts or other complicating issues are involved, the advertising should be reviewed at a convened meeting of the IRB.

FDA expects IRBs to review the advertising to assure that it is not unduly coercive and does not promise a certainty of cure beyond what is outlined in the consent and the protocol. This is especially critical when a study may involve subjects who are likely to be vulnerable to undue influence. [21 CFR §§ 50.20, 50.25, 56.111(a)(3), 56.111(b) and 812.20(b)(11).]

When direct advertising is to be used, the IRB should review the information contained in the advertisement and the mode of its communication, to determine that the procedure for recruiting subjects is not coercive and does not state or imply a certainty of favorable outcome or other benefits beyond what is outlined in the consent document and the protocol. The IRB should review the final copy of printed advertisements to evaluate the relative size of type used and other visual effects. When advertisements are to be taped for broadcast, the IRB should review the final audio/video tape. The IRB may review and approve the wording of the advertisement prior to taping to preclude re-taping because of inappropriate wording. The review of the final taped message prepared from IRB-approved text may be accomplished through expedited procedures. The IRB may wish to caution the clinical investigators to obtain IRB approval of message text prior to taping, in order to avoid re-taping because of inappropriate wording.

No claims should be made, either explicitly or implicitly, that the drug, biologic or device is safe or effective for the purposes under investigation, or that the test article is known to be equivalent or superior to any other drug, biologic or device. Such representation would not only be misleading to subjects but would also be a violation of the Agency's regulations concerning the promotion of investigational drugs [21 CFR § 312.7(a)] and of investigational devices [21 CFR § 812.7(d)].

Advertising for recruitment into investigational drug, biologic or device studies should not use terms such as "new treatment," "new medication" or "new drug" without explaining that the test article is investigational. A phrase such as "receive new treatments" leads study subjects to believe they will be receiving newly improved products of proven worth.

Advertisements should not promise "free medical treatment," when the intent is only to say subjects will not be charged for taking part in the investigation. Advertisements may state that subjects will be paid, but should not emphasize the payment or the amount to be paid, by such means as larger or bold type.

Generally, FDA believes that any advertisement to recruit subjects should be limited to the information the prospective subjects need to determine their eligibility and interest. When appropriately worded, the following items may be included in advertisements. It should be noted, however, that FDA does not require inclusion of all of the listed items.

1. the name and address of the clinical investigator and/or research facility;

2. the condition under study and/or the purpose of the research;

3. in summary form, the criteria that will be used to determine eligibility for the study;

4. a brief list of participation benefits, if any (e.g., a no-cost health examination);

5. the time or other commitment required of the subjects; and

6. the location of the research and the person or office to contact for further information.

B. Receptionist Scripts

The first contact prospective study subjects make is often with a receptionist who follows a script to determine basic eligibility for the specific study. The IRB should assure the procedures followed adequately protect the rights and welfare of the prospective subjects. In some cases personal and sensitive information is gathered about the individual. The IRB should have assurance that the information will be appropriately handled. A simple statement such as "confidentiality will be maintained" does not adequately inform the IRB of the procedures that will be used.

Examples of issues that are appropriate for IRB review: What happens to personal information if the caller ends the interview or simply hangs up? Are the data gathered by a marketing company? If so, are names, etc. sold to others? Are names of non-eligibles maintained in case they would qualify for another study? Are paper copies of records shredded or are readable copies put out as trash? The acceptability of the procedures would depend on the sensitivity of the data gathered, including personal, medical and financial.

NOTES AND QUESTIONS

1. What is the significance of the use of the word "should" in the initial paragraph? ("The IRB *should* review the methods and material that investigators propose to use to recruit subjects.") Although the *Information Sheets* suggest that the IRB has unlimited authority to "review the methods and material that investigators propose to recruit subjects," is it fair to say that the review process appears to be merely a recommendation and not a mandate? Certainly it does not explain *how* those methods should be reviewed.

2. In addition to failing to offer guidance on how recruiting practices should be evaluated, the *Information Sheets* provide no direction on many of the recruitment practices currently in use. For example, they fail to provide guidance to physician-investigators on how to handle the dual role of physician-investigator when recruiting their own patients. Likewise, they do not discuss the types and degrees of financial incentives that constitute a potential conflict of interest. By contrast, as discussed in Chapter 5, in the FDA's guidelines for the submission of new drug applications, investigators are specifically required to disclose certain types of financial arrangements with sponsors, including compensation that could be affected by the study outcome, proprietary interests in the tested product, and equity interests in the sponsor. *See* Chapter 5, at page 218.

3. Assume that the physician practice group at the institution with which you are affiliated as a member of its Board of Trustees wishes to advertise on the Internet. The physician practice group believes it will draw more research opportunities if it advertises. The advertisement titled "Looking for Trials" presented on page 373 above is discussed at a Board meeting. What would be your reaction and why?

[2] OHRP

INSTITUTIONAL REVIEW BOARD GUIDEBOOK
Chapter 3, Basic IRB Review — Section C. Selection of Subjects
U.S. DEPT. OF HEALTH AND HUMAN SERVICES,
OFFICE FOR PROTECTION FROM RESEARCH RISKS
(1993)

To encourage a broad cross-section of research subjects, IRBs might consider the manner in which subjects will be recruited. Will notices appear only on the bulletin boards of the psychology department or the medical school? Will investigators personally recruit subjects only in community health clinics? If a new treatment is available only in the research context, and it is a scarce resource (in that only a small proportion of those who could benefit from the therapy can be accepted as research subjects), the IRB should try to devise procedures to ensure that subjects from a variety of locations and circumstances have an equal chance of being selected. This becomes particularly important when the intervention is a life-saving procedure (e.g., organ transplant or germ-free environment).

IRBs should consider means for reducing the pressures on certain classes of subjects to participate in research. Patients should be reassured during the consent process that no benefits to which they are otherwise entitled, and no care or concern on the part of the health care providers, will be jeopardized by a decision not to participate in research. In cases where the principal investigator is the potential subject's physician, the IRB might find it preferable for someone other than the physician-investigator to discuss participation with the potential subject or to solicit the patient's consent. In other cases, the possibility of pressure may be reduced by consulting beforehand with representatives of the proposed subject group. . . .

Chapter 4 Considerations of Research Design—Section I. Identification and Recruitment of Subjects

This Section deals specifically with practical aspects of how investigators go about identifying and recruiting individual subjects, and IRB considerations related to these activities. These considerations are especially important in *epidemiologic* research. . . .

IRB Considerations

Using Records to Identify Subjects. IRBs are responsible for ensuring the equitable selection of research subjects. In fulfilling this responsibility, IRBs should review the methods that investigators use to recruit subjects.

Subjects with specific diseases or conditions are often identified as potential subjects through some type of record (e.g., registries for cancer cases, surgical or X-ray log books, employment or school records). *Controls* may come from the same population as the subjects (which is always the case in a randomized clinical trial), be persons with unrelated conditions or be volunteers from the general population. Potential subjects may be identified through records maintained at hospitals or physicians' private offices. If potential subjects are identified through medical records, log books, physicians' records, or other records that are not public documents, the IRB should make certain that the following conditions have been met: (1) the investigator is allowed access to such records by the institution or the physician; and (2) responsibility for *confidentiality* and protection of *privacy* is clearly accepted by the investigator.

Sometimes, as in epidemiologic research, it is necessary for an investigator to review thousands of medical records to identify a very small number of subjects who are suitable for a study. . . . Where the records are not computerized, however, IRBs will have to decide under what conditions a scientist may scan thousands of medical or other private records while searching for a small number of appropriate subjects. One factor to consider would be the sensitivity of the information likely to be contained in the records. For example, did the patients have broken ankles or abortions? Were they treated for strep throat or venereal disease? Another factor to consider is the type of information the investigator wishes to obtain from those who are selected as suitable subjects for the study.

. . . In the event that names are sought from physicians' private offices, the patient's physician should request permission from the patient to release his or her name.

For a hospital-based study, most IRBs require that a potential subject's physician give approval before the subject is contacted, particularly when there may be medical or emotional contraindications to participation. If the subject is in the hospital, someone on the hospital staff may inform the patient that he or she is going to be invited to participate in a study, or, more often, an interviewer may approach the subject directly after consultation with his or her physician.

If the subject has left the hospital, various options may be considered. (For each option, most IRBs require that the potential subject's physician give approval before the subject is contacted.) For instance, the investigator may send a letter describing the purpose of the study and requesting that the subject return a postcard indicating whether he or she would like to participate. The effectiveness of this method depends on how many of the postcards are returned.

A second option is to invite participation by letter, and for the subject to send back a postcard (or to telephone) only if he or she does not wish to participate. If no postcard is returned, the subject may then be contacted by an interviewer. This method is less preferable, as it requires that potential subjects take positive action to avoid being made part of a study rather than the other way around. Subjects may become unwitting participants if, for example, they never receive the letter, don't read English, or are simply confused by the instructions. This approach also raises *privacy* concerns for certain types of research (e.g., research involving sexually transmitted diseases or psychiatric illness, or drug or alcohol abuse).

A third approach that is often used is for the patient's physician to send a letter informing the subject about the study and inviting the patient to participate. This method may work well if the study is being undertaken by a relatively small number of physicians who are willing to cooperate with the investigator. Response rates are likely to be high, since the subject often considers it significant that the letter has come from his or her own physician. IRBs should consider whether use of this method will subject potential participants to coercion or undue influence. Finally, the investigator can send a letter to the potential subject explaining the purpose of the study, and then an interviewer can call to invite the potential subject to participate. By permitting interchange between the subject and interviewer, this method allows the subject to make an informed decision about participation. Although there is the risk of coercion by the interviewer, in general this method helps the subject better understand what the purposes of the research are, why his or her participation is important, what procedures are used to protect confidentiality, and what would be asked of him or her as a participant. This approach usually secures the highest response rate; however, people may be offended, especially in research on sensitive topics, by the investigator's having direct access to their name, address, and phone number. IRBs should be sensitive to this concern.

NOTES AND QUESTIONS

1. The above-quoted guidance was written before current federal privacy regulations were enacted. Both the security and privacy provisions of those

regulations now have a significant effect on researchers' ability to identify potential subjects by searching through medical records. For further discussion of this issue, see Chapter 10, at page 459.

2. As the IRB Guidebook notes, there can be both good and bad aspects to allowing the initial contact about a study (such as a letter describing the study) to come from someone other than a person's own physician. While this practice reduces the possibility that the person may feel pressure to enroll in a study if asked to do so by their own doctor, the person might be troubled that someone other than their physician has been given information about their medical problem. The federal privacy regulations tend to reinforce the importance of the privacy issues, encouraging contacts to be made by the subjects' own physicians. If it were up to you, how would you balance these competing concerns?

[C] Institutional Policies

ADVERTISEMENT AND REIMBURSEMENT POLICY
ALBERT EINSTEIN COLLEGE OF MEDICINE ("AECOM")

The purpose of the guidelines is twofold: (a) to ensure adequate disclosure of information to prospective patients or research subjects; and (b) to guard against offers of undue inducement to participate in clinical investigations or seek medical services.

Approval of Advertisement

The [Committee on Clinical Investigation, also known as the] CCI/IRB, *prior to use*, must approve any announcement designed to recruit research participants for a particular study. If available a copy should be submitted to the Committee along with the research protocol. Otherwise, the advertisement may be submitted at any time prior to use. The policy conforms to federal guidelines, and compliance is mandatory. Subsequent to review, the CCI/IRB will provide investigators with a written approval and stamped approved advertisement.

How to Submit

All advertisements, such as: bulletin board postings, newspaper ads, radio announcements, publications, e-mail and world wide web announcements must be submitted to the CCI/IRB with the "Request for Advertisement Approval" form.

General Disclosure

An advertisement or announcement should state its general purpose, for example, whether it is recruiting individuals for a study, offering to provide care for patients, etc. *It should be written in clear, simple English, understandable to lay people.* It should state which hospital or group is conducting the study or offering to provide care.

Specific Disclosure

An advertisement or announcement should specify what type of care is to be provided and at what cost. If "Free" care is offered, the announcement should state whether all patients are entitled to that care or whether certain eligibility conditions must be met. Clearly state who is being recruited; e.g., normal healthy volunteers, or others. Provide a brief, simple indication of what will be required of subjects. If remuneration is offered, give actual or at least ball park amounts; e.g., up to. . . . Payment guidelines are available through the CCI/IRB Administration offices.

Financial Inducements

An advertisement or announcement must specify precisely what care or service will be provided free of charge. The announcement *may not* state a financial equivalent of the "free" care provided (as in the example, "$1,000 worth of free medical care").

Helpful Hints when writing your advertisement

• Clearly state the project is research.

• Err on the side of underestimating benefits and overestimating risks.

• Do not make claims of safety, equivalence, or superiority.

• Avoid phrases like "new treatment," "new medicine," or "new drug."

• Do not use dollar signs or focus on monetary issues.

• Avoid catch phrases such as exciting, fast, cutting-edge, and free.

Additionally, the CCI provides a sample recruitment letter, provided below, to assist physicians who seek to recruit their patients into a research study:

Dear _____:

As your doctor, I am writing to let you know that a research study is being planned that may be of interest to you. It is possible that you may be eligible to participate in this study. Your eligibility can only be determined by the investigators of this study.

Please be aware that, even if you are eligible, your participation in this or any research study is completely voluntary. There will be no consequences to you whatever if you choose not to participate, and your regular medical care will not be affected by that choice. If you do choose to participate, the study will involve [_____ examples: blood tests, x-rays, biopsies, interviews, drugs, medical visits_____].

In order to determine your eligibility and your interest in participating, [_____ name and role in study] will be [calling][writing] you directly. You may choose not to [speak with him/her] [respond to the letter]. If you do [speak][respond], any questions you have about the study will be answered.

If you would prefer not to be contacted at all, please call [number] and provide your name, and the information that you would NOT like to be contacted about this research study.

Of course, if you have any questions for me, please contact me.

[The remainder of the policy discusses AECOM guidelines on payments to research participants, set out later in this chapter.]

NOTES AND QUESTIONS

1. The FDA guidance stated that an advertisement "should not promise 'free medical treatment,' when the intent is only to say that subjects will not be charged for taking part in the investigation." The AECOM guidance states that "[i]f 'Free' care is offered, the announcement should state whether all patients are entitled to that care or whether certain eligibility conditions must be met." Are these two sets of guidelines consistent? If you were a researcher at AECOM and were creating an advertisement for a study that involved the provision of certain types of medical care at no cost to subjects, how would you describe that aspect of the study in the ad?

2. The AECOM guidelines, consistent with the FDA guidance, note that advertising materials should not state that subjects will be given a specified dollar amount (e.g., $1,000) of free medical care. What is the purpose of this prohibition? Is it an appropriate policy? Note that there is not any prohibition against actually providing very substantial amounts of free medical care in a study. Indeed, many studies, including those at the federal government's prestigious National Institutes of Health, provide tens of thousands of dollars of free care. The prohibition is merely against advertising that a study involves a specific dollar amount of free care, not against providing the free care.

[D] Recruiting Normal Healthy Subjects

Federal regulations afford no special protections for healthy people who are asked to participate in research studies. As you read the following excerpt, think about whether such "normal healthy subjects" are more vulnerable or less vulnerable than patients who are recruited to participate in clinical research.

SAFEGUARDING HEALTH RESEARCH SUBJECTS: PROTECTING VOLUNTEERS FROM HARM NEW YORK STATE DEPARTMENT OF HEALTH, WORKGROUP ON IRB GUIDELINES
(1999)
www.health.state.ny.us/nysdoh/provider/volunteer/intro.htm

What is meant by the term "normal healthy subject"?

The term applies to research subjects who are free from diseases or medical conditions that might be affected by or have an impact on the research. The term is used generally to distinguish such subjects from those who are participating in research specifically because they have a condition or disease that the research is intended to ameliorate directly or indirectly. It also is used to distinguish such subjects from ones who are excluded from a study because they have a condition or disease that might be affected negatively by participation in the study. For example, in a sleep study in which subjects are awakened every hour to see the effects on their sleep activity and awake functioning, individuals with acne or a dental bridge would probably be considered normal healthy subjects. However, if the study involved having an orotracheal tube in place while falling asleep, the individual with a dental bridge might not be considered a normal healthy subject. Thus, the term normal healthy subject is relative, defined according to the inclusionary and exclusionary criteria of a specific protocol. . . .

Normal healthy subjects have a special vulnerability that is based on their apparent invulnerability. Researchers, for the most part, recognize the need to maximize protection of patient-subjects who are participating in research. Patients are already weakened or in some way debilitated by their condition. As a result, researchers exercise special cautions not to aggravate the patient-subject's health status. . . .

[S]ubjects coming to a medical facility to participate in research in an office staffed by nurses, physicians, and other care-providers may not be able to relinquish the expectation of direct benefit even when they are not patients and the researcher is not their personal health care provider. As a result, they may experience a "therapeutic illusion."

Therein lies the crux of the challenge for IRBs, researchers, and research institutions — how to ensure that a normal healthy research subject is cognizant of the risks of participating in the research and of the fact that promoting the subject's well-being is not the researcher's basic objective.

INSTITUTIONAL REVIEW BOARD GUIDEBOOK
Chapter 6, Special Classes of Subjects—Section J.
Students, Employees and Normal Volunteers
U.S. DEPT. OF HEALTH AND HUMAN SERVICES,
OFFICE FOR PROTECTION FROM RESEARCH RISKS
(1993)

Normal Volunteers. Strange as it may seem at first, special concerns surround the involvement of normal (i.e., healthy) persons who volunteer to participate in research. Primarily, the principles involved are beneficence and respect for persons. In the Belmont Report, the National Commission for the Protection of Human Subjects of Biomedical and Behavioral Research stated the two general rules that describe beneficent actions as: (1) do not harm; and (2) maximize possible benefits and minimize possible harms. Volunteers for whom no therapeutic benefit can result from participation in research should, therefore, be exposed to risks that are minimized to the greatest extent possible. While the minimization of risks is an important requisite for any research involving human participants, the altruistic motivation of the normal volunteer's agreement to participate (i.e., of contributing to scientific knowledge for the benefit of society) heightens the concern for the risks to which such participants should ethically be exposed.

The principle of respect for persons requires that research participants are, where capable of doing so, allowed to act autonomously and to express their right of self-determination. These principles are effectuated through the process of informed consent, which involves providing subjects with all relevant information about the study, including the risks and benefits involved, in clear and simple language, and ensuring that the information is understood and appreciated. Furthermore, the agreement to participate must be voluntary; the consent negotiations must be free from elements of coercion or undue inducement to participate. In research involving normal volunteers, particularly where the research involves more than minimal risk, IRBs must ensure that any monetary payments to subjects are not so great as to constitute an undue inducement. This issue may be particularly difficult for IRBs to deal with. Since subjects who volunteer to participate in such studies are usually compensated for their time and discomfort, IRBs should seriously scrutinize the payment schedules to ensure that any compensation offered is commensurate with the time, discomfort, and risk involved. Even so, where a research procedure involves serious discomfort and/or the real, though slight, possibility of serious harm (e.g., studies that involve the insertion and positioning of catheters in veins or the heart), one can easily imagine that the motivation of persons who volunteer to participate may be monetary. IRBs should pay particular attention to the proposed study population and whether it may comprise persons who are likely to be vulnerable to coercion or undue influence, such as persons who are educationally or economically disadvantaged. The federal regulations require that IRBs employ special safeguards under such circumstances [45 C.F.R. § 46.111(b)].

One area where normal volunteers are employed in research is in Phase 1 drug trials. The justification for the involvement of normal, healthy subjects is the need for volunteers whose experience with the trial materials is more easily analyzed because of the existence of fewer confounding factors. While Phase 1 trials are the first use of experimental drugs and devices in humans, preliminary studies involving animals provide investigators with data indicating a high likelihood of safe use in humans. Studies have indicated that the risk of injury from participating in Phase 1 studies is small, about the same as the risk of being injured while working as an office secretary. The likelihood of risk, including the availability of animal data, should be scrutinized by IRBs.

Normal volunteers, like students and employees, should be recruited through general announcements or advertisements, rather than through individual solicitations. Personal solicitations increase the likelihood that participation will be the result of undue influence, either because of the relationship between the recruiter and the prospective subject, or methods of communication employed by the recruiter that may act to persuade prospective subjects to participate, thus compromising the voluntariness of the agreement to participate.

Investigators and IRBs should carefully consider what will happen if and when a normal volunteer should become sick or be injured during the research. As with any research involving human subjects, such issues should be clearly spelled out in the informed consent document, and should be reviewed carefully with the prospective subject. For example, subjects should be told: whether any medical treatments will be made available should injury occur and, if so, what they consist of; whom to contact should a research-related injury occur; and that they may discontinue participation at any time without penalty or loss of benefits to which they would otherwise be entitled [45 CFR § 46.116(a)(6-8)]. In addition, where appropriate subjects should be told whether they will be dropped from the study in the event of injury or illness, and whether they will be required to pay for treatment of research-related injuries or illness [45 CFR § 46.116(b)(2-3)]. Where illness in healthy volunteers does occur, particularly during a drug study, investigation by an independent physician may be warranted. . . .

NOTES AND QUESTIONS

1. Consider the hypothetical problem presented as Note 4 on page 376. Assume that the principal investigator wants to use normal healthy research subjects in his trial. He wishes to recruit subjects from his own patient base who do not have any symptoms of the disease, and to enroll those subjects in Phase 1 of the study trial. The investigator believes this is the best method for recruitment because he will know the entire medical history of each subject. If you were a member of the IRB, would you permit this type of recruitment, either

with or without restrictions on the methods the investigator uses to solicit participation? Do in-person solicitations by investigators increase, decrease, or have no effect on the likelihood of undue influence?

2. Do you agree with the New York State Department of Health workgroup that normal healthy subjects are likely to experience a "therapeutic illusion"? Consider, for example, healthy individuals who volunteer for a Phase 1 study of a new pain reliever. If they are not experiencing pain, why would they be under the illusion that the drug might benefit them?

3. Hoi Yan (Nicole) Wan was a healthy nineteen-year old sophomore at the University of Rochester. In an effort to earn $150 in pocket money, she volunteered for a medical experiment conducted at the university. The researchers were investigating the impact of air pollution and second-hand smoke on healthy lungs. The study involved a bronchoscopy, a standard test to diagnose lung infections and tumors. A flexible tube was inserted through her mouth, down her windpipe and into her lungs, in order to retrieve cells. Before the tube was inserted, lidocaine, a local anesthetic used to control gagging, was sprayed into subjects' windpipes. On March 31, 1996, two days after Ms. Wan enrolled in the study, she died after suffering a heart attack. The medical examiner determined that the cause of her death was a lethal level of lidocaine. *See* New York State Department of Health, *Press Release: Case Report on Death of University of Rochester Student Issued,* available at http://www.health. state.ny.us/nysdoh/consumer/pressrel/96/wan.htm.

After Ms. Wan's death, the New York State Department of Health conducted an internal and external investigation. It concluded that the attending physician had failed to monitor Ms. Wan properly after the procedure by discharging her despite her complaints of chest pain, weakness, and coughing up blood. In addition, the investigation determined that the attending physician had allowed an intern to give Wan four times what the Department of Health investigators determined had been the maximum dose of lidocaine approved by the IRB. The Department noted that, while lidocaine generally is a safe topical anesthetic, it can have toxic effects when too high a dose is administered.

4. The procedures performed on Nicole Wan were not at all experimental. In fact, they were quite routine, having been used as part of the standard care of patients for more than one hundred years. Robert Helms, *Experimentation: Reality and the Lie, from* GUINEA PIG ZERO #8, available at www.guineapigzero.com/DIEPPEX.html; Elisabeth Rosenthal, *New York Seeks to Tighten Rules on Medical Research*, N.Y. TIMES, September 27, 1996:B4; David J. Morrow, *Swallowing Bitter Pills for Pay: The Trials of Guinea Pigs*, NEW YORK TIMES, September 29, 1996, Sec. 3, p. 1.

Do you think that Ms. Wan was aware that she might die as a result of participating in this study?

5. Perhaps the most prominent recent instance of harm to a normal healthy volunteer is the case of 24-year-old Ellen Roche, who died as a result of partic-

ipating in a study at Johns Hopkins University in which she inhaled hexamethonium, which was designed to create a simulated asthma attack. Ms. Roche was an employee in the same department as the researcher, raising the issue discussed in the next section of this chapter. For further details on this incident, see Chapter 4, at page 182.

6. There have been a number of lawsuits involving normal healthy volunteers who ended up being harmed as a result of participation in research studies. *See,* e.g., Vodopest v. MacGregor, 913 P.2d 779 (Wash. 1996) (mountain expedition to study new treatment for high altitude sickness); Payette v. Rockefeller University, 643 N.Y.S.2d 79 (N.Y. App. Div. 1996) (radioactive iodine given to subjects to determine how a diet changed their cholesterol levels).

7. For further discussion of recruitment of normal healthy volunteers, see Carl L. Tishler & Suzanne Bartholomae, *The Recruitment of Normal Healthy Volunteers: A Review of the Literature on the Use of Financial Incentives,* 42 J. CLIN. PHARMACOL. 365 (2002).

[E] Soliciting Students or Employees of Researchers

INSTITUTIONAL REVIEW BOARD GUIDEBOOK
Chapter 6, Special Classes of Subjects—
Section J. Students, Employees and Normal Volunteers
U.S. DEPT. OF HEALTH AND HUMAN SERVICES
OFFICE FOR PROTECTION FROM RESEARCH RISKS
(1993)

Students. Universities, and the association of investigators with them, provide investigators with a ready pool of research subjects: students. Many IRBs have faced the question of whether and in what way students may participate in research. Two questions that have been posed are whether students — medical students, in particular — should be allowed to participate in biomedical research (and whether special protections should be adopted to restrict their participation), and whether participation in research can appropriately be included as a course component for course credit. The latter practice is commonly employed in psychology departments.

The problem with student participation in research conducted at the university is the possibility that their agreement to participate will not be freely given. Students may volunteer to participate out of a belief that doing so will place them in good favor with faculty (e.g., that participating will result in receiving better grades, recommendations, employment, or the like), or that failure to participate will negatively affect their relationship with the investigator or faculty generally (i.e., by seeming "uncooperative," not part of the scientific community). Prohibiting all student participation in research, however, may be an overprotective reaction. An alternative way to protect against coercion is to require that faculty-investigators advertise for subjects generally (e.g., through notices posted in the school or department) rather than recruit individual students directly. As with any research involving a potentially vulnerable subject population, IRBs should pay special attention to the potential for coercion or undue influence and consider ways in which the possibility of exploitation can be reduced or eliminated.

Whether medical students in particular require special protections has been hotly debated. Some universities have either prohibited their participation or severely restricted it to, for instance, research involving minimal risk and minimal interruption of time. Strong arguments have been made against such protections, including claims that as future physicians (and possibly researchers) they may be obliged to participate. Angoff has argued that protecting medical students to a greater degree than protecting other normal volunteers smacks of elitism. [He] states, "One may wonder why it is acceptable to ask the masses to accept risk in the name of science but not the very people whose futures are linked to the successful perpetuation of biomedical research." Others have argued that medical students are in a particularly good position to participate in some biomedical research because of their ability to comprehend the procedures involved in studies and evaluate the risks involved, which may not be possible to achieve with other normal volunteers. Angoff and others have also argued that it is acceptable to pay medical students as one would any research participant.

Requiring participation in research for course credit (or extra credit) is also controversial, though common in the social and behavioral sciences. The justification offered for requiring student participation is educational benefit. Clearly, however, participation of students is seen by faculty-investigators as necessary to the conduct of their research. Grant budgets often do not allow investigators to pay subjects; giving course credit or extra credit is a means of obtaining sufficient participation rates. Again, the issue for IRBs is whether such arrangements for selecting subjects is fair and noncoercive.

Participation in studies might be mandatory or for extra credit. Students in beginning psychology courses, for instance, might be required to serve as subjects for a given number of hours of research or in a given number of research projects. Or they might be given the option of participating for additional grade credit. Several mechanisms have been suggested for diminishing or eliminating the coercive aspect of student participation for course credit that IRBs might find useful. Gamble describes a departmental guideline for research involving students where extra credit is offered for participation. Students are to be given other options for fulfilling the research component that were comparable in terms of time, effort, and educational benefit: "for example, short papers, special projects, book reports, and brief quizzes on additional readings." He raises concerns about the comparability of such alternatives with participating in research (e.g., that if they participate in studies, all they have to do is show up and spend the time, but if they choose to write a paper, it gets graded, and if they do extra readings, they have to be tested on them), and concludes that paying student subjects as researchers would any other subject is the only way to protect students' freedom of choice to participate. Cohen describes a similar policy that seems to meet these concerns. To fulfill the research component, students can either participate in five hours of research, write a brief research paper, or attend faculty research colloquia. The paper is not graded, and students who attend the colloquia have only to show up. If students do choose to participate in studies, the policy seeks to increase the likelihood that participation is freely chosen by requiring: that students be given several studies to choose from and may not be required to volunteer for any particular study; that the studies must not involve more than minimal risk; that students can withdraw from the study at any time without losing the extra credit.

Another concern raised by the involvement of students as subjects is confidentiality. As with research involving human subjects generally, IRBs should be aware that research involving the collection of data on sensitive subjects such as mental health, sexual activity, or the use of illicit drugs or alcohol presents risks to subjects of which they should be made aware and from which they should be protected, to the greatest extent possible. The close environment of the university amplifies this problem.

Where students are likely to be participating in research, IRBs should consider including a student member or consulting with students where appropriate.

Employees. The issues with respect to employees as research subjects are essentially identical to those involving students as research subjects: coercion or undue influence, and confidentiality. As medical students have seemed ideal subjects by biomedical researchers, employees of drug companies have been seen by investigators as ideal subjects in some ways, because of their ability to comprehend the protocol and to understand the importance of the research and compliance with the protocol. Meyers provides a good summary of the structure of employee volunteer research programs. As student participation raises questions of the ability to exercise free choice because of the possibility that grades or other important factors will be affected by decisions to participate, employee research programs raise the possibility that the decision will affect performance evaluations or job advancement. It may also be difficult to maintain the confidentiality of personal medical information or research data when the subjects are also employees, particularly when the employer is also a medical institution.

NOTES AND QUESTIONS

1. The University of Minnesota IRB, among others, has created institutional policies governing the use of students in research studies. First, it recommends that investigators avoid using their own students if another group is equally suited. When students participate in research, it provides the following guidelines:

- Students should be given the opportunity to decline participation without jeopardy.

- Unless the research question is directly related to class material, or the study process is being used as a teaching opportunity, such as in a research methods class, the IRB discourages the use of class time to recruit subjects or class time to complete study instruments.

- Use of extra credit points as a reward for research participation should be limited to specific circumstances where the research is closely tied to the course subject matter. The number of points awarded should not be sufficient to augment a student's grade by a whole step, e.g. from B to A.

- The use of financial rewards should be limited to dollar amounts that are proportionate to the inconvenience of participation.

- Whenever possible, a teaching opportunity in the form of an "educational debriefing" should be employed. Students should know something about the IRB review process, the rationale for the study, the process of data collection, and the intent of the researcher.

The University of Minnesota IRB also recommends guidelines for recruiting employees. First, the investigator must offer "a rationale other than convenience" for selecting a colleague or subordinate as a research subject. The investigator must also demonstrate that the recruitment method does not lead the subject to fear retribution for failing to participate. Furthermore, the University of Minnesota IRB recommends recruitment through bulletin board advertisements, approved by the IRB, or through a third party not in a power relationship with the employee. *See Protecting Human Subjects Guide*, available at http://www.research.umn.edu/irb/guide/Protecting%20Human%20Subjects%20Guide.pdf.

2. A psychology professor who studies memory issues wishes to recruit freshmen and sophomore college students from one of the classes he teaches at the university. Students who participate will earn extra credit points toward their final grade. As a member of the IRB, would you permit this recruitment strategy? Why or why not? What if participation was a course requirement, but alternatively students could fulfill the requirement by writing a brief paper on an issue concerning the ethics of research in psychology? Would it matter if students could earn extra credit points by participating as research subjects in any one of a number of projects conducted by various members of the psychology department?

3. Considering the hypothetical above, would your answer be different if the researcher plans to recruit from introductory English classes taught by a friend in the English department, with students again earning extra credit in the English course? Without the possibility of earning extra credit? Would you recommend any special precautions in this case?

§ 8.02 PAYING SUBJECTS

Although a long-standing practice in the United States, paying subjects remains a contentious issue among researchers. Those in favor argue that payment is appropriate to compensate subjects for their time and trouble, and that it is a good thing for society to encourage activities that are helpful to its members. Pragmatically, they claim that it is a necessary means to increase recruitment of subjects and that payment likely will increase subject compliance with the research protocol. Those opposed to payment cite principles such as the importance of avoiding undue influence and the value of encouraging altruism.

Questions regarding when, why, and how much to pay research subjects continue to fuel debate within the research community. There is concern that money may compromise the voluntariness of subjects' decisions to participate in research or their willingness to examine the study's risks and benefits. In addition, there are fears that payments target economically vulnerable populations, thus violating the principle that particular groups should not bear disproportionate risks from scientific research.

[A] Agency Guidance

Nowhere in the sections of the Code of Federal Regulations that govern research with human subjects is the word "payment" mentioned. The only regulatory provision arguably relevant to the issue is the requirement that investigators seek subjects' consent "under circumstances that provide the prospective subject or the representative sufficient opportunity to consider whether or not to participate and that minimize the possibility of coercion or undue influence." 45 C.F.R. § 46.116.

The federal agencies responsible for overseeing human subject research have done little to fill this regulatory void. The FDA Information Sheets address the issue only briefly. OHRP Guidelines, while providing some assistance on the matter, fail to state much that could be considered definitive.

[1] FDA

INFORMATION SHEETS: GUIDANCE FOR INSTITUTIONAL REVIEW BOARDS AND CLINICAL INVESTIGATORS
Payment to Research Subjects
FOOD AND DRUG ADMINISTRATION
(1998)

It is not uncommon for subjects to be paid for their participation in research, especially in the early phases of investigational drug, biologic or device development. Payment to research subjects for participation in studies is not considered a benefit; it is a recruitment incentive. Financial incentives are often used when health benefits to subjects are remote or non-existent. The amount and schedule of all payments should be presented to the IRB at the time of initial review. The IRB should review both the amount of payment and the proposed method and timing of disbursement to assure that neither are coercive or present undue influence.

Any credit for payment should accrue as the study progresses and not be contingent upon the subject completing the entire study. Unless it creates undue inconvenience or a coercive practice, payment to subjects who withdraw from the study may be made at the time they would have completed the study (or completed a phase of the study) had they not withdrawn. For example, in a study lasting only a few days, an IRB may find it permissible to allow a single payment date at the end of the study, even to subjects who had withdrawn before that date.

While the entire payment should not be contingent upon completion of the entire study, payment of a small proportion as an incentive for completion of the study is acceptable to FDA, providing that such incentive is not coercive. The IRB should determine that the amount paid as a bonus for completion is reasonable and not so large as to unduly induce subjects to stay in the study when they would otherwise have withdrawn. All information concerning payment, including the amount and schedule of payment(s), should be set forth in the informed consent document.

NOTES AND QUESTIONS

1. Why does the FDA characterize payments to subjects as a "recruitment incentive" rather than a "benefit"?

2. The FDA emphasizes the need to avoid both "coercive" practices and "undue influence." What is the difference between these two concepts?

3. A study involves having a healthy subject undergo a bronchoscopy once a month for a year. The subject will receive $200 for each of the first four bronchoscopies, $300 for each of the next four bronchoscopies, and $400 for each of the final four bronchoscopies. Subjects who complete all twelve bronchoscopies will receive an additional payment of $1,000. If you were on an IRB asked to review this study, would you approve it? What changes might you require?

[2] OHRP

INSTITUTIONAL REVIEW BOARD GUIDEBOOK
Chapter 3, Basic IRB Review—
Section G. Incentives for Participation
U.S. DEPT. OF HEALTH AND HUMAN SERVICES
OFFICE FOR PROTECTION FROM RESEARCH RISKS
(1993)

Introduction

. . . Although payments are usually monetary, both patients and normal healthy volunteers may be offered other rewards in lieu of or in addition to money. Free medical care, extra vacation time, and academic rewards (in the form of a grade or a letter of recommendation) are examples of alternative rewards. Regardless of the form of remuneration, the issues for IRBs remain the same. IRBs must consider whether paid participants in research are recruited fairly, informed adequately, and paid appropriately. Taking into consideration the subjects' medical, employment, and educational status, and their financial, emotional and community resources, the IRB must determine whether the rewards offered for participation in research constitute undue inducement.

Overview

Federal regulations governing research with human subjects contain no specific guidance for IRB review of payment practices. One of the primary responsibilities of IRBs, however, is to ensure that a subject's decision to participate in research will be truly voluntary, and that consent will be sought "only under circumstances that provide the prospective subject . . . sufficient opportunity to consider whether or not to participate and that minimize the possibility of coercion or undue influence" [21 CFR § 50.20]. . . .

Clear cases of coercion (i.e., actual threats) are readily identifiable; it is more difficult to recognize undue inducement. An offer one could not refuse is essentially coercive (or "undue"). Undue inducements may be troublesome because: (1) offers that are too attractive may blind prospective subjects to the risks or impair their ability to exercise proper judgment; and (2) they may prompt subjects to lie or conceal information that, if known, would disqualify them from enrolling — or continuing — as participants in a research project.

IRB Considerations

IRBs must attempt to make sure that prospective subjects realize that their participation is voluntary, and that choosing not to participate will not adversely affect their relationship with the institution or its staff in any way. To make this determination, IRBs should know who the subjects will be, what incentives are being offered, and the conditions under which the offer will be made.

Some institutions have adopted policies regarding the recruitment and payment of volunteers. In general, they attempt to minimize the possibility of coercion or undue influence by requesting that subjects be recruited by open, written invitation rather than by personal solicitation. Institutions try to ensure that the consent document contains a detailed account of the terms of payment, including a description of the conditions under which a subject would receive partial or no payment (for example, what will happen if they withdraw part way through the research).

Determining the appropriateness of the incentive is another matter. For research that requires subjects to undergo only minor inconvenience or discomfort, a modest payment will usually be adequate. Reimbursement for travel, babysitting, and so forth may also be provided. In more complex research projects, IRBs tend to base their assessment on the prevailing payment practices within their institution or general locale. Volunteers are often compensated for their participation according to an established fee schedule, based upon the complexity of the study, the type and number of procedures to be performed, the time involved, and the anticipated discomfort or inconvenience. Standard payments may be established for each tissue or fluid sample collected, depending on the type of sample (blood, urine, or saliva) and the time (day or evening) the sample is to be collected. Alternatively, subjects may be paid an hourly rate or a fixed amount, depending on the duration of the study and whether the study requires admission to research ward. Extra payments are usually provided for a variety of additional inconveniences (e.g., the imposition of dietary restrictions). Payments may vary according to a number of factors, and, therefore, IRBs may need to become familiar with the accepted standards within their community as well as the anticipated discomforts and inconveniences involved in a particular study to judge appropriateness of payments. Some institutions have a ceiling on the amount an individual may earn in any one study or during a given length of time (e.g., per year, per semester).

One of the most perplexing problems for IRBs is how to assess the appropriateness of payment offers for experiments that involve the assumption of risk or significant discomfort. On a practical level, it is probably impossible for an IRB to determine what amount of money or type of reward would unduly influence a particular individual to accept a given degree of risk. . . . The appropriateness of proposed payments is a matter each institution must address in formulating its policies.

IRB members tend to approach the problem of assuming risk for pay from one of two positions. One side argues that normal healthy volunteers are able to exercise free choice, and that, since judging the acceptability of risk and weighing the benefits is a personal matter, IRBs should refrain from imposing their own views on potential subjects. On this view, IRB responsibility should be confined to ensuring that consent is properly informed. Other IRB members argue that the IRB should protect potential subjects from inducements that may affect their ability to make an informed, voluntary choice. It should be noted that, in this context, incentives need not be financial to cause problems. Free health care for persons with limited resources and major medical problems may be a significant inducement to participate in research (even if the research activity is nontherapeutic). There is no consensus as to whether this kind of inducement is unacceptable. In assessing this potential problem, IRBs might consider whether only the destitute agree to volunteer or if people who can obtain good medical care on their own agree to participate as well. IRBs may need to monitor subject recruitment to make such determinations.

Points to Consider

1. Are all conditions in keeping with standards for voluntary and informed consent?

2. Are the incentives offered reasonable, based upon the complexities and inconveniences of the study and the particular subject population?

3. Are there special standards that the IRB ought to apply to the review of research in which volunteers are asked to assume significant risk?

4. Should the IRB monitor subject recruitment to determine whether coercion or undue influence is a problem?

NOTES AND QUESTIONS

1. Do you think poor communities are likely to support or oppose high payments to research subjects? Is this question relevant to the development of payment policies?

2. What do you think of the following argument?

Some researchers would find it worthwhile to pay inducements in order to attract enough subjects. Those who would accept this reward would not do so unless it were worth it to them. As a result of offering the reward, the researchers get the subjects they want. As a result of participating, the subjects get the reward they want. Both are better off. No one is worse off. Inducement is thus a good thing. This . . . makes a *prima facie* case for inducement.

Martin Wilkinson & Andrew Moore, *Inducement in Research*, 11 BIOETHICS 373 (1997).

3. There are a number of arguments that have been raised against paying subjects. One relates to the fact that research typically requires exposing subjects to unknown risks. Given the unknown nature of the risks, a subject's decision to participate is often a difficult one. Paying them money to be in a study complicates what is already a difficult decision. A separate argument is that it is unjust to offer payments to subjects because the practice encourages the poorest and least sophisticated members of our society to bear a disproportionate share of research risks. "An acceptance of inducement to participate in

research would further increase the inequity of research conducted on the impecunious for the benefit of the well-off." Moreover, "the reason that inducement is particularly of concern is that those most susceptible to inducement may be the least able to assess the aims and technical information relating to the research and to decide on whether or not the risk is worth taking. It is already the poor and socially disadvantaged who volunteer for most research yet it is typically the better off members of society who benefit from research." Paul McNeill, *A Response to Wilkinson and Moore, Paying People to Participate in Research: Why Not?* 11 BIOETHICS 390 (1997).

4. Although there is much debate about making cash payments to research subjects, there is relatively less debate about what some might consider a much more significant type of payment: free medical care. In many studies, subjects receive tens or even hundreds of thousands of dollars in free care. Should researchers be permitted to offer free medical care to subjects? Or should such "hidden" payments be subjected to the same principles that are applied in scrutinizing cash payments? Consider this debate in the context of the fact that, in 2003, more than twenty percent of working adults in the United States lacked health insurance coverage. *See More Adults Lacked Coverage in 2003 Than in 1997, CDC Reports*, 9 HEALTH CARE DAILY (BNA), July 9, 2004.

5. Terrence Ackerman argues that paying subjects can be justified by society's obligation "to encourage forms of social cooperation useful in meeting the essential needs of its members." He argues that, for two reasons, payment ought not be restricted according to the risks subjects incur or the amount of payment that may be offered: (1) we pay people to engage in other dangerous activities, such as firefighting and the military, as they, too, are socially beneficial; and (2) we permit people to be very well paid for dangerous work that is not essential to the welfare of society (e.g., race car drivers and trapeze artists). *See* Terence F. Ackerman, *An Ethical Framework for the Practice of Paying Research Subjects*, 11 IRB, July-August 1989, at 1. Others, by contrast, take the position that society should be promoting participation in research as an altruistic and socially responsible activity, and that consequently payment is unethical. *See, e.g.*, Jeanne M. Sears, *Payment of Research Subjects: A Broader Perspective*, 1 AM. J. BIOETHICS, Spring 2001, at 66.

6. Christine Grady and her colleagues at the National Institutes of Health's Department of Clinical Bioethics reviewed policies and practices regarding payment of participants and explored the influence of payment on research participants' perceptions and decisions to enroll or remain in research. Based on her research, Grady defends the notion of paying subjects for their participation. By way of analogy, she notes that, while individuals may be attracted to a job by a higher salary, a variety of other factors, such as likely satisfaction, fitness, location, etc., will affect the ultimate decision. She argues that an amount of money that is not excessive and is calculated on the basis of time or contribution may, rather than constituting an undue inducement, be an indication of respect for research subjects' efforts. She stresses the need to be sure that

potential subjects, particularly those who may perceive that they have no other choice but to participate — whether because they need the money, the "treatment," or something else the research would provide — understand the nature, risks, benefits, alternatives, and requirements of the research protocol and provide informed consent to participate. *See* Christine Grady, *Money for Research Participation: Does it Jeopardize Informed Consent?* 1 AM. J. BIOETHICS, Spring 2001, at 40. The same issue of the journal in which Dr. Grady's article appeared contains sixteen brief responses to the article.

7. A recent study asked 126 patients with hypertension to answer questions about their willingness to enroll in a hypothetical trial of a new antihypertensive drug. Patients were randomized to different arms of the hypothetical trial, each of which involved different levels of risk and different payment amounts. The researchers assumed that high payments would constitute "undue" inducement if there were "significant negative interactions between risk and payment" — in other words, if the influence of risk on individuals' willingness to participate was weaker as the payment levels increased. Similarly, high payments would constitute "unjust" inducement if there were "significant negative interactions between payment and income" — in other words, if the influence of payments on willingness to participate was higher among poorer patients. The researchers found neither correlation, leading them to conclude that, although "higher payment motivates research participation," there was "no evidence that commonly used payment levels represent undue or unjust inducements." Scott D. Halpern et al., *Empirical Assessment of Whether Moderate Payments Are Undue or Unjust Inducements for Participation in Clinical Trials,* 164 ARCHIVES INTERNAL MED. 801 (2004). Does this study provide empirical evidence that concerns about undue or unjust enrichment are misplaced?

8. Ezekiel Emanuel has argued that, because the federal regulations allow studies to be conducted only after an IRB has determined that they do not expose subjects to excessive risks, concerns about the danger that offering payments to subjects might create undue inducement are unwarranted. In his view, no amount of money can be unduly coercive, as the subject is only being exposed to a reasonable level of risk. *See* Ezekiel J. Emanuel, *Ending Concerns About Undue Inducement,* 32 J.L. MED. & ETHICS 100 (2004). Do you agree?

9. Some commentators argue that paying subjects might be an effective way to dispel the "therapeutic misconception," i.e., the tendency of subjects to believe that participating in research is no different from receiving care in the context of an ordinary physician-patient relationship. *See, e.g.,* Franklin G. Miller & Howard Brody, *A Critique of Clinical Equipoise: Therapeutic Misconception in the Ethics of Clinical Trials,* HASTINGS CENTER REP., May-June 2003, at 19, 26; for further discussion of the therapeutic misconception, see Chapter 7, at page 355. This rationale would support payments even in studies that offer subjects a prospect of direct medical benefits. Do you agree that subjects who are paid

to receive an experimental drug in a clinical trial are less likely to downplay the risks or overestimate the benefits?

10. Additional issues arise when the subject of a study is a minor. If a payment is made to the child's parent, it is possible that the money will improperly influence the parent's decision to enroll the child in the study. On the other hand, it is difficult to structure a payment so that it truly benefits the child, because presumably a parent can always respond by decreasing other payments the child might receive (such as an allowance). For further discussion of these issues, see Chapter 13, at page 537.

[B] Determining an Appropriate Level of Payment

Several models exist for determining the appropriate level of payments to subjects. Neal Dickert and Christine Grady identified three models of payment: the market model, the wage payment model, and the reimbursement model. *See* Neal Dickert & Christine Grady, *What Is the Price of a Research Subject? Approaches to Payment for Research Participation*, 341 NEW ENG. J. MED. 198 (1999).

The Market Model

The market model assumes that most participants enroll in studies for financial reasons and therefore relies on the principle of supply and demand to determine appropriate payment amounts. The likely result of using this model would be high payments for participation in research in which there is little or no prospect of direct benefit, combined with risky or uncomfortable procedures. High payments would also be likely if researchers need to recruit subjects quickly or if eligibility criteria are very narrow, so that few individuals qualify. Large completion bonuses and other payments to encourage protocol compliance would be permitted. On the other hand, payments would be low or non-existent where individuals are enthusiastic to enroll. *See* Dickert and Grady, *supra*.

Consistent with this approach, one commentator argues that, at least with respect to healthy subjects,

> if the main reason for enrolling in a study is to earn money then participation should be treated as a form of labor, and informed consent should be viewed as a kind of contract where subjects exchange their labor for financial rewards. If subjects can agree to a contract for labor — e.g. they are legally competent and they can make informed choices — and the contract is fair and discloses materially relevant information, then there is no compelling reason to regulate or standardize their wages in order to avoid undue influence.

David E. Resnik, *Research Participation and Financial Inducements*, 1 AM. J. BIOETHICS, Spring 2001, at 54, 55. Thus, as long as the researcher pays at least minimum wage, there should be no limit on what a subject can earn beyond what the market will bear. Subjects in Phase 1 clinical trials, for example, should be treated like other laborers in high-risk occupations where it would be unfair to set an upper limit on wages.

The Wage-Payment Model

The wage-payment, or labor, model rests on the belief that research participation is a form of unskilled labor that may involve some risk but that usually does not involve actual labor. Under this model, the compensation offered to study participants is standardized among different protocols and computed so that it is comparable to other similar unskilled but essential jobs available in the community. To the extent that the procedures may require endurance of uncomfortable procedures, the payment may be increased somewhat. A completion bonus could be paid, but should not be a large part of the payment, given that the underlying theory is that payment is for the time spent as a subject. *See* Dickert and Grady, *supra*.

The Reimbursement Model

The third model, known as the reimbursement model, simply provides payment to cover the subjects' expenses. Unlike the market and wage-payment models, it bases compensation on the notion that "research participation should not require financial sacrifice but should be 'revenue neutral' for participants." Dickert and Grady, *supra*. There are two potential approaches to this model. According to one approach, participants would receive reimbursement only for travel, meals, and parking. A second approach would compensate them for their time away from work at their normal rate of pay, in addition to expense reimbursement. Under this model, subjects would not make a profit, they would not be paid for any discomfort they would endure, nor would their payment be a function of either the market for research participation or the market for unskilled work. The amount paid would differ from subject to subject.

NOTES AND QUESTIONS

1. Which of the three models do you prefer? Why?

2. Which model would be most likely to attract volunteers from the middle and upper classes, so as to satisfy the goal of ensuring that the risks of research be shared by all?

3. Should payments vary based on a subject's income? If so, should a poor person be paid less or more than a rich person? Which of the models described by Dickert and Grady would permit differences in payments based on a person's income?

4. Think about the differences between (a) studies involving healthy volunteers, with no prospect of direct benefit, (b) studies involving people with medical problems, with no prospect of direct benefit, and (c) studies involving people with medical problems, where participation may offer them a chance of receiv-

ing a type of treatment not available outside of the study. Should there be differences in the amounts paid to people in these different types of studies? What arguments support such differences?

5. Would it be ethical for sponsors to offer subjects a percentage of any revenue generated from products developed as a result of the research? Is it unethical for the sponsor not to do so? For further discussion of this issue, see Chapter 17, at page 729.

6. After setting out their three models, Dickert and Grady apply them to a study that offered no prospect of direct benefits to subjects. The study extended over twelve days and included eight clinic visits, totaling twenty-nine hours (two lasting the entire day). Subjects were required to take a drug and a narcotic pain medication that could cause diarrhea, nausea, and other side effects, as well as undergo serial blood collections. Under the market model, Dickert and Grady estimate a total payment of $1,125. Under the wage-payment model, the total payment would be $390. The reimbursement of expenses model would yield a total payment of $195, while adding reimbursement of regular wages would yield an additional payment of $1,645 for a professor and $398 for a student.

7. Ultimately, Dickert and Grady advocate the use of the wage-payment model because, in their view, it reduces worries about undue inducement, produces beneficial effects by standardizing payments, and comports with the principle that similar people should be treated similarly. In a response to the authors, Carol Saunders and Alan Sugar argue in favor of a fourth "fair-share" model, under which payment to subjects would be based on a percentage of the per-patient compensation to the investigator or institution. Thus, they suggest, if a Phase 1 study has a payment schedule of $8,000 per subject who completes the study, remuneration of the subject should be based on some percentage (e.g., ten percent) of that total. *See* Carol A. Saunders and Alan M. Sugar, *Correspondence, What's the Price of a Research Subject?* 341 NEW ENG. J. MED. 1550 (1999). What is your reaction to such an approach?

8. Consider again the hypothetical problem presented in note 3 at page 381. Assume that the investigator submits the following advertisement for approval. As a member of the IRB, what recommendations would you make?

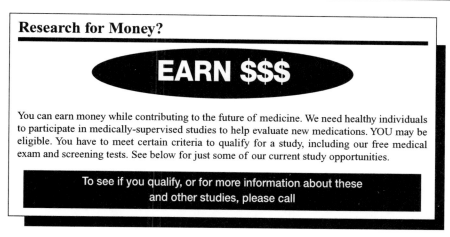

Source: OFFICE OF INSPECTOR GENERAL, DEPARTMENT OF HEALTH AND HUMAN SERVICES, RECRUITING HUMAN SUBJECTS: PRESSURES IN INDUSTRY SPONSORED CLINICAL RESEARCH 21 (2000).

[C] Structuring Payments

As noted earlier, the OHRP Guidelines recommend that IRBs establish a fee schedule that takes into account the complexity of a study, the number of procedures performed, the time involved, and the likely discomfort or inconvenience. The following is an example of one such fee schedule.

RESEARCH PARTICIPATION FEE SCHEDULE
(ALBERT EINSTEIN COLLEGE OF MEDICINE)

The following guidelines are suggested as fair compensation for those who volunteer as research subjects at Montefiore Medical Center. The chief purpose is to avoid excessive payments that might unduly influence subjects to participate, in conformity with federal regulations that prohibit coercion or undue influence in recruiting research subjects.

The pay scales contain two separate categories: an hourly or daily rate of compensation; and a dollar amount that varies according to the type of procedure (risk, discomfort, and inconvenience index). The amounts for hourly/daily rates, and for each procedure done in the course of a study are added together to arrive at the total. The maximum compensation allowed for participation in a study is $750. Any exceptions to the maximum amount in these guidelines must be brought to the Institutional Review Board (IRB) for approval.

Hourly or Daily Rate		
Outpatient	$25 (1st Hour)	$10 (Each additional hour up to 8 hours)	$95 (maximum per day)
Inpatient	$14 - $25 daily rate, plus travel	
Escort Fee	$25 (This fee covers need for children too young to travel for either inpatient or outpatient studies, thus requiring adult supervision. Volunteers are entitled to standard volunteer fees.)	

	Risks, Discomfort, and Inconvenience Index	Dollar Amounts
Level I	Overnight fasting, 24 hour urine collections, venipunctures, limited number, EEG, evoked potential studies psychologic testing, restricted diet, less than one week, routine eye, hearing tests, treadmill (healthy physiology study)	$ 0 - 10
Level II	Immunizations, skin biopsies, restricted diet, over one week, IV drug administration, less than 8 hours, gastric intubation, multiple venipunctures, or more than one day of multiple punctures	$10 - 20
Level III	Lumbar puncture, muscle biopsies, prolonged IV testing, over 8 hours metabolic diet, over one week arterial puncture, isotope administration, experimental drugs, treadmill (cardiac testing)	$20 - 30
Level IV	Right heart catheterization, other invasive procedures that carry high risk	$40 - 50

NOTES AND QUESTIONS

1. Should research institutions develop payment schedules? If so, is the Albert Einstein payment schedule a good model for them to use? If payment models are a good idea, should their development be left to individual institutions, as opposed to regional or national organizations and/or federal agencies?

2. Which of the models discussed in the previous section does the Albert Einstein payment schedule reflect?

3. Examine each of the dollar amounts listed in this payment schedule. Do you think any of them should be lowered or increased, and if so, by how much? What rationale leads you to conclude that a particular payment is too low or too high?

4. An eight-week study involves randomizing subjects with high blood pressure between getting a new type of blood pressure pill or getting a placebo. The people getting the new pill may experience a variety of possible side effects, such

as dizziness, lightheadedness, fainting, slow heart rate, and heart palpitations. The people getting the placebo risk having a heart attack or stroke due to inadequate treatment of their high blood pressure. Is a $500 payment to the subjects so great as to constitute undue inducement? Should the income of the subject matter? *See* David Casarett et al., *Paying Hypertension Research Subjects: Fair Compensation or Undue Inducement?* 17 J. GENERAL INTERNAL MED. 650 (2002).

5. An analysis of existing institutional guidance regarding payments to research subjects indicated that, of thirty-two geographically diverse organizations involved in biomedical research, only 37.5 percent had written guidelines about paying subjects, although all but one reported having rules of thumb. Only 18.8 percent could confidently estimate the percentage of studies that paid subjects. *See* Neal Dickert et al., *Paying Research Subjects: An Analysis of Current Policies*, 136 ANN. INTERN. MED. 368 (2002).

Chapter 9

RESEARCH AND JUSTICE: PROMOTING THE INCLUSION OF WOMEN AND MINORITIES

Most of this book has been concerned with the need to protect the rights and interests of individuals who are subjects or potential subjects in a research study. In this chapter, we broaden our perspective, redirecting our attention from the individual to the group. The focus here is on whether particular groups have suffered more than their reasonable share of the burdens of research, or been denied their fair share of the benefits. We focus on women and minorities in this chapter because, unlike the other groups discussed in this book (e.g., children, prisoners, incapacitated adults), women and minorities are generally not considered "vulnerable" populations in need of heightened protection in research, at least in most respects. While bias and discrimination certainly do exist, there are no legal impediments to the ability of women and members of racial minority groups to act autonomously, as there are for prisoners and other institutionalized persons. Moreover, unlike children or incapacitated adults, there is nothing inherent in the status of being a woman or a member of a racial minority group that makes these individuals less capable than white males of providing informed consent to participate in research. Nonetheless, there is substantial evidence that these two populations are often excluded from research and that the medical care they receive may be less adequate than that provided for other populations. Therefore, the historical under-inclusion of women and minorities in research raises "purer" justice issues than the exclusion of populations thought to be especially susceptible to exploitation and abuse.

§ 9.01 THE CONCEPT OF JUSTICE IN RESEARCH WITH HUMAN SUBJECTS

THE BELMONT REPORT
NATIONAL COMMISSION FOR THE PROTECTION OF HUMAN SUBJECTS OF BIOMEDICAL AND BEHAVIORAL RESEARCH
(1979)

B. Basic Ethical Principles

The expression "basic ethical principles" refers to those general judgments that serve as a basic justification for the many particular ethical prescriptions and evaluations of human actions. Three basic principles, among those generally accepted in our cultural tradition, are particularly relevant to the ethics of research involving human subjects: the principles of respect of persons, benef-icence and justice. . . .

3. *Justice* — Who ought to receive the benefits of research and bear its bur-dens? This is a question of justice, in the sense of "fairness in distribution" or "what is deserved." An injustice occurs when some benefit to which a person is entitled is denied without good reason or when some burden is imposed unduly. Another way of conceiving the principle of justice is that equals ought to be treated equally. . . . Who is equal and who is unequal? What considerations jus-tify departure from equal distribution? Almost all commentators allow that distinctions based on experience, age, deprivation, competence, merit and posi-tion do sometimes constitute criteria justifying differential treatment for certain purposes. . . .

Questions of justice have long been associated with social practices such as punishment, taxation and political representation. Until recently these ques-tions have not generally been associated with scientific research. However, they are foreshadowed even in the earliest reflections on the ethics of research involving human subjects. For example, during the nineteenth and early twen-tieth centuries the burdens of serving as research subjects fell largely upon poor ward patients, while the benefits of improved medical care flowed primarily to private patients. Subsequently, the exploitation of unwilling prisoners as research subjects in Nazi concentration camps was condemned as a particularly flagrant injustice. In this country, in the 1940s, the Tuskegee syphilis study used disadvantaged, rural black men to study the untreated course of a disease that is by no means confined to that population. These subjects were deprived of demonstrably effective treatment in order not to interrupt the project, long after such treatment became generally available.

Against this historical background, it can be seen how conceptions of justice are relevant to research involving human subjects. For example, the selection of research subjects needs to be scrutinized in order to determine whether some classes (e.g., welfare patients, particular racial and ethnic minorities, or persons confined to institutions) are being systematically selected simply because of their easy availability, their compromised position, or their manipulability, rather than for reasons directly related to the problem being studied. Finally, whenever research supported by public funds leads to the development of ther-apeutic devices and procedures, justice demands both that these not provide advantages only to those who can afford them and that such research should not unduly involve persons from groups unlikely to be among the beneficiaries of subsequent applications of the research. . . .

C. Applications

. . . 3. *Selection of Subjects.* Just as the principle of respect for persons finds expression in the requirements for consent, and the principle of beneficence in risk/benefit assessment, the principle of justice gives rise to moral requirements that there be fair procedures and outcomes in the selection of research subjects.

Justice is relevant to the selection of subjects of research at two levels: the social and the individual. Individual justice in the selection of subjects would require that researchers exhibit fairness: thus, they should not offer potentially beneficial research only to some patients who are in their favor or select only "undesirable" persons for risky research. Social justice requires that distinctions be drawn between classes of subjects that ought, and ought not, to participate in any particular kind of research, based on the ability of members of that class to bear burdens and on the appropriateness of placing further burdens on already burdened persons. Thus, it can be considered a matter of social justice that there is an order of preference in the selection of classes of subjects (e.g., adults before children) and that some classes of potential subjects (e.g., the institutionalized mentally infirm or prisoners) may be involved as research subjects, if at all, only on certain conditions.

Injustice may appear in the selection of subjects, even if individual subjects are selected fairly by investigators and treated fairly in the course of research. Thus injustice arises from social, racial, sexual and cultural biases institutionalized in society. Thus, even if individual researchers are treating their research subjects fairly, and even if IRBs are taking care to assure that subjects are selected fairly within a particular institution, unjust social patterns may nevertheless appear in the overall distribution of the burdens and benefits of research. Although individual institutions or investigators may not be able to resolve a problem that is pervasive in their social setting, they can consider distributive justice in selecting research subjects.

Some populations, especially institutionalized ones, are already burdened in many ways by their infirmities and environments. When research is proposed that involves risks and does not include a therapeutic component, other less burdened classes of persons should be called upon first to accept these risks of research, except where the research is directly related to the specific conditions of the class involved. Also, even though public funds for research may often flow in the same directions as public funds for health care, it seems unfair that populations dependent on public health care constitute a pool of preferred research subjects if more advantaged populations are likely to be the recipients of the benefits.

One special instance of injustice results from the involvement of vulnerable subjects. Certain groups, such as racial minorities, the economically disadvantaged, the very sick, and the institutionalized may continually be sought as research subjects, owing to their ready availability in settings where research is conducted. Given their dependent status and their frequently compromised capacity for free consent, they should be protected against the danger of being involved in research solely for administrative convenience, or because they are easy to manipulate as a result of their illness or socioeconomic condition.

45 CFR § 46.111(a)(3):
CRITERIA FOR IRB APPROVAL OF RESEARCH

(a) In order to approve research covered by this policy the IRB shall determine that all of the following requirements are satisfied:

> ... (3) Selection of subjects is equitable. In making this assessment the IRB should take into account the purposes of the research and the setting in which the research will be conducted and should be particularly cognizant of the special problems of research involving vulnerable populations, such as children, prisoners, pregnant women, mentally disabled persons, or economically or educationally disadvantaged persons.

INSTITUTIONAL REVIEW BOARD GUIDEBOOK
Chapter 3, Basic IRB Review —
Section C. Selection of Subjects
U.S. DEPT. OF HEALTH AND HUMAN SERVICES
OFFICE FOR PROTECTION FROM RESEARCH RISKS
(1993)

The requirement for an equitable selection of subjects helps ensure that the burdens and benefits of research will be fairly distributed. ...

Easy availability, compromised position, and susceptibility to manipulation often overlap. For example, psychology students are readily available for psychological research, medical students are readily available for medical research, prisoners, patients in mental institutions, and military personnel are readily available for a variety of research activities, and employees of drug manufacturing companies are readily available for pharmaceutical research. Subjects selected from these populations are also compromised to the extent that their jobs, promotions, grades, etc., are dependent upon those who might be recruiting them for research. This circumstance makes them susceptible to manipulation.

Prisoners and patients in mental institutions are confined under the strict control of people whom they must please and to whom they must appear cooperative and rational if they are to earn their release. These potential subjects may believe, probably as a result of their dependent situation, that agreeing to participate in research will be viewed positively by their wardens, psychiatrists, or social workers. They are also readily available in large numbers, and, therefore, have historically been involved as subjects of drug research that is totally unrelated to the basis of their confinement. Mental patients and prisoners have accepted the risks of research in disproportionate numbers, while the benefits of the research in which they participated went to all segments of the population. ...

Patients may also be susceptible to real or imaginary pressure to participate. If an investigator also serves as a patient's primary physician, he or she

may feel obliged to participate in the research out of a desire to please, grati-
tude, or fear that failure to do so will result in hostility or abandonment.
Patients who are dependent upon a particular facility for their care (e.g., Veterans Hospitals, Indian Health Service Hospitals, or community health clinics)
may feel that they will be treated less well or with less favor if they refuse to
participate in research.

With these caveats in mind, investigators and IRBs must be careful not to
overprotect vulnerable populations so that they are excluded from participating
in research in which they wish to participate, particularly where the research
involves therapies for conditions with no available treatments (such as HIV). So
too, patients with serious or poorly understood disorders may want to participate frequently in research designed to provide a better understanding of their
condition. The fact that the subject may be either a patient of the principal
investigator or a patient in the clinic or hospital where the investigator conducts
the research should not preclude them from the opportunity to choose to participate as often as they wish.

Just as the inclusion of disproportionate numbers of racial or ethnic minorities in research studies might overburden these groups without affording them
the benefits that will result from the research, so will underrepresentation of
these groups in study populations ensure that they will not benefit from the
research. . . .

IRB Considerations

. . . IRBs should consider the extent to which a proposed subject population
is already burdened by poverty, illness, poor education, or chronic disabilities in
deciding whether they are a suitable subject population.

When determining whether the burdens of research are being distributed
equitably, it is appropriate for an IRB to consider more than the risks associated
with the research procedures. It may be appropriate to consider such things as
inconvenience (i.e., the time required, travel involved, restrictions on diet, or
other activities), discomfort, and embarrassment as burdens of participating in
research.

To encourage a broad cross-section of research subjects, IRBs might consider
the manner in which subjects will be recruited. Will notices appear only on the
bulletin boards of the psychology department or the medical school? Will investigators personally recruit subjects only in community health clinics? If a new
treatment is available only in the research context, and it is a scarce resource
(in that only a small proportion of those who could benefit from the therapy can
be accepted as research subjects), the IRB should try to devise procedures to
ensure that subjects from a variety of locations and circumstances have an
equal chance of being selected. This becomes particularly important when the
intervention is a life-saving procedure (e.g., organ transplant or germ-free environment).

. . . Those who accept the risks or burdens of being research subjects should be the ones who share in its benefits whenever possible. One group of subjects should not be asked always to bear the risks of research for the benefit of others. Those who have participated as research subjects should have the first opportunity to receive a therapy that the research has demonstrated to be safe and effective (e.g., subjects of clinical trials who were either in a control group or recipients of a therapy that proved not to be superior should be offered the treatment that the trial demonstrated to be preferable). The study design should provide for the adequate representation of women and minorities in the study population so that the findings will be meaningful for those groups and they can, therefore, share in the benefits of the research. Adequate representation of women and minorities is particularly important in studies of diseases, disorders, and conditions that disproportionately affect them. Note that risk/benefit assessments are relevant to subject selection.

Points to Consider

1. Will the burdens of participating in the research fall on those most likely to benefit from the research?

2. Will the solicitation of subjects avoid placing a disproportionate share of the burdens of research on any single group?

3. Does the nature of the research require or justify using the proposed subject population?

4. Are there any groups of people who might be more susceptible to the risks presented by the study and who therefore ought to be excluded from the research? Are the procedures for identifying such individuals adequate?

5. To the extent that benefits to the subjects are anticipated, are they distributed fairly? Do other groups of potential subjects have a greater need to receive any of the anticipated benefits?

6. To the extent that participation in the study is burdensome, are these burdens distributed fairly? Is the proposed subject population already so burdened that it would be unfair to ask them to accept an extra burden?

7. Will any special physiological, psychological, or social characteristics of the subject group pose special risks for them?

8. Would it be possible to conduct the study with other, less vulnerable subjects? What additional expense or inconvenience would that entail? Does the convenience of the researcher or possible improvement in the quality of the research justify the involvement of subjects who may either be susceptible to pressure or who are already burdened?

9. Has the selection process *overprotected* potential subjects who are considered vulnerable (e.g., children, cognitively impaired, economically or educationally disadvantaged persons, patients of researchers, seriously ill persons) so that they are denied opportunities to participate in research?

10. If the subjects are susceptible to pressures, are there mechanisms that might be used to reduce the pressures or minimize their impact?

NOTES AND QUESTIONS

1. The *Belmont Report* states, "IRBs should consider the extent to which a proposed subject population is already burdened by poverty, illness, poor education, or chronic disabilities in deciding whether they are a suitable subject population." Practically and realistically, how does an IRB go about making such a determination? This question is particularly challenging in institutions that serve a variety of different populations. In such a setting, is it likely that the IRB will include members familiar with all of the populations from which subjects might be drawn?

2. If IRBs solicit the views of nonmember consultants when the membership lacks sufficient expertise to evaluate the scientific merit of studies, should they also seek outside opinions when they are unfamiliar with the expected subject population? As you will see in Chapter 15, IRBs that review research involving prisoners are required to have at least one member who is a prisoner or a prisoner representative. *See* 45 C.F.R. § 46.304(b); *see also* Chapter 15, at page 643. Why do you think no similar requirement exists for any other population?

3. The only aspect of the human subject protection regulations that speaks directly to the issue of justice is the brief provision in 45 CFR § 46.111(a)(3) quoted above. Does the lack of additional elaboration send a message that justice considerations are less important than the principles of respect for persons and beneficence, the two other basic principles identified in the *Belmont Report*?

§ 9.02 JUSTICE AND WOMEN

[A] Federal Policy Before 1993

Guideline for the Study and Evaluation of Gender Differences in the Clinical Evaluation of Drugs (Part VI) U.S. Dept. of Health and Human Services, Public Health Service, Food and Drug Administration
58 Fed. Reg. 39406, 39407-8 (1994)

A. The 1977 Guideline — "General Considerations for the Clinical Evaluation of Drugs"

The 1977 guideline set forth a policy on, among other things, the inclusion of women of childbearing potential in clinical trials. The policy stated that, in general, women of childbearing potential should be excluded from the earliest studies of a new drug, that is, phase 1 and early phase 2 studies. [For a discussion of the various phases of pharmaceutical research, see Chapter 3, at page 150.]

If adequate information on effectiveness and relative safety were amassed during phase 1 and early phase 2, the guideline stated that women of childbearing potential could be included in subsequent studies of effectiveness, that is, later phase 2 and phase 3 studies, so long as animal teratogenicity and the female part of animal fertility studies had been completed. The policy did not specifically address the manner in which the early human evidence of safety and effectiveness and the results of animal reproduction studies should be used to make decisions about participation of women in later trials, leaving these considerations to the usual risk-benefit assessment made by the patient, physician, and IRB, with subsequent FDA review.

In the 1977 guideline, the term "women of childbearing potential" was defined very strictly, essentially referring to all premenopausal women physiologically capable of becoming pregnant, including women on oral, injectable, or mechanical contraceptives, single women, celibate women, and women whose partners had been sterilized by vasectomy. There was no provision for the use of pregnancy testing to identify women who could participate in studies without a risk of fetal exposure. The 1977 guideline also noted, however, that women of childbearing potential could receive investigational drugs in the earliest phases of testing, even in the absence of adequate reproduction studies in animals, when the drugs were intended for life-saving or life-prolonging treatment.

The effect of the 1977 guideline has been that women generally have not been included in phase 1 nontherapeutic studies or in the earliest controlled effectiveness studies (i.e., early phase 2), except for studies of life-threatening illnesses, such as acquired immune deficiency syndrome (AIDS) and cancer.

NOTES AND QUESTIONS

1. Recall the discussion in Chapter 1 of the thalidomide and diethylstilbestrol (DES) scandals. *See* Chapter 1, at page 35. Do those events explain the restrictiveness of the 1977 guidelines? What other factors might also have been involved?

2. As Karen Rothenberg points out, the 1977 guidelines did not preclude manufacturers from marketing drugs that pregnant women might use; they simply prevented them from determining whether those drugs were safe for use during pregnancy. Thus, ironically, the FDA could approve drugs, the toxicity of which was unknown in women and fetuses, for use on the very populations it sought to protect — pregnant women and women of childbearing potential. "Moreover," she argues, "by following FDA guidelines and attempting to 'protect' women of childbearing potential (and themselves from liability for research

injuries), drug manufacturers could find themselves exposed to even greater potential liability should the adverse effects of a drug be discovered after it was marketed to the general public." Karen H. Rothenberg, *Gender Matters: Implications for Clinical Research and Women's Health Care*, 32 Hous. L. Rev. 1201, 1235-36 (1996). Note that similar criticisms have been raised about drug companies' historic unwillingness to conduct pediatric research. *See* Chapter 13, at page 531.

3. For many years, the National Institutes of Health (NIH) had a policy similar to that of the FDA, but in 1986, the NIH issued and implemented guidelines urging (but not mandating) funding applicants to include women in clinical research and requiring a clear rationale if women were to be excluded. *See* Rothenberg, *supra*, at 1230 (citing U.S. Dep't of Health & Human Servs., 15 NIH GUIDE FOR GRANTS AND CONTRACTS 1 (1986)). Subsequently, as noted below, a 1994 NIH policy toughened the requirement significantly.

Wanted: Single, White Male for Medical Research
Rebecca Dresser
22 HASTINGS CENTER REPT., JAN-FEB, 1992, at 6

In June 1990, congressional investigators issued a startling report. The General Accounting Office revealed that despite a 1986 federal policy to the contrary, women continued to be seriously underrepresented in biomedical research study populations. According to the National Institutes of Health, this practice "has resulted in significant gaps in [our] knowledge" of diseases that affect both men and women. In short, many of the important human health data generated by the modern biomedical research revolution are data about men.

The failure to include women in research populations is ubiquitous. An NIH-sponsored study showing that heart attacks were reduced when subjects took one aspirin every other day was conducted on men, and the relationship between low cholesterol diets and cardiovascular disease has been almost exclusively studied in men. Yet coronary heart disease is the leading cause of death in women. Similarly, the first twenty years of a major federal study on health and aging included only men. Yet two-thirds of the elderly population are women. The recent announcement that aspirin can help prevent migraine headaches is based on data from males only, even though women suffer from migraines up to three times as often as men.

The list goes on: studies on AIDS treatment frequently omit women, the fastest growing infected population. An investigation of the possible relationship between caffeine and heart disease involved 45,589 male research subjects. Most amazing is the pilot project on the impact of obesity on breast and uterine cancer conducted — you guessed it — solely on men. Moreover, the customary research subject not only is male, but is a white male. African-Americans, Latinos, and other racial and ethnic groups have typically been excluded from studies, again in spite of a formal NIH guideline encouraging the inclusion of such groups in study populations. Children and elderly persons also have received short shrift, particularly in the testing of new drugs. And in basic research, even female rats are frequently excluded as research subjects!

The physiology of women and men differs in ways that can affect how disease and treatment manifest themselves. Beyond the obviously sex-linked diseases such as uterine and prostate cancer, there is evidence that heart disease, AIDS, depression, and numerous other ostensibly "general-neutral" conditions are expressed differently in women and men. A similar situation exists among different racial and ethnic groups. Lupus, for example, reportedly affects one in 750 women generally, but its incidence is one in 245 among African-American women and one in 500 among Latinas. Such differences make it inappropriate simply to generalize findings based on one gender or racial group to all human beings. As a result of the past over-representation of white men in research populations, physicians now frequently lack adequate evidence on whether women and people of color will be helped, harmed, or not affected at all by numerous therapies now endorsed as promoting "human health."

NIH officials have admitted that the agency's policy on expanding study populations was inadequately publicized as well as substantively feeble, simply recommending that investigators proposing studies "consider" the inclusion of women and minority groups. In the four years that elapsed between the policy's announcement and the GAO report, NIH continued to review numerous proposals that either gave no information on the gender of their study populations, or proposed all-male studies without a rationale for doing so. . . .

In a country that prides itself on its progress in promoting gender and racial equality, how could the federal government sanction such a nakedly discriminatory practice? Why wasn't the original NIH policy more strongly worded and more effectively implemented? Moreover, why was a special NIH policy necessary at all? Why didn't the researchers themselves adopt a more inclusive practice? And finally, why didn't the institutional review boards charged with research oversight demand a more inclusive approach? . . .

Alleged Justifications for the Exclusionary Practice

Some scientists and officials have explained that there often is "scientific" justification for studying only white males. Clean, simple data are needed for studies; the more alike the subjects, the more any variation can be attributed to the experimental intervention. Including women would "complicate" a study due to the hormone changes of the menstrual cycle. I have two responses to this claim. First, even if it is scientifically justifiable to study humans who have a similar physiology, why study white men? Perhaps the choice of racial group can be supported by its dominant proportion in the U.S. population, but not so for the choice of gender. In this country, women are numerically in the majority. Why then the choice of the minority white male? Why is it female, but not male, hormones that "complicate" research? Second, focusing on one type of human physiology reduces the generalizability of the experimental data. Although there is probably a place for such narrowly focused projects, why have they so rarely been conducted on anyone but white men? Again, what accounts for the relative infrequency of studies on homogeneous populations of other kinds of people?

One can also challenge the notion that a study conducted on physiologically close subjects is usually the "best" scientific approach. Such a judgment divorces the concept of scientific merit from its broader context. A project may be designed with the greatest of scientific elegance, but if the data it produces have little value to society, it is not necessarily a meritorious project. Merit, at least in the context of government funding decisions, is tied to a proposal's promise of benefit to society. If NIH's goal is to award support to the projects most likely to advance our knowledge of important human health concerns, it would seem that white-male-only clinical investigations of widespread conditions such as coronary artery disease and aging would have less merit than studies that provided data with broader applicability. . . .

Two other explanations have been offered for the practice of excluding women from study populations. One is concern for the condition of women who could become pregnant while enrolled as research subjects. Threats of miscarriage, birth defects, and so forth are cited as justifications for omitting women. Exclusion is appropriate, it is alleged, to protect potentially pregnant women and their potential children. . . . Certainly caution is warranted here. But is maternal-fetal protection always a valid reason for failing to include female subjects?

Our nation has a long history of excluding women from various activities on grounds that participation would harm the "weaker sex," and thus often denying women the significant benefits of participation. Likewise, the failure to conduct biomedical research on women denies them the benefits of research. The vast majority of women who are not pregnant cannot with sufficient confidence take advantage of numerous health recommendations that have emerged from men-only research studies. In the name of potential protection for potentially pregnant women and their fetuses, all women have lost opportunities to improve and extend their lives.

Complete exclusion of women subjects is an unnecessarily blunt instrument to accomplish the goal of maternal-fetal protection. The exclusionary approach, as Carol Levine notes, "assumes that all women are alike, that all women are sexually active, and that all are unreliable in their contraceptive practices." To the contrary, as one physician pointed out, "Most female cardiac patients are not planning to get pregnant." Neither are the women likely to be subjects in an aging study!

If a study poses a legitimate threat to the potential offspring of women participants, two options come to mind. One is simply to exclude fertile women of reproductive age. Again, however, this seems overbroad; indeed, this is the approach the Supreme Court recently struck down in *Johnson Controls* as violating federal law prohibiting sex discrimination in the workplace. It would be better to adopt a more nuanced approach. In her recent article on the underrepresentation of women in HIV/AIDS research, for example, Levine endorses a three-tiered categorization system to address the problem. Many, perhaps most, human studies fail to pose a foreseeable risk to future children. The unknown and unforeseeable teratogenic risk that accompanies practically any physiological intervention fails to justify excluding fertile women from studies in this category. Similarly, women should have the opportunity to enroll in studies that present known risks to future children, but also have the potential for significantly benefiting the research participants. In these two categories of research, adequate disclosure of the risks and potential benefits of research participation, together with the availability of highly reliable contraceptives and abortion, would give women a reasonable choice regarding whether to accept the risks of participating. The possibility that a few women might become pregnant, might choose against abortion, and might have a child who is harmed by exposure to an experimental intervention is too small to justify the current exclusionary practices. The risk of tort liability in such cases is also small. Women who consent to the risk of harm to potential offspring and who decide against abortion when they become unexpectedly pregnant would be unlikely to recover damages. Any injured children might themselves have a claim, however. Perhaps some form of legislative immunity is needed here. But it should be recognized that the current approach also fails to protect health professionals and drug manufacturers against liability. The present practice merely moves the source of the claims to the damaged future children of women patients who receive drugs and other treatments in the clinical setting.

A third research category is more complicated, however. Levine argues that sexually active fertile women should be excluded from studies that present both a known significant risk to potential offspring and minimal or unknown benefit to women subjects, because parents have a moral responsibility to make reasonable efforts to protect their future children's health and the knowledge sought from such studies is obtainable through other means. Given the ever-present danger of contraceptive failure, the misunderstandings "informed" subjects may have about a protocol's risks and potential benefits, and the possibility that subjects' awareness or appreciation of their exposure to risk could decline over time, it is better to conduct such studies on other groups, Levine contends. If early results reveal a possible substantial benefit for women participants, she suggests that the intervention could be made available to individual women off-protocol.

This would be appropriate, in my view, as long as the same approach is applied to sexually active fertile men. Researchers have been extremely concerned about reproductive risks to women, while largely neglecting the reproductive risks research participation may pose to men. There is growing evidence that many substances may be damaging to sperm, thereby creating the possibility of birth defects in offspring. The emphasis on reproductive hazards to women thus is an unjustifiably narrow means of protecting children's health. If society deems the health of potential future children to justify the blanket exclusion of fertile women from certain research protocols, the exclusion should cover all fertile subjects whose offspring could be endangered, not just female ones. Furthermore, men's lengthier reproductive capacity could lead to their exclusion from risky studies for many more years than women.

The final rationale for women's exclusion from study populations involves alleged recruitment difficulties. For example, researchers in the aspirin and heart disease study claimed that they wanted to include women, but were unable to find enough potential subjects to do so. Their study population was physicians over age forty, they explained, and women comprised only ten percent of this group. Moreover, according to one NIH official, it was doubtful that a sufficient number of women would be "interested in participating and be content to go through the hassle of taking a placebo." In other heart disease studies, researchers have asserted that they could not locate enough women with the condition. Although this is partly due to the lower overall incidence and later development of this disease among women, it turns out that another factor is the medical community's failure to recognize serious heart disease in women.

Blaming the scarcity of potential women subjects for the exclusionary practice is unacceptable. In effect, this adds insult to injury by building on past bias to justify its perpetuation in a different realm. The traditional exclusion of women from the medical profession is the source of the small number of middle-aged women physicians. Health stereotypes about women — "women just don't get heart disease"; "women somaticize their emotional problems" — are one source of physicians' failure to recognize heart disease in women. As one physician put it,

> If a fifty-year-old man goes to the doctor complaining of chest pains, the next day he will be on a treadmill taking a stress test. If a fifty-year-old woman goes to the doctor and complains of chest pains, she will be told to go home and rest.

When heart disease studies exclude women, they only reinforce physicians' misplaced assumptions. And why was it assumed that women would be less interested than men in "go[ing] through the hassle of taking a placebo?" Women who were adequately informed of their risk of heart disease would have as much incentive as men to participate in the study.

Biomedical research studies should be designed to surmount the alleged difficulties in recruiting women. If enough female physicians are not available, why not study female nurses, or some other reasonably accessible group of women? (A recent observational study suggesting that low-dose aspirin could reduce cardiovascular disease in women was conducted on female nurses, but the authors emphasize the need for a randomized, controlled clinical trial to verify that a benefit exists, rule out serious risks, and determine an appropriate dose for women.) If scientists conducting heart disease research are afraid that physicians will not refer enough women patients, then extra recruiting measures should be taken to ensure that they do. Research costs may go up, but the benefits of including women subjects are worth the expense.

What's Wrong with Exclusion

The current disparity between the health information we have about white males and the information we have about women and people of color contravenes basic ethical principles governing human experimentation. Most clearly violated is the principle of beneficence, which holds that biomedical research should be designed to maximize benefit and minimize harm. Proposals promising to advance knowledge of important human health and welfare concerns should receive funding priority. Awarding support to studies on white males withholds research benefits from other groups of people and possibly exposes such people to risk when they and their physicians follow recommendations based on data from white male subjects. When diseases disproportionately affecting women and people of color are given low funding priority, knowledge that could alter current ineffective or detrimental routine medical care is never produced.

The harm produced by the exclusionary practices is not easily dismissed. Simple extrapolation from white males to everyone else can be dangerous. One study, for example, found that due to physiological differences, African-Americans given the "normal" dose of lithium (established in trials on white men) frequently experienced toxic reactions, heightening their already high risk of renal failure. The male-only studies of heart disease and cholesterol led the American Heart Association to recommend a diet that could actually exacerbate the risk of heart disease for women. Oral contraceptives can cause excessive cholesterol levels, yet it has not been systematically demonstrated that the cholesterol-lowering medication proven effective in men works when taken in conjunction with oral contraceptives. The current lack of knowledge on the connection between diet and breast cancer denies women a potential opportunity to protect themselves against a frequently lethal disease that strikes one in nine women. Antiseizure and antidepressant drugs may require different doses over the menstrual cycle to achieve their desired effect, and the failure to calibrate asthma medication to this cycle may contribute to the existing premenstrual rise in asthma deaths.

Scientists and policymakers must recognize that the choice is not whether to protect women and people of color from research risks. Instead, the choice is whether to expose some consenting members of these groups to risk in the closely monitored research setting, or to expose many more of them to risk in the clinical setting without these safeguards, which is the result of the current approach.

The present situation also is unjust. The justice principle mandates fair distribution of the benefits and burdens of biomedical research. But instead, taxpayers excluded from study populations have been charged for research without the assurance that they will share in any health benefits it might produce. Historically disadvantaged groups have subsidized health benefits for the more privileged, while being denied similar benefits for themselves. . . .

The Hidden Roots of Exclusion

How did white males come to be the prototype of the human research subject? Like the pronoun "he," it was taken for granted that the white male subject stood for all of us. In her examination of how the law treats differences among people, Martha Minow suggests some reasons for this. As individuals, she points out, we are all different from everyone else in countless ways. In society, however, certain differences are deemed relevant to how people are regarded. The choice of which differences "matter" inevitably reflects and reinforces existing social structures, and normality and abnormality are determined by the most powerful social group's (usually unstated) point of reference. Accordingly, "women are different in relation to the unstated male norm. Blacks, Mormons, Jews, and Arabs are different in relation to the unstated white Christian norm." Members of the dominant group making decisions in reliance on this norm may discount or be oblivious to the influence of their particular perspective. To the contrary, they see themselves as "objective," and the existing social structure as "natural."

It is easy to see this process at work in the research setting. NIH officials and biomedical researchers have, consciously or unconsciously, defined the white male as the normal, representative human being. From this perspective, the goal of advancing human health can be achieved by studying the white male human model. Physical differences between males and females, or between whites and people of color, are unacknowledged or irrelevant in this world view. Including women and people of color would simply complicate the work, thus making it more difficult and costly, which would detract from the researchers' mission of improving human health and welfare. According to this worldview, "special money" must be raised to study women and people of color, so that the "regular money" can be reserved for "normal" research.

Perhaps there was also a more insidious influence on the decisions about study populations. At least some scientists and government officials might have believed it was not important even to find out whether data from studies on white males applied to women and people of color. We cannot dismiss the possibility that the exclusionary practice reflected implicit social worth judgments on who ought to have priority in obtaining the fruits of biomedical research. An emphasis on the economic costs of human disease could also have inadvertently contributed to the view that research should focus on the "normal" economic contributor, that is, the young or middle-aged white male.

In attempting to trace the origins of the exclusionary practice, we must consider as well the identity of the major players in the research establishment. Science has been and to some extent still is largely populated by white males. . . . A white male-dominated group will assess the nation's biomedical research priorities from a particular vantage point. Decisions by such a group could intentionally or inadvertently undervalue the health concerns of "outsiders." When one researcher asked investigators about the exclusion of African-Americans from clinical trials, many responded that they simply had "never thought about" the matter. Congresswoman Olympia Snow put it succinctly in her comment on the choice to study men to assess obesity's impact on breast and uterine cancer: "Somehow, I find it hard to believe that the male-dominated medical community would tolerate a study of prostate cancer that used only women as research subjects." . . .

The Lessons of Exclusion

. . . The immediate task for scientists and government officials involves revamping study design and reordering funding priorities to remedy past exclusionary practices. The NIH and other funding agencies should back up their paper policies with concrete implementation measures, including the added financial expenditures that may be necessary to ensure more representative study populations. There is also a need for more carefully reasoned policies governing the inclusion of women — and men — of reproductive potential in clinical research. Institutional review boards ought to consider explicitly the composition of proposed study populations in determining whether the selection of subjects is equitable. But the remedies also extend beyond this realm. One task is to continue and to redouble the effort to reduce the disproportionate representation of white men in important scientific and policy positions. Diversity among powerful decisionmakers is one of the best methods to guard against conscious as well as unconscious discriminatory practices.

Second is the challenge to use the emerging knowledge about biological differences for the benefit of historically disadvantaged groups. Perhaps we have come far enough to recognize such differences without transforming them into tools for maintaining the traditional social hierarchy. Particular biological characteristics of women and members of nonwhite racial and ethnic groups must not be viewed through the narrow prism of the status quo, which too frequently labels "difference" as "problem." From a wider perspective, the contributions of people who are "different" can in some cases be "better." Moreover, sometimes, as Martha Minow has noted, it is the system that should adjust to embrace the difference. The goal is to move beyond the restrictive traditional patterns of labeling difference toward a richer, more expansive view.

NOTES AND QUESTIONS

1. Dresser's analysis demonstrates the interrelationship between the principles of autonomy and justice: Excluding women from research is unjust, she suggests, because it deprives them of the opportunity to exercise their autonomy in deciding whether to participate.

2. Dresser refers to the *Johnson Controls* case, which was decided by the U.S. Supreme Court in 1991. The case addressed the validity of a company policy under which all fertile women were barred from jobs in which they would be exposed to amounts of lead greater than that set by the federal Occupational Safety and Health Administration for women planning to have children. The

provision was challenged under Title VII of the Civil Rights Act and the Pregnancy Discrimination Act. The court concluded that the policy resulted in an unlawful discriminatory classification based on gender. It held that neither employers nor the courts should be making such decisions regarding future children, but that the women who conceive and bear the children should make them. *See* International Union, United Automobile, Aerospace and Agricultural Implement Workers of America, et al. v. Johnson Controls, 499 U.S. 187 (1991). As Rothenberg observes,

> While the *Johnson Controls* Court framed its discussion in the context of discrimination in the workplace, the decision nevertheless supports the policy position that excluding women from clinical trials by virtue of their reproductive health is discrimination against women as women. . . . Although the early rationale for excluding women from clinical trials was based historically on ethical concerns designed to protect fetuses those same concerns have served to restrict women's access to important clinical research on women's health and to potential treatment alternatives. . . .

> There is a real need for society to acknowledge that women are to be trusted in the decisions that they make for themselves and others. Women, as competent individuals, should be free to incorporate their own values and preferences into medical decisions that affect their bodily integrity. This would seem to place women, even those who are pregnant, in the best position to decide the advisability of entering a clinical trial. For women with AIDS, and for women with rare diseases, participation in a clinical trial represents a good in and of itself, in that access to the trial may literally be synonymous with the only available treatment. In addition, clinical trials provide good primary health care to women whose access to health care maybe otherwise limited.

Rothenberg, *supra*, at 1243-45.

3. If, as the Supreme Court suggested in *Johnson Controls*, women are entitled to make their own decisions about the risks to which their future children should be exposed, is there any justification for excluding women from the third category of research discussed in Dresser's article — "studies that present both a known significant risk to potential offspring and minimal or unknown benefit to women subjects"? Is it appropriate to impose greater limits on women's decisions regarding research participation than on women's decisions about the type of workplace risks they are willing to accept?

4. Note that, once a woman is pregnant, her decisions about research participation are governed by Subpart B of the federal regulations. *See* Chapter 16, at page 656.

[B] Revisions in Government Policies

[1] FDA

Guideline for the Study and Evaluation of Gender Differences in the Clinical Evaluation of Drugs (Part VI) Department of Health and Human Services, Public Health Service, Food and Drug Administration
58 FED. REG. 39406, 39408-11 (1993)

C. Current FDA Position on Participation of Women of Childbearing Potential in Early Clinical Studies

The agency has reconsidered the 1977 guideline and has concluded that it should be revised. This does not reflect a lack of concern for potential fetal exposure or indifference to potential fetal damage, but rather the agency's opinion that (1) exclusion of women from early trials is not medically necessary because the risk of fetal exposure can be minimized by patient behavior and laboratory testing, and (2) initial determinations about whether that risk is adequately addressed are properly left to patients, physicians, local IRBs, and sponsors, with appropriate review and guidance by FDA, as are all other aspects of the safety of proposed investigations.

The agency is, therefore, withdrawing the restriction on the participation of women of childbearing potential in early clinical trials, including clinical pharmacology studies (e.g., dose tolerance, bioavailability, and mechanism of action studies), and early therapeutic studies. It is expected that, in accordance with good medical practice, appropriate precautions against becoming pregnant and exposing a fetus to a potentially dangerous agent during the course of study will be taken by women participating in clinical trials. It is also expected that women will receive adequate counseling about the importance of such precautions, that efforts will be made to be sure that a woman entering a trial is not pregnant at the time the trial begins (i.e., a pregnancy test detecting the beta subunit of the hCG molecule is negative), and that the woman participant is fully informed about the current state of the animal reproduction studies and any other information about the teratogenic potential of the drug. As is the case for all studies carried out under an investigational new drug application (IND), the adequacy of the precautions taken will be considered by FDA in its review of protocols. In situations where enrollment continues over a prolonged period (unlikely for early clinical studies) and significant new information about teratogenicity becomes available, the sponsor has the responsibility to transmit this information quickly to the investigator and to current as well as potential study participants in the informed consent process.

The agency recognizes that this change in FDA's policy will not, by itself, cause drug companies or IRBs to alter restrictions they might impose on the participation of women of childbearing potential. We do not at this time perceive a regulatory basis for requiring routinely that women in general or women of childbearing potential be included in particular trials, such as phase 1 studies. However, as this guideline delineates, careful characterization of drug effects by gender is expected by the agency, and FDA is determined to remove the unnecessary Federal impediment to inclusion of women in the earliest stages of drug development. The agency is confident that the interplay of ethical, social, medical, legal and political forces will allow greater participation of women in the early stages of clinical trials.

In some cases, there may be a basis for requiring participation of women in early studies. When the disease under study is serious and affects women, and especially when a promising drug for the disease is being developed and made available rapidly under FDA's accelerated approval or early access procedures, a case can be made for requiring that women participate in clinical studies at an early stage. When such a drug becomes available under expanded access mechanisms (for example, treatment IND or parallel track) or is marketed rapidly under subpart E procedures (because an effect on survival or irreversible morbidity has been shown in the earliest controlled trials), it is medically important that a representative sample of the entire population likely to receive the drug has been studied, including representatives of both genders. Under these circumstances, clinical protocols should not place unwarranted restrictions on the participation of women. . . .

Guideline for the Study and Evaluation of Gender Differences in the Clinical Evaluation of Drugs

C. Inclusion of Both Genders in Clinical Studies

The patients included in clinical studies should, in general, reflect the population that will receive the drug when it is marketed. For most drugs, therefore, representatives of both genders should be included in clinical trials in numbers adequate to allow detection of clinically significant gender-related differences in drug response. Although it may be reasonable to exclude certain patients at early stages because of characteristics that might make evaluation of therapy more difficult (e.g., patients on concomitant therapy), such exclusions should usually be abandoned as soon as possible in later development so that possible drug-drug and drug-disease interactions can be detected. Thus, for example, there is ordinarily no good reason to exclude women using oral contraceptives or estrogen replacement from trials. Rather, they should be included and differences in responses between them and patients not on such therapy examined. Pharmacokinetic interaction studies (or screening approaches) to look at the interactions resulting from concomitant treatment are also useful.

Ordinarily, patients of both genders should be included in the same trials. This permits direct comparisons of genders within the studies. In some cases, however, it may be appropriate to conduct studies in a single gender, e.g., to evaluate the effects of phases of the menstrual cycle on drug response.

Although clinical or pharmacokinetic data collected during phase 3 may provide evidence of gender-related differences, these data may become available too late to affect the design and dose-selection of the pivotal controlled trials. Inclusion of women in the earliest phases of clinical development, particularly in early pharmacokinetic studies, is, therefore, encouraged so that information on gender differences may be used to refine the design of later trials. Note that the strict limitation on the participation of women of childbearing potential in phase 1 and early phase 2 trials that was imposed by the 1977 guideline entitled, "General Considerations for the Clinical Evaluation of Drugs," has been eliminated. . . .

G. Precautions in Clinical Trials Including Women of Childbearing Potential

Appropriate precautions should be taken in clinical studies to guard against inadvertent exposure of fetuses to potentially toxic agents and to inform subjects and patients of potential risk and the need for precautions. In all cases, the informed consent document and investigator's brochure should include all available information regarding the potential risk of fetal toxicity. If animal reproductive toxicity studies are complete, the results should be presented, with some explanation of their significance in humans. If these studies have not been completed, other pertinent information should be provided, such as a general assessment of fetal toxicity in drugs with related structures or pharmacologic effects. If no relevant information is available, the informed consent should explicitly note the potential for fetal risk.

In general, it is expected that reproductive toxicity studies will be completed before there is large-scale exposure of women of childbearing potential, i.e., usually by the end of phase 2 and before any expanded access program is implemented.

Except in the case of trials intended for the study of drug effects during pregnancy, clinical protocols should also include measures that will minimize the possibility of fetal exposure to the investigational drug. These would ordinarily include providing for the use of a reliable method of contraception (or abstinence) for the duration of drug exposure (which may exceed the length of the study), use of pregnancy testing (beta HCG) to detect unsuspected pregnancy prior to initiation of study treatment, and timing of studies (easier with studies of short duration) to coincide with, or immediately follow, menstruation. Female subjects should be referred to a study physician or other counselor knowledgeable in the selection and use of contraceptive approaches.

H. Potential Effects on Fertility

Where abnormalities of reproductive organs or their function (spermatogenesis or ovulation) have been observed in experimental animals, the decision to include patients of reproductive age in a clinical study should be based on a careful risk-benefit evaluation, taking into account the nature of the abnormalities, the dosage needed to induce them, the consistency of findings in different species, the severity of the illness being treated, the potential importance of the drug, the availability of alternative treatment, and the duration of therapy. Where patients of reproductive potential are included in studies of drugs showing reproductive toxicity in animals, the clinical studies should include appropriate monitoring and/or laboratory studies to allow detection of these effects. Long-term follow-up will usually be needed to evaluate the effects of such drugs in humans.

NOTES AND QUESTIONS

1. The change in policy was published as a "guideline" rather than a regulation. Consequently, its force is merely advisory.

2. Note the language that "We do not at this time perceive a regulatory basis for requiring routinely that women in general or women of childbearing potential be included in particular trials, such as phase 1 studies." Why do you suppose that such a mandate was not promulgated?

3. Under the *Guideline*, sponsors may initiate Phase 1 and Phase 2 studies prior to the completion of complete reproductive toxicity studies. Does this undermine the *Guideline*'s pledge "to remove the unnecessary Federal impediment to inclusion of women in the earliest stages of drug development"? Isn't completion of reproductive toxicity studies necessary to provide information to women who might otherwise consider participating in earlier phase trials?

4. Note that at the end of Section C of the excerpt above, there is recognition of the fact that "[a]lthough clinical or pharmacokinetic data collected during phase 3 may provide evidence of gender-related differences, these data may become available too late to affect the design and dose-selection of the pivotal controlled trials." What are the implications of such a delay on both the development of the phase 3 study and on the ultimate marketing of the drug, assuming that such marketing actually is approved?

[2] NIH

NIH Guidelines on the Inclusion of Women and Minorities as Subjects in Clinical Research
National Institutes of Health
59 FED. REG. 14508, 14509 (1994)

II. Background:

The NIH Revitalization Act of 1993, PL 103-43, signed by President Clinton on June 10, 1993, directs the NIH to establish guidelines for inclusion of women and minorities in clinical research. . . .

III. Policy

A. *Research Involving Human Subjects*

It is the policy of NIH that women and members of minority groups and their subpopulations must be included in all NIH-supported biomedical and behavioral research projects involving human subjects, unless a clear and compelling rationale and justification establishes to the satisfaction of the relevant Institute/Center Director that inclusion is inappropriate with respect to the health of the subjects or the purpose of the research. Exclusion under other circumstances may be made by the Director of NIH, upon the recommendation of an Institute/Center Director based on a compelling rationale and justification. Cost is not an acceptable reason for exclusion except when the study would duplicate data from other sources. Women of childbearing potential should not be routinely excluded from participation in clinical research. All NIH-supported biomedical and behavioral research involving human subjects is defined as clinical research. This policy applies to research subjects of all ages.

The inclusion of women and members of minority groups and their subpopulations must be addressed in developing a research design appropriate to the scientific objectives of the study. The research plan should describe the composition of the proposed study population in terms of gender and racial/ethnic group, and provide a rationale for selection of such subjects. Such a plan should contain a description of the proposed outreach programs for recruiting women and minorities as participants.

B. *Clinical Trials*

Under the statute, when a Phase III clinical trial is proposed, evidence must be reviewed to show whether or not clinically important gender or race/ethnicity differences in the intervention effect are to be expected. This evidence may include, but is not limited to, data derived from prior animal studies, clinical observations, metabolic studies, genetic studies, pharmacology studies, and observational, natural history, epidemiology and other relevant studies.

As such, investigators must consider the following when planning a Phase III clinical trial for NIH support.

If the data from prior studies strongly indicate the existence of significant differences of clinical or public health importance in intervention effect among subgroups (gender and/or racial/ethnic subgroups), the primary question(s) to be addressed by the proposed Phase III trial and the design of that trial must specifically accommodate this. For example, if men and women are thought to respond differently to an intervention, then the Phase III trial must be designed to answer two separate primary questions, one for men and the other for women, with adequate sample size for each.

If the data from prior studies strongly support no significant differences of clinical or public health importance in intervention effect between subgroups, then gender or race/ethnicity will not be required as subject selection criteria. However, the inclusion of gender or racial/ethnic subgroups is still strongly encouraged.

If the data from prior studies neither support strongly nor negate strongly the existence of significant differences of clinical or public health importance in intervention effect between subgroups, then the Phase III trial will be required to include sufficient and appropriate entry of gender and racial/ethnic subgroups, so that valid analysis of the intervention effect in subgroups can be performed. However, the trial will not be required to provide high statistical power for each subgroup.

C. Funding

NIH funding components will not award any grant, cooperative agreement or contract or support any intramural project to be conducted or funded in Fiscal Year 1995 and thereafter which does not comply with this policy. For research awards that are covered by this policy, awardees will report annually on enrollment of women and men, and on the race and ethnicity of research participants.

NOTES AND QUESTIONS

1. Do you agree that cost is never an acceptable reason for excluding women from research? Will the result be that priority will be given to costly "inclusive" projects, thus limiting the number of studies that NIH can fund? *See* Rothenberg, *supra*, at 1235-36.

2. Might there be non-monetary costs to including members of both sexes in some studies? Given the possible differences between how a treatment affects men and women, it might well require more subjects — and thus take more time — to produce a statistically significant result than if members of only one sex were studied. Is there a way to avoid this delay? What would be the consequences of doing most studies initially on only members of one sex, but making

sure that about one-half of all studies are male-only and one-half are female-only?

3. The Funding section of the NIH Guidelines seems to take a more aggressive approach to the inclusion of women than the FDA Guidelines issued at approximately the same time. Can you speculate why this occurred?

4. In 1990, the Office of Research on Women's Health (ORWH) was established within the Office of the Director of NIH. Among its missions are strengthening and enhancing research related to diseases, disorders and conditions that affect women, ensuring that research conducted and supported by NIH adequately addresses issues regarding women's health, and ensuring that women are appropriately represented in biomedical and biobehavioral research supported by NIH, and supporting research on women's health issues. *See* NATIONAL INSTITUTES OF HEALTH, OFFICE OF RESEARCH ON WOMEN'S HEALTH, available at http://www4.od.nih.gov/orwh/.

[3] Further FDA Revisions

In 1998, the FDA issued its most recent set of Guidelines. These required new drug applications (NDAs) to document effectiveness and safety data for demographic subgroups, "specifically, gender, age, and racial subgroups." The commentary indicated that some sponsors had not collected data that could be analyzed by subgroup, and detailed possible penalties for further exclusion from clinical trials of various subgroups, including women of childbearing potential. Thus, for example, it observed that final approval of a new drug could be withheld if the research leading up to the application did not provide analysis by gender.

It explicitly noted that it was not requiring sponsors to conduct additional studies or collect additional data, nor was it requiring the inclusion of a particular number of individuals from specific subgroups in any study or overall. It was simply asking that researchers keep better records on the various categories into which subjects fell (race, gender, etc.) so that additional analyses, focused on the various subgroups, could be conducted. *See* Food and Drug Administration, *Investigational New Drug Applications and New Drug Applications: Final Rule*, 63 FED. REG. 6854-62 (1998).

Six years later, a group of researchers concluded that, "[d]espite this growing body of federal guidelines and laws related to equitable representation of women in clinical research, there is evidence that some industry-sponsored research continues to exclude WCP [women of childbearing potential] from participation." Gary T. Chiodo et al., *Research Ethics: Continued Exclusion of Women in Clinical Research: Industry Winks at the FDA*, 3 MEDICAL RESEARCH L. & POL'Y (BNA) 180 (2004). Chiodo and colleagues describe two clinical studies developed by different pharmaceutical company sponsors, which, they conclude:

are ethically troubling and contradict the FDA's clear guidance regarding the inclusion of WCP in clinical trials. . . . In both cases, the sponsors stated that the reproductive risks were unknown. This statement was a misrepresentation of the data submitted (primarily animal data), which included teratogenicity studies. . . . The sponsors warned investigators that these drugs must be assumed to be teratogenic yet no submitted data supported these assumptions. Moreover, both sponsors have other approved and currently marketed drugs that have known teratogenicity, carry pregnancy-risk category ratings, and advise physicians that reproductive risk may be mitigated by pregnancy testing and reasonable contraceptive efforts. Clearly, the advice to physicians regarding these approved drugs indicates that the sponsors appreciate and accept the autonomy of WCP when it comes to purchasing these products.

Id. What do you think is driving the continued exclusion of women of child-bearing potential from clinical trials?

§ 9.03 JUSTICE AND RACIAL AND ETHNIC MINORITIES

INSTITUTIONAL REVIEW BOARD GUIDEBOOK
Chapter 6, Special Classes of Subjects — Section I. Minorities
U.S. DEPT. OF HEALTH AND HUMAN SERVICES
OFFICE FOR PROTECTION FROM RESEARCH RISKS
(1993)

Introduction

The participation in research by members of racial and ethnic minority groups raises concerns about appropriate levels of inclusion and generalizability of study results; the issues are parallel to those raised with respect to the inclusion of women in studies. In addition, the involvement of minorities raises concerns about the selection of subjects, the possibility of special vulnerability on the part of some prospective subjects, and about consent and the relative strengths or weaknesses of vulnerable groups in the consent process.

IRB Considerations

The federal regulations require the equitable selection of subjects. In addition, NIH requires that applicants for all research grants, cooperative agreements, and contracts involving human subjects include minorities (and women) in study populations "so that research findings can be of benefit to *all* persons at risk of the disease, disorder or condition under study; special emphasis should be placed on the need for inclusion of minorities and women in studies of diseases, disorders and conditions which disproportionately affect them." Investigators must provide a "clear compelling rationale for their exclusion or under-representation." . . .

The inclusion of minorities in research is important, both to ensure that they receive an equal share of the benefits of research and to ensure that they do not bear a disproportionate burden. Most diseases affect all population groups, minority and nonminority alike. For generalizability purposes, investigators must include the widest possible range of population groups. Sometimes, however, minorities are subject to a differential risk. Some research, for example, relates to conditions that specifically affect various minority groups (e.g., sickle cell anemia or Tay Sachs disease), so that involvement of the relevant minority groups is imperative. Other research focuses on characteristics of diseases or effectiveness of therapies in particular populations (e.g., HIV transmission, treatment for hypertension), and may also concern conditions or disorders that disproportionately affect certain racial or ethnic groups. Exclusion or inappropriate representation of these groups, by design or inadvertence, would be unjust. Further, to the extent that participation in research offers direct benefits to the subjects (in HIV research, for example, the receipt of a promising new drug), underrepresentation of minorities denies them, in a systematic way, the opportunity to benefit. . . .

The manner in which subjects are selected bears directly on the problem of inclusion of minorities. The choice of a geographic area for recruitment may affect the representation of racial and ethnic groups in study populations. Also, to the extent that minorities are reliant on public rather than private health care systems, recruitment of subjects from private physicians will tend to exclude minorities and recruitment from public health clinics will tend to over-include them. In fact, recruiting subjects from any health care system assumes that appropriate subjects have access to and exercise their ability to access a health care system, which may contribute to the homogeneity of the study population. Some writers have suggested that investigators change recruitment strategies so that they recruit subjects through community-based institutions such as churches and neighborhood organizations, rather than solely through health care institutions. In many studies, several institutions collaborate, thereby enrolling subjects from different geographic locations. Such collaborations may also provide a mechanism for ensuring appropriate representation of women and minorities in the study population. . . .

Research designs that include diverse study populations are . . . highly desirable. IRBs should require investigators to justify protocols that call for homogeneous study populations. They should also be aware of the implications of various recruiting strategies, and be prepared to suggest alternative recruitment methods so as to ensure an appropriately diverse or focused subject population. In doing so, the IRB should also be aware of the special needs of prospective subjects, such as the provision of child care or transportation.

In addition to ensuring adequate appropriate representation of minorities in study populations (and guarding against inappropriate overburdening of minorities), IRBs must ensure that any special vulnerabilities of subjects are accounted for and handled appropriately. To the extent that prospective minority study populations are also economically or educationally disadvantaged, IRBs should safeguard their rights and welfare by making sure that any possible coercion or undue influence is eliminated (e.g., compensation that is not commensurate with the risk, discomfort, or inconvenience involved, or recruiting in institutional settings where voluntary participation might be compromised).

IRBs should also safeguard the consent process (and, indeed, the entire research relationship) to ensure open and free communication between the researcher and the prospective subject. Consent documents must be written in language easily understandable to subjects; the possibility of illiteracy should be accounted for, as should the need for communicating in foreign languages. The informed consent documents should be available in English and other languages as appropriate to the subject population(s). Foreign language consent documents should be developed using quality control procedures such as translation from English to the other language and then back to English, to ensure that the information is correctly conveyed. The role of cultural norms of subjects should also be addressed. The involvement of representatives from the target population(s) may also be pertinent to IRB review.

IRBs should keep in mind that the goal here is to ensure that minorities share fairly the benefits and burdens of the research enterprise. In offering protection, however, IRBs should avoid paternalism and stereotyping.

Points to Consider

1. Is the subject population appropriately drawn? Will minority subjects likely be appropriately and adequately represented? If not, is the homogeneity of the study population justified?

2. Are subject recruitment strategies appropriate for obtaining a diverse subject population?

3. Have the special needs of prospective subjects been addressed (e.g., child care, transportation)?

4. Has the possibility of undue influence or coercion been eliminated?

5. Does the proposed consent process ensure open and effective communication between the researcher and prospective subjects? Are the consent documents written in language that will be easily accessible to subjects? Are documents in foreign languages necessary? Is foreign language facility on the part of the research staff necessary (both for obtaining consent and conducting the research)?

NIH Guidelines on the Inclusion of Women and Minorities as Subjects in Clinical Research
National Institutes of Health
59 FED. REG. 14,508, 14,509 (1994)

D. Issues Concerning Appropriate Representation of Minority Groups and Subpopulations in All Research Involving Human Subjects Including Phase III Clinical Trials

While the inclusion of minority subpopulations in research is a complex and challenging issue, it nonetheless provides the opportunity for researchers to collect data on subpopulations where knowledge gaps exist. Researchers must consider the inclusion of subpopulations in all stages of research design. In meeting this objective, they should be aware of concurrent research that addresses specific subpopulations, and consider potential collaborations which may result in complementary subpopulation data.

At the present time, there are gaps in baseline and other types of data necessary for research involving certain minority groups and/or subpopulations of minority groups. In these areas, it would be appropriate for researchers to obtain such data, including baseline data, by studying a single minority group.

It would also be appropriate for researchers to test survey instruments, recruitment procedures, and other methodologies used in the majority or other population(s) with the objective of assessing their feasibility, applicability, and cultural competence/relevance to a particular minority group or subpopulation. This testing may provide data on the validity of the methodologies across groups. Likewise, if an intervention has been tried in the majority population and not in certain minority groups, it would be appropriate to assess the intervention effect on a single minority group and compare the effect to that obtained in the majority population. These types of studies will advance scientific research and assist in closing knowledge gaps.

A complex issue arises over how broad or narrow the division into different subgroups should be, given the purpose of the research. Division into many racial/ethnic subgroups is tempting in view of the cultural and biological differences that exist among these groups and the possibility that some of these differences may in fact impact in some way upon the scientific question. Alternatively, from a practical perspective, a limit has to be placed on the number of such subgroups that can realistically be studied in detail for each intervention that is researched. The investigator should clearly address the rationale for inclusion or exclusion of subgroups in terms of the purpose of the research. Emphasis should be placed upon inclusion of subpopulations in which the disease manifests itself or the intervention operates in an appreciable different way. Investigators should report the subpopulations included in the study.

An important issue is the appropriate representation of minority groups in research, especially in geographical locations which may have limited numbers of racial/ethnic population groups available for study. The investigator must address this issue in terms of the purpose of the research, and other factors, such as the size of the study, relevant characteristics of the disease, disorder or condition, and the feasibility of making a collaboration or consortium or other arrangements to include minority groups. A justification is required if there is limited representation. Peer reviewers and NIH staff will consider the justification in their evaluations of the project.

NIH interprets the statute in a manner that leads to feasible and real improvements in the representativeness of different racial/ethnic groups in research and places emphasis on research in those subpopulations that are disproportionately affected by certain diseases or disorders.

NOTES AND QUESTIONS

1. A 2002 issue of the *New England Journal of Medicine* contained two articles suggesting that blacks do not respond to antihypertensive therapies as well as whites. That and other data led an editorial commentator in the same issue to observe that: "Racial and ethnic differences in drug responses have now been well described for a range of drugs and reflect genetic differences, environmental differences (including shared cultural and dietary habits), and fundamental differences in the pathogenesis of diseases." Alastair Wood, *Racial Differences in the Response to Drugs — Pointers to Genetic Differences*, 344 NEW ENG. J. MED. 1393 (2001). Similarly, studies have found that Asians metabolize the substance propranolol (another drug used to treat hypertension) at faster rates. *See* Paul Cotton, *Is There Still Too Much Extrapolation From Data on Middle-aged White Men?* 265 JAMA 1049 (1990). See also articles cited in Barbara A. Noah, *The Participation of Underrepresented Minorities in Clinical Research*, 29 AM. J.L. & MED. 221, 233 n. 74 (2003).

2. Is it appropriate to conduct research specifically focused on race or ethnicity? In a 2001 editorial in the *New England Journal of Medicine*, Dr. Robert Schwartz argued that "attributing differences in a biologic end point to race is not only imprecise but also of no proven value in treating an individual patient." Emphasizing that "race is a social construct, not a scientific classification," he argued that race-based research "mistakenly assumes an inherent biologic difference between black-skinned and white-skinned people. It falls into error by attributing a complex physiological or clinical phenomenon to arbitrary aspects of external appearance." Robert S. Schwartz, *Racial Profiling in Medical Research*, 344 N. ENG. J. MED. 1392 (2001). Similarly, Erik Lillquist and Charles Sullivan write that race, "even when defined solely by ancestry, is generally meaningless as an independent concept in genetics: there is no set of genes that can tell us whether an individual is or is not a member of a particular race." Erik Lillquist and Charles A. Sullivan, *The Law and Genetics of Racial Profiling in Medicine*, 39 HARV. C.R.-C.L. L. REV. 391, 409 (2004). In fact, they point out, "with only a few exceptions, the variation *within* a race for a given trait is

much greater than the variation *across* races." *Id.* For these and other reasons, they suggest that "[c]omplete exclusion of racial groups from [clinical] trials based on race has little merit." They give the example of the African American Heart Failure Trial, a study designed to evaluate the efficacy of BiDil as a treatment for heart failure in African Americans:

> While there may be preliminary data suggesting that BiDil is more effective in African Americans than whites, the reasons for these differences are unclear. One report suggests that African Americans may "have a greater deficiency of nitric oxide generation that is restored by BiDil." Assuming such a biochemical pathway is the reason, a number of white patients, as well as Asian patients, may share the deficiency that BiDil restores. Simply because, on average, such deficiencies are less frequent among white (or perhaps Asian) patients does not mean they do not exist. Instead, . . . they almost assuredly *do* exist, just in lower frequencies.

Id. at 478. Do you agree that it is inappropriate to design a clinical trial for members of particular racial groups if those individuals are, "on average," more likely than members of other races to benefit from the drug being studied? Do studies that are "race-based in the sense that race is a criteria for admission" violate 42 U.S.C. § 1981, which prohibits racial discrimination in the formation of contracts? If the NIH funds such a study, or if the FDA authorizes the investigational use of a drug solely for members of a particular race, would those agencies run afoul of either the Equal Protection clause or Title VI of the Civil Rights Act of 1964, which prohibits race discrimination in federally funded programs? *See id.* at 462-65 (suggesting numerous legal problems with "racial profiling" in clinical research).

3. Preliminary results in the BiDil study were so successful that the data safety and monitoring board halted the research, reasoning that "it would be unethical to continue giving some patients a placebo because those getting the drug were living significantly longer." Andrew Pollack, *Drug Approved for Heart Failure in Black Patients*, N.Y. TIMES, July 20, 2004. Would including whites and Asians in the study population have made it more difficult to demonstrate this result? Is the answer to that question relevant to assessing the appropriateness of limiting the study to African Americans?

4. A 2003 issue of the *New England Journal of Medicine* contains a series of articles debating race-based clinical research. *See* Esteban González Burchard et al., *The Importance of Race and Ethnic Background in Biomedical Research and Clinical Practice,* 348 N. ENG. J. MED. 1170-1175 (2003) (arguing that evidence of race-correlated gene variants exists and that only by recording race can racially biased health policy and practices be uncovered); Richard S. Cooper et al., *Race and Genomics,* 348 N. ENG. J. MED. 1166-1170 (2003) (finding little evidence that the risk of common diseases is determined by race-correlated gene variants and arguing that the potential for abuse is a reason to disregard race in genetic and medical studies); Elizabeth G. Phimister, *Medicine and the Racial*

Divide, 348 N. ENG. J. MED. 1081-1082 (2003) (concluding that it would be "unwise to abandon the practice of recording race when we have barely begun to understand the architecture of the human genome and its implications for new strategies for the identification of gene variants that protect against, or confer susceptibility to, common diseases and modify the effects of drugs.").

5. There is substantial evidence that whites and minorities enroll in clinical research at different rates. Gifford and colleagues, utilizing nationally representative data from the HIV Costs and Services Utilization Study, concluded that there were marked race-based disparities among patients with HIV in terms of their enrollment in both medication trials and expanded access programs. They estimated that, in 1996, forty-four percent of all AIDS cases reported to CDC were by whites and thirty-seven percent were non-Hispanic blacks, yet forty-nine percent of HIV cases receiving treatment involved whites and only thirty-three percent involved blacks. More dramatically, sixty-two percent of patients receiving care who were enrolled in medication trials where white, while only twenty-three percent were black. Among the group of patients who had ever used experimental medications, sixty-nine percent were white and only seventeen percent were black. The study also found that non-Hispanic blacks were more likely than other patients to withdraw from or stop participating in trials at an approximately eighteen-month follow-up time.

> The authors concluded that most of the differences in participation rates were attributable to differences in the rates at which experimental medications were sought. They found that fewer than half as many black patients as white patients attempted to obtain experimental HIV medications. This suggested to them that there is less awareness and a more widespread negative attitude about research in minority communities. However, even among the group of patients who sought experimental medications, non-Hispanic whites received them more often than non-Hispanic blacks (77% vs. 69%).

Allen L. Gifford et al., *Participation in Research and Access to Experimental Treatments by HIV-Infected Patients,* 346 N. ENG. J. MED. 1373-1382 (2002).

6. What conclusions might be drawn from these data? In an editorial accompanying the study, Talmadge E. King suggested that

> [p]roviders who were experienced in the treatment of HIV infection (and were therefore most likely to be involved in or to know about clinical trials) cared for most of the patients in this cohort. Thus, one inference might be that either overt prejudices or subconscious perceptions on the part of these physicians influenced access to HIV-related clinical trials.

Talmadge E. King, *Racial Disparities in Clinical Trials,* 356 N. ENG. J. MED 1400 (2002). King suggested that health care providers' prejudicial attitudes toward minority groups — especially blacks — might influence treatment decisions and result in patient mistrust of the physician and a disinclination to comply with treatment or to enter a clinical trial.

King also observed that researchers often would intentionally avoid recruiting members of minority groups for clinical trials because of fears of poor compliance. He notes that there were other impediments to participation by such patients (e.g., homelessness, lack of transportation, limited income, lack of child care, active drug use, limited English fluency or health literacy). Although many of those limits could readily be overcome, he argues, it is rare that clinical trials are designed to deal with these issues. Finally, he states that researchers may "have a narrow view of the sort of person who makes a good participant in an HIV-related clinical trial: a white, college-educated, employed, housed, homosexual man. As a result, they have a more difficult time recruiting patients for such trials." *Id.*; *see also* Wafaa El-Sadr and Linnea Capps, *The Challenge of Minority Recruitment in Clinical Trials for AIDS*, 267 JAMA 954 (1992).

Concerns regarding compliance are not limited to HIV-related research, as sponsors and investigators across the board put a premium on expediency and efficiency at a minimum cost. Consequently, they discourage recruitment of marginalized populations, who are assumed to be less likely to adhere to dosing schedules or nutritional requirements, or who may have language or transportation barriers or fewer childcare or other resources, all of which may reduce the likelihood of protocol compliance. *See* Noah, *supra*, at 226-228.

7. Insurance considerations also contribute to the under-participation in research by minorities. While clinical trials frequently offer free or reduced cost access to experimental treatments, they typically do not cover the costs of necessary hospitalizations or routine care associated with the research. Moreover, those without insurance are less likely to utilize primary care physicians, who often play key roles in facilitating clinical trial participation. *See* Noah, *supra*.

8. Giselle Corbie-Smith and colleagues conducted two studies examining African Americans' attitudes toward clinical trials. The first study involved a series of focus group interviews conducted in 1997 with African American adults identified in outpatient settings in an urban public hospital. The participants expressed concerns that: (a) African Americans historically having been used as "guinea pigs" in research, and (b) even if there were positive results from research, African Americans would not necessarily benefit from them because of racial discrimination and poverty. Respondents drew parallels with the clinical care they received in public health care facilities, noting that the prevalence of inexperienced young physicians and interns was like "being experimented on." They generally believed that the purpose of consent documents was to protect hospitals and doctors from legal responsibility rather than to inform patients and research subjects about the nature of treatment, and that lawyers and doctors colluded to make legal remedies impossible. *See* Giselle Corbie-Smith et al., *Attitudes and Beliefs of African Americans Toward Participation*

in Medical Research, 14 J. GEN. INTERN. MED. 537 (1999).

Focus group members suggested that there is a need for more honest and respectful communication by physicians and other research personnel, and that researchers should recognize the desire to receive information from multiple points of view (for example, by ensuring that there is time to go to the library and to talk with friends or family members). They also emphasized the value of video presentations about procedures prior to the completion of the consent process. Respondents requested assurance that the physicians conducting research would be available for questions for the duration of the study, and that early education in elementary and secondary schools include information about why research is important and how science is conducted. *See id.* at 539-542.

Corbie-Smith and other colleagues followed up on the focus group study with a national telephone survey examining the knowledge, attitudes and beliefs of Americans toward physicians and participation in clinical research. This second study focused on distinctions between African American and white respondents, where the principal outcome measure was an index of distrust. The researchers determined that African American respondents were far more likely than white respondents not to trust that their physician would fully explain research participation (41.7% vs. 23.4%), less likely to believe that they could freely ask their physician questions (15.2% to 7.6%), more likely to disagree that their physician would not ask them to become involved in research if the doctor thought it would harm them (37.2% vs. 19.7%), and more likely to say that they believed that their physicians sometimes exposed them to unnecessary risks (45.5% vs. 34.8%). African Americans also were more likely to believe that someone like them would be used as a guinea pig without his or her consent (51.9% vs. 7.2%), that physicians often prescribed medication as a way of experimenting on people without consent (62.8% vs. 38.4%), and that their physicians had, in fact, given them treatment as part of an experiment without their permission (24.5% vs. 8.3%). *See* Giselle Corbie-Smith et al., *Distrust, Race and Research*, 162 ARCH. INTERN. MED. 2458 (2002).

In speculating on the results of the survey, the authors indicated that (a) researchers should think about recruiting African-Americans for clinical trials as an ongoing process of engagement, dialogue and feedback; (b) repeated interactions in long-term relationships not linked to recruiting subjects are necessary, and (c) it would be wise to include members of the target community in study design and in planning and evaluating recruitment strategies. *Id.* at 2462. [For further discussion of the inclusion of study communities in research review, see Chapter 17, at page 710.]

10. In 2000, the federal Minority Health and Health Disparities Research and Education Act established the National Center on Minority Health and Health Disparities and charged it with conducting and supporting basic, clinical, social science and behavioral research directed to promoting minority health and eliminating health disparities. One of its missions is to increase the participation of minorities and other medically underserved populations in clinical

research. *See* NATIONAL INSTITUTES OF HEALTH, NATIONAL CENTER ON MINORITY HEALTH AND HEALTH DISPARITIES, available at www.nih.gov/about/almanac/organ-ization/NCMHD.htm.

Chapter 10

CONFIDENTIALITY

Medical researchers often have access to sensitive personal information, and the disclosure of this information may entail significant personal, legal, or economic risks for subjects or their family members. This chapter examines policies governing the protection of information generated during the course of research, as well as restrictions on researchers' use or disclosure of medical information obtained from clinical records or other sources.

§ 10.01 OVERVIEW OF MEDICAL CONFIDENTIALITY

[A] Confidentiality as an Ethical Principle

THE HIPPOCRATIC OATH

Whatever in connection with my professional practice or not in connection with it I see or hear in the life of men which ought not to be spoken abroad I will not divulge as recommending that all such should be kept secret.

CURRENT OPINIONS OF THE JUDICIAL COUNCIL OF THE AMERICAN MEDICAL ASSOCIATION CANON 5.05

[T]he information disclosed to a physician during the course of the relationship between physician and patient is confidential to the greatest possible degree. . . . The physician should not reveal confidential communications or information without the express consent of the patient, unless required to do so by law.

PRINCIPLES OF BIOMEDICAL ETHICS TOM L. BEAUCHAMP & JAMES F. CHILDRESS 306-08 (5th ed. 2001)

We can easily imagine a society that does not recognize any obligations of confidentiality. Indeed, many of the goods of medicine and research could be realized without rules of confidentiality. On what basis, then, can we justify a system of extensive protections of confidentiality? We believe that three types of argument justify (prima facie) rules to protect confidentiality: (1) consequence-based arguments, (2) rights-based autonomy and privacy arguments, and (3) fidelity-based arguments. These arguments also address legitimate exceptions to rules of confidentiality.

Consequentialist arguments. If patients could not trust physicians to conceal some information from third parties, patients would be reluctant to disclose full and forthright information or to authorize a complete examination and a full battery of tests. Without such information, physicians would not be able to make accurate diagnoses and prognoses or to recommend the best course of treatment. Although such consequentialist arguments establish a need for some rule of confidentiality, consequentialists disagree among themselves about which rule should be adopted, and about the rule's scope and weight.

Consequentialist arguments also support exceptions to the rule of confidentiality. In *Tarasoff* [*see infra*, page 447], both the majority opinion, which affirmed that therapists have an obligation to warn third parties of their patients' threatened violence, and the dissenting opinion, which denied such an obligation, used consequentialist arguments. Their debate hinged on different predictions and assessments of the consequences of (1) a rule that *required* therapists to breach confidentiality by warning intended victims of a client's threatened violence, and (2) a rule that *allowed* therapists to breach confidentiality in the face of some peril to a member of the public. The majority opinion pointed to the victims who would be saved, such as the young woman who had been killed in this case, and contended that a professional's obligation to disclose information to third parties could be justified by the need to protect such potential victims. By contrast, the minority opinion contended that if it were common practice to override obligations of confidentiality, the fiduciary relation between the patient and doctor would soon erode and collapse. Patients would lose confidence in psychotherapists and would refrain from disclosing information crucial to effective therapy. As a result, violent assaults would increase because dangerous persons would refuse to seek psychiatric aid or to disclose relevant information, such as their violent fantasies. Hence, the debate about different rules of confidentiality hinges in part on empirical claims about which rule more effectively protects the interests of other persons.

In the case of other legally accepted and mandated exceptions to confidentiality — such as requirements to report contagious diseases, child abuse, and gunshot wounds — no substantial evidence exists that these requirements have either reduced prospective patients' willingness to seek treatment and to cooperate with physicians or significantly impaired the physician-patient relationship. Even in the aggregate, such reports are relatively isolated events with little effect on others' conduct.

A consequentialist justification for *nonabsolute* rules of confidentiality therefore has strong support. However, to accept this justification is not to overlook the fact that, when physicians breach medical confidentiality, they infringe their patients' rights whenever they have made a promise to keep confidentiality and their relationship was cemented by trust. Such an infringement has negative effects for confiders, and those effects can be outweighed only by substantial threats to others, to the public interest, or to the patient. A physician who breaks confidence cannot ignore the potential for eroding the system of medical confidentiality, trust, and fidelity. A consequentialist justification for breaching confidentiality can thus meet its own high standards only if it considers all such consequences.

Arguments from autonomy and privacy rights. A second approach to the justification of rules and rights of confidentiality looks to respect for autonomy and privacy. The argument for privacy in the previous section can here be extended to confidentiality, breaches of which have often been viewed primarily as violations of privacy and personal autonomy. It is true that such breaches acquire a special importance when disclosures of information subject a patient to legal jeopardy, loss of friends and lovers, emotional devastation, discrimination, loss of employment, and the like. However, an argument that uses an autonomy or privacy rationale does not appeal to these consequences. The thesis is that the values of the exercise of autonomy and privacy themselves support the rules of confidentiality.

Fidelity-based arguments. Another obligation . . . is fidelity in the physician-patient relationship. The physician's obligation to live up to the patient's reasonable expectations of privacy and confidentiality is one way to specify the general obligation of fidelity. Medical practice requires the patient to disclose private and sensitive information to the physician, and a failure of fidelity thus tears at a significant dimension of the patient-physician relationship. Part of the binding force of confidentiality derives from the health care professional's implicit or explicit promise to the person seeking help. For example, if the professional's public oath or the accepted code of professional ethics pledges confidentiality, and if the professional does not expressly disavow confidentiality to the patient, the patient has a right to expect it.

Like the first argument, the second and third arguments do not support absolute rules of confidentiality. When rules of confidentiality are used as absolute shields, they can eventuate in outrageous and preventable injuries and losses. The best approach is to treat rules of confidentiality as prima facie in ethics as in law. However, we will need a proper understanding of the circumstances under which other obligations validly override obligations of confidentiality.

[B] Legal Sources of Medical Confidentiality

[1] State Laws

INFORMATION PRIVACY LAW
DANIEL J. SOLOVE & MARC ROTENBERG
207-09 (2003)

Privacy Torts. . . . Many courts have found that the disclosure of medical information can give rise to a claim for public disclosure of private facts. In *Urbaniak v. Newton* (Cal. App. 1991), the court held that the disclosure of a patient's HIV status was "clearly a 'private fact' of which the disclosure may 'be offensive and objectionable to a reasonable [person] of ordinary sensibilities.'" *See also Susan S. v. Israels* (Cal. Ct. App. 1997) (public disclosure action for disclosure of mental health records). In *Doe v. Mills* (Mich. App. 1995), a group of abortion protestors held up large signs displaying the names of the plaintiffs outside the abortion clinic where they were getting abortions. The court held that the plaintiffs could bring a claim for public disclosure. . . . Likewise, in *Y.G. & L.G. v. Jewish Hospital of St. Louis* (Mo. App. 1990), the court held that the plaintiffs had a viable public disclosure claim against a television station that broadcast the plaintiffs' involvement in a hospital's *in vitro* fertilization plan: "The *in vitro* program and its success may well have been matters of public interest, but the identity of the plaintiffs participating in the program was, we conclude, a private matter."

Tort Law Regulation of Patient-Physician Confidentiality. In addition to the privacy torts, a number of states recognize tort liability for instances where physicians disclose a patient's medical information. . . .

Research Disclosure Laws. A number of states regulate the use of medical data for research purposes. For example, California generally prohibits non-consensual disclosure of alcohol and drug abuse data but permits such non-consensual disclosure for the purpose of conducting research provided that the individual cannot be identified. *See* Cal. Health & Safety Code § 11977.

Medical Confidentiality Laws. Many states have specific statutes providing civil and criminal protection against the disclosure of medical information. Some laws restrict disclosure of medical data by particular entities: government agencies, HMOs, insurance companies, employers, pharmacists, and health data clearinghouses. Other laws prohibit the disclosure by any entity of particular types of medical data, such as AIDS/HIV, alcohol or drug abuse, mental health, and genetic information. *See, e.g.*, CAL. HEALTH & SAFETY CODE § 199.21 (prohibiting disclosure of HIV test results); N.Y. PUB. HEALTH L. § 17 (prohibiting the nonconsensual disclosure of medical records of minors relating to sexually transmitted diseases and abortion; even the disclosure to parents is pro-

hibited without consent); PA. CONS. STAT. § 1690.108 (prohibiting the disclosure of all records prepared during alcohol or drug abuse treatment). . . .

Comprehensive Health Privacy Laws. Most states do not have a comprehensive law governing medical privacy. According to the Health Privacy Project
Report, only three states have a comprehensive law: Hawaii, Rhode Island,
and Wisconsin.

NOTES AND QUESTIONS

1. It is a common misperception that the physician-patient privilege guarantees the privacy of medical information. In fact, the scope of the physician-
patient privilege is quite narrow. First, the privilege does not apply outside the
context of a judicial proceeding; "it is only a testimonial privilege, not a general
obligation to maintain confidentiality." BARRY R. FURROW ET AL., HEALTH LAW:
CASES, MATERIALS AND PROBLEMS 323 (5th ed. 2004). Second, the privilege does
not exist in all jurisdictions, and, where it does exist, it is subject to numerous
exceptions and is easily waived. *See id.*

2. State-law confidentiality protections are not absolute. All states have
statutes that require physicians to report certain types of patient information
to the police or public health authorities, including gunshot or knife wounds, *see,
e.g.*, N.Y. PENAL LAW § 265.25, HIV infection, *see e.g.*, ALA. CODE § 22-11A-2, and
suspected child abuse, *see, e.g.*, FLA. STAT. ANN. § 39.201. In addition, physicians
have long had a duty to warn family members of patients who are diagnosed
with contagious diseases. *See, e.g.*, Skillings v. Allen, 173 N.W. 663 (Minn. 1919)
(scarlet fever). In many states, this duty to warn has been extended to other
types of risks. *See, e.g.*, Tarasoff v. Regents of the University of California, 551
P.2d 334 (Cal. 1976) (finding that, when a patient makes a credible threat of violence against an identifiable individual, a therapist has a duty to breach confidentiality and exercise reasonable care to warn the potential victim); Safer v.
Pack, 677 A.2d 1188 (N.J. Super. 1996) (suggesting that physicians may have a
duty to warn family about patients' genetic diseases if the information can help
the family members avert serious harm).

3. For a complete discussion of rules of privilege and confidentiality, see FAY
A. ROSOVSKY, CONSENT TO TREATMENT: A PRACTICAL GUIDE (2003).

[2] Federal Law

Until recently, the confidentiality of medical information was primarily a
matter of state law. That changed in April 2003, when privacy regulations
promulgated under the Health Insurance Portability and Accountability Act of
1996 (HIPAA) went into effect. *See* 45 C.F.R. Parts 160-164. The HIPAA privacy
regulations provide broad confidentiality protections to "individually identifiable
health information" maintained by any "health plan," "health care clearing-

house," or "health care provider" that processes or transmits health care information electronically in certain types of insurance-related transactions. Under the regulations, health care information may be used without consent for "treatment, payment, and health care operations," but in most cases it may not be used or disclosed for other purposes without obtaining the permission of the individual who is the subject of the information. Exceptions to the confidentiality requirements, however, ensure that HIPAA will not interfere with most of the state-law disclosure obligations discussed above. For a concise summary of the complex regulatory requirements, see SOLOVE & ROTENBERG, *supra*, at 210-17.

HIPAA does not authorize individuals to sue for damages based on a violation of the regulatory requirements. Instead, the regulations provide for criminal penalties and civil fines. However, some commentators believe that, despite the absence of a private right of action, the rules "are likely to be adopted by state common law courts to establish a national minimum standard for liability for breach of confidentiality under state law." Peter Winn, *Confidentiality in Cyberspace: The HIPAA Privacy Rules and the Common Law*, 33 RUTGERS L.J. 617, 619 (2002).

In addition to HIPAA, a handful of other federal statutes protect the confidentiality of specific types of medical information. *See, e.g.*, 42 U.S.C. § 290dd-2 (protecting the confidentiality of substance abuse treatment records).

§ 10.02 CONFIDENTIALITY ISSUES IN RESEARCH

[A] Maintaining the Confidentiality of Research Data

[1] General Issues

45 C.F.R. § 46.111

(a) In order to approve research covered by this policy the IRB shall determine that all of the following requirements are satisfied:

... (7) When appropriate, there are adequate provisions to protect the privacy of subjects and to maintain the confidentiality of data.

IRB GUIDEBOOK
Chapter 3D
U.S. DEPT. OF HEALTH AND HUMAN SERVICES
OFFICE FOR PROTECTION FROM RESEARCH RISKS
(1993)

A major set of concerns about confidentiality pertains to the methods used to ensure that information obtained by researchers about their subjects is not improperly divulged. Perhaps because the creation and handling of confidential records is routine in medical institutions, discussions of confidentiality as a special ethical responsibility of researchers have been more prominent in the social sciences than in the biomedical sciences. Nevertheless, the need for confidentiality exists in virtually all studies in which data are collected about identified subjects. It is in the interest of researchers — and essential to the conduct of research on sensitive topics — that researchers be able to offer subjects some assurance of confidentiality. These assurances should be given honestly, which sometimes requires the researcher and the IRB to make explicit provisions for preventing breaches of confidentiality.

In most research, assuring confidentiality is only a matter of following some routine practices: substituting codes for identifiers, removing face sheets (containing such items as names and addresses) from survey instruments containing data, properly disposing of computer sheets and other papers, limiting access to identified data, impressing on the research staff the importance of confidentiality, and storing research records in locked cabinets. Most researchers are familiar with the routine precautions that should be taken to maintain the confidentiality of data. More elaborate procedures may be needed in some studies, either to give subjects the confidence they need to participate and answer questions honestly, or to enable researchers to offer strong, truthful assurances of confidentiality. Such elaborate procedures may be particularly necessary for studies in which data are collected on sensitive matters such as sexual behavior or criminal activities.

In studies where subjects are selected because of a sensitive, stigmatizing, or illegal characteristic (e.g., persons who have sexually abused children, sought treatment in a drug abuse program, or who have tested positive for HIV), keeping the identity of participants confidential may be as or more important than keeping the data obtained about the participants confidential. In such instances, any written record linking subjects to the study can create a threat to confidentiality. Having the subjects of these studies sign consent forms may increase the risk of a breach of confidentiality, because the consent form itself constitutes a record, complete with signature, that identifies particular individuals of the group studied. The Federal Policy allows IRBs to waive the requirement for the investigator to obtain a signed consent form where it will be the only record linking subjects to the research, and where a breach of confidentiality presents the principal risk of harm that might result from the research. FDA regulations allow IRBs to waive the signed consent form requirement only when the research presents no more than minimal risk and involves procedures that do not normally require consent when performed outside the research context. If both FDA regulations and the Federal Policy apply to a protocol, the IRB must meet the requirements of both. In this instance, documentation of informed consent can be waived only if the consent form is the sole record linking subjects to the research, the research involves minimal risk, breach of confidentiality is the principal risk of harm and the procedure involved in the research is one that does not normally require consent when performed outside the research context. (Note that the foregoing waiver provisions apply to documentation of informed consent and not waiver of the requirement to obtain informed consent.) . . .

For studies in which the data to be obtained concern illegal or stigmatizing activities but which are not eligible for . . . statutory shields against subpoena [these statutory shields are discussed *infra*, at page 452], careful attention should be given to a series of decisions related to confidentiality: (1) whether the researcher will record subject identifiers at all (including on consent forms); (2) if identifiers are to be collected, whether they will be retained after the data are coded; (3) if identifiers are not destroyed, how are they to be maintained; and (4) what subjects should be told about these matters as part of the informed consent process. Some researchers enlist a third party (sometimes in another country) to act as a custodian of keys to coded identifiers or lists of participants. This approach may provide some protection for the data, but may expose the researcher to legal risks. Where such steps are contemplated, investigators should seek competent legal advice regarding the advisability of such arrangements.

Clearly, different types of studies entail different confidentiality problems. A variety of methods for protecting confidentiality are available for different situations, including situations in which there is a danger of deductive identification of otherwise anonymous subjects on the basis of separate elements of data (e.g., birth date, occupation, and zip code). A substantial and highly specialized literature has developed on methods for safeguarding confidentiality. Among the available methods for assuring confidentiality are statistical techniques and physical or computerized methods for maintaining the security of stored data. The more sensitive the data being collected, the more important it is for the researcher and the IRB to be familiar with the state of the art in protecting confidentiality.

NOTES AND QUESTIONS

1. Publication of research results can sometimes lead to breaches of subject confidentiality. One survey conducted in 1991 found that only seven out of seventy-five journals that publish case reports required informed consent for publication from the subjects of the reports, and that only thirteen of the journals had written confidentiality rules. *See* Magne Nylenna & Povl Riis, *Identification of Patients in Medical Publications: Need for Informed Consent*, 302 BRIT. MED.

J. 1182 (1991); for further discussion of case reports, see Chapter 3, at page 108. In a 1998 study, one hundred thirty-one journals reported that they do not obtain informed consent for the publication of pedigree diagrams, which provide information that can sometimes reveal the identity of the individuals depicted in the diagrams. Of the forty-three journals that did obtain consent to publication of pedigrees, only twenty-eight percent obtained consent from all of the family members depicted in the pedigree. See Jeffrey R. Botkin et al., *Privacy and Confidentiality in the Publication of Pedigrees: A Survey of Investigators and Biomedical Journals*, 279 JAMA 1808 (1998). Other than pedigree studies, when else might research generate personal information about individuals who are not participating in the study? These issues, including the question of when such nonparticipants should be considered "human subjects" under the regulations, are examined further in Chapter 17, in the context of genetics research. See Chapter 17, at page 705.

2. Private parties sometimes seek access to research data in connection with civil litigation. In such situations, Rule 26 of the Federal Rules of Civil Procedure directs courts to "balance privacy interests of individuals whose identities may be disclosed in the litigation against the parties' interests in the administration of justice; Rule 26 allows the courts to fashion creative protective orders that permit necessary discovery while limiting infringements on privacy." Lawrence O. Gostin, *Health Information Privacy*, 80 CORNELL L. REV. 451, 502 (1995). When might parties plausibly seek nonpublic data about human subjects from biomedical researchers? Consider the case of Dr. Sheldon Zink, a University of Pennsylvania medical anthropologist conducting ethnographic research on the Abiomed Artificial Heart clinical trial. After a patient in the trial died, a lawsuit was initiated, and a subpoena was issued for Dr. Zink's research materials. The parties seeking the materials hoped to find "evidence that the patient had been aware of the risks of an experimental transplant." Katie Wilson, *Subpoena of Confidential Research: Implications for Informed Consent*, ASBH EXCHANGE, Fall 2003, at 5, available at http://www.asbh.org/resources/exchange/2003/ASBXFal3.pdf. In 1993, Rik Scarce, a sociologist, was jailed for six months after refusing to comply with a subpoena requesting confidential information from a study on environmental activists. See id. (observing that cases like Scarce's suggest that "[s]ome researchers are promising human subjects a confidentiality they can guarantee only if the researchers are willing to go to jail"). An important mechanism for protecting research data from subpoenas, known as a "Certificate of Confidentiality," is discussed in the next section of this chapter.

3. The federal Freedom of Information Act (FOIA) gives the public the right to obtain access to information held by federal agencies. See 5 U.S.C. § 552. Although an exemption to FOIA protects "personnel and medical files and similar files the disclosures of which would constitute a clearly unwarranted invasion of personal privacy," id. at § 552(b)(6), the exemption is not absolute. Instead, "the agency itself has the discretion, not a duty, to withhold disclosure. Further, the judgment of the agency is subject to judicial review under an

unpredictable balancing test that is not always favorable to the individual's assertion of privacy." Gostin, *supra*, at 502-03. FOIA requests can be used not only for research data directly created by federal agencies, but also for any data that were created in a federally funded study if those data have been used to support the creation of federal rules and policies. *See* OMB Circular A-110, *Uniform Administrative Requirements for Grants and Agreements with Institutions of Higher Education, Hospitals, and Other Non-Profit Organizations*, 64 FED. REG. 54926, Oct. 8, 1999; *see also* Richard Shelby, *Accountability and Transparency: Public Access to Federally Funded Research Data*, 37 HARV. J. LEGIS. 369 (2000) (describing the history and implications of OMB Circular A-110). Is it appropriate to give the public access to research data generated through public funding? Aside from privacy concerns, why else might investigators be reluctant to disclose raw research data?

4. Most states protect the confidentiality of hospital quality assurance (or "peer review") committees' proceedings in at least some circumstances. *See* FURROW ET AL., *supra* at 216. "While IRBs serve a different function from traditional peer review committees, these protections may apply to IRBs if the state's peer review statute is broad enough. If this is the case, the protections afforded peer review may shield IRBs and their members from liability — as well as shield IRB records and documents from discovery or admission into evidence." Mary R. Anderlik & Nanette Elster, *Lawsuits Against IRBs: Accountability or Incongruity?* 29 J. L. MED. & ETHICS 220, 225 (2001); *see also* Doe v. Illinois Masonic Medical Center, 696 N.E.2d 707 (Ill. Ct. App. 1st Dist. 1998) (interpreting state Medical Studies Act to protect the confidentiality of IRB records). Despite these legal protections, some IRBs have voluntarily decided to make all of their meetings open to the public. *See* Jesse A. Goldner, *An Overview of Legal Controls on Human Experimentation and the Regulatory Implications of Taking Professor Katz Seriously*, 38 ST. LOUIS U.L.J. 63, 109-10 (1993). Why do you think some IRBs choose to open their meetings while others do not? What are the advantages and drawbacks to treating IRB deliberations as confidential?

[2] Certificates of Confidentiality

As explained in the previous sections, existing law permits, or even requires, the disclosure of research data in a variety of circumstances. However, researchers who want to provide additional protection for subjects' identifiable records have an option: they can obtain a "certificate of confidentiality" from the Secretary of DHHS.

United States Code, Title 42, Public Health and Welfare
Section 6A: The Public Health Service, General Powers and Duties
42 U.S.C. § 241(D): Research and Investigations Generally

The Secretary may authorize persons engaged in biomedical, behavioral, clinical, or other research (including research on mental health, including research on the use and effect of alcohol or other psychoactive drugs) to protect the privacy of individuals who are the subject of such research by withholding from all persons not connected with the conduct of such research the names or other identifying characteristics of such individuals. Persons so authorized to protect the privacy of such individuals may not be compelled in any Federal, State or local civil, criminal, administrative, legislative, or other proceedings to identify such individuals.

Certificates of Confidentiality: Background Information
National Institutes of Health,
Office of Extramural Research
http://grants.nih.gov/grants/policy/coc/background.htm

Certificates can be used for biomedical, behavioral, clinical or other types of research that are sensitive. By sensitive, we mean that disclosure of identifying information could have adverse consequences for subjects or damage their financial standing, employability, insurability, or reputation.

Examples of sensitive research activities include but are not limited to the following:

- Collecting genetic information;

- Collecting information on psychological well-being of subjects;

- Collecting information on subjects' sexual attitudes, preferences or practices;

- Collecting data on substance abuse or other illegal risk behaviors;

- Studies where subjects may be involved in litigation related to exposures under study (e.g., breast implants, environmental or occupational exposures).

In general, certificates are issued for single, well-defined research projects rather than groups or classes of projects. In some instances, they can be issued for cooperative multi-site projects. A coordinating center or "lead" institution designated by the NIH program officer can apply on behalf of all institutions associated with the multi-site project. The lead institution must ensure that all participating institutions conform to the application assurances and inform participants appropriately about the Certificate, its protections, and the circumstances in which voluntary disclosures would be made. . . .

Some projects are ineligible for a Certificate of Confidentiality. Not eligible for a Certificate are projects that are:

- not research;

- not collecting personally identifiable information;

- not reviewed and approved by the IRB as required by these guidelines; or

- collecting information that if disclosed would not significantly harm or damage the participant.

While Certificates protect against involuntary disclosure, investigators should note that research subjects might voluntarily disclose their research data or information. Subjects may disclose information to physicians or other third parties. They may also authorize in writing the investigator to release the information to insurers, employers, or other third parties. In such cases, researchers may not use the Certificate to refuse disclosure. Moreover, researchers are not prevented from the voluntary disclosure of matters such as child abuse, reportable communicable diseases, or subject's threatened violence to self or others. . . . However, if the researcher intends to make any voluntary disclosures, the consent form must specify such disclosure.

Certificates do not authorize researchers to refuse to disclose information about subjects if authorized DHHS personnel request such information for an audit or program evaluation. Neither can researchers refuse to disclose such information if it is required to be disclosed by the Federal Food, Drug, and Cosmetic Act.

NOTES AND QUESTIONS

1. Certificates of confidentiality are not limited to research supported with federal funds. *See* NATIONAL INSTITUTES OF HEALTH, OFFICE OF EXTRAMURAL RESEARCH, FREQUENTLY ASKED QUESTIONS ON CERTIFICATES OF CONFIDENTIALITY, March 15, 2002, available at http://grants.nih.gov/grants/policy/coc/faqs.htm.

2. While certificates of confidentiality do not prevent researchers from voluntarily disclosing information about subjects, if researchers promise subjects that they will not disclose confidential information to third parties, they "will be bound by that promise, as a matter of the research contract between subject and researcher." Mark Barnes & Sara Krauss, *The Effect of HIPAA on Human Subjects Research*, 10 HEALTH L. REP. (BNA) 1026, 1032 (2001).

3. The NIH background information excerpted above states that researchers may *voluntarily* report "matters such as child abuse, reportable communicable diseases, or subject's threatened violence to self or others." As discussed earlier

in this chapter, however, state laws may *require* the reporting of such matters in certain circumstances. *See supra*, page 447. How can the goal of protecting the confidentiality of research subjects be reconciled with the desire to ensure the prompt reporting of communicable diseases and threats of violence to the appropriate authorities? An August 1991 memorandum from the Assistant Secretary for Health at NIH provides the following answer to this question with respect to communicable disease reporting:

> This policy applies to issuance of certificates of confidentiality to projects that intend routinely to determine whether its subjects have communicable diseases and that are required to report them under State law.
>
> 1. In projects in which subjects are referred by treating physicians, a certificate will be issued only if the applicant provides written assurance that the project will accept individuals as subjects only if referring physicians assure the project that they have complied (and will continue to comply) with applicable State communicable disease reporting requirements with respect to the referred subjects.
>
> In instances in which physicians conducting research also see their subjects in a clinical care, non-research, relationship, the protections of the certificate do not apply to the non-research relationship, and those physicians are the referring physicians for the purposes of this policy.
>
> 2. In research projects covered by this policy to which the preceding paragraph does not apply (i.e., there is no referring physician), the applicant must describe in writing the agreement that the applicant has made with the health department to cooperate with the health department in ways that serve the purposes of communicable disease reporting requirements. That may include disclosure of identifiable information about subjects, or it may include other forms of cooperation not involving such disclosure.
>
> In the absence of such an agreement, a certificate may be issued only if the applicant provides, in writing, justification setting out specific reasons, related to confidentiality requirements of the research, that preclude such cooperation. Authority to issue certificates in such circumstances is retained by the Assistant Secretary for Health.
>
> 3. Any disclosure of identifiable information about subjects must be in accord with the rules for protection of research subjects and any other legal limitation that may exist, and must be explained clearly to the subjects in advance.

NATIONAL INSTITUTES OF HEALTH, OFFICE OF EXTRAMURAL RESEARCH, MEMORANDUM FROM THE ASSISTANT SECRETARY FOR HEALTH ON CERTIFICATES OF CONFIDENTIALITY — DISEASE REPORTING, August 9, 1991, available at http://grants1.nih.gov/grants/policy/coc/cd_policy.htm. Does this policy adequately balance the various interests at stake? What do you think is meant by the statement in the second numbered paragraph regarding "other forms of cooperation not involving such disclosure"?

[B] Overseeing the Use and Disclosure of Medical Records

[1] Human Subject Protection Regulations

IRB GUIDEBOOK
Chapter 3D
U.S. DEPT. OF HEALTH AND HUMAN SERVICES
OFFICE FOR PROTECTION FROM RESEARCH RISKS
(1993)

To identify suitable subjects, researchers must sometimes approach institutions (e.g., hospitals or schools) seeking information generally regarded as confidential (e.g., the identity of patients treated for a particular condition or students meeting a particular criterion). In some circumstances, the researcher needs information that would make it possible to contact suitable subjects to obtain further data. In other circumstances, no contact with subjects is contemplated because the information to be obtained from the records is sufficient (or will be combined with data from other sources). In these cases, personal identifiers may not need to be recorded by the researchers, or, if recorded, can be destroyed at some stage of the research. All of these factors are relevant to IRB assessments of privacy and confidentiality issues in research.

When patients give information about themselves to a doctor or hospital for the purpose of facilitating diagnosis or treatment of disease, they do so in a relationship of trust. They generally expect that the information will be shared only as necessary for their health care or reimbursement by their insurance company or other third party payer; patients would not expect information that identifies them to be passed on in casual conversations at cocktail parties or made available to journalists or to university students writing papers. Nor do they necessarily intend that the information will be shared with even their closest family members. Health care providers should respect the patient's trust. They should not betray the confidence placed in them. (The same may be said of educators with regard to students, and of employers with regard to employees.) Yet such confidences are not absolute; patient records are commonly used for a variety of purposes other than the care of a particular patient for the management of the organization through quality assurance programs and for utilization review. To say that an organization has an obligation to keep certain patient information confidential does not resolve the question of what uses are appropriate for those records.

Clearly, some important research cannot be conducted unless an investigator gains access to many records (sometimes thousands). In epidemiological studies, scientists may seek to determine, for example, whether certain industrial or environmental contaminants are associated with an increase in birth defects or deaths from cancer. In their search they might wish to review thousands of hospital or employment records to identify infants born with a defect, patients suffering from a particular form of cancer, or workers exposed to a particular substance. Without access to such records, an investigator cannot identify potential subjects or match the relevant records.

It is not possible to specify precisely when an institution should honor a researcher's request to examine records or when an IRB should approve this potential invasion of privacy. In 1977, the Privacy Protection Study Commission concluded that medical records can legitimately be used for biomedical or epidemiological research without the individual's explicit authorization, provided that the medical care provider maintaining the record:

(i) determines that such use or disclosure does not violate any limitations under which the record or information was collected;

(ii) ascertains that use or disclosure in individually identifiable form is necessary to accomplish the research or statistical purpose for which use or disclosure is to be made;

(iii) determines that the importance of the research or statistical purpose for which any use or disclosure is to be made is such as to warrant the risk to the individual from additional exposure of the record or information contained therein;

(iv) requires that adequate safeguards to protect the record or information from unauthorized disclosure be established and maintained by the user or recipient, including a program for removal or destruction of identifiers; and

(v) obtains consent in writing before any further use or redisclosure of the record or information in individually identifiable form is permitted.

The National Commission endorsed this recommendation, and concluded that in studies of documents, records, or pathological specimens where the subjects are identified, informed consent may be waived if the IRB determines that the subject's interests are adequately protected and the importance of the research justifies the invasion of privacy.[1] Unless otherwise required by the head of the department or agency funding or conducting the research, federal regulations (except those promulgated by the FDA) exempt from review all research involving the collection or study of existing data, documents, records, pathological specimens, or diagnostic specimens from IRB review if the sources are publicly

---

[1] See 45 C.F.R. § 46.116(d); see also Chapter 7, at page 313.

available or if the information is recorded by the investigator in a manner that does not allow subjects to be identified, either directly or through identifiers that are linked to them.[2]

In cases where researchers gain access to identified records without the individual's explicit permission, methods for reducing the associated privacy problems should be considered. For instance, an institution possessing records on suitable subjects may be willing to contact them and ask their permission to release their names to the researcher. Depending on the purpose of the research, the possible biases that this approach would create may be unacceptable, but in other studies it may prove feasible. Another approach is for institutions to make known the uses to which its records may be put in advance, so that individuals will be aware that their records may be used in research. Some institutions provide an opportunity for people to consent (or withhold consent) to use at the time of the initial creation of the record. Other institutions have been reluctant to do this because of either logistical difficulties or systematic biases that might be built into subsequent research. Still another approach, which may be feasible on occasion, is for the researcher to become an employee of, or consultant to, the institution and thereby gain proper access to the records. Various other creative solutions may be negotiated among researchers, institutions, and IRBs. No firm rule can be stated; this is one of many areas in which IRBs must exercise common sense and sound judgment.

NOTES AND QUESTIONS

1. What "systematic biases" might be created by giving individuals the opportunity to consent to the future use of their medical records in biomedical research?

2. What expectations do patients normally have about the use of their records for purposes other than the provision of medical care, third-party payor requirements and, perhaps, internal quality assurance or improvement? If patients do not expect that their records will be used for research in the absence of explicit authorization, is it appropriate to use them without specifically informing the patient? Are such uses inconsistent with the spirit of the Privacy Protection Study Commission's recommendations?

3. According to one survey, most people value the opportunity to decide whether their medical records should be used in research. When asked whether "medical researchers should be able to get [patients'] medical records without [the patients'] permission 'if it will help them to do research that will advance medical knowledge in the future,'" a majority of respondents (60.4%) said no. However, seventy-one percent approved of such a database when told "that only those whom *they* authorized could gain access to the database and that

---

[2] *See* 45 C.F.R. § 46.101(b)(4); *see also* Chapter 3, at page 123, Chapter 17, at page 706.

security measures actually worked." Nancy E. Kass et al., *The Use of Medical Records in Research: What Do Patients Want?* 31 J. L. MED. & ETHICS 429 (2003).

4. The IRB Guidebook notes that, by becoming an employee of, or consultant to, the research institution, an individual may "thereby gain proper access to" individuals' medical records. Is it ethically appropriate to enter into an employment or consultancy arrangement with researchers solely to enable them to gain access to private information that would otherwise be unavailable to them? Do patients expect that their records will be reviewed by such employees or consultants? Might they be concerned about such uses of their medical records even if the information is recorded by the researcher without identifiers? Consider the possibility that the researcher may be a social acquaintance, a neighbor, or a co-worker of a patient.

5. For further discussion of the nonconsensual use of patient information in biomedical research, see Chapter 17, at page 718 (discussing researchers' use of genetic information).

[2] HIPAA Regulations

The implementation of the HIPAA privacy regulations in April 2003 added a new layer of regulatory complexity to research with identifiable medical records. For organizations subject to the regulations, most uses of "protected health information" (PHI) require the patient's prior written authorization. PHI includes most "individually identifiable health information," the definition of which is sufficiently broad to encompass virtually all medical records likely to be of interest to researchers. (For the specific regulatory definition, see 45 C.F.R. § 160.103.) Note that, under the regulations, health information is considered "individually identifiable" if it contains any one of 18 categories of patient-specific information. Thus, simply removing the patient's name, address, and phone number will usually not be sufficient to remove a record from the scope of the regulatory requirements.

Researchers must comply with one of the following procedures before using PHI in research:

- *Obtain a HIPAA authorization for the use and disclosure of PHI*. In most situations, researchers should obtain the subject's written authorization for the use and disclosure of PHI. The authorization, which may be incorporated into the general research consent form, must include the following information: (a) a specific description of the information to be disclosed; (b) the person or entity to whom disclosure will be made; (c) the specific purpose of the use or disclosure; (d) an expiration date or an expiration event for use of the information, or the statement that the authorization has no expiration date; (e) a statement of the individual's rights to revoke authorization in writing and an explanation of how the authorization may be revoked; (f) a statement that information used or disclosed pursuant to the authorization may be subject to redisclosure by the recipient and no longer be protected by the HIPAA privacy requirements; (g) any restrictions placed on the subject's access to the information, and a statement that access to the information will be granted upon completion of the research. *See* 45 C.F.R. § 164.508(c). In addition, subjects should be given a notice of the institution's privacy practices. *See* 45 C.F.R. § 164.520.

- ***Obtain a waiver or alteration of the HIPAA authorization requirement.*** Waivers or alterations of the authorization requirement may be sought from either the IRB or the institution's "privacy board," depending on institutional policy. Alterations or waivers are available if the study meets the following conditions: (a) the use or disclosure of PHI involves no more than minimal risk to the subjects; (b) the research could not practicably be conducted without the waiver or alteration; and (c) the research could not practicably be conducted without access to and use of the PHI. In determining whether the use or disclosure of PHI involves no more than minimal risk, the IRB or privacy board must consider whether there is (i) an adequate plan to protect subject identifiers from improper use or disclosure; (ii) an adequate plan to destroy the identifiers at the earliest opportunity consistent with the conduct of the research, unless there is a health or research justification for retaining the identifiers, or such retention is otherwise required by law; and (iii) adequate written assurance that the PHI will not be re-used or disclosed except as required by law, for authorized oversight of the research project, or for other research for which the use or disclosure of PHI would be permitted by the regulations. *See* 45 C.F.R. § 164.512(i)(2)(ii).

- ***Comply with the rules authorizing the review of PHI "preparatory to research."*** Researchers may review PHI in order to prepare a research protocol or for other purposes preparatory to research. The researcher must file a request for access to the information with an office designated by the institution (often, the medical records department), representing that (a) the request is sought solely to review PHI preparatory to research; (b) no PHI will be removed from the institution in the course of the review; and (c) the PHI for which use or access is sought is necessary for the research purposes. *See* 45 C.F.R. § 164.512(i)(1)(ii). The "preparatory to research" provisions allow researchers who are employees of the covered entity or members of the covered entity's workforce to use or disclose PHI in order to identify and contact prospective research subjects. However, the provisions do not allow the use or disclosure of PHI to outside researchers.

- **Comply with the rules authorizing access to PHI of deceased persons.** Research using a deceased person's PHI is permitted if the researcher files a request for access to the information that includes: (a) a representation that the use or disclosure sought is solely for research on the PHI of decedents; (b) documentation of the death of such individuals; and (c) representation that the use or disclosure of the information is necessary for research purposes. *See* 45 C.F.R. § 164.512(i)(1)(iii).

- **Create a "limited data set," which can be used and disclosed without an authorization or waiver.** A "limited data set" consists of data that has had most, but not all, identifying information removed. Unlike fully de-identified information, a "limited data set" may include dates related to the individual (such as date of birth or dates of hospital admission and discharge), geographic information other than street address (such as zip code), and a unique identifying code. The regulations permit researchers to use or disclose limited data sets without complying with the usual requirements for the use or disclosure of PHI. The option is available only if the researcher has signed a data use agreement with the institution, which places limits on who may receive the information and how it may be used. *See* 45 C.F.R. § 164.514(e)(2).

See generally E.D. Prentice et al., *Nebraska Medical Center IRB Primer on the HIPAA Privacy Rule*, 2 MED. RESEARCH L. & POL'Y REP. (BNA) 117 (2003).

NOTES AND QUESTIONS

1. Note that HIPAA applies not only to researchers' use and disclosure of pre-existing medical records, but also to the use and disclosure of the data generated during the study itself.

2. If the subject has not authorized the disclosure of her PHI, the disclosure must be limited to the minimum necessary to accomplish the purposes of the disclosure. *See* 45 C.F.R. §§ 164.502(b), 164.514(d). However, "the Privacy Rule permits the covered entity to rely, when reasonable, on a request for disclosure of PHI as the minimum necessary . . . when disclosing PHI to researchers who have documentation of an IRB or Privacy Board waiver or alteration of Authorization . . ." DEPARTMENT OF HEALTH AND HUMAN SERVICES, PROTECTING PERSONAL HEALTH INFORMATION IN RESEARCH: UNDERSTANDING THE HIPAA PRIVACY RULE, NIH Pub. No. 03-5388, at 19, available at http://privacyruleand research.nih.gov/pr_02.asp.

3. Researchers need not obtain subjects' permission to comply with laws that require the disclosure of PHI, including laws requiring the reporting of adverse events to the FDA. *See* 45 C.F.R. § 164.512(b)(1)(iii).

4. HIPAA requires that an "accounting" be given to individuals when their PHI is used or disclosed without their consent. *See* 45 C.F.R. § 164.528(b). The accounting requirement applies whenever researchers use or disclose PHI without a written authorization. It does not apply to research involving the use of a limited data set. *See* Prentice et al., *supra*.

5. According to commentary to the regulations issued by DHHS, if a subject revokes a HIPAA authorization after the clinical portion of a study is completed but before the researchers have finished analyzing the data, the researchers may continue to use and disclose the data "to account for [the] subject's withdrawal from the research study, as necessary to incorporate the information as part of a marketing application submitted to the FDA, to conduct investigations of scientific misconduct, or to report adverse events." 67 FED. REG. 53182, 53225 (Aug. 14, 2002). DHHS based this position on language in the regulations that permits covered entities to use or disclose data after the revocation of an authorization to the extent the covered entity had "taken action in reliance thereon." 45 C.F.R. § 164.508(b)(5)(i). *See* Mark Barnes & Clinton Hermes, *Clinical Research After the August 2002 Privacy Rule Amendments*, 1 MED. RESEARCH L. & POL'Y REP. (BNA) 406, 407 (2002) (noting that, "while the scope of this exception should have been explicitly reflected in the text of the regulations, the ambiguity of the 'in reliance' language (which, standing alone, is almost devoid of content in the absence of HHS interpretation), coupled with the commentary's examples, should provide some comfort for researchers and drug and device company research sponsors").

6. DHHS has stated that providers may discuss with their patients the option of enrolling in a clinical trial, but they may not disclose PHI to third parties for recruitment purposes without first obtaining the individual's authorization or a waiver of authorization from an IRB or Privacy Board. As Mark Barnes and Clinton Hermes explain:

> While the commentary does not directly address whether treating physicians may disclose their patients' PHI to other workforce members within a single covered entity (for example, to other employees of the same hospital, which would be a 'use' and not a 'disclosure' under HIPAA) for purposes of recommending patients in clinical trials, such a use is not directly supported by the regulations and would be inconsistent with prevailing pre-HIPAA privacy practices for research recruitment.

Barnes & Hermes, *supra*, at 409.

7. In light of the HIPAA regulations, the fact that research is exempt from the human subject protection regulations does not necessarily mean that it can escape the review of an IRB or Privacy Board. *See* Mark Barnes & Katherine E. Gallin, *"Exempt" Research after the Privacy Rule*, 25 IRB, July-Aug. 2003, at 5. Consider, for example, a study involving existing, identifiable data that will be "recorded by the investigator in such a manner that subjects cannot be identi-

fied, directly or through identifiers linked to the subjects." While such a study would be exempt from the human subject protection regulations under 45 C.F.R. § 46.101(b)(4), the researchers' review of the data before it is anonymized would still trigger HIPAA's requirements governing the use or disclosure of PHI.

8. Note that creating a database itself constitutes "research" under the HIPAA privacy regulations. Thus, researchers may not place subjects' PHI in a database without obtaining subjects' specific authorization. Additional authorizations (or waivers) would be necessary before using information in the database in future research projects. "Under federal guidance, it is insufficient, and impermissible, to obtain a blanket authorization from subjects authorizing the use and disclosure of the subjects' PHI for unspecified future research purposes." Mark Barnes & Kate Gallin Heffernan, *The "Future Uses" Dilemma: Secondary Uses of Data and Materials by Researchers and Commercial Research Sponsors*, 3 MED. RESEARCH L. & POL'Y REP. (BNA) 440 (2004).

9. The HIPAA privacy regulations generally do not apply to commercial research sponsors. Thus:

> [O]nce PHI is disclosed by a covered entity to a non-covered third party such as a commercial research sponsor, the information is no longer subject to HIPAA's requirements. A statement to this effect must be included in any research authorization form signed by a research subject permitting the use and disclosure of his or her PHI for the purposes of a research study. Research subjects are thereby put on notice that if they authorize the covered institution or investigator to disclose their PHI to a third party who is not covered by HIPAA — for example the sponsor of the research study — the law provides no protection to that information once it is in the hands of the non-covered party.

Barnes & Heffernan, *supra*. The fact that sponsors are not subject to HIPAA means that they are free to use subjects' identifiable medical information in subsequent research projects without obtaining additional authorizations. They are also not obligated to honor requests by the subjects to revoke their initial authorizations.

> This, then, is the box into which HIPAA, assisted by research regulations, has backed IRBs and investigators: they are required to be specific about uses, disclosures, and purposes that are unknowable at the time the consents and authorizations are acquired, and required to inform subjects of a right to revoke their authorization, while knowing full well that the bulk of "future use" databases maintained by sponsors need not honor any such request.

Id. What should subjects be told about this state of affairs? Is there anything that researcher institutions can do to limit sponsors' subsequent use of subjects' identifiable tissue samples?

10. When a group of Canadian researchers sought to develop a national registry of stroke victims, including information about the patients' symptoms and clinical course, they found that, despite "concerted effort[s] to obtain written informed consent for participation, the overall participation rate never exceeded half of the eligible patients." Moreover, the patients who agreed to participate in the registry were not representative of the eligible population; those who were sicker or more impaired were disproportionately left out. Jack V. Tu et al., *Impracticability of Informed Consent in the Registry of the Canadian Stroke Network*, 350 NEW ENG. J. MED. 1414 (2004). An editorial accompanying this study lamented the fact that "data repositories are now at risk of significant bias because concern about privacy has led to the requirement that consent be obtained before an individual person's data can be used." Julie R. Ingelfinger & Jeffrey M. Drazen, *Registry Research and Medical Privacy*, 350 NEW ENG. J. MED. 1452 (2004). Under both the Common Rule and HIPAA, is there any way that researchers can create registries without obtaining patients' specific authorization?

11. For DHHS guidance on navigating the complex HIPAA privacy requirements, see http://privacyruleandresearch.nih.gov/irbandprivacyrule.asp.

Chapter 11

MONITORING OF ONGOING RESEARCH

The need to protect human subjects does not end with an IRB's initial approval of a study. A number of procedures have been developed to make sure that protections remain in place even after a study has been approved and researchers have begun enrolling subjects. These include additional duties imposed on IRBs — including requirements to perform continuing review of studies and to review adverse events — and a somewhat different type of review by entities known as data and safety monitoring boards.

§ 11.01 CONTINUING REVIEW

Not only must most studies be approved by an IRB before they begin, but the IRB's approval also must be renewed at least once a year. This aspect of an IRB's work is referred to as "continuing review." Although there is probably agreement on the need for some type of continuing review of studies, there remains quite a bit of controversy regarding what IRBs are supposed to be doing when they perform such review.

45 C.F.R. § 46.109(e): IRB REVIEW OF RESEARCH

This provision is reproduced in Appendix A, at page A-9. Please review it before proceeding.

GUIDANCE ON CONTINUING REVIEW
OFFICE FOR HUMAN RESEARCH PROTECTIONS
(2002)
http://www.hhs.gov/ohrp/humansubjects/guidance/contrev2002.htm

The HHS regulations for the protection of human subjects (45 CFR Part 46) require that, among other things, (1) institutions have written procedures which the IRB will follow for (a) conducting its continuing review of research and for reporting its findings and actions to investigators and the institution, and (b) determining which projects require review more often than annually (45 CFR 46.103(b)(4)); . . . and (3) an IRB conducts continuing review of research at intervals appropriate to the degree of risk, but not less often than once a year (45 CFR 46.109(e)).

WHAT CONSTITUTES SUBSTANTIVE AND MEANINGFUL CONTINUING REVIEW?

Continuing review of research must be substantive and meaningful. In accordance with HHS regulations at 45 CFR 46.108(b) and at 46.115(a)(2), continuing review by the convened IRB, with recorded vote on each study, is required unless the research is otherwise appropriate for expedited review under Section 46.110 (see below). Furthermore, HHS regulations at 45 CFR 46.111 set forth the criteria that must be satisfied in order for the IRB to approve research. These criteria include, among other things, determinations by the IRB regarding risks, potential benefits, informed consent, and safeguards for human subjects. The IRB must ensure that these criteria are satisfied at the time of both initial and continuing review. The procedures for continuing review by the convened IRB may include a primary reviewer system.

In conducting continuing review of research not eligible for expedited review, all IRB members should at least receive and review a protocol summary and a status report on the progress of the research, including:

- The number of subjects accrued;

- A summary of adverse events and any unanticipated problems involving risks to subjects or others and any withdrawal of subjects from the research or complaints about the research since the last IRB review;

- A summary of any relevant recent literature, interim findings, and amendments or modifications to the research since the last review;

- Any relevant multi-center trial reports;

- Any other relevant information, especially information about risks associated with the research; and

- A copy of the current informed consent document and any newly proposed consent document. . . .

When reviewing the current informed consent document(s), the IRB should ensure the following:

- The currently approved or proposed consent document is still accurate and complete;

- Any significant new findings that may relate to the subject's willingness to continue participation are provided to the subject in accordance with HHS regulations at 45 CFR 46.116(b)(5). . . .

What are Some Additional Considerations for Continuing Review in Multi-Center Trials Monitored by a DSMB, DMC, Other Similar Body, or Sponsor?

As noted above, continuing review of research by the IRB should include consideration of adverse events, interim findings, and any recent literature that may be relevant to the research.

OHRP recognizes that such information may not be readily available to local investigators participating in multi-center clinical trials or to their local IRBs. However, OHRP notes that such trials are often subject to oversight by a Data and Safety Monitoring Board (DSMB), Data Monitoring Committee (DMC), other similar body, or sponsor whose responsibilities include review of adverse events, interim findings, and relevant literature. [DSMBs are discussed *infra*, at page 475.]

In such circumstances, IRBs conducting continuing review of research may rely on a current statement from the DSMB or sponsor indicating that it has reviewed study-wide adverse events, interim findings, and any recent literature that may be relevant to the research, in lieu of requiring that this information be submitted directly to the IRB. The IRB must still receive and review reports of local, on-site adverse events and unanticipated problems involving risks to subjects or others and any other information needed to ensure that its continuing review is substantive and meaningful. In addition, institutions and IRBs may require additional information for continuing review at their discretion. . . .

How is the Continuing Review Date Determined?

HHS regulations at 45 CFR 46.108(b) and 109(e) require, respectively, that (1) except when an expedited review procedure is used, each IRB must review proposed research at convened meetings at which a majority of the members of the IRB are present, including at least one member whose primary concerns are in nonscientific areas; and (2) an IRB must conduct continuing review of research at intervals appropriate to the degree of risk, but not less frequently than once per year. The IRB should decide the frequency of continuing review for each study protocol necessary to ensure the continued protection of the rights and welfare of research subjects.

Several scenarios for determining the date of continuing review apply for protocols reviewed by the IRB at a convened meeting. To determine the date by which continuing review must occur, focus on the date of the convened meeting at which IRB approval occurs. (These examples presume the IRB has determined that it will conduct continuing review no sooner than within 1 year).

> Scenario 1: The IRB reviews and approves a protocol without any conditions at a convened meeting on October 1, 2002. Continuing review must occur within 1 year of the date of the meeting, that is, by October 1, 2003.

Scenario 2: The IRB reviews a protocol at a convened meeting on October 1, 2002, and approves the protocol contingent on specific minor conditions the IRB chair or his/her designee can verify. On October 31, 2002, the IRB chair or designee confirms that the required minor changes were made. Continuing review must occur within 1 year of the date of the convened IRB meeting at which the IRB reviewed and approved the protocol, that is, by October 1, 2003.

Scenario 3: The IRB reviews a study at a convened meeting on October 1, 2002, and has serious concerns or lacks significant information that requires IRB review of the study at subsequent convened meetings on October 15 and October 29, 2002. At their October 29, 2002 meeting, the IRB completes its review and approves the study. Continuing review must occur within 1 year of the date of the convened meeting at which the IRB reviewed and approved the protocol, that is, by October 29, 2003. . . .

Review of a change in a protocol ordinarily does not alter the date by which continuing review must occur. This is because continuing review is review of the full protocol, not simply a change to it.

The regulations make no provision for any grace period extending the conduct of research beyond the expiration date of IRB approval. Therefore, continuing review and re-approval of research must occur on or before the date when IRB approval expires. OHRP recognizes the logistical advantages of keeping the IRB approval period constant from year to year throughout the life of each project. When continuing review occurs annually and the IRB performs continuing review within 30 days before the IRB approval period expires, the IRB may retain the anniversary date as the date by which the continuing review must occur. This would be, for example, October 1, 2003, in the above Scenarios 1 and 2, and October 29, 2003, in Scenario 3, even if the continuing reviews took place up to 30 days prior to these dates.

WHAT OCCURS IF THERE IS A LAPSE IN CONTINUING REVIEW?

The IRB and investigators must plan ahead to meet required continuing review dates. If an investigator has failed to provide continuing review information to the IRB or the IRB has not reviewed and approved a research study by the continuing review date specified by the IRB, the research must stop, unless the IRB finds that it is in the best interests of individual subjects to continue participating in the research interventions or interactions. Enrollment of new subjects cannot occur after the expiration of IRB approval.

When continuing review of a research protocol does not occur prior to the end of the approval period specified by the IRB, IRB approval expires automatically. Such expiration of IRB approval does not need to be reported to OHRP as a suspension of IRB approval under HHS regulations.

NOTES AND QUESTIONS

1. As the OHRP guidance document notes, an IRB is required to have written procedures describing which studies need to be reviewed more often than once a year. What criteria should an IRB use in determining which studies fit into this category? Draft the language for a short paragraph that an IRB could use as part of its written procedures to satisfy this OHRP requirement.

2. Assume, in Scenario 1 above, that an IRB was following the OHRP rule that allows the IRB to maintain a consistent anniversary date for continuing review. If the IRB reviewed the study on September 5, 2003, what is the last day in 2004 by which the IRB must again review the study? Is this set of circumstances consistent with what section 46.109(e) requires?

3. The portions of this document dealing with multi-center studies are relatively new, and respond in part to complaints by IRBs that they are not sure what to do with multi-center studies. Imagine that a study is being conducted in fifty separate sites, enrolling hundreds of patients, and your IRB is at one of the smaller sites, which has enrolled only one patient. To what extent should your IRB be looking at what is happening in this study in all of the other locations? The growing use of data and safety monitoring boards (DSMBs), discussed in more detail later in this chapter, is one attempt to lessen the burden placed on IRBs in such studies. Note that the OHRP guidance relating to review of multi-center studies applies only to studies in which there is a DSMB or similar group monitoring the study. If there is no such group, what is OHRP's view of the IRB's duty to review events taking place at other study sites?

4. In portions of the document that have not been reprinted above, OHRP discusses instances in which continuing review can be performed using "expedited" review procedures. As discussed in Chapter 4, expedited review allows a study to be reviewed by the Chair of the IRB or by one or more designated members, instead of at a convened meeting of the IRB. *See* Chapter 4, at page 195. Expedited continuing review can be performed where the study would have qualified for expedited review the first time it was reviewed by the IRB. In addition, even if the study initially would not have qualified for expedited review, there are several circumstances in which continuing review can nonetheless be conducted with expedited review procedures: (a) the study is closed to enrollment of new subjects, all subjects have completed any interventions (e.g., drug or other treatments or procedures), and only follow-up data collection on what happens to subjects is taking place; (b) no subjects have yet been enrolled and no new risks have been identified; (c) the only remaining research activities are data analysis; or (d) for research that does not involve either an Investigational New Drug application (IND) or Investigational Device Exemption (IDE) from the FDA, if the IRB at a previous convened meeting has determined that the study involves only minimal risk. These rules are discussed in section F and in Research Categories (8) and (9) of Department of Health and Human Services, *Categories of Research That May Be Reviewed by the Institutional Review*

Board (IRB) through an Expedited Review Procedure, 63 FED. REG. 60364 (1998), which is reproduced in Appendix B. In addition, OHRP has provided a decision chart on this topic. *See* OFFICE FOR HUMAN RESEARCH PROTECTIONS, CHART 9: MAY THE IRB CONTINUING REVIEW BE DONE BY EXPEDITED PROCEDURES? available at http://www.hhs.gov/ohrp/humansubjects/guidance/decisioncharts.htm.

5. The regulations provide that expedited review procedures can be used to review a "minor change" in an approved study. See 45 C.F.R. § 46.110(b)(2). What sort of changes should be considered "minor" under this rule? Would a change in one of the co-investigators be considered minor? What factors should be considered in making such an assessment? What if a principal investigator leaves the institution and the sponsor is willing to have a former co-investigator become the principal investigator? Note that, as stated in the OHRP guidance document, approval of a change in a protocol — whether by an expedited procedure or at a meeting of the IRB — does not change the timing of when continuing review takes place. Continuing review is considered a review of the entire study, whereas when a change is approved, the review might be limited to only the issues raised by that particular change.

6. As noted above, continuing review is one of the most contentious aspects of IRBs' work. When OHRP audits an institution, one of its common findings is that the IRB is not paying enough attention to continuing review, and that such review was not "substantive and meaningful." Many IRB members would likely respond that, as currently designed, the continuing review process requires IRBs to spend too much of their time reviewing written answers by investigators to a variety of not-that-important questions, and that such review has little impact on the well-being of subjects. Moreover, to make continuing review meaningful — such as by requiring actual audits of ongoing studies — would require a huge change in the nature of the activities that IRBs currently conduct, including major changes in funding and staffing. For a discussion of these issues, see Sharona Hoffman, *Continued Concern: Human Subject Protection, The Institutional Review Board, and Continuing Review*, 68 TENN. L. REV. 725 (2001).

§ 11.02 ADVERSE EVENT REPORTING

In the discussion of continuing review in the previous section, it was noted that OHRP requires IRBs to look at "adverse events" that took place in a study since the last review by the IRB. An adverse event is, in very general terms, some sort of a bad thing that happened to a subject while participating in a study, such as an allergic reaction to a drug. There are a number of rules, from a variety of federal agencies, that require such events to be reported to IRBs. But the world of adverse event reporting is filled with a great deal of confusion about what constitutes an adverse event, which ones have to be reported to IRBs, how quickly they have to be reported, and what IRBs are supposed to be doing with these reports.

45 C.F.R. § 46.103(b)(5): WRITTEN PROCEDURES FOR ENSURING PROMPT REPORTING

This provision is reproduced in Appendix A, at page A-6. Please review it before proceeding.

21 C.F.R. § 312.32: INVESTIGATIONAL NEW DRUG SAFETY REPORTS

(a) *Definitions.* The following definitions of terms apply to this section:

Associated with the use of the drug. There is a reasonable possibility that the experience may have been caused by the drug.

Disability. A substantial disruption of a person's ability to conduct normal life functions.

Life-threatening adverse drug experience. Any adverse drug experience that places the patient or subject, in the view of the investigator, at immediate risk of death from the reaction as it occurred, i.e., it does not include a reaction that, had it occurred in a more severe form, might have caused death.

Serious adverse drug experience: Any adverse drug experience occurring at any dose that results in any of the following outcomes: Death, a life-threatening adverse drug experience, inpatient hospitalization or prolongation of existing hospitalization, a persistent or significant disability/incapacity, or a congenital anomaly/birth defect. Important medical events that may not result in death, be life-threatening, or require hospitalization may be considered a serious adverse drug experience when, based upon appropriate medical judgment, they may jeopardize the patient or subject and may require medical or surgical intervention to prevent one of the outcomes listed in this definition. Examples of such medical events include allergic bronchospasm requiring intensive treatment in an emergency room or at home, blood dyscrasias or convulsions that do not result in inpatient hospitalization, or the development of drug dependency or drug abuse.

Unexpected adverse drug experience: Any adverse drug experience, the specificity or severity of which is not consistent with the current investigator brochure; or, if an investigator brochure is not required or available, the specificity or severity of which is not consistent with the risk information described in the general investigational plan or elsewhere in the current application, as amended. For example, under this definition, hepatic necrosis would be unexpected (by virtue of greater severity) if the investigator brochure only referred to elevated hepatic enzymes or hepatitis. Similarly, cerebral thromboembolism and cerebral vasculitis would be unexpected (by virtue of greater specificity) if the investigator brochure only listed cerebral vascular accidents. "Unexpected," as used in this definition, refers to an adverse drug experience that has not been previously observed (e.g., included in the investigator brochure) rather than from the perspective of such experience not being anticipated from the pharmacological properties of the pharmaceutical product.

[Similar definitions are provided for medical devices (21 C.F.R. §812.3(s)) and for biological products (21 C.F.R. § 600.80 (a)).]

IRB Review of Adverse Events in Investigational Drug Studies
Ernest D. Prentice & Bruce G. Gordon
19 IRB, Nov.-Dec. 1997, at 1

IRB review of adverse events (AEs) that occur in investigational drug studies is necessarily part of the process of continuing review. . . . While most IRBs perform a scheduled continuing review no more often than annually, IRBs also have an obligation to perform a more or less continuous, ongoing assessment of AEs. Unanticipated AEs may alter the risk-benefit relationship of the research or they may precipitate disclosure requirements where current and even previously enrolled research subjects must be advised of a heretofore unknown risk. . . .

The IRB is required by 45 CFR 46.103(b)(5) . . . to establish a procedure for "prompt reporting to the IRB . . . of any unanticipated problems involving risk to the subjects or others. . . ."

. . . In consideration of the criteria "unanticipated" and "involving risk" it would seem that any AE not previously reported or noted in the investigator's brochure (and presumably in the consent document) that poses any risk, however small, should be reported to that IRB. Therefore, in the absence of any criteria based upon level of risk, even a minor new drug reaction should be reported to the IRB without delay. While the regulations do not specify a reporting time frame in terms of days, it is appropriate for an IRB to establish notification requirements according to the seriousness of the AE. For example, the sudden, unexpected death of a subject while on protocol should be reported within a short time period such as 24 hours, whereas a minor side effect such as a limited skin rash could reasonably be reported within 48 hours or even later. . . .

[T]he National Cancer Institute (NCI) and cooperative research groups have their own reporting requirements . . . The NCI requires investigators . . . to promptly report . . . any "previously unknown toxicities and life-threatening or fatal toxicities regardless of whether previously unknown." . . .

[The FDA's rules relating to Investigational New Drug (IND) applications] require the sponsor to notify "all participating investigators in a written IND safety report of any adverse experience associated with the use of the drug that is both serious and unexpected" within 10 working days. While this regulation does not require the sponsor to notify IRBs at participating study sites, it is routine for sponsors either to instruct investigators to provide their IRB with a copy of the safety report or to send a copy of the report directly to the IRB. . . .

Beginning in the 1990s, IRBs at major academic medical centers have been increasingly inundated with safety reports from sponsors that are not restricted to a description of AEs which are serious *and* unexpected. . . . [I]t would appear that the pharmaceutical industry, with encouragement and/or tacit endorsement from the FDA, has decided that IRBs should at least be notified of reported AEs regardless of the nature of the event. One reason may be the pharmaceutical industry's fear of litigation. . . .

View from the IRB

IRB review of AEs is largely driven by FDA, sponsors, NCI, and cooperative research groups. In consideration of the variability in AE reporting requirements, it is not surprising that many IRBs are confused about their responsibilities. Unless an IRB adopts a comprehensive approach to the review of AEs there will be inconsistency across the institution's clinical trials in terms of what kinds of AEs are reported to the IRB. . . .

To cope with a virtual flood of safety reports, some IRBs are forced to expend the time, effort and expense necessary to use expert consultants. Other IRBs may perform cursory reviews that offer little if any protection for the human subjects enrolled in the research. Conversely, an IRB may devote an inordinate amount of full board time to the review of AEs. This level of detailed review, however, is often unjustified in light of the fact that both the sponsors and investigators should be thoroughly assessing the significance of AEs in terms of protection of human subject issues. . . . In large-scale clinical trials, this evaluation is performed by data safety monitoring boards (DSMBs). While investigators and IRBs are not privy to the deliberations of DSMBs, it is, nevertheless, comforting to know there is independent, ongoing monitoring of data. Also, FDA reviews the data. Thus AEs are often subject to multiple reviews in addition to the one performed by the IRB. This necessarily raises a question about the extent to which IRBs should be reviewing AEs.

NOTES AND QUESTIONS

1. Having read these excerpts from Prentice and Gordon's article, is it clear to you what types of "adverse events" an investigator is supposed to report to an IRB? If you had to draft, for an IRB's instructions to investigators, the language describing what constitutes a reportable adverse event, what would you write?

2. The Prentice and Gordon article notes that the rules provided by a number of federal agencies require the reporting only of "unexpected" adverse events, thus excluding adverse events that are "expected" (such as known side effects of a drug, already described in the consent form). If "expected" problems

are not reported, how will an increase in the frequency of a known side effect ever be detected? If an investigator notices that a higher-than-expected number of subjects are experiencing a known side effect, must she report that development as an adverse event?

3. Assuming that a particular event must be reported to an IRB, what is the IRB supposed to do when it receives that report? Recall that, in most studies, continuing review takes place only once a year. Yet, presumably, adverse events are reported to the IRB at many different times, sometimes months before the next scheduled review by the IRB. Is someone at the IRB supposed to be looking at the adverse event report when it shows up? If so, who: an administrator? The Chair? A member of the IRB designated by the Chair? A subcommittee of the IRB designated to review adverse events? Or should the adverse event be reviewed by the IRB itself at its next convened meeting? (The Prentice and Gordon article, in portions not excerpted here, suggests that the full IRB should review all adverse events that are both serious and unanticipated.)

4. The Prentice and Gordon article notes that there is a lack of clarity about when adverse events should be reported to an IRB. The authors suggest that a sudden, unexpected death should be reported in 24 hours, while a rash could be reported in 48 hours, or "even later." How much later? If you were writing the procedures for an IRB, what time limits would you propose for reporting adverse events that relate to minor risks? Does it make sense to have each IRB setting its own policies for when adverse events should be reported?

5. Should it make a difference if the adverse event relates to a subject at the IRB's own institution, as opposed to a subject at some other site in a multi-site study? In 1999, the NIH issued guidance to researchers about reporting adverse events to IRBs in NIH-sponsored multi-center research studies. The guidance document noted that:

> [A]n IRB may receive individual adverse event reports from sites other than its own. Such off-site reports may not be presented in a useful format and duplicate reports are received, sometimes, months apart. The receipt of reports that are not aggregated (no numerators or denominators are included) and that come from disparate sources contributes to confusion and added workload of the IRB. More importantly, the format of the reports jeopardizes the IRB's ability to make an informed judgment on the appropriate action, if any, to be taken.

The guidance document indicated that, if it is in compliance with a particular IRB's policies, reporting of adverse events from other sites to that IRB could be performed by having the DSMB that reviews that study forward to the IRB its analysis of the adverse events. Under those circumstances, the investigator would not be required to report such adverse events to the IRB. NATIONAL INSTITUTES OF HEALTH, GUIDANCE ON REPORTING ADVERSE EVENTS TO INSTITUTIONAL REVIEW BOARDS IN NIH-SUPPORTED MULTICENTER CLINICAL TRIALS (1999), available at http://grants2.nih.gov/grants/guide/notice-files/not99-107.html.

6. Although the focus of this chapter is on the continuing review of a study by IRBs and other entities, it must be remembered that the researcher has the primary duty to protect the well-being of each subject. The researcher should remove subjects from a study whenever the occurrence of an adverse event or any other circumstances suggest that continued participation by a subject is too risky. A well-written research protocol should spell out in some detail the circumstances in which a subject's participation in the study will be terminated. For further discussion of researchers' obligations to remove subjects from a study, see Chapter 12, at page 505.

§ 11.03 DATA AND SAFETY MONITORING BOARDS

Although IRBs are required to receive and review adverse events, there is a growing recognition that IRBs often are not well qualified to do the types of analysis that are needed to evaluate the significance of these events. *See* Elizabeth Bankert & Robert Amdur, *The IRB Is Not a Data and Safety Monitoring Board*, 22 IRB, Nov.-Dec. 2000, at 9. That analysis generally requires a very high level of knowledge about the medical problem being studied, substantial training in statistics, and quite a bit of time and effort doing the necessary calculations. Such tasks are more commonly being assumed by entities known as data and safety monitoring boards or committees (DSMBs or DSMCs). Unlike IRBs, which generally review all the studies being conducted at a particular institution, a separate DSMB is usually created for each study that requires one.

Data Safety and Monitoring Boards
Arthur S. Slutsky & James V. Lavery
350 NEW ENG. J. MED. 1143 (2004)

Data safety and monitoring boards, also known by other names (e.g., data monitoring committees), were first introduced in the 1960s as a mechanism for monitoring interim data in clinical trials in order to ensure the safety of the participating subjects. The key concept was to recruit board members who were experts in the field of interest but not otherwise intimately involved in the study (that is, not organizers, sponsors, or investigators), so that they could be objective in their assessment of issues that arose during the study. Over the past decade, the use of data and safety monitoring boards has increased substantially, for a number of reasons. These include the greater number of trials with end points such as death from any cause or death due to cardiovascular disease, more trials funded or sponsored by government agencies that require boards as part of their design, and greater awareness of methodologic issues in trial design, especially with respect to the potential bias that can result when trials are stopped early because of evidence that one treatment has greater efficacy or causes greater harm than another.

. . . Their principal role is to assure the safety of patients, which they do by analyzing adverse events and by performing interim analyses of the clinical outcome data.

GUIDELINES ON DATA SAFETY MONITORING FOR HUMAN SUBJECTS RESEARCH
SAINT LOUIS UNIVERSITY [SLU] INSTITUTIONAL REVIEW BOARD
http://www.slu.edu/research/irb/documents/
DataSafetyMonitoring11_4_03.doc

A. *Introduction*

Ethical considerations and guidelines promulgated by Federal agencies and professional organizations require oversight and adequate monitoring of ongoing clinical trials. In cases of federally funded or industry-sponsored multicenter research, clinical trial monitors and the establishment of and efforts by external Data Safety Monitoring Committees (DSMCs) typically provide some degree of oversight. This situation is addressed in Section C.3 of these guidelines. The remaining guidelines below provide a mechanism for investigators involved with other interventional biomedical research to determine whether research subject monitoring carried out by individuals not directly affiliated with the protocol is needed, and what type of oversight would be appropriate for any particular study.

B. *Determination of Whether Research Subject Data Safety Monitoring Is Required*

1. *No safety monitoring plan will be required if the proposed research:*

- is a descriptive study and does not involve vulnerable populations nor presents risks to subjects in the event of loss of confidentiality;

- does not use a drug or device in an unapproved manner and does not involve a new investigational procedure; or

- reviews retrospective data or is a non-interventional follow up such that subjects are not likely to be placed at risk of physical, psychological, financial, or other harm.

When a research proposal involves a clinical intervention and is considered to pose greater than minimal risk to subjects (as described below), the principal investigator will provide a data safety monitoring plan, which must include predetermined safety considerations with "decision points," and either a Data Safety Monitor (DSM) or a Data Safety Monitoring Committee (DSMC).

2. *A Data Safety Monitor (DSM) will likely be required in any of the following situations:*

- The study is a pilot study of a novel treatment, such that there is little prior information on clinical safety; or

- The study, of any phase, is one in which there is evidence that the protocol raises concerns about the potential for serious end organ irreversible toxicity; or

- The study involves vulnerable populations, or

- The study presents significant risks to subjects in the event of a loss of confidentiality; or

- The study is a single center trial utilizing high-risk interventions (e.g. gene therapy, cancer treatments, AIDS treatments).

3. *A Data Safety Monitoring Committee (DSMC) (sometimes known as Data Safety Monitoring Board or DSMB) will likely be required* when the protocol presents greater than minimal risk to subjects, and entails any of the following situations. The study is a:

- Multicenter phase 3 study using investigational new drugs (IND) or devices (IDE), which evaluate interventions intended to prolong life or reduce the risk of major adverse health outcomes such as cardio-vascular events or recurrent cancer; or

- Multicenter trial in which mortality or major morbidity is a primary or secondary endpoint; or

- Multicenter trial in which any group is at relatively high risk of death or morbidity due to their underlying conditions, and where a medical intervention with subjects might increase such risk or cause unanticipated adverse events; or

- Multicenter or single center study performed in an emergency (life-threatening) setting in which informed consent has been waived (see 21 CFR 50.24(a)(7)(iv)).

C. *Requirements for a Data Safety-Monitoring Plan*

1. *All plans must include each of the following elements:*

- A determination of the appropriate interval for safety review; and

- A mechanism for review of safety data including adherence to the consent process, and monitoring of the data records and case report forms; and

- Procedures to assure that Serious Adverse Events (SAEs) will be provided in a timely manner to appropriate recipient agencies and to the IRB; and

- Specific predetermined criteria for stopping the study (predetermined "decision points") should that become necessary; and

- Identification of the individual or a listing of the committee members who will review the study's case report forms and consent documents to verify adherence to the study protocol. . . . ; and

- A description of how the data will be assessed to determine that there are no significant new interventions, procedures, or safety concerns that would affect the subjects' willingness to participate, without modification of the consent form; and

- Where applicable, a mechanism to immediately notify all study sites regarding findings relevant to the safety of study participants.

For guidelines and a sample of a generic monitoring plan, see the following websites: http://www.niams.nih.gov/rtac/clinical/dsmb3.html

http://www.cancer.gov/clinicaltrials/conducting/dsm-guidelines

2. Additional Requirements for a Local DSMC

When a local DSMC is required, the investigator will be responsible for establishing such a Committee. The DSMC must meet all of the following requirements:

- be composed of no less than three members possessing the qualifications and expertise to supervise the study; and

- have one member who is a biostatistician; and

- have no members affiliated with the study; and

- produce a semiannual report for the IRB.

3. Information Regarding DSMC on Multicenter Studies

There may be instances when the IRB will request from an SLU Principal Investigator, who is a sub-investigator in a multicenter project, information about the master protocol's study monitoring plan. When the IRB determines both that there is significant risk to subjects enrolled in a multicenter protocol, and that a DSMC is required, the SLU Principal Investigator will confirm that:

- for an industry-sponsored protocol, the proposal has a DSMC, or equivalent mechanism.

- for an NIH Sponsored Cooperative Group protocol, there is a DSMC in place.

Ethical Issues Arising When Interim Data in Clinical Trials Is Restricted to Independent Data Monitoring Committees
Robert J. Wells, Peter S. Gartside & Christine McHenry
22 IRB, Jan.-Feb. 2000, at 7

Over the past 20 years the use of independent data monitoring committees (DMCs) or data safety monitoring boards (DSMBs) to monitor and administer clinical trials has become quite common. Currently, they are mandated by federal policy for many U.S. government-sponsored trials. Inherent in the operation of these committees as established is that some information (interim data) from the trial is available only to members of the DMC. This information is not available to the group that designed the trial, the clinicians/researchers responsible for the medical care of the patients/subjects, or to the actual or potential patients/subjects in the trial. . . .

Clinical trials are designed to address important questions in medicine. Many times the question involves which of several potential available therapies is superior in terms of survival, lack of major complications, and, more recently, cost. In many cases, they involve prospective randomization among multiple therapeutic options. Often, the trials accrue patients over several years and may require up to seven to ten years of follow-up before a conclusion about the relative merits of the therapies tested is reached. During this time "trends" may develop that favor one or another of the therapies. For the purpose of this paper, *trend* is defined as a difference in a key outcome favoring one therapy that does not reach or exceed the pre-established rules to stop a trial. By convention, a p [probability] value of <0.05 is necessary to conclude at the end of a trial that one therapy is superior to another, while a much lower p value is necessary to reach the same conclusion on the basis of an interim analysis.

The membership of DMCs usually consists of knowledgeable individuals in the field studied (cancer specialists if the trial involves cancer, for example), statisticians, and more recently ethicists, government agency representatives, and "consumer" or patient representatives. They generally have no connection to the group who developed the trial. . . . As currently established, the DMC is the only body that is allowed to review complete information about a study as it accrues patients over time. The group that developed and is executing the trial may get some information about toxicity caused by their trial, but outcome results — including the relative outcomes in multiarm trials — is restricted to the DMC.

The rationale for establishing a DMC is that the group that developed the trial might be less objective than an independent body in the early detection of toxicity or efficacy. . . . [I]t was felt that if the group that developed the study . . . knew about interim data as it accrued, they might question the validity of their initial impression that there were no important differences among the therapies under study. Patient accrual would then decrease because the clinicians involved would not offer the study to their patients. Instead they would pick the "best" treatment as established by early data trends and thus interfere with the eventual demonstration of the superiority of one therapy over another.

. . . [C]onsider the following example. Assume that a clinical trial is well designed to determine which of two therapies, therapy A or therapy B, is superior. . . . In addition, assume that when 50% of the projected patients are enrolled two years into a planned four-year accrual period an interim analysis is performed and that this analysis shows therapy A is doing better than therapy B by the key end point of survival (p=0.10). The DMC, who will be the only people to see this information, would allow the study to continue unchanged since the difference seen reached neither the significance level that would allow a valid scientific determination of the superiority of therapy A at the end of the study (p<0.05) nor the more stringent difference used for early termination of the study (usually p<0.01 or 0.02) at interim analysis points. While it is true that scientific superiority of therapy A over B by current standards has not been demonstrated, potential patients and their clinicians have a keen interest in these results.

These data also can be used to estimate the relative risk of one therapy being found inferior, superior, or equal to another. For instance, in the example used (therapy A better than B with p=0.10 at 50% accrual) the probability of A being proven superior with p<0.05 at the end of the trial is 0.169, the probability of B being proven superior is 0.00002, and the chance of neither being superior is 0.8309. The relative risk of a patient getting inferior treatment . . . is 8,450 times higher if the patient is treated with therapy B. If clinicians and patients were aware of this information, many probably would find this relative risk too high and elect not to participate in the trial; they would simply choose therapy A over therapy B. Their decision would reduce further patient accrual.

NOTES AND QUESTIONS

1. As these readings note, one of the reasons that the use of DSMBs is growing rapidly is that federal agencies that fund research increasingly require them. The National Institutes of Health (NIH) require that a DSMB monitor each phase 3 study. For phase 1 and 2 studies, there is no automatic requirement to have a DSMB, although there must still be a detailed plan for monitoring data, which should be reviewed by an IRB. The NIH notes that a DSMB may be appropriate even in phase 1 and 2 studies if the studies have multiple clinical sites, are masked (blinded), or employ particularly high-risk interventions or vulnerable populations. See NATIONAL INSTITUTES OF HEALTH, FURTHER GUIDANCE ON A DATA AND SAFETY MONITORING FOR PHASE I AND PHASE II TRIALS, June 5, 2000, http//grants.nih.gov/grants/guide/notice-files/NOT-OD-00-038.html. The National Cancer Institute (and other divisions of the NIH) also has detailed requirements about the use of DSMBs, which appear at http://www.nci.nih.gov/clinicaltrials/conducting/dsm-guidelines.

2. As noted in Chapter 12, there have been a number of lawsuits filed in which IRB members have been named as defendants. *See* Chapter 12, at page 498. Is it likely that a member of a DSMB also could be sued as a result of an adverse outcome in a clinical investigation? If so, describe the likely elements of a cause of action in such an instance. While IRB members often will be indemnified by the institution on whose board they serve, is there any similar protection for DSMB members? If not, short of resignation, is there anything that such a DSMB member could do to protect him- or herself from liability?

3. As the Wells article notes, if a DSMB reviews interim results from a study and finds that the study results have not yet reached the level of statistical significance needed to stop the study, then the study will be permitted to continue. This can happen even though the results may be strongly leaning in favor of one outcome (such as that drug B is no better than drug A, and may be worse). Although subjects might very much want to know this information, it will almost never be given to them, because doing so could cause many of them to drop out of the study. What makes it ethical to deny them this information (or are current practices not ethical)? The Slutsky and Lavery article recommends certain types of disclosures to be made to prospective subjects in consent forms regarding the release of interim data. What types of disclosures do you think are appropriate?

4. How often is a DSMB supposed to be reviewing adverse events from a particular study? Is someone on the DSMB supposed to promptly make some sort of analysis of those events, rather than waiting for when the DSMB has its "regular" meetings (which, depending on the study, may only be once or twice a year)? If so, what are they to look for? Note, as discussed earlier in this chapter, how DSMB review to some extent is replacing IRB review of adverse events in multicenter studies. Does that circumstance help you answer this question? In a multicenter trial, is the IRB for the site where the adverse event takes place the only entity with a duty to promptly review the event?

5. For guidance on the functions of DSMBs, see SUSAN S. ELLENBERG ET AL., DATA MONITORING COMMITTEES IN CLINICAL TRIALS: A PRACTICAL PERSPECTIVE (2002).

**NBCC RAISES CONCERNS ABOUT HALTING
OF LETROZOLE CLINICAL TRIAL
NATIONAL BREAST CANCER COALITION**
(2003)

You have probably heard about the National Cancer Institute press release today [October 9, 2003] of the results of a breast cancer trial. Unfortunately, the National Cancer Institute has again stopped a breast cancer trial early, on the basis of interim results. A multicenter randomized placebo-controlled clinical trial of Letrozole indicated that after five years of Tamoxifen therapy, and an average of 2.4 years of follow-up, the risk of breast cancer recurrence was lower in the Letrozole group. Recurrence included local, contralateral and metastatic events.

Why are we concerned?

We certainly hope that long term this therapy helps women with breast cancer. However, this trial should not have been stopped. We don't know the long term side effects, which could outweigh the benefit of fewer recurrences. More importantly, recurrence is an interim outcome measure, and is not the correct end point for this trial. The study should not have been stopped unless a marked mortality benefit was shown for one of the two interventions or if it had been futile to continue, because no difference between the two groups was likely to emerge.

Putting the Letrozole findings in context.

You should recall the lumpectomy vs. mastectomy trials. All data combined indicate that having a mastectomy results in fewer recurrences than lumpectomy. Yet, over the long term, women die at the same rate regardless of which surgery they receive. If we had relied on recurrence data for assessing the relative values of the two surgeries, women would still be getting mastectomy and not lumpectomy. It is extremely important that we understand how to analyze clinical trials in order to evaluate information we receive from the research and provider communities. NBCC is in the process of releasing a fact sheet on study end points that will help advocates going forward.

Background information on the Letrozole trial.

For your information, the Letrozole trial was a double blind, placebo controlled study designed to determine whether giving patients the aromatase inhibitor, Letrozole, for 5 years after they had already completed approximately 5 years of Tamoxifen therapy would improve recurrence or survival. It looked at 5187 women who were postmenopausal, had early stage breast cancer, and had completed Tamoxifen therapy. Half got Letrozole and half got placebo. When the interim analysis was performed, the DSMB found that 132 women in the placebo group had experienced a disease recurrence, while only 75 of the women in the Letrozole group had experienced recurrence. A total of 42 women in the placebo group and 31 women in the Letrozole group had died (p=0.25 for overall survival). The median follow up was 2.4 years. The Kaplan Meier estimates for four-year disease free survival were 93% in the Letrozole group and 87% in the placebo group (P<0.001). Based upon the reductions in recurrence and the Kaplan Meier survival estimates, the DSMB decided to halt the trial, unblind the study, and notify the women.

What should you do?

The press releases from NCI quote the investigators as saying that based upon these findings, women should discuss 5 years of Letrozole with their doctor after completing Tamoxifen therapy. The biggest issues here are that the follow up is extremely short and the end point of recurrence is not meaningful. Letrozole is an aromatase inhibitor like Anastrazole, and we don't have the data yet to know what the long term effects of this treatment might be, particularly in terms of osteoporosis or cognition. We will need to continue to follow these women to determine the full side effects and benefits of this treatment. In the meantime, women need to know that we don't fully understand the long term effects of this drug yet.

NOTES AND QUESTIONS

1. In most instances, as part of designing a study, researchers will be required to specify in their protocol under what conditions a study will be ended "early" as a result of a DSMB's analysis of what has been happening in the study. In the case of the Letrozole study, these so-called "stopping rules" did indeed say that the study would be terminated if a specified statistical difference was reached between the time to cancer recurrence in the two groups, and that difference had been reached. In an editorial in the *New England Journal of Medicine*, the writers noted that the decision of the DSMB was thus justified. They reached that conclusion "reluctantly," however, echoing the concerns of the National Breast Cancer Coalition in noting that the primary reason for conducting the study — to see if using Letrozole actually caused the women to live longer — had not been fulfilled. *See* John Bryant & Norman Wolmark, *Letrozole after Tamoxifen for Breast Cancer — What is the Price of Success?* 349 NEW. ENG. J. MED. 1855 (2003). They suggested that future studies should possibly have stopping rules in the protocol that do not permit the study to be stopped early if doing so would "compromise" a primary purpose of the study, unless the study was being stopped due to safety concerns (e.g., that the drug being studied was causing too many side effects).

2. The *New England Journal of Medicine* editorial writers also noted a second reason for the DSMB having stopped the study early: that it would have been unethical not to do so, because the consent form included the statement, "If new side effects or information about my disease or treatment are discovered during the study, I will be told." Do you agree with that conclusion? (Note that study subjects generally are not told about the criteria in the protocol for stopping the study early.) If this was an ethical problem in this study, what if the stopping rules in the protocol had been different, and did not require the study to be stopped until a difference in survival between the two groups had been adequately proven? Would that have been ethical, assuming the consent form still contained the same statement about advising subjects of new information?

3. In a recent article, a gynecologic oncologist has suggested that consent forms should "explicitly state the criteria to be used for early study closure, thereby permitting the patient to make an informed decision regarding study participation." Stephen A. Cannistra, *The Ethics of Early Stopping Rules: Who Is Protecting Whom?* 22 J. CLINICAL ONCOLOGY 1542 (2004). Would such a dis-

closure be helpful? Imagine that the Letrozole study had been conducted with a revised stopping rule, one that said the trial would be stopped early only if a difference in survival (at the 5% level of statistical significance) had been demonstrated between the two arms. In what way might a subject use that information (as opposed to a more general comment in the consent form that subjects will not be told of interim results that may strongly suggest that one arm is better than another)?

4. Would it have been possible, in the Letrozole study, for the DSMB to have decided not to stop the trial, but merely to disclose to the current study participants what the interim analysis showed, and let each of them decide whether or not they wanted to continue to be in the study?

5. For additional discussions of the appropriateness of ending the Letrozole study early, see Editorial, *Halting a Breast Cancer Study*, N.Y. TIMES, Oct. 12, 2003, Sec. 4, at 10 (suggesting that early termination of the study might have been wrong, given that the study had not yet determined if Letrozole actually saved lives); Richard A. Friedman, *Long-Term Questions Linger in Halted Breast Cancer Trial*, N.Y. TIMES, Oct. 21, 2003, at F5.

6. Should there be any limitations on a sponsor's ability to terminate a study for reasons unrelated to subject protection? In the 1990s, a large study was conducted to see whether a relatively new type of medication for treating high blood pressure (a member of a class of drugs described as calcium channel blockers) was better than older and cheaper types of medications (beta blockers and diuretics). The study planned to enroll more than 15,000 subjects over several years, at sites located in fifteen countries. It was stopped two years prior to its planned end point by its pharmaceutical company sponsor for what were described as "business considerations." The DSMB monitoring this study had recommended that it be continued, because none of the end points specified in the protocol had been reached. The drug company's action resulted in an editorial in *JAMA*, claiming that ending a study early for purely commercial reasons appeared to be unethical and in violation of at least one international code of research ethics (the Declaration of Helsinki). *See* Bruce M. Psaty & Drummond Rennie, *Stopping Medical Research to Save Money: A Broken Pact With Researchers and Patients*, 289 JAMA 2128 (2003). The *JAMA* editorial claimed that the study sponsor broke the "covenant of mutual rights and responsibilities [between researchers and subjects that was] established during the informed consent process," because the subjects had agreed to be in the study with the understanding that they would be contributing to increasing medical knowledge. Do you agree with their conclusions? Should an early termination of a study for business reasons be viewed as a violation of the Common Rule (and if so, which provisions)? It is now common for many consent forms to include a provision specifying that a study sponsor may terminate a study "for any reason." If that clause had been in the consent form for the high blood pressure study, would it alter your assessment of the appropriateness of the sponsor's decision to terminate the study early?

7. People suffering from chronic fatigue syndrome participated in a study of a new drug, Ampligen, that had not yet been FDA approved. The study randomized subjects between the drug and placebo. The subjects were told that, after the randomized study ended, they would be permitted to enroll in a follow-up study where everyone would get the drug until it received FDA approval. After the initial results of the randomized study, the FDA rejected the company's application to give the drug to a broader group, noting that it caused "serious and potentially life-threatening reactions." However, the FDA had no objection to having the proposed follow-up study take place with the subjects who had been in the initial study. The company decided it did not want to do the follow-up study, and the subjects sued because they wanted to be treated with the drug. Did the company have a legal obligation to conduct that study? *See* Dahl v. HEM Pharmaceutical Corp., 1996 U.S. App. LEXIS 2549 (9th Cir. 1996).

Chapter 12

COMPENSATION FOR RESEARCH INJURIES

Although many other countries have developed comprehensive compensation systems for individuals who are injured as a result of participating in research, no such system exists in the United States. Instead, injured subjects must either rely on compensation mechanisms voluntarily adopted by some research institutions and sponsors, seek payment for their expenses from their own health and/or disability insurance, or, if they believe their injuries were the result of negligence or other misconduct, pursue damages through the tort system. Many subjects end up bearing some or all of the costs associated with their injuries themselves.

This chapter examines the ethical, legal, and policy issues surrounding existing compensation mechanisms for human research subjects, as well as proposals to establish a comprehensive no-fault compensation system as a matter of federal law. As you read these materials, think about the advantages and drawbacks of conditioning compensation on proof of negligence or other research-related misconduct, as opposed to awarding compensation to injured subjects in all cases. Consider also the role that various institutions should play in a compensation system, including research institutions and sponsors, insurers, administrative agencies, and the courts.

§ 12.01 ETHICAL CONSIDERATIONS

COMPENSATION FOR RESEARCH INJURIES
PRESIDENT'S COMMISSION FOR THE STUDY
OF ETHICAL PROBLEMS IN MEDICINE AND BIOMEDICAL
AND BEHAVIORAL RESEARCH
50-60 (1982)

The basic case for a program of compensation for injured subjects can be stated briefly: Medical and scientific experimentation, even if carefully and cautiously conducted, carries certain inherent dangers. Experimentation has its victims, people who would not have suffered injury and disability were it not for society's desire for the fruits of research. Society does not have the privilege of asking whether this price should be paid: it is being paid. In the absence of a program of compensation of subjects, those who are injured bear both the physical burdens and the associated financial costs. The question of justice is why it should be these persons, rather than others, who are to be expected to absorb the financial, as well as the unavoidable human costs of the societal research enterprise which benefits everyone.

The argument in favor of compensating injured subjects proceeds from a simple rule of thumb for determining the justice of the distribution of burdens and benefits in contexts like that of medical research: those who receive the benefits should be those who undertake the risks. In some medical research, the subjects are patients who volunteer precisely because the experiment offers the greatest chance of cure; prospective benefits outweigh prospective risks and distributive justice is not a major concern. When, however, as is often the case in research with human subjects, those who bear the risks are not the direct beneficiaries of the research, it is felt that the scales of justice are out of balance. Institutional Review Boards and other protective mechanisms have been designed to ensure that the balance is thrown off-center as little as possible, consistent with the goal of permitting promising research to continue. Compensation may be regarded as a means of restoring the balance after the fact, when the residuum of risk not eliminated by the protective devices has eventuated in injury. Like the protective devices, compensation is a further means of limiting the burdens borne by individual subjects in research.

The Argument from Fairness. The ethical norm underlying most of the literature favoring a program of compensation is that of fairness, a key element in the concept of justice. One formulation of a principle of fairness was provided to the Commission, following the philosophers Hart and Rawls:

> If there is a "mutually beneficial scheme of social cooperation," then "a person who has accepted the benefits of the scheme is bound by a duty of fair play to do his part and not to take advantage of the free benefits by not cooperating."

Stated as such, this is a principle of distributive justice: it dictates an assignment of benefits and burdens that is held to be just. This principle is invoked, for example, by moral and political theorists to justify the extraction of taxes from those who may never have signed an actual agreement to contribute to the state's budget. The idea is simply that if one benefits while others take their turns, then one too must take his or her turn. . . . In the research context, it is the government, representing the society, which must "take its turn." The research subject has contributed by exposing himself to risks, and the government must do its part. . . .

[An] important precedent is the Veterans' Compensation for Service-Connected Disability or Death Program. The obligation here is toward those

> who have entered into a special relationship of service to the American society, and who are, therefore, entitled to special compensation in the event of a service-connected disability. In short, the American society has recognized a special obligation to compensate veterans for injuries sustained in connection with their service since society is both sponsor and beneficiary of their services.

Further, soldiers

> . . . could sustain compensable injury — even serious injury or death — without anyone being guilty of negligence or any other tort. . . . [S]ociety, through its governmental agents, has intervened in the lives of the injured individuals, and therefore society may be said to have an obligation to repair (so far as possible) injury done to individuals, whether they are volunteers or draftees, in connection with their service to society.

> . . . Though these principles of fairness do not command universal assent among contemporary moral or political theorists, they have received considerable support in leading theories of distributive justice. They provide a moral basis for government mechanisms necessary for the harmonious functioning of large and complex societies, which must proceed in the absence of an actual contract and which would be crippled if denied the means for dealing with the problems of "free riders" who would take advantage of others' contributions to the public good.

The point of the argument from fairness, then, is that the potential beneficiaries of medical research — which includes the entire citizenry — ought not have a "free ride" at the expense of injured research subjects. If the human costs of research are low — say, a matter of a little time and inconvenience — then the allocation of costs is not a serious ethical issue. When, however, higher costs are occasionally imposed, as in the case of injured subjects, the question "Who pays?" becomes important. Research subjects are already doing more than their share, merely by the fact of having volunteered. Those who are injured bear the greatest burden of all. According to this view, certainly, they are the *least* appropriate parties to have to bear the financial costs of injury. Let those costs be shouldered by the potential beneficiaries who have contributed neither time nor health to the research effort. The society ought to meet this expense, through government action if necessary, in order to compensate the injured subjects.

The Gift of Security: Consenting Subjects as Free Agents. There is, however, another view which denies that a failure to compensate injured research subjects is necessarily an injustice. This view attempts to rebut the argument from fairness by stressing the possibility of informed consent to the risk of injury. Professor H. Tristram Engelhardt, who in his essay for the [Department of Health, Education, and Welfare] Task Force [examining research compensation] argued in favor of compensation, stated that

> [F]ree and informed consent would seem in most cases equivalent to waiver of any moral basis for a claim to recover for damages. Respect for freedom of the individual would include, so this argument would go, respect for that individual's freedom to choose to risk and suffer the consequences. When a human subject, who is sufficiently informed and who is free to choose, chooses in the absence of coercion to participate in an experiment, it would appear that the subject has given up any

strict moral claim to compensation for damages incident to being a subject in an experiment.

Similarly, Childress admits that

[t]o show that an injured party voluntarily assumed a risk is often a defense against that party's claim for reparative or compensatory justice.

The moral principle underlying these statements is often given in its Latin formulation: *volenti non fit injuria* — there is no injury [for which another party is responsible] to one who consents. Its application in the research context appears straightforward: the subject is told of the risks; he consents to joining the experiment even though those risks are present, and he has not been promised any compensation. Why, then, would society be obligated to compensate in the case of injury?

The Task Force, after much debate, took a strong stand on this question:

Informed consent in the research setting functions as a recognition of and a protection for a person's integrity and autonomy, but does not imply a waiver of the right of the person to compensation in the event of injury. . . . Even if a subject perfectly understands a research procedure and agrees to participate in that procedure, the subject's consent does not, in and of itself, include, explicitly or implicitly, a waiver of compensation. [V]olunteers may give informed consent to participation in biomedical and behavioral research without thereby surrendering the right to be compensated should injury occur.

But if, as the Task Force stated, one ought to respect the autonomy of the potential subject, it is at least initially difficult to understand why there is a moral requirement to compensate a subject who consents to participation without the expectation of compensation in case of injury. If "respect for autonomy" requires the subject's consent to be secured before using him or her as a research subject, why would that same "respect" not also require that the subject be permitted to agree to shoulder the risk of injury without the possibility of compensation?

The Task Force, it must be recalled, was speaking of a consent form (and process) that merely listed the risks and benefits of procedures, together with a statement of certain rights of the patient having nothing to do with compensation. Perhaps it could be said of that consent form, and of the process of obtaining consent which the form records, that the signing and consenting did not amount to an assumption of responsibility for risk. Shortly after the Task Force's report, however, institutions receiving Federal funds for research were told to include an explicit statement on their policy of providing or not providing medical care and other compensation. Thus the consent form became something closer to an explicit assumption of risk. And the forms could be made even clearer on this score — for example, with the addition of a sentence such as: "In signing this form I knowingly and freely assume all risks attendant to the non-negligent conduct of this experiment and do not expect, and will not seek to hold others liable for, compensation in case of injury not resulting from negligence." In this latter instance, if not at present, it is difficult to understand a contention that the subject's consent did not entail an assumption of risk.

Thus, there would seem to be an inconsistency in a position that would allow a subject of medical research to volunteer his or her time and comfort but not to assume the risk of possible injury. When the subject agrees to participate in an experiment, he or she voluntarily makes a gift to society of the time and inconvenience involved in participation, and agrees to bear any discomfort, which may be quite substantial. In some cases, subjects are paid for their time and trouble, but often they are not. One does not think that unless they are paid a sum proportional to their contribution, they have been treated unjustly. Indeed, subjects who are not paid may be especially admired. Their participation in the research is simply accepted as a gift.

A subject is, moreover, in a position to give still another gift. This is the gift of security, the assumption of the risk of injury without guarantee of compensation. Some potential subjects might be willing to give only the gift of their time and trouble, but others are willing to give not only that gift but also the gift of security. Why should it be considered unjust to accept the second gift if it is perfectly ethical to accept the first?

Whereas the Task Force asked whether volunteers must be compensated, the "free agent" view asks whether the government should be considered unjust if it refuses to accept volunteers who are unwilling to make the additional gift of their security. The government, that view holds, is under no obligation to accept as research subjects those who will not or cannot waive all rights to compensation if injured. As long as the government's needs can be met by accepting as volunteers only those who can pledge to forswear compensation if injured, there is no injustice done to anyone by failing to compensate injured subjects.

Fairness vs. Consent. These two perspectives on the question of whether failure to compensate injured subjects of medical research is unjust thus lead to quite different conclusions. The argument from fairness holds it to be unfair to impose the financial costs of injury upon those physically injured in the course of altruistic service to the community as research subjects. The second perspective stresses the freedom of citizens to volunteer their security as well as their convenience. As long as subjects make their choices freely, no injustice is done if only those subjects are accepted who assume responsibility for the cost of injuries.

Which of these two perspectives ought to be adopted in the case of research-related injuries? The Commission recognizes that each is worthy of serious consideration, and further recognizes that the divergence of views on the matter of compensation of subjects is but one instance of a divergence in thinking about social justice generally.

The fairness argument, stated in isolation, seems particularly convincing. It is, intuitively, quite unfitting that persons already injured should be saddled with the attendant costs; and it is equally unfitting that potential subjects be asked to agree to assume those costs as a condition of being enrolled in research. This view of justice prevails in many other contexts. Soldiers and other Federal employees, for example, are not asked to waive rights to compensation if injured on the job, even though it might be possible to recruit persons for these positions even were such a waiver required. Indeed, even private employers are not permitted to ask employees to waive coverage under Workmen's Compensation programs. The question of what would constitute a just distribution of burdens and benefits is decided in these other contexts before it is asked whether a waiver could be obtained; what matters is less whether an employee would agree to be denied compensation than whether this should even be asked.

When one fails to compensate injured subjects, though fiscal resources are available, one does not display the virtue of charity. Indeed, since the need arises because these subjects have displayed their concern for others by becoming subjects, a failure to compensate is distinctly uncharitable. The core question, however, is whether failure to compensate is not only uncharitable but unjust. A definitive answer would, it seems, require the Commission to choose between the rival views of justice: one emphasizing the achievement of an equitable pattern of distribution of the benefits and costs of research, the other stressing the transactions of free agents, whatever the resulting distribution. On the former view, the government has a strict obligation to compensate injured subjects, and its present failure to do so constitutes an injustice. On the latter view, uncompensated, injured subjects suffer no injustice so long as they freely and knowingly assumed responsibility for these costs before joining the experiment in which they were injured. Failure to compensate would then at most constitute a deficit in charity or benevolence.

Several serious reservations about the consent that is obtained from subjects make the latter view less convincing to the Commission. First, the consent argument's appeal to the notion of a gift freely offered would be strongest if the research subject were offered at the time he or she agreed to participate the alternatives of either having or not having compensation available should injury result. If subjects then reject the promise of compensation, they would appear to wish to donate both their time and their security. But in the absence of such an offer of future compensation, one cannot conclude that the consent of subjects who wish to aid research indicates their desire to make the additional gift of their security. Moreover, if injured subjects would accept compensation were it offered, then it would appear that they did not wish to make the gift of their security. This is not to say that consent could not be valid without an offer of compensation, but it does suggest that an element of capitalizing on subjects' desire to help science may sometimes occur.

Many subjects will have an altruistic desire to aid research by offering their time, together with a personal desire not to put their security at risk. If the research investigator and the government can afford to offer compensation for injury, but refuse to do so knowing that they will still obtain volunteers, they thereby exploit the altruistic motivation of volunteers: when a subject gives the willing gift of his or her time, the unwilling gift of his or her security is extracted as well. If exploitation is a form of unfair taking advantage of another, then the government or researcher may act unfairly in asking for volunteers while refusing them the possibility of compensation for injury. In particular cases, there may be no ground for concern over the moral sufficiency of consent — for example, when an intelligent, financially secure, educated adult agrees to undertake a small, accurately estimated risk of a minor harm of known character. But rules concerning compensation of subjects will not, as a practical matter, be able to distinguish these simple cases from the more difficult ones and the conditions of less-than-ideal consent are present often enough that the difficulties should be taken into account in formulating policy.

In many experiments, the risks are not well known. A treatment may be so new that the pattern of adverse reactions or side effects has not been established, nor will it be possible to determine whether a given subject is at especially high risk for these harms. Remote risks of serious harms are especially likely to attend experimental procedures. Consent in such cases is necessarily somewhat blind, and true appreciation of risk is doubtful, even for ideally competent subjects. Further, there is accumulating evidence that people do not perform well in calculating the expected utilities of events with small probabilities of occurrence. Events of different orders of magnitude of probability may be given the single rating of "unlikely." Assigning full responsibility to the subject for assumption of remote, but serious, risks of research thus takes on the air of exploitation of known weaknesses.

In the case of remote risks, when subjects agree to participate without compensation for injury, their gift of security is a small one because the substantial harm that might ensue is discounted for its low probability. For the unfortunate few subjects for whom the harm later materializes, however, an uncompensated injury dramatically increases the size of their gift to the research enterprise. While they agreed at the outset to bear the injury without compensation should it occur, one may reasonably conclude that they did not expect it to occur and did not truly intend to make this larger gift. Viewing the exchange in this light helps to account for some lingering sense that even allowing for the subject's valid consent to participate without compensation for injury, it is unfair for them to have to bear such a substantial burden. It may also help explain the strong obligation felt by many people (including many researchers) to provide compensation in order to "repay" this gift . . ., since the gift is not only large but probably more than the subjects initially intended to make.

To these difficulties may be added a host of standard complaints about the consent process. Patients who are subjects are sometimes, despite recitations of subjects' rights, in fear of displeasing their care-givers and hence in a dependent and unfree relationship. Patients are often agitated and distraught because of the very medical condition that qualifies them for an experiment. Moreover, a significant number of subjects, including children, the severely retarded, and the senile, are simply incompetent. The propriety of altruism-by-proxy which may be asked of these subjects is not established, even for the small risks permitted by the HHS regulations.

It can be presumed that under the current regulatory system, consent to treatment in most research involving human subjects meets the standards upon which society insists for valid transactions in other contexts, such as commerce. Indeed, the knowledge, competence, and independence of the contracting parties in society generally are seldom scrutinized as closely as are those qualities of potential subjects in biomedical research. Nevertheless, it is fitting to use a higher moral standard in the research context. The goals of human health and well-being that motivate research ought to be reflected as well in a higher moral standard than the *caveat emptor* of the marketplace.

NOTES AND QUESTIONS

1. How strong is the analogy between research participation and military service? Does the fairness argument depend on the assumption that subjects do not receive sufficient direct benefits from research participation to compensate them for the inherent risks? Is the argument stronger in certain types of research than others?

2. According to the Commission's description of the fairness position, potential beneficiaries of research, "who have contributed neither time nor health to the research effort" should not get a "free ride" by forcing injured subjects to bear all of the costs of their injuries. Is it relevant to the free rider argument that much biomedical research is supported by taxpayer money?

3. The Commission states, "If the research investigator and the government can afford to offer compensation for injury, but refuse to do so knowing that they will still obtain volunteers, they thereby exploit the altruistic motivation of volunteers." How would you determine whether the investigator and the government can "afford" to offer compensation? Would it be necessary to show that that funds currently spent on research are being wasted, or that money used for other, less valuable, purposes can easily be diverted to compensation programs? If the National Institutes of Health has a limited pool of money to award in grants, should it use some of it to cover the costs of compensating injured subjects, even if that means cutting back on the number of projects it supports?

§ 12.02 THE REGULATORY FRAMEWORK

45 C.F.R. § 46.116: GENERAL REQUIREMENTS FOR INFORMED CONSENT

This provision is reproduced in Appendix A, at page A-12. Please review the preamble and subsection (a)(6) before proceeding.

NOTES AND QUESTIONS

1. Is it fair to say that the regulations incorporate the "gift of security" position discussed in the President's Commission excerpt, insofar as they do not require researchers or sponsors to compensate subjects for injuries? If so, why do you think the regulations do not allow subjects to waive the right to sue for negligence?

2. It is important to distinguish researchers' obligations to *compensate* subjects for medical injuries from their duty to *treat* injured subjects. As to this latter duty, consider the following principle of tort law:

> If the actor knows or has reason to know that by his conduct, whether tortuous or innocent, he has caused such bodily harm to another as to make him helpless and in danger of further harm, the actor is under a duty to exercise reasonable care to prevent such further harm.

RESTATEMENT (SECOND) TORTS, § 322. In light of this principle, would a researcher who fails to provide prompt medical treatment to a subject who suffers injuries be liable for any further harm the subject experiences as a result of not receiving appropriate care? What if the subject's injuries do not develop for days, weeks, or years after the study? What if the subjects were informed, at the beginning of the study, that no medical treatments will be available in the event they are injured?

§ 12.03 TORT LIABILITY

Tort law is the body of rules and principles that determine when one person will be required to compensate another for "harmful wrongdoing." DAN B. DOBBS, THE LAW OF TORTS 1 (2000). Unlike much of the law applicable to human subject research, tort law is a matter of state, not federal, law. Although tort cases related to human subject research date back to the 1970s, it was not until the 1990s that research-related tort litigation began to take off. The next section examines the role of tort litigation in human subject research today. For an overview of the early cases, see E. Haavi Morreim, *Medical Research Litigation and Malpractice Tort Doctrines: Courts on a Learning Curve*, 4 HOUSTON J. HEALTH L. & POL'Y 1 (2003).

[A] The Emerging Role of Tort Litigation in Human Subject Research

The Rise of Litigation in Human Subjects Research
Michelle M. Mello, David M. Studdert & Troyen A. Brennan
139 ANN. INT. MED. 40 (2003)

In recent years, three important innovations have occurred in litigation over research-related injuries. First, the types of legal claims have diversified. Second, as a result the number and types of defendants named in these lawsuits have increased. Finally, plaintiffs' attorneys are increasingly using class action techniques to bring claims on behalf of large groups of research subjects. These developments individually and collectively may have significant implications for the future of human subjects research. . . .

The New Legal Claims

Enterprising plaintiffs' attorneys have turned to a daunting array of legal doctrines in framing lawsuits against those who perform and oversee research. A lawsuit that 20 years ago would have been brought as a routine informed consent claim may today include allegations of defective products, fraud, negligent conduct and monitoring of the research, intentional infliction of emotional distress, breach of patients' rights protected by state law, violation of federal regulations, and violation of constitutional rights. This diversification in legal causes of action is not unique to research-related litigation — it is also visible in other tort litigation such as suits brought by health maintenance organization enrollees against health plans that deny them coverage for services. However, it is especially pronounced in the human subjects area. A popular approach in lawsuits alleging injuries in pharmaceutical trials is to combine the traditional informed consent claim with product liability claims against the drug manufacturer. For example, the mother of an infant who died in a trial of the heartburn drug Propulsid recently filed suit against the Children's Hospital of Pittsburgh and Janssen Pharmaceuticals, alleging that she was not informed of risks and adverse events associated with Propulsid and that the drug was defectively designed. This legal tactic recycles one used in some of the earliest human subjects litigation, claims brought by women whose infants were injured by diethylstilbestrol.

Three other recent cases illustrate even greater legal creativity in the drafting of claims. The case of *Gelsinger v. University of Pennsylvania Hospital* arose from the death of 18-year-old Jesse Gelsinger in a phase I gene therapy trial. The Gelsinger family coupled the usual informed consent claim with a product liability claim, and then went further: They alleged that the investigators had committed fraud by not revealing that previous subjects enrolled in the protocol had died and that the principal investigator had a financial relationship with the sponsoring biotechnology company. The parties reached a confidential settlement in November 2000.

Robertson v. Oklahoma, a state court case that grew out of a federal suit dismissed for lack of jurisdiction, involved injuries to subjects in a phase I/II melanoma vaccine trial at the University of Oklahoma Health Sciences Center at Tulsa. The plaintiffs made three main allegations. First, they alleged a lack of informed consent based on the investigators' failure to reveal that the vaccine had not been subjected to animal studies, their failure to disclose all the relevant risks, and their misrepresentation of the vaccine as a potential cure for cancer. Second, they claimed that the trial itself was negligently run — essentially a claim of investigator "malpractice" in the conduct of research — because the investigators enrolled ineligible patients and failed to monitor the subjects' health appropriately. Third, they alleged that investigators fraudulently misrepresented the purpose, risks, and benefits of the study. Some of the defendants reached a settlement with the plaintiffs in July 2002.

The case of *Wright v. Fred Hutchinson Cancer Center* is another interesting cocktail of legal claims; it incorporates the kind of "research malpractice" and fraud claims used in *Robertson,* includes conflict of interest allegations like those in *Gelsinger,* and adds several new theories. In this case, subjects in a trial to prevent graft failure in patients undergoing bone marrow transplantation alleged that the investigators used misleading consent materials and failed to disclose various conflicts of interest. The plaintiffs also claimed that the investigators failed to report deaths appropriately to the IRB and failed to update consent forms as required by the IRB, in essence alleging negligent conduct of the trial. In addition, the plaintiffs in *Wright* posited a "breach of the right to be treated with dignity" under the due process clause of the 14th Amendment to the U.S. Constitution, arguing that international conventions such as the Nuremburg Code and the Declaration of Helsinki substantiated this right. The same group of attorneys have taken these groundbreaking constitutional and international law claims even further in other cases, although it is too early to judge their legal sway. The trial court in *Wright* recently dismissed the constitutional and international law claims made in that case, while a New York district court allowed similar claims to proceed in a case involving a drug trial in Nigeria.

The fraud claims in cases like *Wright* are of particular interest because they give the plaintiffs' attorney significant leverage in court. An allegation of fraud is likely to powerfully affect jurors. While the public may be becoming more cynical about business ethics in the wake of several major corporate scandals, the public is used to thinking of researchers as committed to new knowledge and the welfare of research subjects rather than the pursuit of profits that might come from a successful trial. Such a claim, casting investigators as intentionally leading subjects into danger for their own financial gain, can alter the entire tenor of a case.

Fraud allegations also open the door for enormous damages awards. In tort law, damages may have three components: compensation for economic losses, such as lost wages; damages for pain and suffering; and "punitive" damages. The punitive damages component, which is intended to punish especially blame-worthy defendants, usually accounts for a substantial portion of the multimil-lion-dollar personal injury verdicts that attract media attention. In actuality, punitive damages are rare: They occur in less than 1.5% of medical malpractice verdicts and approximately 5% of plaintiff trial wins overall. However, punitive damage awards are exceptionally common among fraud claims, occurring in about one-fourth of verdicts for the plaintiff. Hence, research subjects who bring successful fraud claims stand a good chance of receiving very large dam-ages awards. This makes research-related litigation very attractive to plaintiffs' attorneys who work on a contingency-fee basis.

The New Defendants

In addition to the proliferation of different types of claims, plaintiffs' attor-neys have innovated by casting their net across a wider range of defendants, including IRBs. The Gelsingers, for instance, sued the university, the hospital, the investigators, and the biotechnology company that sponsored the trial. The *Robertson* plaintiffs sued the hospital, the principal investigator, the pharma-ceutical sponsor, top university officials, the individual members of the IRB, and the university bioethicist who consulted with the IRB. Most recently, a suit brought by the family of a man who died in a trial of the Abiomed artificial heart even named the hospital's patient advocate.

The move to target IRBs has resonated deeply with academic medical centers, their IRB members, and the courts. This strategy formed the centerpiece of the highly publicized decision in *Grimes v. Kennedy-Krieger Institute*. . . . [The *Grimes* decision is excerpted in Chapter 13, at page 567.]

The multiple-defendant strategy used in cases like *Kennedy-Krieger* creates attractive litigation dynamics for the plaintiffs' attorney. Most obviously, it increases the pool of money available to pay a judgment. In addition, the nam-ing of top university officials and individual IRB members raises the profile of the case, attracting media attention and prompting concern on the part of offi-cials and IRB members at other institutions about their personal legal exposure. Finally, suing IRB members opens the door for courts to review the procedures and substance of IRB deliberations, rather than confining their scrutiny to the behavior of the investigators. This represents an important change in the scope of judicial review and regulation of human subjects research.

The New Class Actions

The third major innovation in human subjects research litigation is the use of class action techniques. In a class action lawsuit, a large number of individ-uals who have similar injuries and legal claims sue as a group, seeking a judg-ment or settlement that will apply to the entire class. The use of class action techniques in product liability claims has exploded over the last 30 years. In recent years, class action suits have proven powerful in litigation against drug manufacturers and tobacco companies. Pioneering uses of this strategy in research-related litigation date back to the diethylstilbestrol cases, and class actions are now becoming the norm in human subjects litigation.

Human experimentation injuries are quite amenable to the class action approach. The basic requirements for obtaining court permission to pursue a class action are that the group of plaintiffs is sufficiently numerous, that the commonalities among the plaintiffs outweigh the differences, that the named plaintiffs are typical of the rest of the class, and that the plaintiffs' attorneys can adequately represent the class. The requirement of numerosity is usually met since research protocols involve multiple subjects. Satisfaction of the commonality and typicality requirements tends to follow in cases involving a defectively designed protocol because subjects will probably feel the effects of the defect in similar ways. The representativeness requirement no longer poses a significant barrier because plaintiffs' attorneys have become very skilled in class action techniques and can ably represent large groups of plaintiffs.

The use of class actions has several advantages for plaintiffs' attorneys. With dozens to thousands of plaintiffs, the potential award to plaintiffs becomes much higher, making for higher contingency fees. Indeed, at least one firm has found clinical trials litigation so lucrative that it is marketing a specific practice niche in this area. Plaintiffs' firms can also combine forces and achieve economies of scale in litigation that would otherwise be too costly and cumbersome to pursue.

NOTES AND QUESTIONS

1. The core claim in most of the tort cases related to human subject research is that individuals or organizations involved in designing, conducting, or overseeing studies acted negligently. (Informed consent claims, a central element of many of the recent cases, are treated as a type of negligence claim in most jurisdictions.) Liability for negligence depends on proof that the plaintiff's injuries were the result of the defendant's "unreasonable" conduct.

In most tort cases, the reasonableness of the defendant's conduct is determined by considering "what the reasonably prudent person would do under the circumstances." 3 F. HARPER, F. JAMES, JR. & O. GRAY, THE LAW OF TORTS 389 (2d. ed. 1986). However, in cases alleging professional liability, such as medical malpractice cases, the definition of negligence is different. In place of the generic "reasonable person" standard, the focus is on the "standard of care" of the particular profession. Most jurisdictions define the standard of care in terms of the care "customarily" provided by other members of the profession under similar circumstances. Some jurisdictions have shifted away from an exclusive reliance on professional custom and allow juries to assess the overall reasonableness of the physician's actions. *See* Philip G. Peters, Jr., *The Role of the Jury in Modern Malpractice Law*, 87 IOWA L. REV. 909 (2002). Yet, even under this approach, the customs of the medical profession remain highly relevant to the jury's inquiry.

What role should professional standards of care play in cases involving human subject research? In cases against IRB members, for example, many of the defendants are professionals, whose decisions are likely to be influenced by their training and the norms of their professional communities. Yet, IRBs are comprised of individuals from a variety of professional backgrounds, and some IRB members do not have any professional affiliation at all. In cases alleging IRB negligence, which of the following standards should be applied: (1) the reasonably prudent person standard; (2) the reasonably prudent person standard for nonprofessional members of IRBs, and professional standards of care for the professional members, with the specific standard applied based on the professional affiliations of the particular member; (3) a uniform professional standard of care based on the standards of the "IRB community"? Similar questions arise when bioethicists are sued for negligently advising researchers on how to design a study, as happened in the *Gelsinger* case. *Cf.* Bethany J. Spielman, *Professionalism in Forensic Bioethics*, 30 J. L. MED. & ETHICS 420 (2002) (examining whether bioethicists have sufficiently clear and distinct professional standards to warrant their use as expert witnesses). What are the policy implications of adopting a professional standard of care for IRB members or bioethicists, as opposed to an ordinary reasonable person standard?

The relevance of professional medical standards to cases against physicians conducting human subject research is particularly complicated because research physicians often provide the same medical interventions as nonresearch physicians, but they do so for the purpose of developing generalizable knowledge, not for the benefit of any particular subject. This issue is examined in more detail below, at page 502.

2. While there has yet to be a successful lawsuit against members of an IRB, the mere possibility of being sued as a result of service on a committee that usually involves a great deal of work, and that generally brings relatively few concrete benefits for the members (apart from an occasional free meal), has created some degree of consternation among such members. However, "one legal scholar suggests that the decision to sue IRB members is consistent with a general practice among plaintiffs' attorneys to cast the net as wide as possible, at least initially." Even if these claims are not successful, "naming IRB members as defendants may be a way of intimidating them and undermining their credibility should they ever be called to testify." Mary R. Anderlik & Nanette Elster, *Lawsuits Against IRBs: Accountability or Incongruity?* 29 J. L. MED. ETHICS 220 (2001). Should IRB members ever be required to pay money damages when injuries result from studies the IRB approved? If so, under what conditions should the members be held personally liable for an IRB's decision to approve a study? *See generally* David B. Resnik, *Liability for Institutional Review Boards: From Regulation to Litigation*, 25 J. LEGAL MED. 131 (2004).

3. While some plaintiffs have asserted claims based on alleged violations of the federal research regulations, the regulations do not expressly give subjects the right to sue for damages, nor do they appear to provide an "implied" right to sue. *See* Lori A. Alvino, *Note: Who's Watching the Watchdogs: Responding to the Erosion of Research Ethics by Enforcing Promises*, 103 COLUM. L. REV. 893, 909 n.114 (2003). Assuming the regulations do not themselves form the basis of a claim for damages, how might they still be relevant to a tort suit involving human subject research?

4. As a result of recent lawsuits against individual IRB members, the Institute of Medicine has urged research institutions to "indemnify both internal and external board members" — i.e., to pay for any damages awarded against the members — "to prevent them from being unduly influenced by the personal risks of potential litigation." INSTITUTE OF MEDICINE, RESPONSIBLE RESEARCH: A SYSTEMS APPROACH TO PROTECTING RESEARCH PARTICIPANTS 195 (2003). How might the potential for litigation "unduly influence" an IRB member?

5. More generally, what type of incentive is tort litigation against researchers, research institutions, and others involved in human subject research likely to create? Will it encourage greater attention to human subject protections, or will it lead to a risk-averse climate that slows down the progress of medical discoveries? Might it do both of these things simultaneously?

Similar questions have been raised with respect to the incentives created by the medical malpractice system. For a long time, the primary complaint about the incentives created by malpractice law was that the fear of liability led physicians to practice "defensive medicine," i.e., to order excessive tests or perform unnecessary procedures in an effort to avoid a lawsuit. More recently, the focus has shifted to the impact of the malpractice system on system-wide efforts to reduce medical errors, a concern fueled by a 2000 Institute of Medicine report documenting high rates of medical errors in American hospitals. *See* COMMITTEE ON QUALITY OF HEALTH CARE IN AMERICA, INSTITUTE OF MEDICINE, TO ERR IS HUMAN: BUILDING A SAFER HEALTH SYSTEM (2000). According to some commentators, the malpractice system makes it difficult to implement error-reduction programs because its focus on assigning blame makes physicians reluctant to talk about, and thereby learn from, their inevitable mistakes. *See* David M. Studdert & Troyen A. Brennan, *Toward A Workable Model of "No-Fault" Compensation for Medical Injury in the United States*, 27 AM. J.L. & MED. 225, 228 (2001) ("Both anecdotal and empirical evidence suggest that providers are less willing to disclose information about errors they make or see when a punitive atmosphere prevails."). Of course, the flip side of the incentives argument is that fear of liability will lead physicians to take appropriate precautions to avoid causing injury. Critics of the current system, however, contend that there is only "thin" evidence that the malpractice system actually deters medical mistakes. *See* Michelle A. Mello & Troyen A. Brennan, *Deterrence of Medical Errors: Theory and Evidence for Malpractice Reform*, 80 TEX. L. REV. 1595 (2002).

Does the fact that research is subject to greater prospective oversight than ordinary clinical treatment alter the way in which researchers are likely to respond to tort lawsuits?

[B] Defining Researchers' Duties to Subjects

In malpractice cases related to the provision of ordinary medical treatment, the legal standard governing physicians is relatively clear: Once a physician-patient relationship has been established, the physician is expected to be guided by the medical best interests of the individual patient. In medical research, by contrast, the primary goal is not to promote the best interests of the subjects in the study. Instead, it is to develop generalizable knowledge for the benefit of patients in the future. While participating in research may sometimes be consistent with the medical best interests of individual subjects, in many situations research requires trade-offs between the subject's best interests and the study's scientific goals. For example, in order to avoid the problem of selection bias, researchers assign subjects to different arms of a study randomly, with no effort to determine whether one intervention is better for a particular subject in light of his or her individual needs. Similarly, rather than basing dosages of drugs and timing of interventions on a case-by-case evaluation of each subject's circumstances, researchers must adhere to the requirements of the protocol, which typically do not allow for a great deal of variation. Researchers also may perform invasive procedures on subjects, such as biopsies or lumbar punctures, solely for the purposes of gathering data, with little or no potential to benefit the subject's own health. Indeed, given the numerous ways in which research can conflict with individual subjects' best interests, if physicians conducting research were held to the same legal obligations of treating physicians, much of what they do would have to be considered malpractice per se.

The next excerpt considers how these differences between research and ordinary treatment affect the nature of the legal duties to which researchers should be held.

Duties to Subjects in Clinical Research
Carl H. Coleman
58 VAND. L. REV. 387 (2005)

Physicians who conduct clinical research with human subjects face a profound conflict in professional roles. As physicians, they are committed to promoting the medical best interests of current patients. As researchers, however, their goal is to produce generalizable knowledge by studying the effects of interventions in broad cohorts of subjects. Because producing generalizable knowledge often requires actions that are inconsistent with the medical best interests of the individuals enrolled in a study, these dual objectives often come into conflict. In such situations, where should the physician-researcher's loyalties lie? . . .

At one extreme, courts might conclude that researchers have the same therapeutic obligations to subjects in clinical trials that physicians owe patients receiving ordinary medical treatment, a position advanced by several commentators. . . . According to this approach, researchers providing potentially therapeutic interventions in the context of clinical trials may not deviate from the medical best interests of individual subjects, because to do so would violate the physician's professional obligation to promote the patient-subject's well-being. . . .

[H]owever, the methodological demands of clinical trials often pose unavoidable conflicts with the medical interests of individual subjects. Thus, if taken seriously, the view that researchers' duties are equivalent to those of treating physicians would require a virtual prohibition of clinical research. Moreover, the approach ignores the fact that some individuals might rationally choose to sacrifice the therapeutic commitment of a physician-patient relationship in exchange for other benefits that being in a clinical trial can sometimes entail.

Alternatively, courts could take the opposition position — i.e., that because clinical trials do not constitute a form of medical treatment, researchers have no obligation to promote subjects' individual medical interests. Such an approach would emphasize the researcher's commitment to producing scientifically valid data, a consideration not relevant when physicians provide care outside of research. Because producing scientifically valid data often requires actions inconsistent with subjects' medical interests, courts might conclude that it is illogical to hold researchers to the same therapeutic obligations that apply to treating physicians. Commentators who endorse this approach argue that protecting subjects' individual interests is the function of the informed consent process, and that subjects who have consented to participate in a study should not rely on the researcher to look out for their individual needs.

While this position avoids the restrictiveness of the first approach, the view that researchers have no obligation to protect subjects' medical interests errs too far in the opposite direction. Its reliance on informed consent as the primary mechanism for protecting subjects' welfare ignores the fact that the process of informed consent suffers from significant limitations. In addition, even when the validity of subjects' consent cannot reasonably be doubted, the process of human experimentation implicates interests beyond those of the individuals who agree to be subjects. Regulatory oversight of research addresses some of these issues, but these oversight mechanisms are not designed to identify specific individuals for whom enrolling or continuing in a study poses unacceptable risks. . . .

We are thus left with a dilemma: On the one hand, if clinical research is different from ordinary medical treatment, researchers' deviation from the medical best interests of individual subjects is not necessarily problematic, provided there are valid reasons for conducting the study and the subjects voluntarily agree to assume the risks of foregoing individualized medical care. On the other hand, deficiencies in the process of informed consent to research, combined with the societal interest in overseeing the conduct of medical professionals, suggest that researchers should not be permitted to completely ignore the medical best interests of individual subjects, even if protecting subjects' welfare may impede the production of generalizable knowledge. The challenge is to define researchers' duties in a manner that both recognizes subjects' presumptive authority to consent to deviations from their medical best interests, while carving out a limited duty of therapeutic attentiveness to which all researchers must adhere.

Fortunately, this type of challenge is not unique to human subject research. The function and limits of consent in relationships characterized by trust and dependency also is a familiar theme in the regulation of financial transactions, where the issue frequently arises in dealings between individuals in fiduciary relationships. Consider, for example, a young adult who inherits property in the form of a trust, which will be managed by a trustee until the beneficiary reaches a certain age. The beneficiary stands in a highly vulnerable position vis-à-vis the trustee, given that the trustee has legal title to the property and the authority to manage it, while the beneficiary may lack the maturity, financial acumen, or access to information necessary to determine whether the trustee is managing the property appropriately. The law regulates such situations to ensure that the trustee does not pursue interests at odds with those of the beneficiary, in part by limiting the legal effectiveness of the beneficiary's consent. For example, if the trustee sells trust property to a business in which she has significant interests — potentially benefiting the trustee at the expense of getting the best price for the property — the transaction may be voidable even if the beneficiary consented to it. The law does not bar beneficiaries from consenting to transactions in which trustees pursue conflicting interests, but it requires additional indicia of fairness before the transaction will be upheld. In other fiduciary relationships, the law similarly imposes limits on the beneficiary's power to authorize transactions in which the fiduciary is pursuing competing interests, although the nature and extent of those constraints differs depending on the type of relationship involved.

Admittedly, there are differences between the conflicts that typically arise in relationships governed by fiduciary principles and the conflicts inherent in clinical research. In traditional fiduciary relationships, the underlying purpose of the relationship is to benefit the beneficiary; in research, the primary goal is to develop generalizable knowledge. In addition, conflicts in traditional fiduciary relationships usually involve the fiduciary's effort to derive *personal* advantages at the expense of the beneficiary; in research, the conflict involves the researchers' pursuit of *societal* benefits in a manner that compromises the subject's medical needs. Nonetheless, the law's treatment of the pursuit of self-interest by fiduciaries in financial relationships provides a model for thinking about the power and limits of consent in dependent relationships more generally. For one thing, it calls into question the assumption that individuals in vulnerable relationships are inherently incapable of consenting to actions that are potentially inconsistent with their overall best interests. At the same time, the fact that the legal effectiveness of consent is limited in fiduciary relationships suggests that consent is not necessarily a sufficient safeguard to protect vulnerable individuals from exploitation and abuse. Ultimately, fiduciary principles can help bridge the gap between the all-or-nothing views of researchers' obligations . . ., by providing a framework in which consent, while important, becomes just one of several conditions necessary to justify deviations from the pursuit of subjects' medical well-being.

[In an omitted portion of this article, the author notes that courts and commentators disagree about whether the researcher-subject relationship fits into the usual definition of a fiduciary relationship. However, he concludes that] the critical question is not whether the researcher-subject relationship necessarily *is* a fiduciary relationship, but whether it is sufficiently *similar* to fiduciary relationships to warrant the application of a comparable legal approach. . . . [T]he relationship between researchers and subjects is characterized by the same type of vulnerability, trust, and expectation of protection that underlie the relationship between fiduciaries and beneficiaries. These similarities make fiduciary principles an appropriate model for defining researchers' duties to subjects, even if the researcher-subject relationship is different from traditional fiduciary relationships in certain respects. . . .

[The remainder of this article considers the implications of adopting a fiduciary-like framework to damage claims against researchers.] Consider a study that randomizes subjects between standard treatment and an investigational drug for the treatment of stage IV pancreatic cancer, a condition for which available treatments are not very helpful. After the study begins, one subject experiences severe nausea and has difficulty keeping down food. While other subjects have also experienced some similar symptoms, this subject's experience is particularly severe. Because the study is double-masked, no one knows whether the subject is receiving standard treatment or the investigational drug. If the subject drops out of the study, she can receive individually-tailored treatment that might pose fewer side effects — although it is possible that, if she has been randomized into the standard treatment arm, the treatment she would receive outside the study might not differ greatly from what she is currently receiving. If she continues in the study, however, her nausea and discomfort are likely to continue.

The IRB may well have acted appropriately in authorizing this study, assuming a favorable balance between the study's overall risks and benefits. Nonetheless, the IRB's approval does not free the researcher from considering the implications of continuing in the study for the subject's well-being. If the subject continues in the study, suffers increasing discomfort, and ultimately sues the researchers for causing her injuries, a fiduciary-law approach suggests the following framework for evaluating her claim:

First, the plaintiff would have to show that the decision to continue in the study posed a conflict between her medical best interests and the pursuit of scientific knowledge. In other words, as in a traditional breach-of-fiduciary-duty claim, the plaintiff would have the burden of showing that the researcher was actually faced with a conflict of interest. If no such conflict existed, any claim for breach of the researcher's duties would necessarily fail.

Assuming the plaintiff can make such a showing (which should not be difficult under the hypothetical presented above), the burden of persuasion would shift to the researcher to demonstrate that the subject consented to continue in the study after being fully informed about the risks and alternatives. This requirement mirrors the approach used in breach-of-fiduciary-duty cases involving trustees, both in that it treats consent as an absolute requirement in all situations and that it shifts the burden of persuasion to the defendant once the plaintiff has established that a conflict existed. The trustee approach is appropriate in this context because, as discussed above, the researcher-subject relationship exhibits at least as much vulnerability and dependency as the relationship between trustee and beneficiary.

However, even if the researcher can establish that the subject was given adequate information and expressed her willingness to continue, the inquiry would not end there. Just as a trustee may not engage in unfair transactions even if the beneficiary has consented, the researcher should have a duty to avoid unreasonable risks to the subject's medical interests regardless of whether the subject has knowingly accepted those risks. In other words, under some circumstances the researcher should be required to override a subject's decision to continue in a study, if continuing would pose unreasonable risks to the subject's well-being.

The critical question, of course, is giving content to the concept of "reasonableness" in this context. . . . [T]he standard used in traditional breach-of-fiduciary-duty claims, which focuses on what might have occurred in the absence of the fiduciary's conflict of interest, is inappropriate in research, given that some subjects might reasonably accept some deviations from their medical interests in order to pursue other legitimate goals. Instead, the reasonableness inquiry should turn on the *extent* to which the decision compromised the subject's medical interests in order to pursue the potential for generalizable knowledge. This interpretation of reasonableness would prevent researchers from taking unfair advantage of subjects without denying individuals the autonomy to participate in research for reasons that are important to them.

To achieve this goal, the fact-finder should consider a variety of factors that affect individuals' decisions about participating in research. Thus, it should take into account the possibility that some individuals are genuinely motivated by altruism, as well as the other factors that might lead a reasonable person to continue in a study even when doing so involves risks to their medical well-being. At the same time, it should consider the vulnerability inherent in the researcher-subject relationship, as well as the impact of the therapeutic misconception on the process of consent. Ultimately, the purpose of the inquiry should be to determine whether the decision to continue in the study reflects a reasonable tradeoff between the individuals' medical interests and other goals that a reasonable person might plausibly pursue.

If the researcher cannot satisfy this reasonableness standard, and the plaintiff can show that she actually experienced an injury, the researcher should be permitted to escape liability only by demonstrating that the subject's injuries were not proximately caused by the researcher's deviation from the subject's medical interests. Putting the burden on the researcher to disprove the causal link between the breach of fiduciary duty and the damages suffered by the plaintiff is again modeled on the approach used in cases involving trustees. Essentially, the plaintiff's burden is simply to demonstrate the existence of the conflict and a physical injury; at that point, the defendant bears the burden of persuasion on the elements of consent, reasonableness, and proximate cause.

An important aspect of this approach is that the reasonableness of tradeoffs between the pursuit of generalizable knowledge and the protection of subjects' welfare would be based on a lay community standard, i.e., on the fact-finder's assessment of the tradeoffs a reasonable person would be likely to accept. The use of a lay standard is appropriate in this context because the acceptability of tradeoffs between pursuing generalizable knowledge and protecting subjects' medical interests is primarily a question about ethics and values, which are not matters about which researchers can claim special expertise. Thus, these cases are not like malpractice cases involving ordinary medical treatment, in which the law has traditionally deferred to the medical profession's own assessment of the standard of care. When physicians provide treatment to patients in a non-research setting, the risks and benefits all relate to the consequences of the treatments for the individual patient. Physicians can plausibly claim special expertise in determining the type of treatments most likely to promote the health of their patients, but researchers know nothing more than the rest of us about the ethical acceptability of sacrificing subjects' medical interests for the larger social good.

This distinction between expert professional matters and ordinary questions of reasonableness has already been recognized in the law of informed consent. In *Canterbury v. Spence*, one of the first cases to hold that physicians must inform patients about the risks, benefits, and alternatives that a "reasonable patient" would consider material to a decision, the court emphasized that the professional standard of care should be limited to questions that bring the physician's "medical knowledge and skills peculiarly into play." In rejecting the professional standard for questions related to the disclosure of information, the court found that "[t]he decision to unveil the patient's condition and the chances as to remediation . . . is ofttimes a non-medical judgment." The same can be said for decisions about balancing the pursuit of generalizable knowledge and individual subjects' medical needs.

Applying a lay standard in this context would also create appropriate incentives for researchers. When pursuing scientific rigor poses potential risks to individual subjects, the researcher would have to consider not just her own views on the matter, or the views of her professional colleagues, but how a lay decision-maker is likely to view the reasonableness of asking a subject to accept the particular tradeoff. At the same time, because the standard incorporates the possibility that reasonable people might accept risks to their medical interests under some sets of circumstances, it would not preclude the use of methodological features that require deviations from the medical best interests of subjects, provided those deviations satisfy a reasonableness test.

NOTES AND QUESTIONS

1. Do you agree that researchers should sometimes be required to remove a subject from a study because continuing would pose unreasonable risks to the subject's medical interests — even if the subject has been informed of those risks and would like to continue?

2. Should researchers who enroll their own patients in clinical trials have a greater duty to protect those individuals' individual medical interests than they would have in the absence of a pre-existing therapeutic relationship? What would be the implications of requiring such physicians to adhere to the therapeutic obligations of physicians providing ordinary medical treatment?

3. Should the approach proposed in the preceding excerpt apply in cases alleging that an entire study was negligently designed, as opposed to a claim that a physician-researcher failed to take adequate precautions to protect an individual subject? For example, suppose a research subject tried to kill himself after being taken off his antipsychotic medications during the "washout" phase of a clinical trial. (Recall the UCLA schizophrenia study discussed in Chapter 6, at page 271.) He now claims that the trial was negligently designed because the washout period should have been conducted in an in-patient setting. Should the appropriateness of hospitalizing subjects who are being taken off anti-psychotic medications be evaluated in light of what treating physicians customarily do, what researchers customarily do, or what a lay jury thinks would be reasonable under the circumstances?

4. Research subjects who are injured as a result of taking an investigational drug may be able to bring a products liability lawsuit against the drug's manufacturer. See Gaston v. Hunter, 588 P.2d 326 (Ariz. Ct. App. 1978) (finding that products liability law applies to drugs that are distributed to subjects in clinical trials). However, in most cases such claims are unlikely to succeed. Unless the drugs the plaintiff took were manufactured incorrectly (e.g., there were dangerous impurities in the pills that the plaintiff swallowed), the plaintiff would have to show that the drug was designed defectively or that it was accompanied by inadequate warnings. Proving that a drug is defectively designed is notoriously difficult; according to the Restatement of Torts, a prescription drug or medical device can be considered defective in design only if the risks are so great in light of the potential benefits "that reasonable health care providers, knowing of such foreseeable risks and therapeutic benefits, would not prescribe the drug or medical device for any class of patients." RESTAT. 3D OF

TORTS: PRODUCTS LIABILITY, § 6. Inadequate warning claims are also unlikely to be successful, as many of the risks associated with investigational drugs are unknown. *See generally* Anna C. Mastroianni, *HIV, Women, and Access to Clinical Trials: Tort Liability and Lessons from DES*, 5 DUKE J. GENDER L. & POL'Y 167 (1998) (discussing the application of tort principles to clinical trials).

5. Should cases in which subjects are injured as a result of standard clinical procedures performed in a study, such as biopsies or X rays, be decided according to the standard of care used for physicians performing those procedures in clinical practice? Consider a subject who experiences pain while undergoing a bronchoscopy (a procedure in which a slender tube with a small light on the end is inserted into the patient's bronchi in order to perform an inspection) in a study that is not expected to benefit the subjects directly. The subject is obviously experiencing discomfort, so the researchers give her an additional dose of a local anesthetic. (Recall that this is what happened to Nicole Wan, the University of Rochester student who died during a study in which she had enrolled as a normal healthy volunteer. *See* Chapter 8, at page 390.) Physicians performing bronchoscopies for clinical purposes believe that it is appropriate to provide additional anesthesia to make the procedure more tolerable, despite the increased risks to the patient, because the risks are outweighed by the potential benefits of the procedure for the patient. Here, however, the subject will experience no benefits from the bronchoscopy, because she has no medical need to undergo the procedure. If the subject is injured as a result of the increased anesthetic, does the fact that increasing the dose of anesthetic would be considered acceptable outside of research mean that the researchers' actions were not negligent?

6. If a researcher's failure to adhere to the protocol causes an injury, should the protocol violation be considered negligence per se?

7. In *Grimes v. Kennedy Krieger Inst.*, 782 A.2d 807 (Md. 2001) (discussed more extensively in Chapter 13, at page 567), researchers were attempting to determine the effectiveness of modified forms of lead abatement in inner-city households, given that the prevailing methods were so expensive that landlords did not use them. During the course of the study, they discovered that some houses that had undergone modified lead abatement had higher-than-normal lead levels, but they did not inform the residents of those test results. Several months later, a child in one of the houses was found to have elevated lead levels in her blood. Her mother brought suit against the researchers, arguing that the researchers should have told the family of the earlier results from testing the house. The court concluded that a "special relationship . . . can result from the relationship between researcher and subject," and that this relationship may require the researcher to warn subjects "regarding dangers present when the researcher has knowledge of the potential for harm to the subject and the subject is unaware of the danger." *Id.* at 818, 846.

8. As discussed in Chapter 6, research can impose risks on third parties not involved in the study. For example, in a study testing a new drug with unknown

side effects, a subject might become unconscious while driving a car and injure a third party. *See* Chapter 6, at page 279. In a study in which individuals with schizophrenia are taken off their medications, subjects could become homicidal. If a third party sues a researcher for injuries resulting from the research, how should courts evaluate the claim? Outside of research, some courts have held that physicians have legally enforceable obligations to any third party who is foreseeably endangered by the physician's conduct. *See, e.g., Welke v. Kuzilla*, 375 N.W.2d 403 (Mich. Ct. App. 1985) (holding that the estate of a woman killed in a car accident could assert a claim against the physician who prescribed medication to the driver of the other car, on the theory that the medication precipitated the accident). Other courts have been unwilling to extend physicians' legal duties so far. *See, e.g.,* Kirk v. Michael Reese Hosp., 513 N.E.2d 387 (Ill. 1987) (rejecting claims against a physician under circumstances similar to *Welke* and holding that "a plaintiff cannot maintain a medical malpractice action absent a direct physician-patient relationship between the doctor and plaintiff or a special relationship . . . between the patient and the plaintiff"). Which approach do you find preferable? Should the scope of researchers' duties to third parties necessarily be equivalent to the scope of nonresearch physicians' duties?

[C] Additional Issues in Informed Consent Cases

In informed consent cases not involving medical treatment, most jurisdictions require plaintiffs to satisfy a three-part test. First, the plaintiff must establish that the physician failed to disclose adequate information about the risks, benefits, or alternatives of the treatment. In about one-half of the states, the adequacy of information is determined by asking what a reasonable practitioner would have disclosed under the circumstances. The jury makes this determination by evaluating expert medical testimony. In most other states, the jury determines what constitutes adequate information by asking what a reasonable person in the patient's circumstances would want to know, an assessment that does not depend on what type of information is customarily disclosed. Second, the plaintiff must show that the possible consequences of the treatment that were not disclosed — such as the risk of a particular complication — actually materialized. Finally, the plaintiff must prove that, if the physician had made an adequate disclosure, a reasonable person in the patient's position would not have undergone the procedure. *See generally* Aaron D. Twerski & Neil B. Cohen, *Informed Decision Making and the Law of Torts: The Myth of Justiciable Causation*, 1988 U. ILL. L. REV. 607. These burdens are often quite difficult to satisfy, and for that reason most informed consent claims are not successful. This is particularly true when the patient has received what the medical community considers to be the best option for treating a serious disease or condition. Under those circumstances, regardless of how much information the physician has withheld from the patient, it may be impossible to convince a jury that a reasonable person would have rejected the treatment if she were fully informed.

The next excerpt argues that courts should apply different standards to evaluating informed consent claims related to human subject research.

Medical Research Litigation and Malpractice Tort Doctrines: Courts on a Learning Curve
E. Haavi Morreim
4 HOUSTON J. HEALTH L. & POL'Y 1 (2003)

Duty of Care: Scope of Disclosure

. . . Neither of the traditional malpractice standards is adequate for research. A physician-based standard could embrace little or no disclosure if physicians' prevailing practice were to keep patients in the dark. The "reasonable patient" standard has little applicability because the decision to enter research is highly individual. Research does not aim to benefit any individual patient, and people can have a wide variety of reasons for entering research, from altruism to financial gain to a desperate, last-ditch hope for cure. The *Belmont Report* itself came to this conclusion back in 1979, finding both of the conventional disclosure standards "insufficient since the research subject, being in essence a volunteer, may wish to know considerably more about risks gratuitously undertaken than do patients who deliver themselves into the hand of a clinician for needed care." . . .

Accordingly, research requires a distinctive standard of disclosure. It will be based heavily on federal regulations that require an array of facts to be disclosed, such as the purposes, duration and procedures of the research; any reasonably foreseeable risks or discomforts; potential benefits to the enrollee or to others; available alternatives to the research trial; and other specified information.

Additionally, the disclosure standard for research should include a subjective element in deference to individuals' varying needs for personally important information. Consent forms virtually always incorporate this element by inviting prospective enrollees to ask questions. At the same time, such a subjective element should not usher in a requirement that investigators be mind-readers who can anticipate every distinctive concern that each potential research enrollee might have.

Given this tension, a reasonable standard of disclosure might have several elements. First, per the *Belmont Report*, a "reasonable volunteer" standard would require telling patients clearly that the study is not geared toward their personal benefit, and that their participation would be a voluntary activity dedicated to furthering scientific knowledge.

Second, many of the particulars that must be disclosed would be identified according to regulatory requirements, with the caveat that tort law should probably expect those requirements to be met whether or not the particular research project in question is technically subject to federal regulation.

Third, to balance subjects' need for personalized disclosure with investigators' need for clear expectations, the research standard of disclosure might include a rebuttable presumption. The information provided on the consent form should be presumed adequate except where the prospective enrollee has explicitly asked for additional information, as where someone might inquire about the physician's level of experience, or where a Jehovah's Witness might ask about the use of blood products. Once the physician is explicitly on notice that a particular kind of information is important to the prospective participant, his duty to disclose would expand to encompass it. This rebuttable presumption will prove important in assessing causality, an issue addressed below.

Injury

. . . Unfortunately, existing tort law may be inadequate to identify the kinds of injuries that may be especially important in the research setting. After all, so long as courts consider a breach of informed consent in research to be simply another instance of informed consent as a medical malpractice tort, they will require — and will only recognize — the kinds of injuries familiar in medical malpractice actions. Medical malpractice ordinarily requires some sort of physical injury in order to conclude that a remedy is warranted. Many jurisdictions recognize some non-physical injuries, such as emotional distress, but commonly even these must be linked to a physical injury or the threat of one. On this approach, if a duped or ill-informed research subject does not incur physical or other specifically accepted harms, there is no tort. And yet in research, such limits would seem seriously inappropriate. . . .

Even for ordinary medical care, a number of scholars have recommended that serious deficiencies of informed consent be deemed a distinct dignitary tort. . . . If this is a problem in ordinary medicine, it is even more so in the research setting.

People who are imminently dying pose a particularly poignant illustration, because a requirement of physical injury is nearly impossible to satisfy. In *Heinrich v. Sweet*, the First Circuit ultimately determined that people with terminal brain cancer had no cause of action for wrongful death when they were allegedly subjected to experimental radiation treatments, because there was no evidence that the experiment hastened these patients' already-imminent deaths. In cases like this, where the only documentable harm is deprivation of the right to make an informed choice, courts' denial of dignitary violations as a distinct injury can effectively preclude recovery even in egregious cases. . . .

During the late 1990s and early 2000s, a series of lawsuits against several major research institutions attempted to bring dignity torts into the research arena by arguing that the Nuremburg Code and the Declaration of Helsinki warrant a dignity tort when research subjects are inadequately informed about the protocol's objectives and risks. More grandly stated, unconsented or inadequately informed participation in research might be deemed a crime against humanity. These suits typically also argued that violations of federal regulations governing the treatment of human research subjects should be seen as a tort against the research subjects. . . .

Courts have not been receptive to importing international ethics codes into U.S. law. Just one court has indicated any willingness to regard the Nuremberg Code or the Declaration as U.S. law. The Maryland Court of Appeals, arguing that there is a special relationship between investigator and subject, acknowledged that although no United States court "has ever awarded damages to an injured experimental subject, or punished an experimenter, on the basis of a violation of the Nuremberg Code," nevertheless the Code was intended for international application and has never been rejected in the U.S. Even here, the court's interest in the Code appears as dicta rather than black-letter law. [The Maryland case, *Grimes v. Kennedy Krieger Institute*, is excerpted in Chapter 13, at page 567.]

Otherwise, courts have found that the Code and similar documents provide ideals, not hard law. One federal district court opined that, although international law is "an inseparable part of American jurisprudence . . . none of the cases cited by the plaintiffs recognizes a general private right of action under international law." Several other courts have likewise cited the Nuremberg Code and Helsinki Accords, but not as domestic law. Rather, these documents are typically cited in . . . civil rights claims as evidence that surely people who committed research abuses such as the radiation research of the 1940s, '50s and '60s should have known that people have a right to be free from unconsented research. . . . In that spirit, courts ruling on the latest cases have tended to discard the Nuremberg-based dignity claims as not cognizable under federal law.

Despite the current impediments to recognizing dignity torts and other special injuries in the research setting, there is reason to think that courts might evolve toward somewhat greater acceptance. At least one court has recognized dignitary injuries in ordinary medical care. When a state statute required the Louisiana Supreme Court to deny battery in a case where the surgeon simply ignored his promise to use a specific surgical technique the patient had requested, the Court nevertheless held that

> this case is different from the usual lack of informed consent cases where the doctor failed to inform the patient of a material risk and the risk materialized to cause physical damages. Here, the doctor's failure to inform the patient adequately did not cause the patient to undergo a risk that materialized and caused physical damages. Rather, the doctor's breach of duty caused plaintiff to undergo a medical procedure to which the patient expressly objected and for which the doctor failed to provide adequate information in response to the patient's request, thereby causing damages to plaintiff's dignity, privacy and emotional well-being. The doctor, rather than explaining the advantages and disadvantages of the patient's express request, patronized his patient and mentally

reserved the right to decide to disregard the patient's expressed wishes. Even the dissenting judge in the court of appeal noted that plaintiff is entitled to an award of damages for being deprived the opportunity of self-determination in regard to subjecting himself to an unwanted procedure.

The court went on to find that "in this type of case, damages for deprivation of self-determination, insult to personal integrity, invasion of privacy, anxiety, worry and mental distress are actual and compensatory. The primary concern in this injury to the personality is vindication of a valuable, though intangible, right, the mere invasion of which constitutes harm for which damages are recoverable."

If such a purely dignitary injury can be acknowledged in ordinary medical care, surely it should be even more readily available in research, where a person seeking help for his illness can potentially be turned into a research subject without his full understanding and consent. In the case of *Diaz v. Tampa General Hospital*, such reasoning led to a high-dollar settlement in a case where no physical injury was ever claimed. Rather, plaintiffs argued that sophisticated consent forms were tantamount to inadequate informed consent for pregnant women whose socioeconomic and cultural status impeded their comprehending the information they were given.

In the final analysis, courts need to recognize that "patients can be harmed when they are prevented from making decisions about their own care, even when, or perhaps especially when, no physical harm occurs." When inadequacies of information have inappropriately steered a patient's decision about whether to participate in research, courts should be willing in at least some instances to see this as an injury in itself.

Causality

An informed consent tort does not require simply a breach of duty and an injury. The former must cause the latter. However, as with the duty and injury elements of the tort, causality takes on a distinctive twist in research. Even as informed consent doctrine evolved toward the patient-based disclosure standard in the early 1970s, courts favored an objective approach. Rather than expecting physicians to guess each patient's informational preferences, courts asked physicians only to disclose what the reasonable and prudent person in this patient's situation would want to know.

Those same pivotal cases also instituted an objective standard for causality. It is a standard that most courts follow whether they use a physician-based or patient-based standard of disclosure. Thus, the inadequacy of disclosure is said to cause the injury only if the reasonable and prudent person in the patient's position would have refused the intervention if given adequate information. Courts adopted this objective approach largely out of fairness to physicians who would otherwise be vulnerable to patients' hindsight regrets, and out of deference to juries who would otherwise confront difficult hypothetical questions about what this particular person might or might not have done if given different information.

Unfortunately, this objective causality standard overlooks the obvious problem that even for ordinary medical care, people can weigh information very differently in light of their own values and then, ever so reasonably and prudently, come to markedly different decisions. However we might resolve this issue for ordinary care, courts should recognize a more subjective causality standard for research for two reasons.

First, it is neither "reasonable" nor "unreasonable" to enter a research study, as a one-size-fits-all judgment. . . . [U]nlike ordinary medical care, research does not aim to benefit any particular person. The protocol may hope to benefit groups of people, and individuals may hope for and receive a benefit. But benefiting any specific enrollee is never the goal of a research protocol. Since research cannot promise to promote any individual's self-interest, the across-the-board "reasonableness" judgments of the kind required for objective findings of causality make little sense. The decision is as individual as the decision whether or not to buy a lottery ticket.

Second, the only relatively assured outcome of research participation is the altruism of helping others (assuming the project is scientifically meritorious and soundly designed). Here especially, the decision is intensely personal, and there can be no single, objectively "reasonable" or intrinsically "prudent" decision.

Case law favors this critique. In *Zalazar v. Vercimak*, a woman sought cosmetic surgery to remove bags under her eyes. Although she was illiterate, no one read to her the consent form describing the procedure's significant risks. An Illinois appellate court found that an objective, "reasonable patient" standard of causality should not be used in a case of aesthetic surgery. Unlike the situation in which a patient seeks needed medical treatment for an illness or injury,

> the choice plaintiff made was a subjective, personal one that only she could make. . . . We believe no expert or other third party could possibly assert how a reasonable person in the plaintiff's position would have weighed the risks and complications of the surgery, and whether such individual would have decided against or gone ahead with the four-lid blepharoplasty had the proper disclosures been made.

The court continued: "Indeed, where a surgical procedure involves no medical benefit to the patient and the decision is so subjective, the admissibility of the expert's opinion is questionable." . . .

If the foregoing discussion is correct, causality analysis should not treat research decisions like ordinary medical treatment decisions. They are highly personal, not suitably subjected to an evaluation of whether the "reasonable" person would think it "prudent" to enter research. Just as with a decision to have cosmetic surgery, the question is what the individual person would want.

Admittedly, there remains the concern that a subjective standard of causality could hold physicians hostage to patients' bitter hindsight. However, several responses seem reasonable. First, the investigator should ensure that the prospective enrollee has ample opportunity to ask questions that could flag the issues he considers personally important. An animal-rights activist, given the opportunity to ask about any animal studies that preceded the trial he is being invited to enter, can place the investigator on notice that if this person is not given full disclosure on that issue, he may later be able to say that he would not have entered a trial, had he known more about its use of laboratory animals.

Second, juries must routinely grapple with factual questions about litigants' motives and intentions. After noting that the objective standard of causality does not adequately honor patients' autonomy, the Oklahoma Supreme Court held that

> this basic right to know and decide is the reason for the full-disclosure rule. Accordingly, we decline to jeopardize this right by the imposition of the "reasonable man" standard. . . . Although it might be said this approach places a physician at the mercy of a patient's hindsight, a careful practitioner can always protect himself by insuring that he has adequately informed each patient he treats.

Similarly, the *Zalazar* court ruling in the case of aesthetic surgery acknowledged that

> We recognize that our holding today places a burden on a defendant-physician to probe the subjective decision-making process of cosmetic surgery plaintiff-patients complaining of lack of informed consent, but we deem the subjective standard preferable to the insurmountable burden that the objective standard poses for the plaintiff-patient in such cases. Also, we note that documentation of the informed consent procedure via video tape or other means would not appear to be unreasonably burdensome, considering the regularity with which photography is utilized in connection with surgical procedures.

Third, the plaintiff bears the burden of proof in tort litigation. As a practical matter, this will mean that if the plaintiff did not ask questions about special issues that were important to him personally, he cannot readily cite those personal issues in asserting that his injury was caused by the defendant's failure to inform him regarding a matter about which he himself failed to ask. As Morin notes, causation issues cannot be resolved until the scope of the disclosure duty is circumscribed; only if the information should have been disclosed can it be said the patient's decision would have differed. If the plaintiff receives broad, otherwise adequate general information but then failed to ask questions about issues personally important to him, such as the use of animals in this research, he will be hard-pressed to argue the investigator had a duty of disclosure or breached that duty. At that point, the investigator's failure to disclose a specific fact that went beyond the general duty to disclose would not be the cause of the patient's injury. Thus, even under a subjective standard the plaintiff must antecedently have made it clear that he wanted certain kinds of additional information, if he is to successfully claim he has been harmed for lack of that information.

NOTES AND QUESTIONS

1. Is it appropriate to rely on the federal informed consent regulations to evaluate the adequacy of researchers' disclosures even when the research is not "technically subject to the regulations"?

2. One commentator has argued that physicians should not only be required to tailor their disclosures to patient-specific issues about which they are actually aware (as suggested in the excerpt), but that they also should have an affirmative obligation to *inquire* about patients' subjective treatment goals. *See* Robert Gatter, *Informed Consent and the Forgotten Duty of Physician Inquiry*, 31 Loy. U. Chi. L.J. 557 (2000). Should such a "duty of inquiry" be required in research? If so, what should researchers ask prospective subjects?

3. The *Diaz* case, mentioned in the preceding excerpt, involved pregnant women at risk of premature delivery, who alleged that they were enrolled in research without their knowledge or consent. The research, which was designed to reduce respiratory problems in premature infants, required the women to undergo repeat amniocenteses to test for signs of infection, a procedure that carries a small but real risk of causing a miscarriage. The study was uncovered when one of the nurses at the hospital asked why so many poor, non-English speaking women were undergoing as many as ten amniocenteses. *See* Peter Aronson, *A Medical Indignity*, Nat'l L.J., March 27, 2000, at A1.

4. If courts recognize a cause of action for "dignitary harms" when research is conducted without adequate consent but no physical harm results, will they be forced to recognize a similar claim outside the research context? Or might it be appropriate to limit the claim to cases involving research?

> The argument for recognizing a cause of action based on the failure to obtain proper consent, even in the absence of any physical harm, is stronger in research than in ordinary medical treatment. In the clinical setting, obtaining informed consent is certainly an important ethical and legal requirement, but it is not the only basis for justifying a physician's provision of medical treatment. In addition to the patient's consent, the physician's actions are justified by the principle of beneficence: by providing treatment that meets the prevailing standard of care, the physician is helping to promote the patient's medical well-being. In research, by contrast, consent is usually the *only* justification for performing risky interventions that have no potential to benefit the subject's individual medical interests. Absent consent, imposing risks on subjects for the benefit of others would be a flagrant violation of per-

sonal dignity, as it would violate the maxim that people should be treated as ends in themselves and not simply as means. Thus, nonconsensual research is a far greater violation of personal dignity than nonconsensual treatment, and therefore justifies a remedy even if one does not exist for nonconsensual treatment that does not directly cause physical harm.

Coleman, *supra.*

5. Research conducted without any consent whatsoever (as opposed to consent that was insufficiently informed) may constitute a battery. *See* Mink v. University of Chicago, 460 F. Supp. 713 (N.D. Ill. 1978) (finding that plaintiffs had stated a claim for battery by alleging that they were given DES as part of a medical experiment without their knowledge or consent). In a battery claim, the plaintiff is not required to prove that the defendant's actions caused any physical injuries; proof of an "offensive" touching is sufficient to support at least nominal damages. *See id.* at 717-18.

6. Morreim argues that the objective causation standard typically used in informed consent cases is inappropriate in cases involving human subject research because "it is neither 'reasonable' nor 'unreasonable' to enter a research study," and therefore "across-the-board 'reasonableness' judgments of the kind required for objective findings of causality make little sense." Of course, the same can be said for many decisions about ordinary medical treatment. Consider, for example, the difficulty of determining whether the "reasonable person" would undergo chemotherapy with a 50-50 chance of prolonging life by a few months but a near-certain reduction in the patient's quality of life. Is the only solution to move to a purely subjective standard for determining causation? What if courts instructed juries to determine whether a reasonable person *might* have refused the intervention if full information were provided, rather than asking what the reasonable person *would* have done? Would this formulation of the question be consistent with an objective standard of causation? Would it satisfy the plaintiff's requirement to prove that her injuries were "more likely than not" caused by the defendant's negligence?

7. Does the obligation to obtain informed consent extend only to the individual researcher, or does it also extend to the hospital in which the research is conducted? Outside of research, most courts that have considered the question have rejected efforts to hold hospitals liable for failing to obtain a patient's informed consent. *See,* e.g., Mele v. Sherman Hosp., 838 F.2d 923 (7th Cir. 1988). However, there is some support for holding hospitals liable for failure to obtain the informed consent of a research subject. *See* Kus v. Sherman Hosp., 268 Ill. App. 3d 771 (2d Dist. 1995). Should hospitals have a duty to ensure that a research subject has provided informed consent if they do not have a duty to ensure that patients have consented to nonresearch interventions?

§ 12.04 NO-FAULT COMPENSATION

No-fault compensation, as the name suggests, enables injured persons to receive financial compensation without having to establish that their injuries were the result of another person's fault. No-fault compensation is not a part of the tort system but an alternative to it. It operates through administrative mechanisms rather than civil litigation, awards are typically based on standard compensation formulas rather than jury determinations, and the amount of recovery tends to be much lower than plaintiffs can receive through the tort system. *See generally* Randall R. Bovbjerg & Frank A. Sloan, NO-FAULT FOR MEDICAL INJURY: THEORY AND EVIDENCE, 67 U. CIN. L. REV. 53 (1998).

The primary example of no-fault compensation in this country is worker's compensation. Developed in the early part of the twentieth century, worker's compensation guarantees workers who suffer on-the-job injuries relatively quick and certain recovery, but the trade-off is that workers are precluded from suing their employers for tort damages. Unlike worker's compensation, other no-fault compensation systems give injured parties the option of pursuing either no-fault compensation or tort litigation. For example, the National Childhood Vaccine Injury Act, 42 U.S.C. §§ 300aa-1 to 300aa-34, which establishes a no-fault compensation program for children who suffer vaccine-related injuries, prohibits those who accept an award from bringing a tort suit, but individuals are free to seek tort damages if they forego compensation under the program. Similarly, Congress provided an optional no-fault compensation package to survivors of individuals killed in the terrorist attacks of September 11, 2001; those who accept the compensation are precluded from suing the airlines whose planes were hijacked in the attacks. *See* 49 U.S.C. § 40101. Some no-fault systems combine mandatory and optional elements. Many states, for example, have mandatory no-fault compensation schemes for automobile accidents that give individuals the option of pursuing tort litigation in cases involving substantial physical harm. *See* Gary T. Schwartz, *Auto No-Fault and First-Party Insurance: Advantages and Problems*, 73 S. CAL. L. REV. 611 (2000).

While no-fault compensation is not the norm for injuries stemming from medical treatment or research in the United States, a few states have established no-fault systems for particular areas of medicine. For example, Virginia and Florida have no-fault compensation programs for certain birth-related injuries. *See* Studdert & Brennan, *supra*, at 239. In several other countries, no-fault compensation programs cover all types of medical injuries, completely displacing the medical malpractice system. *See id.* Many other countries also have no-fault compensation programs for research-related injuries. *See* INSTITUTE OF MEDICINE, RESPONSIBLE RESEARCH: A SYSTEMS APPROACH TO PROTECTING RESEARCH PARTICIPANTS 189 (2003).

In the absence of comprehensive no-fault compensation for either medical treatment or research, some institutions have voluntarily adopted their own compensation programs. The following section examines one such program.

[A] Voluntary No-Fault Compensation Schemes

HUMAN SUBJECTS MANUAL
UNIVERSITY OF WASHINGTON
(1999)
http://depts.washington.edu/hsd/INFO/hsman.htm, Page VII.8

G. Compensation for Adverse Events

The University's policy on compensation for adverse events to human subjects is intended primarily to provide necessary medical care to subjects who sustain bodily injury as a direct result of participation in a research project.

"Adverse Effect" is defined to mean bodily injury. Except in special circumstances, the term does not include impairment of mental processes or emotional distress, nor does it encompass effects resulting from: (1) injuries from diagnostic or therapeutic procedures, either standard or experimental, performed as part of patient management; (2) the normal course of a disease or condition; or (3) non-compliance with study procedures.

The program operates on a "no-fault" basis; that is, the claimant does not need to establish negligence. Rather, the claimant or the investigator must only demonstrate only [sic] that the subject has suffered an adverse effect as a result of participation in a University-sponsored study. The program is included as part of the University's overall general liability self-insurance program.

If an investigator believes an adverse effect has occurred, he or she should immediately prepare a report summarizing the background, nature, and result. A form for this purpose may be obtained by telephoning the Human Subjects Division. The report will be submitted to the Human Subjects Division and the Office of Risk Management, which may consult with the Attorney General's Division and to the Human Subjects Review Committee in making a determination as to the applicability of the compensation program.

A report must be submitted within one year of the occurrence of the adverse effect, but as soon as possible after the researcher becomes aware of the event. In a case of latent disability, the time for filing the report does not begin until the subject or the subject's legal representative is aware or reasonably should be aware of the causal relationship of the disability to his or her participation in the research. This allowance takes into account an adverse effect to a fetus.

The compensation program for adverse effects may not apply to research carried out by investigators under grants administered through other institutions; and it is not effective for research carried out in foreign countries. However, adverse effects should be reported to the HSD whether or not the investigator believes that the compensation plan may be applicable.

It is the position of the University of Washington that subjects and their third-party payers or governmental programs should not be held accountable for the costs of treating adverse effects incurred as a result of taking part in clinical trials sponsored by commercial companies.

The terms of the agreement under which the trial is conducted shall determine whether the sponsor or the University of Washington is financially responsible for the treatment of adverse effects. With rare exception, the agreement will specify that the University will hold the sponsor harmless from adverse effects resulting from the negligence of University employees, including failure to adhere to the protocol, while the sponsor will hold the University harmless from adverse effects resulting from the prescribed use of the test article or protocol. It is possible, though unusual, that both University negligence and sponsor negligence could concurrently cause adverse effect, in which both parties share financial responsibility.

The consent form should include information that physical injuries to the subject that are a direct result of study procedures will be treated at no cost to the subject.Wherever possible, the consent form should state that the sponsor is the responsible party. For example:

> "If you have a physical injury as a direct result of this study, we will treat you or refer you for treatment. The X company, the sponsor of this study, will pay for this treatment."

In cases in which the sponsor does not wish to be named, acceptable wording is as follows:

> "If you have a physical injury as a direct result of this study, we will treat you or refer you for treatment. The treatment will be given at no cost to you."

In rare instances in which the University's compensation plan does not apply, or when the sponsor has made no provision for treating adverse events, the subject or the subject's health insurer may be the payer of last resort. In this case, the consent process should include this information, along with the proviso that insurers may not be willing to pay for treatment of adverse events resulting from treatment provided in the research context. The Human Subjects Review Committee may request a pre-approval procedure to make sure that the insurer will pay for these costs before the subject is enrolled in the study.

NOTES AND QUESTIONS

1. The University of Washington's compensation program for research subjects was developed in the 1970s and remains exceptionally generous, as compared to voluntary compensation programs at other institutions. According to a 2003 report by the Institute of Medicine, while "many research organizations conducting clinical trials agree to provide short-term medical care (during the course of the study) for research-related injuries," few provide coverage for long-term medical costs or lost earnings resulting from adverse events. INSTITUTE

OF MEDICINE, *supra*, at 188. Why do you think the University of Washington decided to provide coverage for long-term medical costs when most other research institutions do not?

2. According to a 1998 estimate by University of Washington officials, the compensation program paid $2,300 to $5,000 annually for research-related injuries. Although the compensation program does not prevent injured parties from suing for negligence — remember, under the federal regulations, institutions may not require individuals to waive their right to sue — individuals who have their medical expenses covered under the program may have less motivation to sue the University.

3. What are the precise obligations the institution assumes by telling subjects, "If you have a physical injury as a direct result of this study, we will treat you or refer you for treatment," as suggested by the policy? If the subject goes to his or her own doctor or an emergency room without first contacting the University, must the University reimburse the subject for her out-of-pocket expenses? Must it indemnify the doctor or hospital that provided the treatment?

[B] Proposals for Comprehensive No-Fault Compensation Systems

Since the President's Commission 1982 report excerpted at the beginning of this chapter, there have been repeated calls for the federal government to create a comprehensive no-fault compensation system for individuals who suffer injuries in the course of biomedical research, similar to systems that currently exist in many European countries and in New Zealand. The Institute of Medicine — an arm of the National Academy of Sciences, a private, nonprofit organization that operates under a congressional mandate to advise the federal government on scientific and technical matters — added its prestigious voice to this movement in 2003.

RESPONSIBLE RESEARCH: A SYSTEMS APPROACH TO PROTECTING RESEARCH PARTICIPANTS INSTITUTE OF MEDICINE, NATIONAL ACADEMY OF SCIENCES
(2003)

Because the contributions of science benefit society as a whole, it seems indisputable that society is obligated to assure that the few who are harmed in government-sponsored scientific research are appropriately compensated for study-related injuries. As the Department of Health, Education, and Welfare (DHEW) Taskforce, which focused solely on federally funded research, noted in 1977, "Because society is both the beneficiary and the sponsor of research, compensatory justice may come into play for the redress of injuries suffered by persons in connection with biomedical or behavioral research conducted, supported, or regulated by the Federal Government." The costs of the loss should not fall on the research participant.

The same argument applies to privately funded research, perhaps to an even greater extent, as the economic survival of a company depends largely on the availability of participants to test new therapies, drugs, and other products. Because the participants are ultimately contributing to the profits of the company, any costs that result from the research should be the responsibility of the sponsor. Furthermore, whether a study is privately or publicly sponsored, the results are intended to eventually benefit all of society. . . .

The first step, which should be taken as soon as possible, would implement a compensation program along the lines recommended by [the National Bioethics Advisory Commission] as a requirement for [human research participant protection program] accreditation. Accredited research organizations would be expected to identify, characterize, and report research-related injuries and to cover costs of medical care and rehabilitation that are attributable to research-related injury. Meanwhile, voluntary efforts would be simultaneously undertaken by NIH and private sponsors to establish demonstration programs that would also cover lost income due to temporary or permanent disability or death under various plans for valuation and payment. After three to five years of experience and data collection, the entire compensation effort would be evaluated, including an assessment of whether the fee scale(s) used in the demonstration programs are perceived as fair and easy to administer by those who are affected by it. The assessment should provide a basis for informed judgments about the best approach to take, including the best model for measuring work-related disability.

Under the approach envisioned by the committee, the responsibility for compensation would fall initially on the institution or organization actually accountable for conducting the research, and its terms would be specified in the documentation accompanying the participant's agreement to participate. Presumably, most research organizations will attempt to insure themselves against such losses, and a market for such insurance may eventually emerge, especially after the necessary data have been compiled. In the context of pharmaceutical research, the allocation of responsibility for compensation between the sponsoring company and the research organization will presumably be determined by contract. This strategy embraces the basic approach of the Association of the British Pharmaceutical Industry.

Alternatively, the government could establish a federal compensation program, which could be included as a direct cost within grants, a surcharge on medical bills, or money from general revenues.

NOTES AND QUESTIONS

1. As mentioned in the excerpt, the National Bioethics Advisory Commission (NBAC), which operated during the Clinton administration, also urged the fed-

eral government to adopt a no-fault compensation system for subjects in medical research. *See* NATIONAL BIOETHICS ADVISORY COMMISSION, 1 ETHICAL AND POLICY ISSUES IN RESEARCH INVOLVING HUMAN PARTICIPANTS 126 (2001). However, NBAC's proposal was limited to the medical and rehabilitative costs resulting from participation in research, in contrast to the Institute of Medicine's call for "full recovery for economic loss, including work-related disability, and in appropriate cases, for lost earnings of a deceased participant." INSTITUTE OF MEDICINE, *supra*, at 193. Why do you think NBAC did not propose compensation for subjects' full economic losses?

2. The Institute of Medicine suggested that its proposed no-fault compensation scheme would not completely displace the option of tort litigation. Instead, "when the participant alleges that the injury was caused by a possibly defective product or possible negligence in the design and conduct of the study, the tort system is likely to remain the appropriate channel for redress, serving as a back up to the no-fault compensation agreement for cases in which elements of liability can be proved." INSTITUTE OF MEDICINE, *supra*, at 191. What are the advantages and drawbacks of this model, as compared to the model of worker's compensation systems, which limit injured parties to no-fault compensation without giving them the option of seeking tort damages in court?

3. Any no-fault system for compensating individuals who sustain injuries from medical treatment or research must confront the difficult problem of determining causation — i.e., distinguishing individuals whose injuries are *the result of* their medical treatment or participation in research from those who are simply experiencing the natural progression of their underlying disease. In their proposal for a "workable model" of no-fault compensation for medical injuries, David Studdert and Troyen Brennan argue that the most appropriate test for determining causation is that used by the Swedish compensation system, which requires claimants to prove that their injuries were "avoidable." *See* Studdert and Brennan, *supra*, at 232. How does the concept of "avoidability" relate to the issue of causation? Does a finding of avoidability depend on assuming a particular level of skill of the physicians or researchers, or a particular level of available resources? If so, in what way does an avoidability standard differ from the negligence standard traditionally used in malpractice cases? Can you think of an alternative to the avoidability standard that would still limit recovery to injuries "caused" by the physicians or researchers, as opposed to injuries attributable to the patient or subject's underlying disease?

4. What do you think are the primary barriers to implementing a no-fault compensation system for injuries to research subjects? Are they technical issues, such as determining which injuries would be eligible for compensation or setting the appropriate amount of awards, or are they more political in nature? Are they any different from the issues that complicate malpractice reform outside the area of human subject research?

PART III
REVIEWING RESEARCH PROPOSALS: SPECIAL SITUATIONS

Chapter 13

RESEARCH WITH CHILDREN

This chapter considers the issues that are raised when planning for and conducting research with children, a category of human subjects who generally cannot provide legally and ethically adequate informed consent. The issues raised by involving children in research are complicated by the fact that there are various sub-groups represented under this general heading. Clearly, neonates and small children cannot participate in decisions about research. By contrast, eight- and nine-year-olds may not be able to evaluate the options and choose the right course, but they often will be capable of expressing an opinion. In addition to having opinions about the desirability of participating in a study, they may be capable of helping to structure the way that the study is conducted. For example, children can participate in decisions about how and where to get their medications — whether to sit on the bed or in the playroom; whether to have the needle before or after story time. Researchers and clinicians have found that this bit of control often makes the experience very different for the child. Some older teens may actually be capable of providing a robust form of "assent," although they may nonetheless be legally precluded from making a binding decision.

The Department of Health and Human Services (DHHS) regulations on research with human subjects contain a special subpart governing research with children. While this subpart is not formally part of the Common Rule, it has also been adopted by the FDA, and it will be the rare study that is subject to the Common Rule and not also to this subpart. For some categories of research, this subpart includes upper limits on the level of risk to which children can be exposed. As you read these materials, consider how the regulations governing research with children differ from those applicable to human subject research generally, what policy decisions underlie those differences, and whether those differences are legally and ethically justifiable.

§ 13.01 RESEARCH WITH CHILDREN: PAST AND PRESENT

Research with Children
Leonard H. Glantz
24 Am. J.L. & Med. 213 (1998)

The first tests of immunization were performed on slaves and children. Edward Jenner vaccinated his one-year-old son with cowpox to see if it offered immunity to smallpox. His next subject was an eight-year-old child who was challenged with an inoculation of smallpox material in order to determine if the inoculation was effective. In 1802, Jenner's vaccine was tested on forty-eight children living in an almshouse. All the children were challenged with smallpox to see if they were effectively immunized.

Following the exploitation of children as laborers in the Industrial Revolution, the 1900s saw an increased interest in child welfare along with an increased desire to learn more about children's health problems. In the first decade of the 1900s, Alfred Hess, a respected pediatrician, became the medical director of the Hebrew Infant Asylum in New York. He noted that conducting research in an asylum was ideal because it approximated those "conditions which are insisted on in considering the course of experimental infection among laboratory animals, but which can rarely be controlled in a study of infection in man."

The germ theory was tested by intentionally infecting both adults and children with diseases. The health officer at a Hawaiian leprosarium injected six girls under his care with the syphilis virus. Dr. Henry Heiman reported that he was able to successfully produce gonorrhea in a four-year-old "idiot" with chronic epilepsy as well as in a sixteen-year-old male "idiot."

The invention of the X ray prompted much research in children and adults. Physicians used X rays to study the normal development of children and adults, including the fetus in utero.

In 1896, Dr. Arthur Wentworth published a paper describing spinal taps he performed on twenty-nine children at Children's Hospital in Boston to determine if the procedure was harmful. He determined they were safe. However, John Roberts, a Philadelphia physician, noting that these procedures were with "no therapeutic indications for the operation" and for "purely and avowedly experimental" reasons, labeled Wentworth's use of these procedures "human vivisection."

In 1941, Francis Payton Rous, editor of the Journal of Experimental Medicine, rejected a manuscript from a physician and wrote to the author, "the inoculation of a twelve month old infant with herpes . . . was an abuse of power, an infringement of the rights of an individual, and not excusable because the illness which followed had implications for science." The fact that "a child was 'offered as a volunteer' — whatever that may mean — does not palliate the action." This statement represents an important turning point in the discussion of research with children. It is one of the first statements to acknowledge that children themselves have rights as individuals and that the thought that one could be "offered as a volunteer" was a contradiction in terms.

In one of the initial research projects designed to determine if phenylalanine accumulations caused phenylketonuria (PKU), a metabolic disorder that causes mental retardation, the researchers first put a two-year-old girl with PKU on a diet low in phenylalinine. A gradual improvement resulted over a few months. Due to the importance of establishing the role of phenylalinine in this condition, the researchers decided to add phenylalanine to the child's special diet without telling the child's mother so that any change could be noted by her without bias. The mother reported a definite deterioration; within a few days, she reported that her daughter lost all the ground that had been gained in the past ten months. This was then repeated with the same child. From the 1950s through the 1970s, a research team at the Willowbrook State School systematically infected mentally retarded children with strains of hepatitis. [For further discussion of the Willowbrook studies, see Chapter 1, at page 39.] . . .

Other examples could be given here but are not necessary. It is clear that children have been misused as research subjects and the very fact that they were children would seem to have made them more likely to be abused as research subjects.

Speed, Safety, and Dignity: Pediatric Pharmaceutical Development in an Age of Optimism
Randall Baldwin Clark
9 U. CHI. L. SCH. ROUNDTABLE 1 (2002)

The most obvious and important problem is the frankly and inevitably utilitarian justification for pediatric research. That pediatricians might have the ability — when the time comes — to cure the generations of children who are not yet ill, researchers must now ask the presently sick to suffer certain discomfort and run the risk of injury or death. The recent federal pediatric pharmaceutical development initiatives force us to ask, once again, if this calculation still comports with our moral sensibilities: Should the health and dignity of the children who currently suffer be sacrificed to the health of the many more who will later fall ill?

Less obvious, less important, but more pertinent to the present-day structuring of our institutions is the challenge that the [recent federal efforts to promote pediatric research pose] to the federal rule that has strictly limited the nature of pediatric experimentation over the last two decades. In the 1970s, largely in response to the revelation that the consulting physician to the Willowbrook School, an overcrowded state-run home for the mentally disabled, had deliberately infected healthy children with hepatitis to learn more about the disease's aetiology, Congress authorized the Department of Health, Education, and Welfare ("DHEW") to regulate experimentation on children. Though the final rule ("Subpart D") does not categorically prohibit pediatric experimentation, it does present itself to the research community as an attempt to limit the participation of children in clinical research trials. . . .

The impending collision between these two regimes prompts many questions. On the one hand, caregivers will want assurances that children's interests are in fact promoted: Will pediatricians acquire useful pharmacological tools in a timely manner? Will child subjects be safe? Will societal regard for the dignity of children be preserved? On the other, the research community will want to discern the boundaries of the law: How far can an aggressive researcher push the envelope? When must the institutional review board ("IRB") deny authorization? What sort of protocol can government regulators cite as a violation? Finally, our legislators will want to figure out how to revise the law so as to satisfy both groups: How can we clarify boundaries for the research community and accommodate the speedy, safe, and dignified advance of pediatric medicine?

NOTES AND QUESTIONS

1. How do you think the researchers described in Glantz's historical overview justified their use of children as human research subjects? Do you agree with Glantz that the fact that the subjects of these studies were children "made them more likely to be abused as research subjects"?

2. In the late 1800s, Alfred Hess, director of the Hebrew Infant Asylum of New York, explained that using institutionalized children as research subjects could provide an enormous benefit to science due to the standardized conditions in institutional settings. *See* Alfred Hess, *The Use of a Series of Vaccines in the Prophylaxis and Treatment of an Epidemic Pertussis,* 63 JAMA 1007 (1914). Assuming he was correct, does his argument constitute a sufficient ethical justification for research with institutionalized children?

3. In its 1977 report on research involving children, the National Commission for the Protection of Human Subjects of Biomedical and Behavioral Research concluded that two factors make research with children ethically permissible: (1) children differ markedly from both adults and nonhuman animals, and that research with those groups is therefore not an adequate substitute for testing in children; and (2) lack of appropriate research in children will increase children's risk of harm from untested practices and treatments. *See* NATIONAL COMMISSION FOR THE PROTECTION OF HUMAN SUBJECTS OF BIOMEDICAL AND BEHAVIORAL RESEARCH, RESEARCH INVOLVING CHILDREN: REPORT AND RECOMMENDATIONS (1977). Does the fact that pediatric research benefits children *as a group* necessarily justify enrolling *a particular child* in research? If not, what additional factors would need to be present to make the decision to enroll a particular child in research ethically acceptable?

4. The philosopher Paul Ramsey believed that children should never be used as research subjects. According to Ramsey, the principle of "respect for persons" requires that research be conducted only with individuals who can provide ethically and legally valid consent. Research with children is unethical, he argued, because it essentially amounts to an "unconsented touching." Paul Ramsey, *The Enforcement of Morals: Nontherapeutic Research on Children,* HASTINGS CENTER REP., Aug. 1976, at 21. In contrast, Richard McCormick argued that we should presume that children would consent to research that "fulfills an important social need and involves no discernible risk." He based this view on

his belief that "respecting persons includes recognizing that they are members of a moral community with its attendant obligations." ROBERT J. LEVINE, ETHICS AND REGULATION OF CLINICAL RESEARCH 2D ED. 237-38 (1986). Who has the better argument? If you agree that research with children can be ethically acceptable, is McCormick's rationale the best justification?

5. The recent history of pediatric testing is Byzantine, to say the least. In the 1990s, the FDA, under then-Commissioner David Kessler, began to respond to pediatricians' concerns that the dearth of information on the use of pharmaceuticals in pediatric treatment effectively made children into "therapeutic orphans." It was generally acknowledged that 80 percent of the medications then being used to treat children had never been adequately tested in research studies involving children. Pediatricians were being forced to use drugs that had only been approved for use in adults, prescribing them "without FDA approval and without good information on dosing and side effects." Sheryl Gay Stolberg, *Children Test New Medicines Despite Doubts*, N.Y. TIMES, Feb. 11, 2001, Sec. 1, at 1. One of the FDA's first efforts to change this state of affairs was a rule proposed in 1992 to encourage pharmaceutical companies to include information about pediatric safety and efficacy on drug labels. The FDA was concerned that pharmaceutical companies were omitting this information because they believed that they could not include it without actually performing clinical trials in children. The proposed rule sought to eliminate this misunderstanding by stating that a manufacturer did not necessarily have to complete pediatric clinical trials to qualify for a pediatric label. The rule became final in 1995. Food and Drug Administration, *Specific Requirements on Content and Format of Labeling for Human Prescription Drugs*, 59 FED. REG. 64,240 (1994). However, the rule appeared to have little actual effect.

A more significant development occurred in November 1997, when Congress passed the FDA Modernization Act (FDAMA), PUB. L. NO. 105-115, 111 STAT. 2296 (codified at 21 U.S.C. §§ 301-392), which provided a six-month patent extension (or "exclusivity period") for manufacturers who tested their drugs in pediatric populations (section 111 of FDAMA, codified at 21 U.S.C. § 355a). This six-month extension created a financial surge for manufacturers. For example, Schering-Plough (faced with no competition from generic drugs) earned an additional $975 million in sales during the six-month pediatric patent extension on its drug Claritin. *See User Fees, Pediatric Exclusivity Keys in FDAMA Reauthorization*, FOOD & DRUG LETTER, June 22, 2001; *see also* FOOD AND DRUG ADMINISTRATION, THE PEDIATRIC EXCLUSIVITY PROVISION: JANUARY 2001 STATUS REPORT TO CONGRESS, available at http://www.fda.gov/cder/pediatric/report-cong01.pdf.

In 1998, concerned about gaps in FDAMA's incentive structure, and hoping to better balance pediatric labeling needs, children's vulnerability, and the desirability of quick drug approval, the FDA promulgated the Regulations Requiring Manufacturers to Assess the Safety and Effectiveness of New Drugs and Biological Products in Pediatric Patients (known as the "Pediatric Rule"),

63 FED. REG. 66,632. The Pediatric Rule allowed the FDA to require testing for products used by a substantial pediatric populace or products that provided a meaningful therapeutic benefit over an existing treatment. Unlike FDAMA, this new rule contained no incentives, just a mandate. A sponsor could request a waiver of the pediatric testing requirement if it could show that the necessary studies would be impossible or highly impractical, or where evidence strongly suggested the product would be unsafe or ineffective in all pediatric age groups. Partial waivers were available for specific sub-populations of children (like adolescents or neonates) under similar circumstances. Unlike the voluntary 1994 rule and FDAMA, the Pediatric Rule authorized the FDA to punish manufacturers for noncompliance.

Even after the passage of FDAMA and the Pediatric Rule, concerns remained about the lack of incentives for drugs whose patents had already expired, especially because six of the ten drugs most widely prescribed to children were older antibiotics. Critics also focused on the fact that providing extended patent protection provided little incentive for manufacturers to test drugs with a small pediatric market, such as neonates, and that the provision prompted drug companies to study only blockbuster drugs that would garner the greatest profits in six months. These criticisms led to the enactment of the Best Pharmaceuticals for Children Act (BPCA), PUB. L. NO. 107-109, 115 STAT. 1408 (2002). The BPCA required the NIH and the FDA to develop a prioritized list of off-patent drugs for which additional studies in pediatric populations should be performed, and provided federal funding to conduct such studies. It also extended the pediatric exclusivity provision for an additional five years, since it had originally been scheduled to expire in 2002.

As these developments in Congress were taking place, the 1998 Pediatric Rule was undergoing a challenge by a coalition of organizations that maintained that mandating pediatric research was beyond the scope of the FDA's authority. In 2002, a federal district court agreed with these organizations and struck down the Pediatric Rule. See Assoc. of American Physicians & Surgeons v. FDA, 226 F. Supp. 2d 204 (D.D.C. 2002). Shortly after this decision was announced, President Bush signed into law the Pediatric Research Equity Act (PREA), PUB. L. NO. 108-155, 117 STAT. 1936 (2003), which explicitly gave the FDA the authority to require manufacturers to undertake pediatric testing (thus rendering the FDA's appeal of the lawsuit moot). Some commentators have criticized PREA for failing to include adequate safeguards to protect child test subjects from harm. See Melissa Healy, *Push to Test Drugs on Kids Comes with Reservations*, CHICAGO TRIBUNE, March 7, 2004.

6. Could the new incentives and requirements for pediatric research create too much pressure on physicians and parents to enroll children in research inappropriately? Philip Walson, a professor at Ohio State University, was quoted in 2000 as noting that, after conducting pediatric research for twenty-five years, "there has been more research done in the past three years than in all the others combined." Stacey Schultz, *Drug Trials Are Clamoring for Kids, But Scru-*

tinize the Study Before Signing Up, U.S. NEWS & WORLD REP., Apr. 17, 2000, at 62. The *U.S. News* article described massive efforts on the part of drug manufacturers to enroll more than 170,000 children in almost 200 studies. It noted the concern of some experts that "the rush to test drugs in kids has led to ethically questionable behavior, such as taking children off a standard medication to study the effects of a newer one." One asthma researcher reported that because the IRB at his institution felt it was unethical to enroll a child in a study if the asthma was already well controlled on current medications, he was unable to recruit a single subject in one particular study. In contrast, a doctor down the street had exceeded his quota, because the IRB at his facility apparently allowed children to discontinue medications in order to enroll in the study. *See id.* Under what conditions should a child be permitted to discontinue an effective medication in order to be enrolled in a study?

7. What if it turns out that only poor people are placing their children in research? Should there be a plan in place to monitor patterns of enrollment?

§ 13.02 THE REGULATORY FRAMEWORK

[A] Decision-Making Authority of Parents and Children

[1] Parental Authority: Permission and Refusal

REQUIREMENTS FOR PERMISSION BY PARENTS OR GUARDIANS
45 C.F.R. §§ 46.408(b), (c), and (d):

These provisions are reproduced in Appendix A, at page A-29. Please read them before proceeding.

Speed, Safety, and Dignity: Pediatric Pharmaceutical Development in an Age of Optimism
Randall Baldwin Clark
9 U. CHI. L. SCH. ROUNDTABLE 1 (2002)

1. The Problem of Proxy Consent

The vexing complication arises . . . from the fact that plenty of medical research occurs which does not hold out the prospect of direct and personal medical benefit. The question that then arises is a terribly challenging one: May parents, those people peculiarly entrusted with the responsibility of protecting their child from the buffetings of the world, consent that he be subjected to potentially harmful procedures from which he will receive no benefit whatsoever? Does the duty to guide and protect preclude this sort of consent? Some parents might be interested in sacrificing their child's health and comfort for the greater good of medicine, but why would the child — utterly unwilling to share his toys — be willing to make repeated and painful donations of his spinal fluid? But the fact remains that the child has no legal voice and, barring unusual circumstances, it is the parent who must speak for him. To what sort of standard should this proxy be held?

Traditional standards for proxy consent in other realms of medical research and care provide some limited guidance. When an adult becomes incompetent, surrogate decisions are often made in accordance with three hierarchically ordered principles. The first, and preferred, option is that the patient's treatment conform to the directives he laid out before the onset of his debilitation. Because the sound — in body and mind — are rarely inclined to imagine the multitude of ways they might become debilitated and thus to lay out adequate guidance, their caregivers must turn to other, less prescriptive methods of guiding the physician. Preferable is the exercise of substituted judgment: What would he want were he now capable of speaking? Least favored is the task of determining what course of treatment is in the "best interests" of the afflicted. Translated into legal jargon, the proxy must here act as a fiduciary.

But when we try to apply each of these standards to the question at hand we see how unique the conundrum is. The first rule is clearly inapplicable, given that a child, prior to finding himself in this situation, has never had legal authority to declare his will. That the second offers a certain appeal — and debilities — is suggested by the debate started in the 1970s between two theologians, Richard McCormick and Paul Ramsey. The basic argument advanced by McCormick for the exercise of substituted judgment holds that parents are indeed capable of assuming, with a certain knowledge of their child's fundamental goodwill, that he would be more than willing — absent the fright of the moment — to act altruistically: "He would choose this were he capable of choice because he 'ought' to do so." The riposte articulated by Ramsey is far more libertarian: "No child or adult incompetent can choose to become a participating member of medical undertakings, and no one else on earth should decide to subject these people to investigations having no relation to their own treatment."

The most illuminating, however, is the third approach, that the proxy must act in the "best interests" of the child. This standard has a certain visceral attraction: Most parents would instinctively say that they always act in the best interests of their children. Not necessarily. Parental dedication to the child's "best interests" is assumed, but this is neither legally nor logically self-evident: The Supreme Court has indicated that a child's interest can be perceived as separable from his parents' estimation thereof.

Careful examination of asserted parental dedication to a child's "best interests" reveals that this parental assertion can be subject to various interpretations, especially in the context of biomedical research. On the one hand, it can be argued that this standard, when interpreted as a "fiduciary duty," is far too exacting for any parent, save the pathologically overbearing. In the day-to-day familial struggle to satisfy adequately the needs of a variety of constituencies

— including but not limited to employers, spouses, friends, community, and, not to be forgotten, other children — every parent inevitably falls far short of acting in the "best interests" of any given child. Kids are dragged on shopping trips, sit in pediatricians' waiting rooms with their siblings, get dumped early in the morning into for-profit day-care centers, are left in the evening with channel surfing baby-sitters, and are ignored by their father at the end of the day as he unwinds in front of the tube with a can of cold beer cradled in his limp hands. Undivided attention, such as a "fiduciary" must give . . . is not the standard by which parents normally act. This standard would, if its implications were teased out, categorically exclude any research on children that does not hold out at least the prospect of some direct benefit for the child in question.

Interpreted slightly more generously, however, "best interests" is a quite capacious standard. While a child's intellectual development might well be best secured by spending his mornings at the local Montessori school rather than being stunted by trips to the store to procure food and clothing, bored by too many hours in doctors' waiting rooms, angered when left with sitters, and saddened by an unfocused father, the aim of each of these things — protection from starvation, exposure, and untreated disease at home, not to mention the preservation of parental sanity — contributes, each in its own way, to the child's long-term "best interests."

Many have argued that a child's participation in medical experimentation is one way in which his "best interests" can be promoted, even if — or perhaps especially if — the intervention holds out no prospect of direct medical benefit for that child. Parents regularly ask their children to give up something they treasure — a favorite toy, the good graces of an exclusive school-yard clique, or their playtime — to provide a more bountiful Christmas to kids on the other side of the tracks, to befriend ostracized classmates, or to cheer up the denizens of the local nursing home. While much of this is requested in the genuine belief that the child's actions might actually make the world a better place, this sort of parental initiative likely aims rather more at the positive psychological development of their own child. As a number of observers of the biomedical research enterprise have noted, it is surely possible that the same instinct can motivate parents to enroll their children in biomedical experiments: This is yet another context in which children might develop the charitable instincts that parents want them to possess.

At least one parent is on record as declaring as much. Upon being told by a researcher that his son's refusal to donate a small sample of blood for research purposes — in spite of the father's clearly articulated desire to the contrary — would be respected as binding, the father angrily exclaimed: "This is my child. I was less concerned with the research involved than with the kind of boy that I was raising. I'll be damned if I was going to allow my child, because of some idiotic concept of children's rights, to assume that he was entitled to be a selfish, narcissistic little bastard."

2. Research Promotion Strategies

That being said, what standard of proxy consent do the regulations present to investigators (and their institutions' lawyers) who wish to maximize the participation of children in their studies? The answer, I think, is that the regulations allow the designers of ambitious research protocols to make one of two moves: to characterize the research as beneficial to the child at hand, or, if that is not possible, beneficial to the practice of pediatric medicine or the development of pediatric bioscience.

Informed Consent, Parental Permission, and Assent in Pediatric Practice
Committee on Bioethics of the American Association of Pediatrics
95 PEDIATRICS 314 (1995)

[This discussion, designed to address pediatric practice, is also relevant to parental decision-making about research.]

PROBLEMS WITH THE CONCEPT OF "CONSENT" BY PROXY

In attempting to adapt the concept of informed consent to pediatrics, many believe that the child's parents or guardians have the authority or "right" to give consent by proxy. Most parents seek to safeguard the welfare and best interests of their children with regard to health care, and as a result proxy consent has seemed to work reasonably well.

However, the concept encompasses many ambiguities. Consent embodies judgments about proposed interventions and, more importantly, consent (literally "to feel or sense with") expresses something for one's self: a person who consents responds based on unique personal beliefs, values, and goals. . . .

PARENTAL PERMISSION AND SHARED RESPONSIBILITY

Decision-making involving the health care of young patients should flow from responsibility shared by physicians and parents. Practitioners should seek the informed permission of parents before medical interventions (except in emergencies when parents cannot be contacted). The informed permission of parents includes all of the elements of standard informed consent. . . .

Usually, parental permission articulates what most agree represents the "best interests of the child." However, the Academy acknowledges that this standard of decision-making does not always prove easy to define. In a pluralistic society, one can find many religious, social, cultural, and philosophic positions on what constitutes acceptable child rearing and child welfare. The law generally provides parents with wide discretionary authority in raising their children. Nonetheless, the need for child abuse and neglect laws and procedures makes it clear that parents sometimes breach their obligations toward their children. Providers of care and services to children have to carefully justify the invasion of privacy and psychological disruption that come with taking legal steps to override parental prerogatives.

NOTES AND QUESTIONS

1. On what basis should parents decide to permit or refuse the enrollment of their children in research? Should they try to place themselves in the "shoes of the child" and see if the intervention would be welcomed or rejected by him or her? Should they attempt to process the particulars through the lens of their own values and experience? What if a particular parent would be willing to undergo some discomfort for the payment of $25? Should he or she be able to extrapolate that particular personal calculus to the child? Does it matter whether the parents intend to give the child any payments received by the researchers?

2. Do you agree with McCormick's view that we can presume that children would act altruistically "absent the fright of the moment"? If not, should parents be permitted to force their children to be altruistic? Do Clark's examples of other ways in which parents attempt to inculcate charitable values in their children support parental decisions to enroll their children in nontherapeutic research? Does it depend on the nature of the research? If so, in what type of studies might "compelled altruism" be more acceptable?

3. The regulations permit parents *or* guardians to grant permission. What assumptions do we make about a parent's relationship to his or her child? Are the same assumptions justified in regard to a guardian? Should the latter have the same powers?

4. Note that, under 45 C.F.R. § 46.408(c), the IRB may waive the requirement of parental permission if it finds that "parental or guardian permission is not a reasonable requirement to protect the subjects," as long as an "appropriate mechanism for protecting the children who will participate as subjects" is substituted and the waiver does not violate other legal provisions. In addition to the example provided in the text of the regulations (neglected or abused children), in what sorts of research might a waiver of the permission requirement be appropriate? What would an "appropriate mechanism" to replace the permission requirement look like?

5. Should parents be given "incentives" or "sweeteners" for entering their children into a clinical trial? For example, should they be offered $25, $50, or $100 for transporting their child to the clinic? What about offering a parent free care if their child is uninsured? Do the arguments for and against paying adult research subjects (discussed in Chapter 8, at page 395) apply equally to the use of incentives in pediatric research? Approximately one in four pediatric research studies offers some sort of payment for participation, with amounts commonly in the range of $200 to $400, and sometimes greater than $1,000. *See* Schultz,

supra at 62. For discussions of these issues, *see,* e.g., David Wendler et al., *The Ethics of Paying for Children's Participation in Research*, 141 J. PEDIATR. 166 (2002); Paul M. Fernhoff, *Paying for Children to Participate in Research: A Slippery Slope or an Enlightened Stairway (Editorial)*, 141 J. PEDIATR. 153 (2002); Kathryn Weise et al., *National Practices Regarding Payment to Research Subjects for Participation in Pediatric Research*, 110 PEDIATRICS 577 (2002).

6. The Institute of Medicine's report on research involving children devotes a chapter to the issue of payments for research participation and summarizes the existing literature. *See* INSTITUTE OF MEDICINE, ETHICAL CONDUCT OF CLINICAL RESEARCH INVOLVING CHILDREN 211-28 (2004). It concludes that it should never be necessary to offer children higher payments for participating in riskier studies (as sometimes happens in research with adults), because the federal regulations generally do not permit children to be enrolled in risky studies. However, the report concludes that it is acceptable to "provide reasonable, age-appropriate compensation for children based on the time involved in research that does not offer the prospect of direct benefit." Is there any reason to be concerned about the incentives this might provide to a child who otherwise does not have a job or other sources of income?

7. What obligations do researchers have when they believe that a parent is making decisions that are not in their child's best interests? What mechanisms exist to ensure that researchers adhere to these obligations?

8. For studies to which Subpart D applies, the regulations essentially create an almost irrebutable presumption that children are incapable of providing informed consent to research. What do we gain and lose by such an approach?

[2] Soliciting a Minor's Assent

45 C.F.R. §§ 46.408(a) and (e):
REQUIREMENTS FOR ASSENT BY CHILDREN

These provisions are reproduced in Appendix A, at page A-29. Please read them before proceeding.

Informed Consent, Parental Permission, and Assent in Pediatric Practice
Committee on Bioethics of the American Association of Pediatrics
95 PEDIATRICS 314 (1995)

Decision-making involving the health care of older children and adolescents should include, to the greatest extent feasible, the assent of the patient as well as the participation of the parents and the physician. Pediatricians should not necessarily treat children as rational, autonomous decision makers, but they should give serious consideration to each patient's developing capacities for participating in decision-making, including rationality and autonomy. If physicians recognize the importance of assent, they empower children to the extent of their capacity. Even in situations in which one should not and does not solicit the agreement or opinion of patients, involving them in discussions about their health care may foster trust and a better physician-patient relationship, and perhaps improve long-term health outcomes.

Assent should include at least the following elements:

- Helping the patient achieve a developmentally appropriate awareness of the nature of his or her condition.

- Telling the patient what he or she can expect with tests and treatment(s).

- Making a clinical assessment of the patient's understanding of the situation and the factors influencing how he or she is responding (including whether there is inappropriate pressure to accept testing or therapy).

- Soliciting an expression of the patient's willingness to accept the proposed care. Regarding this final point, we note that no one should solicit a patient's views without intending to weigh them seriously. In situations in which the patient will have to receive medical care despite his or her objection, the patient should be told that fact and should not be deceived.

As children develop, they should gradually become the primary guardians of personal health and the primary partners in medical decision-making, assuming responsibility from their parents.

Just as is the case with informed consent, the emphasis on obtaining assent should be on the interactive process in which information and values are shared and joint decisions are made. The Academy does not in any way recommend the development of new bureaucratic mechanisms, such as "assent forms," which could never substitute for the relational aspects of consent or assent.

NOTES AND QUESTIONS

1. The regulations permit IRBs to dispense with the assent requirement if "the intervention or procedure involved in the research holds out a prospect of direct benefit that is important to the health or well-being of the children and is available only in the context of the research" — even if the children have the mental capacity to provide assent. Is that appropriate?

2. Assume that a child with cancer has been treated unsuccessfully over the years and has finally decided that he does not want any more treatment. What should happen if the parents want to enroll the child in a protocol examining a promising new intervention that might benefit the child, but the child is unwilling to assent? Would your answer depend on the child's age? If so, how old would the child have to be before you would allow his refusal to trump the parents' decision?

3. Randall Baldwin Clark questions the view that requiring a child's "assent" to research "endows a child-subject with 'additional protection'":

> This provision is unproblematic if one views the opportunity to decline to participate as an indulgence we dispense to children to enable them to exercise their moral agency freely and thereby mature into autonomous and charitable adults. One might then inquire, however, why this requirement can be so easily waived. If, on the other hand, one views the "assent" provision as placing the decisional firewall in the child's control, it becomes quite dubious that child subjects have thereby been granted "additional protection." This can be seen from two points of reference. As previously noted, there are far too many situations in which the IRB may allow the researcher to "waive" the "assent" requirement. Also, we place in the hands of children — whose moral faculties are still developing well into their teen-age years — responsibility for a decision that only mature and responsible adults can reasonably make.

Clark, *supra* at 39–40. Are these objections convincing? Do you agree with Clark's view that there are "far too many situations" in which the assent requirement can be waived?

4. Suppose that researchers intend to enroll both adults and minors in a study, and the IRB has determined that the study meets the criteria for waiving informed consent under the "general" waiver rules of 45 C.F.R. § 46.116(d). How would that determination affect (i) the need to obtain parental permission, and (ii) the need to obtain the assent of the minors?

[3] Allocating Decision-Making Authority in Research with Adolescents

Guidelines for Adolescent Health Research:
A Position Paper of the Society for Adolescent Medicine
John S. Santelli et al.
33 J. ADOLESCENT HEALTH 396 (2003)

Numerous national commissions, panels, and reports have articulated their great concern about adolescent health and the urgent need for research that can guide interventions and inform public policy in this area. Violence, human immunodeficiency virus (HIV) infection and other sexually transmitted diseases (STDs), alcohol and other drug use, and unintended pregnancy pose continuing and serious challenges to the health and well-being of youth in communities across the country. Many potentially deleterious health behaviors begin in adolescence, including sexual activity, smoking and alcohol consumption, illicit drug use, interpersonal violence, and behaviors that cause unintentional injuries. The timing of pubertal development also affects adolescent health behaviors and health status; an historic decline in the age of puberty has been accompanied by social pressures for extended schooling and delayed marriage.

Research with adolescents has produced important benefits for this population in recent years, with significant insights emerging about the ways in which adolescents differ from both children and adults. For example, differences between pediatric and adult patient populations are substantial in drug elimination and therapeutic response. In addition, studies of the Human Papillomavirus have demonstrated an unexpectedly high prevalence in sexually experienced adolescents and have informed clinical practice in screening for cervical cancer. Research into adverse pregnancy outcomes (e.g., low birth weight, infant mortality) of young adolescents has demonstrated that these outcomes are related to social deficits and *not* age or physical maturity and that comprehensive prenatal care can address these deficits and improve outcomes. Finally, research on school and community health education has documented an evolution in program efficacy over the past 25 years; from this research have emerged principles for effective prevention that can be incorporated into programs to prevent HIV infection, other STDs, and unintended pregnancy among teens. Unfortunately, the successes of research involving adolescents are often overshadowed by the gaps in knowledge about this age group that persist. For example, significant deficits remain in our knowledge of the effects of puberty on a drug's action or elimination. In addition, the optimal design of clinical preventive services for adolescents is limited by a lack of health service research data. Furthermore, significant gaps remain in the knowledge needed to create effective HIV prevention for gay and bisexual youth, who are often at exceptionally high risk. Prevention of delinquency and violence and treatment for mental health problems have also been hindered by a dearth of research to guide interventions that will help young people successfully navigate the difficult and sometimes deadly challenges to their future health and productivity. Equally disconcerting is the paucity of information about the factors that support the resiliency of adolescents against psychosocial risks or about how to disseminate successful model programs in prevention to other communities.

Although numerous threats to adolescent health continue to be evident, the ability to conduct research with adolescents remains difficult. A critical problem is the difficulty that researchers and Institutional Review Boards (IRBs) have with interpreting the federal regulations as they apply to research involving adolescents. Not surprisingly, adolescents, as a class, have often been excluded from participation in clinical trials, studies in public health prevention, and other critical research efforts from which this age group would benefit. The result is that treatment options and the design of interventions for adolescents must often be extrapolated from studies involving either children or adults. The wisdom of this approach is suspect, because the period of adolescence is marked by significant changes in physical and psychosocial development that set adolescents apart from their younger and older counterparts. Likewise, the research agenda itself is vulnerable to the influence of political currents; adults are often uncomfortable dealing with adolescents and their health issues.

Researchers and IRBs have reported a wide variation in the interpretation of the federal regulations as they apply to research involving adolescents. Interpretations have been particularly disparate with respect to issues related to an adolescent's capacity to consent to research participation without parental permission, the protection of confidentiality for adolescent research participants, and the conduct of research that addresses "socially sensitive" subjects, such as illicit drug use, violence, and sexuality. These differences are not surprising, because the current federal regulations do not specifically address the inherent differences between adolescents and children. . . .

An important context for these *Guidelines* is the legal status of children and adolescents. The legal status of children has evolved from that of property (chattel) under traditional English common law to persons with limited autonomy. The "personhood" of children was recognized implicitly by states as they enacted child abuse reporting laws and medical consent laws during the 1960s and explicitly by the United States Supreme Court in the 1967 decision *In re Gault*, which extended the due process protection of the Fourteenth Amendment to children as well as adults. These legal changes acknowledge that there is not always a congruence of interests among children, their parents, and the state and seek to protect the welfare of children and adolescents.

NOTES AND QUESTIONS

1. Several federal and state statutes permit children to consent to certain types of medical interventions before they have reached the general age of consent to medical care, including treatment for drug and alcohol abuse, family planning and contraception, and, in some instances, mental health treatment. *See generally* Abigail English & Madlyn Morreale, *A Legal and Policy Framework for Adolescent Health Care: Past, Present, and Future*, 1 HOUSTON J. HEALTH L. & POL'Y 63 (2001). Some of these laws protect minors' rights to make constitutionally protected decisions free of parental interference. *See, e.g.*, Carey v. Population Serv. Int'l, 431 U.S. 678 (1977) (holding that states may not ban the sale of nonprescription contraceptives to minors). Others reflect a policy judgment that requiring minors to involve their parents in certain types of health care decisions may lead them to delay or forego care, thus risking ongoing health problems and, in some cases, creating threats to the public health.

2. Given that minors can consent to family planning services without parental involvement, would a study testing a new form of birth control among high school students be subject to Subpart D? (In answering this question, consider the definition of "children" under 45 C.F.R. § 46.402(a).) What about a study to gather data about behaviors that put adolescents at risk for becoming pregnant, or a study evaluating interventions to reduce risky behaviors? *See* Debra K. Katzman, *Guidelines for Adolescent Health Research*, 33 J. ADOLESCENT HEALTH 410 (2003) (proposing guidelines that would permit minors to consent to such studies without parental involvement).

3. In addition to the types of laws described in the previous two notes, there are other situations in which minors may become legally qualified to make health care decisions. First, a minor can become legally "emancipated" as a result of certain types of events (such as marriage or military service) that demonstrate that she is functioning independent of her parents. The actual events that cause emancipation vary from state to state, and often are not specifically spelled out in any statute. Second, some state courts have recognized the concept of a "mature minor," i.e., a minor who has demonstrated that she is sufficiently mature to make her own health care decisions. If a minor becomes emancipated or is determined to be a mature minor, should that person be allowed to enroll in research without the permission of her parents? Might it make a difference if the study does not offer a prospect of direct benefit to the child? *See, e.g.*, Leonard H. Glantz, *Research with Children*, 24 AM. J.L. & MED. 213, 225-26, 230 (1998); Amy T. Campbell, *State Regulation of Medical Research with Children and Adolescents: An Overview and Analysis*, in INSTITUTE OF MEDICINE, ETHICAL CONDUCT OF CLINICAL RESEARCH INVOLVING CHILDREN 320 (2004).

4. Consider the following quotation from the Society for Adolescent Medicine:

Subpart D often takes a one-size-fits-all approach, and generally fails to acknowledge the changing vulnerability of children to research risk or the changing capacity of children to make autonomous choices. As documented in our position paper, adolescents show considerable capacity to make decisions about research participation. By contrast, the recent adoption by the FDA of Subpart D, while excluding the possibility of a waiver of parental permission, demonstrates an appalling lack of understanding of these realities for adolescent research participants.

Growth into adolescence is marked by an increasing capacity to make independent and intelligent decisions. Developmental psychologists recognize emerging cognitive abilities (i.e., changes in the ability of the human organism to understand increasingly complex and abstract concepts), while ethicists have recognized a related concept, capacity, the ability to provide informed consent (i.e., to appreciate the risks and benefits of participation in research activities and to make reasoned choices). Capacity is linked to both developing cognition and previous life experiences. Research on cognition and capacity suggests that both adolescents and younger children show significant ability to provide informed consent. For mid- and late adolescents (age 14 years or older), understanding of research and the cognitive ability to make decisions about research participation are similar to these abilities in adults.

Testimony by the Society for Adolescent Medicine before the Committee on Clinical Research with Children, Institute of Medicine, National Academy of Sciences (2003).

If, in fact, adolescents are as capable of choosing as this testimony states they are, should parental permission be required for research with adolescents? Should the regulations be amended to require researchers to evaluate each adolescent's decision-making capacity, so that adolescents with capacity could consent to research without parental involvement? Should researchers and IRBs at least have the option of permitting such individualized capacity determination? What public policies and societal conventions would these approaches implicate? Why might parents object to amending the regulations even if they believe their adolescents have decision-making capacity?

5. The testimony goes on to argue that, "for minimal risk research, the assent of the adolescent subject is adequate protection and that parental permission can be waived routinely." Does this suggest a fundamental change in the allocation of decision-making authority among parent, child, pediatrician/ researcher, and the state? Is such a change appropriate?

[B] Categories of Permissible Risks

[1] General Principles

Unlike studies on adult subjects, which only have to satisfy the general risk-benefit balancing set forth in 45 C.F.R. § 46.111(a)(1)-(2), studies involving minors also must fit within one of several "risk" categories. There are three main categories, described in sections 404, 405, and 406 of Subpart D, that are in general designed to impose a limit on the magnitude of the "net" risks (those not offset by benefits from participation) to which a minor can be exposed. The thinking behind these rules is that, even though a parent has given permission, and the minor may have also assented, we are on shakier ethical ground in enrolling such a subject than where a competent adult has made a similar decision regarding his own participation. These three categories, which are discussed in order below, employ a number of vague terms, and are the source of a great deal of confusion and debate. (A fourth category, described in section 407, is a type of catch-all for the rare important study that is not approvable under any of the other three categories; that provision is discussed separately later in this chapter.)

45 C.F.R. § 46.102(i): DEFINITION OF MINIMAL RISK AND § 46.404: RESEARCH NOT INVOLVING GREATER THAN MINIMAL RISK

These provisions are reproduced in Appendix A, at pages A-5 and A-28. Please read them before proceeding.

American Academy of Pediatrics Statement Before the Institute of Medicine Committee on Clinical Research Involving Children: Participation and Protection of Children in Clinical Research
David J. Schonfeld
July 9, 2003
http://www.aap.org/advocacy/washing/david_ schonfeld_testimony.htm

The AAP interprets the definition of minimal risk to be that level of risk associated with the daily activities of a normal, healthy, average child. What constitutes a risk to the child should be evaluated in the broadest context and incorporate known and predictable effects of the treatment and procedures including discomfort, inconvenience, pain, fright, separation from parents and familiar surroundings, and the effects on growth, development, and psychological functioning. Conceptually, the minimal risk standard defines the permissible level of risk in research as equivalent to the socially allowable risks which an average parent would generally permit their children to be exposed to in non-research situations. We recognize that certain groups of children are routinely exposed to greater risks as part of their ordinary lives because of adverse circumstances in which they live (such as children living in poverty or unsafe neighborhoods). However, the level of risk considered minimal in research should not be any different for these children than for others simply because the level of risk faced in their daily experience is greater than that faced by an average child. The Academy agrees with these principles and finds that there is little disagreement among the pediatric community regarding the participation of children as subjects in clinical research when the research involves only minimal risk.

NOTES AND QUESTIONS

1. Compare the definition of "minimal risk" in 45 C.F.R. § 46.102(i), which applies to pediatric research, to the definition of the same term in 45 C.F.R. § 46.303(d), which applies to research with prisoners. How do the two definitions differ? Do the differences suggest that the concept of "minimal risk" means something different for chronically ill children than it does for healthy children? For example, for a child with diabetes or cancer, could some interventions that would be more than minimal risk for a healthy child be so routine as to constitute a minimal risk? Note that, despite the regulatory language, many IRBs believe that it is inappropriate for the sickest children to be exposed to the greatest risks, and therefore apply a uniform definition of "minimal risk" for all children. Is such an approach permissible under the regulations? If you were on an IRB, would you support a uniform or a relative approach to the definition of "minimal risk"?

2. There is some interesting history on this issue. The National Commission for the Protection of Human Subjects of Biomedical and Behavioral Research, whose reports formed the basis for many provisions of the federal regulations, had used language defining minimal risk in terms of "healthy children." NATIONAL COMMISSION FOR THE PROTECTION OF HUMAN SUBJECTS OF BIOMEDICAL AND BEHAVIORAL RESEARCH, RESEARCH IN CHILDREN xix (1977). However, the actual wording in the regulations does not use that language. Moreover, in the preamble to the regulations, it was stated that minimal risk was to be determined in relationship to the risks encountered "in the daily life of the subjects of the research." INSTITUTE OF MEDICINE, ETHICAL CONDUCT OF CLINICAL RESEARCH INVOLVING CHILDREN 121 (2004). Does knowing this history change your views on the questions raised in the previous note?

3. Consider the following findings from a recent study of 188 IRB chairpersons:

Overall, 27% of IRB chairpersons categorized allergy skin testing as too risky for IRB approval without a prospect of direct benefit to the participating children, while 66% deemed such testing safe enough for IRB approval without a prospect of direct benefit. Similarly, 59% would prohibit a pharmacokinetic study with a 1 in 100,000 risk of death as excessively risky, yet 37% would permit such a study as posing minimal risk or a minor increase of minimal risk. While 19% of chairpersons consider a confidential survey of sexual behavior to be too risky for IRB approval, 73% deemed it approvable by an IRB.

Seema Shah et al., *How Do Institutional Review Boards Apply the Federal Risk and Benefit Standards for Pediatric Research?* 291 JAMA 476 (2004). Should we be troubled by these findings, or do they show that IRBs are appropriately applying different local values to minimal risk determinations? (Recall the rationale for local IRBs discussed in Chapter 4, at page 173.) If you believe there should be greater uniformity in IRBs' application of the minimal risk standard, what policy measures might promote such a result? *See, e.g.,* Carl H. Coleman, *Rationalizing Risk Assessment in Human Subject Research*, 46 ARIZ. L. REV. 1 (2004) (proposing measures to promote "principled consistency" in IRB decision-making); INSTITUTE OF MEDICINE, ETHICAL CONDUCT OF CLINICAL RESEARCH INVOLVING CHILDREN 261-65 (2004).

4. A decision chart by Robert Nelson for determining whether a study is approvable under any of the risk categories (sections 404 through 407) appears at page 119 of the Institute of Medicine report, *supra*.

45 C.F.R. § 46.405: RESEARCH INVOLVING GREATER THAN MINIMAL RISK BUT PRESENTING THE PROSPECT OF DIRECT BENEFIT TO THE INDIVIDUAL SUBJECTS

This provision is reproduced in Appendix A, at page A-28. Please read it before proceeding.

NOTES AND QUESTIONS

1. Section 405 is perhaps the most important of the risk categories, because most studies that involve testing some treatment on a child with a medical problem are approved under this category. It will be relatively rare that giving a child a not-fully-proven treatment could be considered a minimal risk activity, or even a "minor increase over minimal risk" (the category to be discussed in the next section). Thus, such studies have to be approved under section 405, which in essence requires that participation in the study be a reasonable choice from the point of view of the child's best interests: the possible benefits have to outweigh the risks. Note that unlike the other risk categories, section 405 does not place any type of upper limit on the amount of risk to which a child may be exposed.

2. Notice that the language of each of the risk categories refers to the risk presented by "an intervention or procedure." This is generally interpreted to mean that *each* intervention or procedure involved in a study approved under section 405 must separately satisfy the criteria of section 405, or alternatively be approvable under one of the other sections of the regulations. In other words, the IRB is not supposed to "add up" the benefits and risks for all the interven-

tions in the study and then apply the tests of section 405. What problems might arise if IRBs were permitted to apply section 405 to the total risks of a study, rather than the risks of each specific intervention or procedure? *See, e.g.*, Ernest D. Prentice et al., *Can Children Be Enrolled in a Placebo-Controlled Randomized Clinical Trial of Synthetic Growth Hormone?* 11 IRB, Jan.-Feb. 1989, at 6 (discussing the use of placebo injections); cf. Chapter 6, at page 292 (discussing a "component" approach to risk-benefit assessment).

3. As discussed in Chapter 3, subjects in Phase 1 drug studies are exposed to a particular dose of a drug primarily to see how high a dose can be given before unacceptable side effects start to appear. *See* Chapter 3, at page 153. Such studies are generally required before any testing for efficacy takes place. In the case of new chemotherapy drugs, which are highly likely to cause many substantial side effects, Phase 1 testing takes place in children with cancer. Would such studies ever be approvable under section 405? *See, e.g.*, Eric Kodish, *Pediatric Ethics and Early-phase Childhood Cancer Research: Conflicted Goals and the Prospect of Benefit*, 10 ACCOUNTABILITY IN RESEARCH 17 (2003).

45 C.F.R. § 46.406: RESEARCH INVOLVING GREATER THAN MINIMAL RISK AND NO PROSPECT OF DIRECT BENEFIT TO INDIVIDUAL SUBJECTS, BUT LIKELY TO YIELD GENERALIZABLE KNOWLEDGE ABOUT THE SUBJECT'S DISORDER OR CONDITION

This provision is reproduced in Appendix A, at page A-28. Please read it before proceeding.

American Academy of Pediatrics Statement Before the Institute of Medicine Committee on Clinical Research Involving Children: Participation and Protection of Children in Clinical Research
David J. Schonfeld
July 9, 2003

The more contentious issue relates to a third category of approvable research that allows children who have an underlying condition (i.e., who are not "healthy") to participate in research that does not hold out the prospect of direct benefit to them. This type of research is approvable if the intervention or procedure is likely to yield generalizable knowledge about the subjects' disorder or condition which is of vital importance for the understanding or amelioration of the disorder or condition, and participation in the research does not expose the child to greater than "a minor increase over minimal risk." While we understand and support the necessity to conduct research to advance our understanding of illness and its treatment, and realize that at times this may involve asking children to assume slightly more than minimal risk even in the absence of the likelihood of personal gain (other than their ability to contribute to the study of a childhood disease), we find the distinction between the "healthy" child and the child with an illness or condition somewhat artificial and the increment in risk from minimal to a minor increase above minimal to be vague.

The over-riding principle behind the "minor increase over minimal risk" standard is the recognition that certain research procedures might be more familiar and less concerning to children that are subjected to similar experiences on a regular basis because of their underlying medical condition. A child who has already undergone the same or comparable diagnostic or therapeutic procedure as part of the management of an underlying medical condition may be in a better position to judge the likely discomfort and inconvenience associated with the procedure. Having tolerated the procedure in the past, the child may be at a lesser personal risk for discomfort or complication as a result of a repeat administration of the procedure for the proposed research project. The complicating factor, though, is that children who undergo such procedures (e.g., a lumbar puncture or bone marrow aspirate), may also be psychologically sensitized to these procedures (because of learned negative associations) and/or have underlying medical conditions that place them at increased physical risk (e.g., children with leukemia who may have an increased risk of infection or bleeding after a bone marrow aspirate as compared to a healthy child). This situation illustrates that children with an underlying medical condition may either be at increased or decreased risk — the presence of an underlying medical condition associated with prior experience with the procedure in question does not, in and of itself, render the child at lesser (or greater) risk.

In considering approval in this category of research, it would seem most appropriate that the IRB ensure that the investigator consider those situations that may increase the discomfort or risk of a particular procedure for a child with an underlying condition (e.g., if a non-diagnostic or non-therapeutic bone marrow aspirate is part of the proposed protocol, children who have a platelet count or white blood cell count below a certain level, or who showed or expressed distress during a prior aspirate) and exclude them from participation. In addition, the investigator should put into place a mechanism for soliciting the child's and parent's input on the likely emotional and psychological distress that a repeat of the procedure may entail for the particular child. Through this approach involving careful consideration of personal risk and conscientious steps to ensure full informed consent and assent for participation, it is likely that some children will be identified who, due to their successful and non-traumatic prior experience with a procedure that many children may find otherwise painful or frightening, are, in fact, only at minimal risk for participation in the proposed study. In this way, studies that would otherwise involve a "minor increase over minimal risk" if applied to the general population, can allow the selective informed participation of children whose prior experiences decrease their personal risk to the level where it can be felt to be minimal.

The AAP would also like to emphasize that we feel it is the duty of the investigator and the IRB to ensure that all potential research risks are minimized to the fullest extent possible. Thus, even in research studies that have risks deemed minimal, every reasonable attempt should be made to minimize the risks even further.

NOTES AND QUESTIONS

1. Consider the following possible justifications for section 406: (1) even if the children in the study are not expected to receive any direct benefits, they may ultimately benefit if the study contributes to the development of effective treatments in the future; (2) we can presume that children with a particular disorder or condition would want to assume some risks for the benefit of other children with the same disorder or condition; (3) treatments for childhood illnesses cannot be developed without testing them on children who have those illnesses; therefore, allowing such testing, even if it involves greater-than-minimal risks, is consistent with the best interests of those children as a group. Are any of these justifications persuasive?

2. In its report on categories of permissible risk in research on children, the National Human Research Protections Advisory Committee (NHRPAC) of the Department of Health and Human Services offered the following example of a study that would be permissible under section 406:

> Children who are obese are at greater risk than normal weight children of developing Type 2 diabetes, associated with resistance to the physiologic action of insulin. Research scientists may propose to examine the time course and mechanism of insulin resistance in obese children who are otherwise healthy. Such studies might use various procedures to assess insulin resistance. These tests would not meet the criteria of minimal risk procedures because the risks and discomforts associated with the tests are greater than ordinarily encountered in the daily lives of normal, healthy, average children.

> However, obesity can be considered a condition that warrants study because of its association with the development of Type 2 diabetes and other serious diseases. Thus, if the IRB determined that the proposed study was likely to yield generalizable knowledge of vital importance about the development of diabetes or the pathophysiology of obesity, that the risk of the procedures performed in the proposed study represent a minor increase over minimal and are commensurate with expected experiences of the subjects, and that the site for the study and the skill and experience of the investigator were appropriate, the study could be approved under 45 C.F.R. § 46.406, research involving greater than minimal risk and no prospect of direct benefit.

NATIONAL HUMAN RESEARCH PROTECTIONS ADVISORY COMMITTEE, FINAL REPORT TO NHRPAC FROM CHILDREN'S WORKGROUP, available at www.hhs.gov/ohrp/nhrpac/documents/nhrpac16.pdf. Is this analysis convincing?

3. As part of that report, NHRPAC also provided specific suggestions regarding the level of risks imposed by some common procedures. It categorized four procedures as falling within the category of a minor increase over minimal risk: urine collection using a catheter, lumbar puncture (a spinal tap), a skin punch biopsy with topical pain relief, and a bone marrow aspirate with topical pain relief. It also noted that insertion of a nasogastric catheter (a flexible tube that is threaded through a person's nostril and down their throat into their stomach) would usually also fit within this category. What do you think of these conclusions?

4. In what way is the parental permission requirement for studies approved under section 406 different from that for studies approved under sections 404 or 405?

[2] Applying the Standards: The Fenfluramine Studies

Research with Children
Leonard H. Glantz
24 AM. J.L. & MED. 213 (1998)

A recently published study provides an example of the vagueness of the concept of minimal risk when applied to research on children. The study subjects were thirty-four impoverished African American and Hispanic boys, ranging from seven to eleven years of age, who were younger brothers of delinquents. . . . [T]he investigators assessed the boys' serotonergic activity based on prior work that supposedly shows a relationship between serotonin levels and aggression. To accomplish this, all boys were free of medications for at least one month, all followed a low-monoamine diet for four days, and all fasted the night before the test (referred to as a "challenge"). On the day of the challenge, the boys received nothing by mouth and an intravenous catheter was inserted at 8:30 A.M. and remained in place for about five and a half hours. Researchers orally administered fenfluramine hydrochloride to the boys at 10:00 A.M. and took blood samples every hour from the catheter. By measuring certain biochemical responses to the fenfluramine challenge, the investigators would be able to make an assessment of the boys' central serotonergic activity. The investigators conducted this research in an attempt "to replicate results that have suggested that aggression in prepubertal children is positively correlated with central serotonergic activity" and to determine if "an association between adverse-rearing conditions and serotonin in children" existed.

Because this study presented no possible benefit to the minor subjects, the question is whether it should have been performed on this group of boys. Is this a minimal risk study or a greater than minimal risk study? The study involves conferring on the boys a psychiatric diagnosis related to aggressiveness that they apparently did not previously carry. Was this diagnosis passed on to the parents? If so, what is the effect on the children of such labeling? This negative diagnosis or labeling was created only for the purpose of furthering research, not for developing a treatment or preventive program for the child. The children were placed on a special diet for four days, a catheter was inserted and remained in place for five and a half hours, and the children were administered a drug that has no pediatric indication solely for the purpose of producing a response to the drug. Is the probability and magnitude of harm not greater than those encountered in the "routine physical or psychological examinations or tests"? In "routine" physical and psychological tests, children are not exposed to substances that cannot possibly be of use in diagnosis and treatment of a condition from which they might suffer. Moreover, the administration of fenfluramine in adults had previously been documented to cause adverse reactions. Certainly this study would not meet Ramsey's criteria for the permissible treatment of children nor would it seem to meet McCormick's less stringent criteria for child involvement in research. Further, the study raises the question of how one keeps children with "oppositional defiant disorder," "conduct disorder" and "attention-deficit hyperactivity disorder" from withdrawing from the study during the many long hours of study. If the study presents more than minimal risk to the child-subjects and is not "likely to yield generalizable knowledge about the subjects' condition which is of vital importance for the understanding or the amelioration of the subject's disorder or condition," then it would clearly be barred under the federal regulations. First, it is not clear that these children have a "disorder or condition," as those terms are used in the regulations. Indeed, it appears the only "diagnosis" these children had was the one conferred on them by the investigators. Second, nothing in this study was designed to be of "vital importance" to the amelioration of a condition or even the understanding of the condition. But the larger question is, Why should a parent have the authority to submit a child to such nonbeneficial procedures? Even if each individual procedure to which the children were subjected presented minimal risk, when a child is subjected to several minimal risk procedures, when does this amount to more than minimal risk? For example, it has been suggested that "when testing a new treatment for meningitis it is acceptable to perform one lumbar puncture on a sick child to satisfy the protocol's scientific needs, but not five." If each procedure is of minimal risk why do five of them constitute more than minimal risk? Part of the answer is that the more often one is exposed to a risk, the greater the chance of the harm it presents occurring. But more important, I believe, the answer is that at some undefined moment, we run into the Ramsey problem: at some point, the totality of these "minor" interventions makes us realize that we are violating our "duty of loyalty" to the child.

There are other examples in which the estimation of risk is difficult to ascertain, but in which the child is used in ways that are not designed to further the child's needs. For example, other investigators conducted a fenfluramine challenge in a study that was entirely nonbeneficial for seven- to eleven-year-old subjects. These children had all previously met the criteria for attention-deficit hyperactivity disorder. In addition to a fenfluramine challenge similar to that just discussed, this study had a one month "washout" period during which time children who were taking medication to treat their attention-deficit disorder were removed from the medication. Assuming that the medication was properly prescribed to treat the children's behavioral problems that would be manifested at school and home, and assuming that these medications were effective, it would seem clear that the risks of removing children from these medications exceeds those of risks encountered in "routine" medical care. Undoubtedly, children are appropriately removed from medications by their physicians because of unacceptable side-effects, or if the child does not require continuing use of the medication. These decisions are made in the best interests of the child, on an individual basis after individual assessment of the appropriateness of the drug discontinuation. In this case, however, the discontinuation of an effective treatment often used in an attempt to improve a child's school performance was not designed or intended to benefit the children in the study, but was required to ensure that the research results were not affected by the presence of these chemicals in the child's body. Because of this, the risk to the children exceeds that found in ordinary medical practice.

NOTES AND QUESTIONS

1. Under which regulatory provision should these studies have been evaluated — section 404, 405, or 406? In the study of the younger brothers of children with behavioral problems, is it possible to identify a "disorder or condition" of the subjects that would justify the application of section 406?

2. What were the risks of the study involving the younger brothers — the risk of developing a headache and nausea or the risk of being labeled a child with a psychiatric illness? What possible harms might result from labeling the child? Could it affect the child's relationship with his parents or siblings? What if the diagnosis is revealed to school authorities and results in the reassignment of the boy to a "special class"? How should an IRB weigh these considerations?

3. How should these protocols be evaluated in terms of their importance to "generalizable knowledge"? What if it were demonstrated that there is indeed a connection between serotonergic levels and aggressive behavior? Is that a significant finding? What scientific benefits might such a finding yield? Would those benefits justify these studies?

4. In at least some of the fenfluramine studies, both the boys and their parents were given incentives to participate. In one of the studies, for example, the boys were given $25 gift certificates to a popular store, and the parents were paid $100. *See* Ann E. Ryan, *Protecting the Rights of Pediatric Research Subjects in the International Conference on Harmonisation of Technical Requirements for Registration of Pharmaceuticals for Human Use*, 23 FORDHAM INT'L. L.J. 848

(2000). Does knowing this affect your evaluation of the acceptability of the study? Would you feel more comfortable if the parents were given nothing for the time they spent monitoring the boys' diets and medications? (Recall the discussion of the role of payments in pediatric research earlier in this chapter.)

[C] DHHS Review of Research Not Otherwise Approvable

45 C.F.R. § 46.407: RESEARCH NOT OTHERWISE APPROVABLE WHICH PRESENTS AN OPPORTUNITY TO UNDERSTAND, PREVENT, OR ALLEVIATE A SERIOUS PROBLEM AFFECTING THE HEALTH OR WELFARE OF CHILDREN

This provision is reproduced in Appendix A, at page A-29. Please read it before proceeding.

————————

Applications for approval of pediatric research under 45 C.F.R. § 407 were rare until recently: before 2000, only two studies had been reviewed under this provision. The requirements for approval under § 407 contain both procedural and interpretative ambiguities. For example: (1) What is the expertise required on the advisory panels? (2) What sort of information should be offered to the public for comment? (3) What if the public disclosure requirements conflict with investigators' intellectual property or commercial interests? (4) Is there *any* upper limit to the risks that can be authorized under § 407, or is the standard simply that risks must be reasonable in relation to the potential scientific merit of the study? (5) How does § 407 conform to other laws and policies, such as the "best interests of the child" standard under family law? *See* Loretta Kopelman and Timothy F. Murphy, *Ethical Concerns about Federal Approval of Risky Pediatric Studies*, 113 PEDIATRICS 1783 (2004).

The excerpts that follow consist of protocols sent by IRBs to DHHS for review under 45 C.F.R. § 46.407. As you read the protocols and commentaries, keep the following two questions in mind: First, should the particular protocol have been approved? Second, does the review process created by Section 407 appear to be a useful way to deal with studies not approvable under Subpart D?

[1] Cystic Fibrosis in Neonates

APPLICATION FOR APPROVAL OF RESEARCH INVOLVING
HUMAN SUBJECTS: CHARACTERIZATION OF MUCUS AND
MUCINS IN BRONCHOALVEOLAR LAVAGE FLUIDS FROM INFANTS
WITH CYSTIC FIBROSIS
(2001)
http://www.hhs.gov/ohrp/panels/407-02pnl/irbappl.pdf

Purpose and Rationale:

Cystic fibrosis (CF) results from mutation in the gene for CFTR, a protein which normally transports chloride ions out of epithelial cells. Children with CF are born with histopathogically normal lungs, but over the first weeks or months of life develop chronic bacterial infections of the conducting airways, along with intensive, neutrophil-dominated inflammation, and obstruction of the airways. It is still unclear exactly how the CFTR defect results in these changes. The best evidence at present favors a "drying" of airway surface liquid (ASL) in the absence of normal CFTR function, due to hyperabsorption of sodium and water secondary to the lack of chloride efflux. This drying severely impairs mucociliary clearance of inhaled bacteria and leads to chronic infection. Data from sputum studies and cell culture models also suggest several abnormalities of mucus biochemistry and expression of mucin peptides in CF. However, it is unclear whether these abnormalities are inherently related to CFTR dysfunction, or are secondary to chronic infection and inflammation.

Due to lack of a completely analogous animal model for CF, direct confirmation of hypotheses on the early events in the lung relies heavily on sampling of ASL from the infant lung using bronchoalveolar lavage fluid (BALF). A precise knowledge of the order of pathogenetic events will greatly focus efforts toward early therapy interrupting the primary processes leading to established infection and inflammation. At present, there is almost no information characterizing mucus or mucins in CF infants prior to the onset of infection and inflammation.

Published BALF studies from our laboratory and others suggest that a short "window" of infection- and inflammation-free lungs occurs in the weeks after birth in children with CF. Preliminary work in our laboratories suggests that mucins can be quantified in BALF using an immunoassay method, and mucus "plugs" can be isolated, fixed, and biochemically characterized by careful processing of BALF samples.

The goals of the proposed study are:

Quantify mucin in BALF and compare quantities before infection vs. after infection onset in CF; and compare CF vs. non-CF.

Correlate mucin quantity with measures of infection (quantitative bacteriology) and inflammation (cell numbers, neutrophil products, inflammatory cytokines).

Isolate mucus plugs and characterize their histology before and after infection, in order to more accurately describe early relationships among mucus obstruction, infection, and inflammation.

Subjects

Infants with a clinical diagnosis of CF in the neonatal period, who are typically immediately referred to the UNC CF Center for further diagnosis and clinical care. . . . As per the expected epidemiology of CF, gender distribution will be equal, and Caucasians will outnumber African-Americans and Hispanics approximately 20:1. . . .

Full description of the study design, methods and procedures

The proposed study is a longitudinal study of BALF changes over the first year of life in infants with CF. Subjects will be tested at 3 time points: 1) after diagnosis, within the first 6 weeks after birth; 2) at 6 months of age; 3) at 12 months of age.

At each study visit, subjects will be asked to come to UNC Children's Hospital where they will undergo flexible fiberoptic bronchoscopy according to standard clinical protocol. Subjects will be held NPO [nothing by mouth (non per os)] for 4 hours prior to time of procedure, and will be processed through pre-care in identical fashion to children undergoing clinically-indicated bronchoscopy. An intravenous line will be placed prior to procedure, and presedation with chloral hydrate will be given p.o. [by mouth]. Once the patient is transported to the bronchoscopy laboratory, baseline monitoring parameters will be established then the subject will receive i.v. fentanyl and versed at standard doses. When sedation is adequate, 2% lidocaine drops and Otrivin drops will be placed in the nose, and the scope passed to the larynx where additional 2% lidocaine will be instilled via the scope onto the vocal cords. The scope will be passed to the trachea and the lower airways briefly examined. BALF will be obtained by instilling 10 ml into the right middle lobe bronchus then suctioning intermittently. Identical procedure will be done in lingula and the 2 samples pooled. Bronchoscope will then be removed and patient recovered from sedation in the bronchoscopy laboratory and PACU as per standard clinical protocol. . . . Parents of subjects will also be asked to complete a questionnaire regarding respiratory symptoms and medication use in the period preceding the procedure. . . .

Full description of risks and measures to minimize risks:

Bronchoscopy can cause some irritation of the walls of the nose, throat or bronchial passage. If this occurs, it can cause some bleeding, cough, or wheezing (1-2% of patients). Pneumothorax and atelectasis can also occur but it is much rarer (less than 1%). These complications are minimized by using a very small bronchoscope (⅛-inch wide) and having the procedure done only by experienced bronchoscopists. The investigators are very experienced at doing this procedure.

The bronchoscope will partially block the breathing passage while the procedure is being done. In some cases this causes significant respiratory distress, but this is rare in the absence of structural airway anomalies, due to the small caliber of the scopes used. Risk is minimized by continuous monitoring of pulse oximetry, respiratory and heart rates, as well as direct visual monitoring by a Respiratory Therapist, as per standard bronchoscopic procedure. If desaturation or bradycardia occurs, the procedure is halted and support given as necessary.

Insertion of the bronchoscope may cause a risk of infection in the lung. The risk of this is very small (less than 1%) because the bronchoscope is sterile, although the bronchoscope may transfer infection from the nose to the lung.

Bronchoscopy can cause a transient slowing of the heart rate in 1-2% of cases. This can occur even if the child's oxygen level is kept high. Risk of complications from this are minimized by continuous heart rate monitoring.

Bronchoalveolar lavage (BAL) can cause transient fever during the 24 hour period following the procedure. This is seen more commonly in young children only when there is a significant amount of inflammation already present in the airways. Fever after bronchoscopy (BAL) is treated with acetaminophen (Tylenol).

Medications used to sedate for bronchoscopy (chloral hydrate, fentanyl, and versed) can be associated with slowing of breathing or apnea, at high doses. This risk is minimized by dosing within standard weight-based guidelines. Complications from this are minimized by the monitoring described above. If desaturation or bradycardia occurs, the procedure is halted and support given as necessary.

Risk for breach of confidentiality is minimized by encoding samples with access to subject's identity limited to the investigators.

Benefits to subjects and/or society

It is widely believed that early treatment of bacterial infections in the CF airway is likely to slow progression of lung disease. Bronchoscopy (BAL) is the only procedure available to obtain reliable microbiologic cultures from the lower airway of young patients with CF. Therefore the culture results obtained as part of this study may be directly beneficial in terms of choosing appropriate antibiotic therapy for pulmonary infections. From a longer term perspective, the results of this study may lead to discovery of important information regarding the pathogenesis of CF lung disease, potentially altering therapeutic strategies in early life.

––––––––––

The following two excerpts are from reviewers commissioned by DHHS to evaluate the protocol:

STATEMENT OF RONALD C. RUBENSTEIN, M.D., PH.D.
http://www.hhs.gov/ohrp/panels/407-02pnl/exp1.pdf

I feel that the selection of subjects is equitable, given that all subjects with CF identified in early infancy will be eligible. I also feel that the risks to the subjects are reasonable (as detailed below) with respect to the importance of knowledge that may reasonably be expected to result from this research, with attention to additional safeguards suggested below aimed at further minimizing risk. I do not feel that bronchoscopy with sedation can be considered minimal risk (§ 46.404). The risk of difficulty breathing with sedation exceeds that which would be inherent in everyday life.

The investigators, and a subcommittee of the CF Foundation Data Safety Monitoring Board has argued that participation in this trial has the prospect of direct benefit for the subjects, and therefore would be approvable under § 46.405. I agree with their contention that bacterial culture of BAL samples is the "gold standard" for assessing microbiologic colonization and infection of the CF lung, and that there is ample evidence that the more usual (and less invasive method) of deep throat culture has high false positive and false negative rates. There is also evolving sentiment in the field, based primarily on anecdotal data at this point, that early, aggressive antimicrobial therapy may be beneficial to subjects with CF by delaying the initiation of the "vicious cycle." However, there is also concern that such early, aggressive antimicrobial therapy may portend a later increase in antibiotic resistance. While I do agree that one bronchoscopy may afford the opportunity to identify an otherwise unsuspected pathogen in the lung of an infant with CF, I am less persuaded that participation in the trial would afford the possibility of direct benefit that is not available outside of the research, and therefore do not feel that this protocol is approvable under § 46.405. . . .

As discussed above, I feel that this study is likely to yield vital generalizable knowledge regarding CF lung disease that would potentially allow amelioration of this disorder in the future. Also, as part of the local practice at the CF Center at the University of North Carolina-Chapel Hill, apparently ~75% of infants less than 1 year of age will undergo bronchoscopy for clinical indications. While this is admittedly higher than many other CF centers, this practice reflects that Center's experience with bronchoscopy in infants and their use of early, aggressive, organism directed antimicrobial therapy in CF with cultures of BAL fluid serving as the best source of material. Thus, undergoing bronchoscopy for a child with CF who is less than 1 year of age as part of a study protocol is reasonably commensurate with the experience of a similar child with CF who is not a part of this study.

Thus, in my opinion, the approvability of this study under 46.406 hinges on whether bronchoscopy with sedation performed 3 times over the first year of life can be considered a minor increase over minimal risk. The position of the IRB at the University of North Carolina-Chapel Hill was that this procedure was more than a minor increase over minimal risk. The investigators have provided complication data for over 2,000 bronchoscopies with sedation performed in children at their center since 1998, with 432 of these performed in children less than 12 months of age. Their complication rate was far less than 1%, with no reported serious complication. Even when only the children <12 months of age were considered, the complications rate remained less than 1%. With the presence of a dedicated, experienced bronchoscopy team, that the investigators who will be performing these procedures are very experienced, and their documented low complication rate with lack of serious complications, that this procedure, can, in my opinion, potentially be considered a minor increase in minimal risk. I therefore feel that, with attention to a number of additional safeguards delineated below, this study would be approvable under § 46.406.

STATEMENT OF JOAN L. HOOPENGARDNER
http://www.hhs.gov/ohrp/panels/407-02pnl/exp2.htm

Prior to my report on the proposed study by Dr. Noah, I would like to provide a little background information. First, I am a parent with an 18-year-old son who has Cystic Fibrosis (CF). He presented meconium ileus at birth and emergency surgery was performed 24 hours later. After numerous tests, he was pronounced "normal" and we were told to go on with our lives. I did not feel comfortable with that diagnosis, and so pursued the issue. Finally, at 3 months of age, he was given the sweat test using the pylocarpine, not the electrodes, and he tested positive for CF. We have continued to visit the CF Centers regularly every 3 months, or more often as needed, for the last 18 years. He has been hospitalized 3 times for pulmonary exacerbations, and has participated in one study already. We have used some of the cutting edge antibiotic treatments and therapies even though there have been no clinical studies done to prove their effectiveness. Basically, I feel that any extra time I can buy my son is worth the risk; if the risk is minimal. Daily life with a child is a constant risk, especially a child with CF. I am my son's advocate. I fight every day to insure that all treat him equally, fairly, and respectfully. This is a difficult battle and one that will never be won until the disease is cured or under control. . . .

I do consider the protocol to be approvable under 45 CFR § 46.406, "Greater than minimal risk and no prospect of direct benefit to individual subjects, but likely to yield generalizable knowledge about the subject's disorder or condition." As previously stated, there is definitely a risk involved with the bronchoscopy, less than 1%, and there appears to be no direct benefit to the individual at this time. However, the data and information gathered will definitely yield new information about the lungs and their fluids in young CF patients. Perhaps this will yield information about the disease that will lead to better treatments and therapies. In any case, there will be knowledge that is previously unavailable on this disorder and condition and is unable to be obtained in any other way.

NOTES AND QUESTIONS

1. Rubenstein acknowledges that the study may identify "an otherwise unsuspected pathogen in the lung of an infant with CF," and that early aggressive treatment of these pathogens "may be beneficial to subjects." Yet he is unwilling to conclude that "participation in the trial would afford the possibility of direct benefit that is not available outside of the research," given the potential for early treatment to increase the infants' resistance to antibiotics. Are his concerns about antibiotic resistance really related to the potential *benefits* of the study, or are they more properly analyzed as a question about the study's *risks*? This question is not merely semantic: If the study is characterized as offering a "prospect of direct benefit to the individual subjects," it falls under 45 C.F.R. § 46.405, which does not contain any absolute upper limit to the level of permissible risk, as do §§ 404 and 406. Is it possible to disentangle the potential risks of an unproven intervention from that intervention's potential to benefit the subjects?

2. Hoopengardner analyzes the issues from a quite different perspective. Does her personal stake in the matter make her better able to protect the rights and interests of neonates, or does it undermine her ability to provide an objective analysis? Is it a good idea to include "patient advocates" like Ms. Hoopengardner as "experts" in § 407 panels?

3. Does Hoopengardner's conclusion that the study may "yield information about the disease that will lead to better treatments and therapies" establish that the study is approvable under 45 C.F.R. § 406?

4. How does one evaluate the risks of a bronchoscopy for a neonate? Neonates have extraordinarily small organs and connective tissue. It takes skill to do a bronchoscopy in such a small baby. Should approval of the study be conditioned on the researchers' credentials or their experience performing bronchoscopies in neonates?

5. In the summary of this proposal (*see* http://www.hhs.gov/ohrp/children/mucus.html), there is a letter stating the recommendation of OHRP, after considering the discussions of the special panel and reviewing the one comment that was received after publication in the *Federal Register*. The agency's conclusion was that the proposal was approvable with certain conditions under Section 407 because it presents a reasonable opportunity to understand, prevent or alleviate a serious problem affecting the health or welfare of children. The conditions include:

(1) clarification in the protocol and parental permission document regarding the presence of an anesthesiologist and regarding who will be present during the procedure and actually performing the procedure; . . .

(3) delineation, in both the protocol and parental permission document, of maximum amounts of sedative agents to be used, explicit descrip-

tion of the sedative drugs to be used and targeted level of sedation, and corresponding discussion of aborting the procedure if the appropriate level of sedation (e.g., moderate or "conscious" sedation) cannot be achieved or is exceeded; . . .

(6) formulation of intra-procedural stopping rules for inclusion in the protocol and parental permission document, with regard to: (a) oxygen saturation (e.g., saturation below 90% with supplemental oxygen); (b) apnea; (c) bradycardia; (d) hypotension (with sedative agents); (e) laryngospasm; (f) bleeding, and clarification that the procedure may be stopped sooner than would be the case in a clinically-indicated bronchoscopy; . . .

(9) inclusion in the protocol of a provision for the involvement of a research subject advocate in the enrollment process, to screen for the possibility of vulnerable parents who do not adequately appreciate the voluntariness of trial enrollment (including the right to withdraw at any time) or how the intervention will be experienced by the child; . . .

(11) provision in the protocol for periodic review by an independent safety monitoring committee comprised of experts in CF and bronchoscopy, with a directive regarding stopping rules that would terminate the study depending on the nature and frequency of complications or adverse events; . . .

(15) fuller description in the parental permission document of procedures and risks attendant to, for example, the 2% lidocaine and the medications used for the procedural sedation (e.g., chest wall rigidity with fentanyl infusion), using language that will be understandable to the parents of expected subjects; . . .

(19) removal of any statement in the parental permission document suggesting that the study provides the possibility of direct benefit to the infant subject (for example, any statement that the findings might assist in determining treatment options for a subject should be removed);

(20) provision to the IRB by the PI of an assurance that the PI will initiate and obtain permission only from the parents of potential subjects for whom he does not provide treatment; and, correspondingly, where the PI is the treating physician of a potential subject, he will make arrangements so that a co-PI takes on the responsibility of presenting and obtaining permission in those situations; . . .

Separately, OHRP noted that four of the six expert panelists either called for IRB consideration of compensation or would have required compensation for subjects who are injured as a result of participation in the research; OHRP did not include that issue in its list of required actions.

What do you think of the conditions OHRP attached to the approval of the protocol? Have they rewritten the protocol? If so, is that their proper role? Should IRBs be making this sort of extensive list of changes and corrections for protocols that they would otherwise reject? Should OHRP seek to negotiate protocol revisions with the researchers and/or the IRB, rather than insisting that they be made in order for the study to proceed?

[2] Smallpox Vaccination in Young Children

A MULTICENTER, RANDOMIZED DOSE RESPONSE STUDY OF THE SAFETY, CLINICAL AND IMMUNE RESPONSES OF DRYVAX® ADMINISTERED TO CHILDREN 2 TO 5 YEARS OF AGE
(2002)
http://www.hhs.gov/ohrp/children/dryvax.html

Background: In light of recent terrorist attacks, particularly those involving the transmission of anthrax from contaminated mail, there has been heightened concern over the use of infectious agents as population weapons. The two agents thought by experts to be potentially most dangerous are smallpox (variola) and anthrax. Both are characterized by features which make them ideal weapons of bioterrorism, including: 1) high mortality rate (up to 30% in unvaccinated persons), 2) stability, 3) transmission by aerosol, 4) capability of large-scale production and storage, 5) potential to cause widespread panic, 6) delayed disease recognition, and 7) a requirement for intense utilization of health-care resources.

At the present time, the only two World Health Organization-approved repositories of smallpox virus are located at the Centers for Disease Control and Prevention (CDC) and the Russian State Research Center on Virology and Biotechnology, Koltsovo, Novosibirsk Region. The number of potential covert stockpiles at other sites is unknown. Following the last known naturally occurring human case of smallpox in 1977, it was resolved by the World Health Assembly that all stocks of smallpox virus be destroyed in June 1999. Subsequently, concerns over the potential use of smallpox for biologic warfare were felt to mandate a need for further study of variola virus, and plans for its destruction have been postponed.

Variola virus infects only humans and is transmitted by aerosol. Prior to 1979, smallpox had worldwide distribution and required an intensive public health vaccination effort to eradicate. The incubation period lasts 7-17 days, after which fever, aching pains and prostration develop. Two to three days later a papular rash develops over the face, hands and forearms, extending to the trunk and lower extremities over the next week. The lesions quickly evolve into pustular vesicles, and finally scab and heal, leaving scars. Unlike varicella, the development and resolution of lesions are synchronous. A more malignant rapidly fatal form of the disease, hemorrhagic smallpox, develops in 5%-10%. Smallpox is transmissible from the time of the appearance of rash until all the scabs separate. The secondary attack rate among unvaccinated household contacts is 25-40%.

Vaccination against smallpox is protective if administered before exposure or within 2-3 days thereafter. Following eradication of smallpox, Dryvax production for general use in the U.S. was discontinued in 1982 and general distribution of smallpox vaccine was discontinued in 1983. Few physicians in the United States have actually seen a case of smallpox, so in the event of an outbreak, smallpox may not be diagnosed until late in the course, after secondary transmission has already occurred. A single case of smallpox would be expected to result in 10-20 more cases through aerosol transmission. Although it is estimated that approximately 20% of the adult population has some residual immunity from prior vaccinations, it is not known how protective this immunity would be in an outbreak. In the event of a bioterrorist threat, to prevent further transmission, infected patients would need to be isolated in negative pressure facilities. Although the probability of such an event is low, the effect in a largely unimmunized population would be significant and could result in millions of deaths in the U.S. alone. . . .

Essentially the entire U.S. population is now susceptible to smallpox and the standards for vaccine safety are now much more stringent than they were 30 years ago. . . . None of [certain specified] adverse events has been found in about 740 adult subjects studied in multicentered Dryvax studies sponsored by the NIH. . . .

One way to increase the available number of doses would be to dilute the vaccine; however, the number of dilutions that could be performed without compromising vaccine immunogenicity and effectiveness is unknown for children.

Abstract of Protocol

Purpose: This study is to evaluate the potency, dose, and safety of vaccinia virus vaccine (Dryvax®) administered to children in the event there is a smallpox terrorist event. The objective of this study is to evaluate the safety and the rate of clinical and immune responses with stockpiled Dryvax vaccine when administered to children 2-5 years of age. It will be evaluated undiluted and at a 1:5 dilution, with 5 skin punctures; additionally, the safety of semi-occlusive dressings to limit self-inoculation and secondary transmission will be evaluated. Revaccination of non-responders will help define the value of a second dose. The vaccine take and immune response rate will be compared between pediatric subjects in the two study groups and by comparisons with results from similar trials conducted in adults.

Research Environment: Two NIH Vaccine and Treatment Evaluation Units (VTEU): 1) UCLA Center for Vaccine Research, and 2) Cincinnati Children's Hospital.

Volunteers: A total of 40 volunteers will participate in the study.

Volunteer Participation: The volunteers will be immunized by scarification with Dryvax on day 0. All volunteers will be observed by their parents/legal guardians at their homes and will be excluded from daycare and school for at least 30 days from the date of immunization and until a scab is well formed. At visit days 6-8, if there is no "take," the subject will be re-vaccinated with the same dose and method of administration of Dryvax as for the first vaccination. Each subject's participation will last for at least 6 months. During this time volunteers will return periodically for dressing changes, assessment of any adverse safety events, and for blood draws to check immune responses. A subset of subjects will have immune responses followed for 3 years.

Variables to be Investigated: Adverse events to and side effects of the vaccine, and clinical and immunogenicity responses, including vaccine "take," antibody responses, intracellular cytokine production and IFN-γ responses to the vaccine.

Risks/Benefits: The risks of participating in this study are those known to exist for vaccination with vaccinia vaccine (Dryvax) and those of blood draw. The benefit to the volunteer is potential protection against smallpox disease if the volunteer has a "take." The benefit to society is to determine whether smallpox vaccine can be diluted to provide an increased number of doses in the event of a release of smallpox into the environment, at the same time providing adequate protection in children.

Confidentiality: Volunteers will have unique study identification numbers and will not be identified by name.

DHHS convened a panel of ten experts to review this protocol. The following are excerpts from the experts' statements: (available at http://hhs.gov/ohrp/children/dryvax.html (select links to experts 1, 3, 4, and 5)):

Mary Faith Marshall, Ph.D. commented: The ethical analysis of the study is complicated by the fact that a second generation vaccine is under development. The new vaccine . . . will be safer and can be mass produced quickly. Clinical trials in adults are apparently underway but not complete. Whether there are plans for trials in children is unknown to this reviewer. The issue, then, is the temporal window between completion of the dose response study under consideration and the availability of pediatric clinical trials of the safer vaccine. Placing healthy children at risk of harm for no individual benefit merits serious ethical consideration. Some might argue that it should never be allowed. The rejoinder to that argument is that, in this context at least, children will become research subjects by default in the event of a bioterrorist attack; subjects in less controlled and safe circumstances.

[Marshall then went on to determine that the study is approvable only under section 407.]

The risk of a biological attack with smallpox as a weapon constitutes a serious problem that would affect the health of children in the U.S. One can assess the seriousness of the problem using the criteria that one uses for assessing risk: probability and magnitude. The probability of a bioterrorist attack is unknown but real. Even a remote probability, however, must be balanced by the magnitude of the problem, or harm that would result from it. A 30% mortality rate among those infected constitutes a serious problem. . . .

The investigators have taken great care in selecting their prospective research population. No subjects or classes of subjects are being selected because of easy availability, compromised position, or manipulability. . . . All children in the U.S. (and other countries) stand to benefit from the research in the event of a bioterrorism attack with smallpox as the weapon.

David Stevens, M.D. concluded that the protocol should be approved under § 407 if it were determined that "a credible risk of a smallpox outbreak now exists." He commented:

[T]he data derived from the study would be extremely valuable and reassuring before beginning a mass vaccination program in the setting of a smallpox case.

The research must be conducted in accordance with sound ethical principles and adequate provisions should be made for soliciting the permission of parents and guardians. Issues raised during the two institutional reviews need to be fully addressed (e.g., risk to the child, parental screening, contact risk, liability, reimbursement for medical care, both parents' consent) before the study is begun. Consent must emphasize the risks to children and to contacts of these children. My belief is that the current consent form . . . with phrases like "as with all vaccines" does not fully convey the serious risks of this vaccine to the parents. Dryvax is currently an investigational drug made from a nonsterile bovine product, administered using new techniques and methods (e.g., semi-permeable occlusive dressing) that might enhance vaccine reactogenicity or secondary complications such as superinfections. The risk to the child of serious injury and even death is low but not remote. The risk of spread to others in the family and outside the family is not negligible. For example, the exact procedure for the semi occlusive dressing (e.g. with sterile gauze first) is not clearly defined in the consent or protocol, nor is how changes of the vaccine site dressings are to be discarded by families and staff. These risks must be made very clear to the parents. . . .

Ellen Wright Clayton, M.D., J.D. stated that the study would "probably [be] approvable under § 46.407." She noted that, although the "risk that smallpox will be used as a biological weapon is small," it "is not zero," and "it does not appear that new vaccine will be available in the foreseeable future. Given the limited quantity of vaccine currently available, it is important to determine the most dilute effective dose so that more children can be vaccinated in the event of attack. The critical distinction . . . is that the relevant benefit to meet the requirements of this subpart is to the health of children generally, not to that of a particular child. Being able to save five times as many children would be an important public health outcome. Even the benefits to children generally would not suffice were it not for the facts that even though this vaccine is quite reactogenic, the incidence of serious adverse effects with long term sequelae appears to be quite low and that this protocol makes every effort to minimize these serious risks. It is reassuring that more dilute vaccine is effective in adults."

Robert S. Baltimore, M.D. opined that the protocol was approvable under § 46.405. He argued that it is impossible to quantify the risk of a smallpox bioterrorist attack but that "there are many individuals who perceive the risk as being great enough for them to demand smallpox vaccine or at least to wish to be vaccinated and have their children vaccinated if the vaccine is available. It is these people who will volunteer for this study. The study will attract such people and they will perceive immunization against variola to be valuable. . . . I distinguish the benefits and risks to the participants in this study to be different from mass vaccination of the general population where I believe the risks outweigh the benefits."

NOTES AND QUESTIONS

1. Nine of the ten reviewers found the proposal approvable, with certain conditions, under section 405 or 407 (eight under section 407, two under 405 and one under either section). One commentator declared it was approvable but did not cite a particular section. Seven of the experts concluded that the protocol was not approvable under any of sections 404, 405, or 406, but that it was approvable under section 407. Do you agree with any of these conclusions? How should an IRB take into account imponderables relating to the possibility of a smallpox attack by terrorists? Did the members of this national panel deal appropriately with such issues?

2. After much debate about this protocol, it ultimately was withdrawn. In January 2003, OHRP concluded that "[s]ince initiating this regulatory review process . . . bioterrorism preparedness plans have evolved such that, under current plans, the potential to use diluted Dryvax in children will no longer exist. In the absence of plans to use diluted Dryvax in children, the Secretary, HHS, and the Commissioner, FDA, have determined that there is not justification for this particular clinical investigation to proceed." Letter from OHRP and FDA to Dr. Stewart Laidlaw, Jan. 24, 2003, available at http://www.hhs.gov/ohrp/dpanel/determ.pdf.

§ 13.03 PEDIATRIC RESEARCH IN THE COURTS: THE KENNEDY KRIEGER CASE

The case excerpted below is based primarily on tort and contract law, not the federal research regulations. Nonetheless, it raises fundamental questions about the assumptions underlying the federal regulations, particularly those related to the scope of parental decision-making authority, the obligations of researchers, and the significance of the informed consent form. As you read this opinion by the Maryland Court of Appeals (the highest court in Maryland), compare the Court's approach to existing federal policy on pediatric research. Which approach do you find more appropriate?

GRIMES v. KENNEDY KRIEGER INSTITUTE, INC.
Maryland Court of Appeals, 782 A.2d 807 (2001)

In these present cases, a prestigious research institute, associated with Johns Hopkins University, based on this record, created a nontherapeutic research program whereby it required certain classes of homes to have only partial lead paint abatement modifications performed, and in at least some instances, including at least one of the cases at bar, arranged for the landlords to receive public funding by way of grants or loans to aid in the modifications. The research institute then encouraged, and in at least one of the cases at bar, required, the landlords to rent the premises to families with young children. In the event young children already resided in one of the study houses, it was contemplated that a child would remain in the premises, and the child was encouraged to remain, in order for his or her blood to be periodically analyzed. In other words, the continuing presence of the children that were the subjects of the study was required in order for the study to be complete. Apparently, the children and their parents involved in the cases . . . were from a lower economic strata and were, at least in one case, minorities. . . .

The purpose of the research was to determine how effective varying degrees of lead paint abatement procedures were. Success was to be determined by periodically, over a two-year period of time, measuring the extent to which lead dust remained in, or returned to, the premises after the varying levels of abatement modifications, and, as most important to our decision, by measuring the extent to which the theretofore healthy children's blood became contaminated with lead, and comparing that contamination with levels of lead dust in the houses over the same periods of time. . . .

Apparently, it was anticipated that the children, who were the human subjects in the program, would, or at least might, accumulate lead in their blood from the dust, thus helping the researchers to determine the extent to which the various partial abatement methods worked. There was no complete and clear explanation in the consent agreements signed by the parents of the children that the research to be conducted was designed, at least in significant part, to measure the success of the abatement procedures by measuring the extent to which the children's blood was being contaminated. It can be argued that the researchers intended that the children be the canaries in the mines but never clearly told the parents. (It was a practice in earlier years, and perhaps even now, for subsurface miners to rely on canaries to determine whether dangerous levels of toxic gases were accumulating in the mines. Canaries were particularly susceptible to such gases. When the canaries began to die, the miners knew that dangerous levels of gases were accumulating.) . . .

Otherwise healthy children, in our view, should not be enticed into living in, or remaining in, potentially lead-tainted housing and intentionally subjected to a research program, which contemplates the probability, or even the possibility, of lead poisoning or even the accumulation of lower levels of lead in blood, in order for the extent of the contamination of the children's blood to be used by scientific researchers to assess the success of lead paint or lead dust abatement measures. Moreover, in our view, parents, whether improperly enticed by trinkets, food stamps, money or other items, have no more right to intentionally and unnecessarily place children in potentially hazardous nontherapeutic research surroundings, than do researchers. In such cases, parental consent, no matter how informed, is insufficient.

. . . Nothing about the research was designed for treatment of the subject children. They were presumed to be healthy at the commencement of the project. As to them, the research was clearly nontherapeutic in nature. The experiment was simply a "for the greater good" project.[6] The specific children's health was put at risk, in order to develop low-cost abatement measures that would help all children, the landlords, and the general public as well. . . .

The research project at issue here, and its apparent protocols, differs in large degree from, but presents similar problems as those in the Tuskegee Syphilis Study conducted from 1932 until 1972, the intentional exposure of soldiers to radiation in the 1940s and 50s, the tests involving the exposure of Navajo miners to radiation and the secret administration of LSD to soldiers by the CIA and the Army in the 1950s and 60s. The research experiments that follow were also prior instances of research subjects being intentionally exposed to infectious or poisonous substances in the name of scientific research. They include the

---

[6] The ultimate goal was to find the cost of the minimal level of effective lead paint or lead dust abatement costs so as to help landlords assess, hopefully positively, the commercial feasibility of attempting to abate lead dust in marginally profitable, lower rent-urban housing, in order to help preserve such housing in the Baltimore housing market. One of the aims was to evaluate low-cost methods of abatement so that some landlords would not abandon their rental units. For those landlords, complete abatement was not deemed economically feasible. The project would be able to assess whether a particular level of partial abatement caused a child's blood lead content to be elevated beyond a level deemed hazardous to the health of children.

The tenants involved, presumably, would be from a lower rent-urban class. At least one of the consenting parents in one of these cases was on public assistance, and was described by her counsel as being a minority. The children of middle class or rich parents apparently were not involved.
. . .

Tuskegee Syphilis Study, . . . the Jewish Hospital study, and several other post-war research projects. Then there are the notorious use of "plague bombs" by the Japanese military in World War II where entire villages were infected in order for the results to be "studied"; and perhaps most notorious, the deliberate use of infection in a nontherapeutic project in order to study the degree of infection and the rapidity of the course of the disease in the Rose and Mrugowsky typhus experiments at Buchenwald concentration camp during World War II. . . .

It is clear to this Court that the scientific and medical communities cannot be permitted to assume sole authority to determine ultimately what is right and appropriate in respect to research projects involving young children free of the limitations and consequences of the application of Maryland law. The Institutional Review Boards, IRBs, are, primarily, in-house organs. In our view, they are not designed, generally, to be sufficiently objective in the sense that they are as sufficiently concerned with the ethicality of the experiments they review as they are with the success of the experiments. . . .

I. The Cases

We now discuss more specifically the two cases before us, and the relevant law.

Two separate negligence actions involving children who allegedly developed elevated levels of lead dust in their blood while participating in a research study with respondent, Kennedy Krieger Institute, Inc., (KKI) are before this Court. Both cases allege that the children were poisoned, or at least exposed to the risk of being poisoned, by lead dust due to negligence on the part of KKI. Specifically, they allege that KKI discovered lead hazards in their respective homes and, having a duty to notify them, failed to warn in a timely manner or otherwise act to prevent the children's exposure to the known presence of lead. Additionally, plaintiffs alleged that they were not fully informed of the risks of the research. . . .

II. Facts & Procedural Background

. . . The research study included five test groups, each consisting of twenty-five houses. The first three groups consisted of houses with a considerable amount of lead dust present therein and each group received assigned amounts of maintenance and repair. The fourth group consisted of houses, which at one time had lead present in the form of lead based paint but had since received a supposedly complete abatement of lead dust. The fifth group consisted of modern houses, which had never had a presence of lead dust. The aim of the research study was to analyze the effectiveness of different degrees of partial lead paint abatement in reducing levels of lead dust present in these houses. The ultimate aim of the research was to find a less than complete level of abatement that would be relatively safe, but economical, so that Baltimore landlords with lower socioeconomical rental units would not abandon the units. The research study was specifically designed, in part, to do less than comprehensive lead paint abatement in order to study the potential effectiveness, if any, over a period of time, of lesser levels of repair and maintenance on the presence of lead dust by measuring the presence of lead in the blood of theretofore (as far as the record of the cases reveals) healthy children. . . .

One way the study was designed to measure the effectiveness of such abatement measures was to measure the lead dust levels in the houses at intervals and to compare them with the levels of lead found, at roughly the same intervals, in the blood of the children living in the respective houses. The project required that small children be present in the houses. To facilitate that purpose, the landlords agreeing to permit their properties to be included in the studies were encouraged, if not required, to rent the properties to tenants who had young children.

In return for permitting the properties to be used and in return for limiting their tenants to families with young children, KKI assisted the landlords in applying for and receiving grants or loans of money to be used to perform the levels of abatement required by KKI for each class, of home.

The research study was to be composed of two main components and a total of five groups of study houses. The first component of the study concerned the first three groups of houses. Houses in each group received different amounts of repair and maintenance. The following three groups of houses within the first component of the research study were:

Group 1—Repair & Maintenance—Level I Properties receiving a minimal level of repair and maintenance ($1,650.00).

Group 2—Repair & Maintenance—Level II Properties receiving a greater level of repair and maintenance ($3,500.00).

Group 3—Repair & Maintenance—Level III Properties receiving an even greater level of repair and maintenance ($6,000.00–$7,000.00). . . .

Measurements of lead in the blood of the children and vacuum dust samples from the houses were to be obtained at the following times: pre-intervention, immediately post intervention, and one, three, six, twelve, eighteen, and twenty-four months post intervention. Measurements of lead in the exterior soil were to be obtained at pre-intervention, immediately post intervention, and twelve and twenty-four months post intervention. Measurements of lead in drinking water were to be obtained at pre-intervention, and twelve and twenty-four months post intervention. Additionally, the parents of the child subjects of the study were to fill out a questionnaire at enrollment and at six-month intervals.

The second component of the research study was composed of two control groups:

Group 4—Properties identified as having previously been completely abated of lead paint which were to receive no additional repair and maintenance.

Group 5—Modern Urban Dwellings—Properties constructed after 1980 and presumed not to have lead-based paint which were to receive no repair and maintenance. . . .

If the children were to leave the houses upon the first manifestation of lead dust, it would be difficult, if not impossible, to test, over time, the rate of the level of lead accumulation in the blood of the children attributable to the manifestation. In other words, if the children were removed from the houses before the lead dust levels in their blood became elevated, the tests would probably fail, or at least the data that would establish the success of the test or of the abatement results, would be of questionable use. Thus, it would benefit the accuracy of the test, and thus KKI, the compensated researcher, if children remained in the houses over the period of the study even after the presence of lead dust in the houses became evident.

B. Case No. 128

. . . Nowhere in the consent form [for the study] was it clearly disclosed to the mother that the researchers contemplated that, as a result of the experiment, the child might accumulate lead in her blood, and that in order for the experiment to succeed it was necessary that the child remain in the house as the lead in the child's blood increased or decreased, so that it could be measured. The Consent Form states in relevant part:

> PURPOSE OF STUDY: As you may know, lead poisoning in children is a problem in Baltimore City and other communities across the country. Lead in paint, house dust and outside soil are major sources of lead exposure for children. Children can also be exposed to lead in drinking water and other sources. We understand that your house is going to have special repairs done in order to reduce exposure to lead in paint and dust. On a random basis, homes will receive one of two levels of repair. We are interested in finding out how well the two levels of repair work. The repairs are not intended, or expected, to completely remove exposure to lead.

> We are now doing a study to learn about how well different practices work for reducing exposure to lead in paint and dust. . . . This study is intended to monitor the effects of the repairs and is not intended to replace the medical care your family obtains. . . .

D. The Trial Courts' Findings

[The Court of Appeals here briefly discussed what happened in the trial court. That court had evaluated the pleadings in the context of a motion for a summary judgment. The task before that court was to determine if, assuming all of the alleged facts are true, there could possibly be a case for liability. The trial court dismissed the charges because it determined as a matter of law that there was no contract between the researchers and their subjects, no special duty owed to those subjects, and thus no facts could support a charge of breach of contract or of negligence. The Court of Appeals, in the remainder of the opinion that follows, ends up overruling that decision and sending the case back for a trial on the facts.]

III. Discussion

A. Standard of Review

... The threshold issues before this Court are whether, in the two cases presented, appellee, KKI, was entitled to summary judgment as a matter of law on the basis that no contract existed and that there is inherently no duty owed to a research subject by a researcher. Perhaps even more important is the ancillary issue of whether a parent in Maryland, under the law of this State, can legally consent to placing a child in a nontherapeutic research study that carries with it any risk of harm to the health of the child. . . .

The purpose of the summary judgment procedure is not to try the case or to decide the factual disputes, but to decide whether there is an issue of fact, which is sufficiently material to be tried. . . .

B. General Discussion

Initially, we note that we know of no law, nor have we been directed to any applicable in Maryland courts, that provides that the parties to a scientific study, because it is a scientific, health-related study, cannot be held to have entered into special relationships with the subjects of the study that can create duties, including duties, the breach of which may give rise to negligence claims. . . . We shall hold initially that the very nature of nontherapeutic scientific research on human subjects can, and normally will, create special relationships out of which duties arise. . . .

[In footnote 32 the Court describes a set of experiments at the University of Iowa at what is now the Wendell Johnson Speech and Hearing Center. Orphans were recruited from the local asylum to try to turn them into stutterers in order to learn more about the disorder. Some of the children were turned into stutterers and remained so throughout their lives. The Court concluded that "[i]nappropriate experimentation in this country involving children as subjects is not new."]

C. Negligence

It is important for us to remember that appellants allege that KKI was negligent. Specifically, they allege that KKI, as a medical researcher, owed a duty of care to them, as subjects in the research study, based on the nature of the agreements between them and also based on the nature of the relationship between the parties. They contend specifically that KKI was negligent because KKI breached its duty to: (1) design a study that did not involve placing children at unnecessary risk; (2) inform participants in the study of results in a timely manner; and (3) to completely and accurately inform participants in the research study of all the hazards and risks involved in the study. . . .

IV. The Special Relationships

A. The Consent Agreement

Contract

Both sets of appellants signed a similar Consent Form prepared by KKI in which KKI expressly promised to: (1) financially compensate (however minimally) appellants for their participation in the study; (2) collect lead dust samples from appellants' homes, analyze the samples, discuss the results with appellants, and discuss steps that could be taken, which could reduce exposure to lead; and (3) collect blood samples from children in the household and provide appellants with the results of the blood tests. In return, appellants agreed to participate in the study, by: (1) allowing KKI into appellants' homes to collect dust samples; (2) periodically filling out questionnaires; and (3) allowing the children's blood to be drawn, tested, and utilized in the study. . . .

By having appellants sign this Consent Form, both KKI and appellants expressly made representations, which, in our view, created a bilateral contract between the parties. At the very least, it suggests that appellants were agreeing with KKI to participate in the research study with the expectation that they would be compensated, albeit, more or less, minimally, be informed of all the information necessary for the subject to freely choose whether to participate, and continue to participate, and receive promptly any information that might bear on their willingness to continue to participate in the study. This includes full, detailed, prompt, and continuing warnings as to all the potential risks and hazards inherent in the research or that arise during the research. KKI, in return, was getting the children to move into the houses and/or to remain there over time, and was given the right to test the children's blood for lead. As consideration to KKI, it got access to the houses and to the blood of the children that had been encouraged to live in a "risk" environment. . . .

B. The Sufficiency of the Consent Form

The consent form did not directly inform the parents of the fact that it was contemplated that some of the children might ingest lead dust particles, and that one of the reasons the blood of the children was to be tested was to evaluate how effective the various abatement measures were.

A reasonable parent would expect to be clearly informed that it was at least contemplated that her child would ingest lead dust particles, and that the degree to which lead dust contaminated the child's blood would be used as one of the ways in which the success of the experiment would be measured. The fact that if such information was furnished, it might be difficult to obtain human subjects for the research, does not affect the need to supply the information, or alter the ethics of failing to provide such information. A human subject is entitled to all material information. The respective parent should also have been clearly informed that in order for the measurements to be most helpful, the child needed to stay in the house until the conclusion of the study. Whether assessed by a subjective or an objective standard, the children, or their surrogates, should have been additionally informed that the researchers anticipated that, as a result of the experiment, it was possible that there might be some accumulation of lead in the blood of the children. The "informed" consent was not valid because full material information was not furnished to the subjects or their parents.

C. Special Relationship

. . . As we indicated earlier, the trial courts appear to have held that special relationships out of which duties arise cannot be created by the relationship between researchers and the subjects of the research. While in some rare cases that may be correct, it is not correct when researchers recruit people, especially children whose consent is furnished indirectly, to participate in nontherapeutic procedures that are potentially hazardous, dangerous, or deleterious to their health. . . .

Institutional volunteers may intend to do good or, as history has proven, even to do evil and may do evil or good depending on the institution and the community they serve. Whether an institutional volunteer in a particular community should be granted exceptions from the application of law is a matter that should be scrutinized closely by an appropriate public policy maker. Generally, but not always, the legislative branch is appropriately the best first forum to consider exceptions to the tort laws of this State — even then it should consider all ramifications of the policy — especially considering the general vulnerability of subjects of such studies — in this case, small children. In the absence of the exercise of legislative policymaking, we hold that special relationships, out of which duties arise, the breach of which can constitute negligence can result from the relationships between researcher and research subjects.

D. The Federal Regulations

A duty may be prescribed by a statute, or a special relationship creating duties may arise from the requirement for compliance with statutory provisions. Although there is no duty of which we are aware prescribed by the Maryland Code in respect to scientific research of the nature here present, federal regulations have been enacted that impose standards of care that attach to federally funded or sponsored research projects that use human subjects. . . .

Clearly, KKI, as a research institution, is required to obtain a human participant's fully informed consent, using sound ethical principles. It is clear from the wording of the applicable federal regulations that this requirement of informed consent continues during the duration of the research study and applies to new or changing risks. In this case, a special relationship out of which duties might arise might be created by reason of the federally imposed regulations. The question becomes whether this duty of informed consent created by federal regulation, as a matter of state law, translates into a duty of care arising out of the unique relationship that is researcher-subject, as opposed to doctor-patient. We answer that question in the affirmative. . . .

V. The Ethical Appropriateness of the Research

[After citing to the Nuremberg Code and the Declaration of Helsinki:]

The determination of whether a duty exists under Maryland law is the ultimate function of various policy considerations as adopted by either the Legislature, or, if it has not spoken, as it has not in respect to this situation, by Maryland courts. In our view, otherwise healthy children should not be the subjects of nontherapeutic experimentation or research that has the potential to be harmful to the child. It is, first and foremost, the responsibility of the researcher and the research entity to see to the harmlessness of such nontherapeutic research. Consent of parents can never relieve the researcher of this duty. We do not feel that it serves proper public policy concerns to permit children to be placed in situations of potential harm, during nontherapeutic procedures, even if parents, or other surrogates, consent. Under these types of circumstances, even where consent is given, albeit inappropriately, policy considerations suggest that there remains a special relationship between researchers and participants to the research study, which imposes a duty of care. This is entirely consistent with the principles found in the Nuremberg Code.

Researchers cannot ever be permitted to completely immunize themselves by reliance on consents, especially when the information furnished to the subject, or the party consenting, is incomplete in a material respect. A researcher's duty is not created by, or extinguished by, the consent of a research subject or by IRB approval. The duty to a vulnerable research subject is independent of consent, although the obtaining of consent is one of the duties a researcher must perform. All of this is especially so when the subjects of research are children. . . .

This duty requires the protection of the research subjects from unreasonable harm and requires the researcher to completely and promptly inform the subjects of potential hazards existing from time to time because of the profound trust that participants place in investigators, institutions, and the research enterprise as a whole to protect them from harm. . . .

The study, by its design, placed and/or retained children in areas where they might come into contact with elevated levels of lead dust. Clearly, KKI contemplated that at least some of the children would develop elevated blood lead levels while participating in the study. . . .

While we acknowledge that foreseeability does not necessarily create a duty, we recognize that potential harm to the children participants of this study was both foreseeable and potentially extreme. A "special relationship" also exists in circumstances where such experiments are conducted.

VI. Parental Consent for Children to Be Subjects of Potentially Hazardous Non-therapeutic Research

The issue of whether a parent can consent to the participation of her or his child in a nontherapeutic health-related study that is known to be potentially hazardous to the health of the child raises serious questions with profound moral and ethical implications. What right does a parent have to knowingly expose a child not in need of therapy to health risks or otherwise knowingly place a child in danger, even if it can be argued it is for the greater good? The issue in these specific contested cases does not relate primarily to the authority of the parent, but to the procedures of KKI and similar entities that may be involved in such health-related studies. The issue of the parents' right to consent on behalf of the children has not been fully presented in either of these cases, but should be of concern not only to lawyers and judges, but to moralists, ethicists, and others. The consenting parents in the contested cases at bar were not the subjects of the experiment; the children were. Additionally, this practice presents the potential problems of children initiating actions in their own names upon reaching majority, if indeed, they have been damaged as a result of being used as guinea pigs in nontherapeutic scientific research. Children, it should be noted, are not in our society the equivalent of rats, hamsters, monkeys, and the like. Because of the overriding importance of this matter and this Court's interest in the welfare of children — we shall address the issue. . . .

It is not in the best interest of a specific child, in a nontherapeutic research project, to be placed in a research environment, which might possibly be, or which proves to be, hazardous to the health of the child. We have long stressed that the "best interests of the child" is the overriding concern of this Court in matters relating to children. Whatever the interests of a parent, and whatever the interests of the general public in fostering research that might, according to a researcher's hypothesis, be for the good of all children, this Court's concern for the particular child and particular case, over-arches all other interests. It is, simply, and we hope, succinctly put, not in the best interest of any healthy child to be intentionally put in a nontherapeutic situation where his or her health may be impaired, in order to test methods that may ultimately benefit all children.

To think otherwise, to turn over human and legal ethical concerns solely to the scientific community, is to risk embarking on slippery slopes, that all too often in the past, here and elsewhere, have resulted in practices we, or any community, should be ever unwilling to accept.

We have little doubt that the general motives of all concerned in these contested cases were, for the most part, proper, albeit in our view not well thought out. The protocols of the research, those of which we have been made aware, were, in any event, unacceptable in a legal context. One simply does not expose otherwise healthy children, incapable of personal assent (consent), to a nontherapeutic research environment that is known at the inception of the research, might cause the children to ingest lead dust. . . .

VII. Conclusion

We hold that in Maryland a parent, appropriate relative, or other applicable surrogate, cannot consent to the participation of a child or other person under legal disability in nontherapeutic research or studies in which there is any risk of injury or damage to the health of the subject.

We hold that informed consent agreements in nontherapeutic research projects, under certain circumstances can constitute contracts; and that, under certain circumstances, such research agreements can, as a matter of law, constitute "special relationships" giving rise to duties, out of the breach of which negligence actions may arise. We also hold that, normally, such special relationships are created between researchers and the human subjects used by the researchers. Additionally, we hold that governmental regulations can create duties on the part of researchers towards human subjects out of which "special relationships" can arise. Likewise, such duties and relationships are consistent with the provisions of the Nuremberg Code.

The determination as to whether a "special relationship" actually exists is to be done on a case by case basis. . . . Accordingly, we vacate the rulings of the Circuit Court for Baltimore City and remand these cases to that court for further proceedings consistent with this opinion.

CONCUR: Raker, J., concurring in result only:

I concur in the Court's judgment because I find that appellants have alleged sufficient facts to establish that there existed a special relationship between the parties in these cases, which created a duty of care that, if breached, gives rise to an action in negligence. . . . I agree with the majority that this duty includes the protection of research subjects from unreasonable harm and requires the researcher to inform research subjects completely and promptly of potential hazards resulting from participation in the study. As a result of the existence of this tort duty, I find it unnecessary to reach the thorny question, not even raised by any of the parties, of whether the informed consent agreements in these cases constitute legally binding contracts. . . .

I cannot join in the majority's sweeping factual determinations that the risks associated with exposing children to lead-based paint were foreseeable and well known to appellees and that appellees contemplated lead contamination in participants' blood; that the children's health was put at risk; that there was no complete and clear explanation in the consent agreements that . . . a certain level of lead accumulation was anticipated; . . . that the consent form was insufficient because it lacked certain specific warnings; . . . that the Institutional Review Board involved in these cases abdicated its responsibility to protect the safety of the research subjects by misconstruing the difference between therapeutic and nontherapeutic research and aiding researchers in circumventing federal regulations; that Institutional Review Boards are not sufficiently objective to regulate the ethics of experimental research; that it is never in the best interest of any child to be placed in a nontherapeutic research study that might be hazardous to the child's health; that there was no therapeutic value in the research for the child subjects involved; that the research did not comply with applicable regulations; or that there was more than a minimal risk involved in this study. I do not here condone the conduct of appellee, and it may well be that the majority's conclusions are warranted by the facts of these cases, but the record before us is limited. Indeed, the majority recognizes that the record is "sparse." The critical point is that these are questions for the jury on remand and are not properly before this Court at this time.

. . . I cannot join the majority in holding that, in Maryland, a parent or guardian cannot consent to the participation of a minor child in a nontherapeutic research study in which there is *any* risk of injury or damage to the health of the child without prior judicial approval and oversight. Nor can I join in the majority's holding that the research conducted in these cases was *per se* inappropriate, unethical, and illegal. Such sweeping holdings are far beyond the question presented in these appeals, and their resolution by the Court, at this time, is inappropriate. I also do not join in what I perceive as the majority's wholesale adoption of the Nuremberg Code into Maryland state tort law. Finally, I do not join in the majority's comparisons between the research at issue in this case and extreme historical abuses, such as those of the Nazis or the Tuskegee Syphilis Study.

ON MOTION FOR RECONSIDERATION

Much of the argument in support of and in opposition to the motion for reconsideration centered on the question of what limitations should govern a parent's authority to provide informed consent for the participation of his or her minor child in a medical study. In the Opinion, we said at one point that a parent "cannot consent to the participation of a child . . . in nontherapeutic research or studies in which there is any risk of injury or damage to the health of the subject." As we think is clear from Section VI of the Opinion, by "any risk," we meant any articulable risk beyond the minimal kind of risk that is inherent in any endeavor. The context of the statement was a non-therapeutic study that promises no medical benefit to the child whatever, so that any balance between risk and benefit is necessarily negative. As we indicated, the determination of whether the study in question offered some benefit, and therefore could be regarded as therapeutic in nature, or involved more than that minimal risk is open for further factual development on remand.

NOTES AND QUESTIONS

1. How would you characterize the tone of the court's opinion? Dispassionate? Concerned? Outraged? What do you think accounts for this tone? Was it justified under the circumstances?

2. Were the children already living in the homes before the study began exposed to any *additional* risks of lead poisoning as a result of the researchers' actions? What about the children who moved into the homes that the researchers had asked the landlords to rent to families with young children? Is it fair to say that children in this latter group were put at risk by the research?

Does the answer depend on what other housing options would have been available to their families at the time? At one point, the court states that "parents . . . have no more right to intentionally and unnecessarily place children in potentially hazardous nontherapuetic research surroundings, than do researchers." What, exactly, did the parents do that placed their children in "potentially hazardous nontherapeutic research surroundings"? Was it their initial decision to move into homes containing lead paint? Or their decision to allow the researchers to remove some of the lead paint and monitor the children's blood levels?

3. Assuming that the federal regulations applied to this study, under which of the risk categories in Subpart D (if any) would this study be approvable? For the children already living in the homes when the study began, would it be appropriate to analyze the study under 45 C.F.R. § 46.405, on the ground that the researchers' efforts to reduce the level of lead in the children's homes offered a prospect of direct benefit to the children? For the children not already living in the homes, would section 406 be applicable, on the theory that the study involved a "minor increase over minimal risk" and that it was "likely to yield generalizable knowledge about the subject's disorder or condition"? *See* Loretta M. Kopelman, *Pediatric Research Regulations Under Legal Scrutiny: Grimes Narrows Their Interpretation*, 30 J.L. MED. & ETHICS 38, 44 (2002) (noting that it would be possible to claim that "[a]ll the children in the lead abatement study . . . [had] a disorder or condition because they either had elevated blood levels of lead or were at risk of having elevated blood-lead levels, given the communities in which they lived," but ultimately rejecting that argument).

4. After *Grimes*, can a researcher in Maryland who is subject to the Common Rule conduct a pediatric study involving more than minimal risk if the study is approvable under 45 C.F.R. § 46.406?

5. At the very beginning of its opinion the court notes that the researchers "required certain classes of homes to have only partial lead paint abatement modifications performed." That wording might be read as suggesting that the researchers *prevented* more extensive lead abatement modifications from taking place. Did the researchers in fact do that? Here is how the Kennedy Krieger Institute describes what happened:

> The Study was designed so that every participating family in [the study] would have the opportunity to live in safer housing than 95% of the non-lead abated housing stock in Baltimore City — and safer than required by then-federal, state or local law. At that time, there were no legal requirements for lead paint hazard intervention or prevention. [The three groups of homes in the study that contained lead paint hazards] all received lead safety interventions designed to reduce lead paint and dust exposure. . . . From KKI's earlier research, KKI knew that all three tiers of intervention reduced lead dust by approximately 80% from that found in untreated properties, that is, the overwhelming

majority of affordable rental stock housing then available in Baltimore's low-income, high-risk neighborhoods.

Lead-Based Paint Study Fact Sheet, available at http://www.hopkinsmedicine.org/press/ 2001/SEPTEMBER/leadfactsheet.htm. Based on these two conflicting descriptions, can you come up with a fair reading of what was really taking place with regard to the lead abatement measures used in these homes?

6. The court concludes that the researchers "enticed families with young children to enter the study." The Benefits section of the consent form stated that the families would receive, in addition to the free blood testing of the children, a $5 payment at the start of the study for answering questions, and a $15 payment twice a year for the time required to complete a questionnaire. Should these payments be viewed as "enticements" to enter the study? Are there other aspects of the study that might be considered "enticements"?

7. Do you think the court would have reached a different conclusion if this study had been conducted only on families already living in homes that had lead contamination? What would your view be about the legitimacy of such a study?

8. The court notes that the researchers "did not rescue the children who were in danger." What specific circumstances is it referring to? A child whose blood levels of lead are rising, but are still below the levels at which any medical treatment is generally required? If a child's blood tests showed a lead level that would generally require medical treatment, do you think the researchers would have told the parents about this result?

9. Note that it is possible to take the position that the risks of the study may have been reasonable, at least for some of the children, but that the study was nonetheless flawed for other reasons — such as the inadequacy of the informed consent process, or the failure to warn the parents of the children's elevated lead levels. Would such an approach have been more appropriate?

10. The trial court had dismissed the case on the ground that the researchers did not have a "special relationship" with the children, and therefore had no duty to warn a parent when test results indicated that a child had an elevated lead level. The Maryland Court of Appeals was very clear in its holding that a special relationship can exist between researchers and subjects in nontherapeutic research, but it did not actually determine that such a relationship existed in this case. Instead, it directed the trial court to resolve that issue when it rehears the case. What factors did the Court of Appeals consider relevant to determining whether a special relationship exists? Is it likely that the trial court, when it revisits the issue, will find that a special relationship existed in this case?

11. What are the implications of characterizing the relationship between the researchers and the children as a "special relationship"? Does it mean that the researchers had a duty to warn the parents of *any* risks to the children that the researchers happened to discover? For example, if a researcher happened to notice that one of the children had symptoms of untreated asthma or dia-

betes, would she have been under a legal duty to warn the child's parents? Diane Hoffmann and Karen Rothenberg argue that the court was not at all clear about the scope of the researchers' duty to warn:

> The Court's phrasing of the duty in the question presented as a "duty to warn [research subjects] regarding dangers present when the researcher has knowledge of the potential for harm to the subject and the subject is unaware of the danger," appears unique in its apparent inclusion of situations where the duty is not based on risks that have arisen as a result of participation in the research. As written, the statement seems to include preexisting risks to the individual subject, which the researcher discovers, that are not caused by participation in the research study. Rather, the risks become known by the researcher during the course of the investigation and may not be known by the subject. In fact, the Court stated that a study in which subjects will interact with "already existing, or potentially existing hazardous conditions" is one in which special relationships would normally be created.
>
> Imposing a "duty to warn" raises questions as to what the researchers should have told the subjects at the start of the study as well as whether the researchers had a duty to inform the subjects much earlier than they did of the results of the dust sample tests. A broad interpretation of such a duty would mean that the researchers: 1) had a duty to warn of risks not necessarily created by the study; and 2) had an obligation to inform subjects of the dust and blood sample test results as soon as possible so that subjects could act on the knowledge conveyed, similar to the obligation that would be imposed on a physician reporting clinical test results to a patient. If this broader duty is what the court had in mind, the case breaks new ground by imposing an obligation on researchers that has not clearly been established elsewhere.

Diane E. Hoffmann & Karen H. Rothenberg, *Whose Duty Is It Anyway? The Kennedy Krieger Opinion and Its Implications for Public Health Research,* 6 J. HEALTH CARE L. & POL'Y 109 (2002).

12. Toward the end of their article, Hoffmann and Rothman speculate about the implications of the decision for other types of research:

> Consider, for example, research on malnutrition. Could a researcher study a population that exposes its children to a diet without certain nutrients or would the researcher be required to tell the subjects of the risks of such a diet and urge them to change their diet or see their physician? If families agreed to be part of the study, when the researchers found, each day, that the child's diet was deficient in essential nutrients, would they be required to tell the family immediately? If they did not tell the family, but later the child was found to have organ damage as a result of their diet, could the parents successfully sue the researchers for failure to tell them of their observational findings that

the child's diet each day had been deficient in these essential nutrients? If the researchers had noted some harmful effects on the health of the children, would they have a duty to tell the parents and urge them to take the children to their family doctor? If the parents did not take the children to the doctor would the researchers have any obligation to report the parents for child neglect?

Alternatively, consider research on the effects of second-hand smoke on children living in housing with parents who smoke. Should it be the obligation of the researchers to inform the parents at the start of the research of the risks to children of second-hand smoke? Should they be required to tell them every time they find a level of smoke in the air that might be hazardous? If the parents do not change their smoking habits, should the researchers be required to report them for child abuse or neglect?

Id. How do you think the *Grimes* court would analyze these scenarios? And what is your view? Should researchers be under a duty to inform the parents about the second-hand smoke risks? What if the study involved following young pregnant women who were heavy smokers: should there at least be a duty to let the women know, as part of the consent process, that smoking can cause serious and permanent harm to a fetus?

13. Hoffmann and Rothenberg note that the duty to warn created by the *Grimes* court does not exist between two people who are not in a special relationship. However, the relationship between a researcher and a subject certainly is special, and, as noted in Chapter 7, researchers have a very high duty of disclosure to subjects, one greater than that imposed on doctors dealing with their patients. Given that, is the *Grimes* court's analysis of the duty to warn as unusual as these commentators suggest? Consider how Hoffmann and Rothenberg's analysis might apply to a modern version of what happened in the Tuskegee study. Imagine that over the course of many years, researchers study the effects of an untreatable disease on a group of poor, African-American men. They make it clear to the subjects that the purpose of the research is not to treat them, but merely to study their health. If during the course of the study, the researchers learned of a treatment for the disease, one that the subjects were not aware of, should they be under a duty to inform the subjects about that new development? How controversial do you think such a duty would be?

14. The majority opinion concludes that the consent form did not "clearly inform" a mother "that it was at least contemplated that her child would ingest lead dust particles." Based on the excerpt from the consent form that appears on page 571, what is your opinion on this issue?

15. The authority of parents to enroll their children in medical research also was at issue in another state court decision, *T.D. v. New York State Office of Mental Health*. In that decision, favorably quoted by the *Grimes* court (in portions of the opinion not reprinted here), a New York appellate court determined

that parents do not have a right to enroll their children in nontherapeutic research studies that involve greater than minimal risk. The court's decision was based on New York and federal constitutional law. That case is excerpted and discussed in greater detail in Chapter 14, at page 621.

Chapter 14

ADULTS WHO LACK DECISION-MAKING CAPACITY

According to the Nuremberg Code, "the voluntary consent of the human subject is absolutely essential." NUREMBERG CODE § 1; *see* Appendix D. A literal application of this provision would preclude any research with individuals who lack the mental capacity to provide informed consent — for example, comatose patients, or persons with mental illnesses that undermine the ability to make meaningful decisions. Such a policy, however, would make it difficult to develop treatments for individuals affected with these conditions. In addition, excluding these individuals from research would deny them the benefits that participating in research sometimes entails.

At the same time, allowing researchers to enroll subjects who lack decision-making capacity raises a host of challenging problems. While some of these problems also arise in pediatric research — another area in which it often is impossible to satisfy the Nuremberg Code's insistence on voluntary consent — society is generally comfortable giving parents the authority to make decisions for their children, at least within limits. With adults who lack decision-making capacity, by contrast, it is uncertain who, if anyone, should be given the authority to make decisions on the individual's behalf. Moreover, it is far from clear that the parent-child relationship is an appropriate framework for devising policies governing adults who lack decision-making capacity. Unlike parents, who have a constitutionally protected interest in making medical decisions for their children, *see, e.g., Parham v. J.R.*, 442 U.S. 584 (1979), family members or guardians cannot claim any "right" to consent to risks on an incapacitated adult's behalf.

Given the ethical complexities of research with adults who lack decision-making capacity, one might think that the federal regulations would contain provisions specifically addressed to this type of research. In fact, however, the regulations contain no such provisions. The lack of regulatory guidance does not mean that research with adults who lack decision-making capacity is not being conducted. On the contrary, the amount of such research has grown exponentially in recent years. Yet much of this research is being conducted without any clear legal authority.

As you read these materials, consider whether researchers should be permitted to conduct research with adults who lack decision-making capacity, particularly research in which the subjects are not expected to receive any direct benefits. If you could develop regulatory standards to guide such research, what would those standards provide? In the absence of federal regulations, what can researchers, IRBs, and others do to ensure that the rights and interests of incapacitated adults are sufficiently protected?

§ 14.01 THE APPROPRIATENESS OF CONDUCTING RESEARCH WITH ADULTS WHO LACK DECISION-MAKING CAPACITY

In the following excerpt, the National Commission for the Protection of Human Subjects of Biomedical and Behavioral Research addresses the problem of research with "those institutionalized as mentally infirm." This report — the only piece of the Commission's work that was never incorporated into the federal regulations — draws on the ethical framework the Commission first articulated in its influential *Belmont Report. See* Appendix F.

REPORT AND RECOMMENDATIONS: RESEARCH INVOLVING THOSE INSTITUTIONALIZED AS MENTALLY INFIRM
NATIONAL COMMISSION FOR THE PROTECTION OF HUMAN SUBJECTS OF BIOMEDICAL AND BEHAVIORAL RESEARCH
(1978)

Beneficence

. . . [T]he principle of beneficence requires that subjects be protected from harm and that there be positive benefits from the research. This means that the possible good to be produced must justify the risk of harm to the subjects. Thus, beneficence requires a careful comparative analysis of possible harms to individual subjects and possible benefits either to the subjects or to others.

This application of risk/benefit analysis to the involvement of those institutionalized as mentally infirm raises no substantial controversy if applied exclusively to research involving interventions from which the subjects may derive direct benefit. The major controversies arise over the involvement of persons for whom the research holds out no immediate prospect of direct benefit.

Robert Veatch and H. Tristram Engelhardt, Jr., both argue that because of certain minimal duties each of us owes to society, we may reasonably be expected to bear minor risks for the general welfare of all. Richard McCormick also emphasizes the duty to benefit others as the specific justification for research with subjects incapable of consent.

Furthermore, since some research involving the mentally infirm cannot be undertaken with any other group, and since this research may yield significant knowledge about the causes and treatment of mental disabilities, it is necessary to consider the consequences of prohibiting such research. Some argue that prohibiting such research might harm the class of mentally infirm persons as a whole by depriving them of benefits they could have received if the research had proceeded. Moreover, it is sometimes unclear whether the subjects of a particular research project will derive some indirect or future benefit from their participation.

The ethical principle of beneficence thus provides several justifications for the general involvement of those institutionalized as mentally infirm in research; however, most who acknowledge the importance of the principle of beneficence are also careful to set limits to what it may justify. David Hume remarked, for example, that one is not obliged to do a small good to society at the expense of a great harm to oneself. . . .

Justice

Questions of justice relevant to the selection of subjects of research occur at two levels — the levels of social justice and individual justice. Social justice demands a consideration of which classes of subjects ought and ought not to participate in research. Specific questions of social justice are: whether there should be an order of preferability in the selection of classes of subjects (e.g., adults before children, the competent before the incompetent), and whether those institutionalized as mentally infirm should be research subjects, and, if so, under what conditions they may be involved. Answers to these questions of social justice require a theory about how to distribute benefits and burdens to various social classes.

Individual justice demands a consideration of which individuals ought and ought not to participate in research. Thus, individual justice requires that after it has been determined that a particular class of subjects such as children or those institutionalized as mentally infirm may legitimately participate in research, it must be determined which specific members of the class may participate. Answers to the questions of individual justice require a theory about how to distribute benefits and burdens to particular individuals. Thus in addition to a theory of social distributive justice, a theory of individual distributive justice is necessary.

Problems of social and individual justice are brought into sharp focus by the Willowbrook studies. [For discussion of the Willowbrook studies, see Chapter 1, at page 39.] The first question, one of social justice, is whether research on an infectious disease should involve those institutionalized as mentally infirm. The American Bar Association (ABA) Commission on the Mentally Disabled has recommended that:

> The proposed research should relate directly to the etiology, pathogenesis, prevention, diagnosis or treatment of mental disability, and should seek only such information as cannot be obtained from other types of subjects.

The ABA Commission further concluded that involving institutionalized persons in research on the causes or treatment of infections such as hepatitis, which can be contracted by anyone, cannot be justified merely on the ground that such infections are widespread in some institutions. It said: "There is no acceptable reason why such research cannot be conducted with [noninstitutionalized] subjects who are free and fully informed." Although the ABA Commission does not attempt to justify its position on philosophical grounds, one could argue that the principle of justice, in a strict interpretation, requires that risks and burdens be distributed equally, so that no class of persons is unjustly required to bear an unequal distribution of burdens. If there are two classes of subjects, one of which is already severely burdened and the other of which is much less burdened, then in order to equalize the distribution of burdens, the latter class ought to accept any additional risks. Because those institutionalized as mentally infirm are already burdened by their disabilities, other less burdened classes of persons should accept the risks of research.

On the other hand, some theories would not prohibit participation of those institutionalized as mentally infirm in such research. One argument based on the considerations advanced by Engelhardt, Veatch and McCormick is the following: All persons insofar as they are members of a social community, have a duty to help others in that community. As an expression of common humanity, every person ought to benefit others and ought to be benefited by others. Because these reciprocal duties of beneficence apply to all persons, an enhancement of benefits for society as a whole will result. Thus, persons who are mentally infirm share to an equal degree with other persons this duty of beneficence; and it might even be argued that it would be a violation of their right to pursue their moral obligations if this class of individuals were categorically excluded from such participation. Research entailing only minimal risk could, according to this theory, legitimately involve those institutionalized as mentally infirm even if other subjects were available — so long as there was equal involvement.

Assuming for the moment that an acceptable theory of social justice would justify at least limited involvement of those institutionalized as mentally infirm in research, it would then be necessary to determine those criteria that are relevant to selecting individual subjects. With respect to a specific research project, it might be asked whether certain persons institutionalized as mentally infirm, perhaps because of the nature of their infirmity, are more likely to be harmed by participating in the research than other individuals. It might also be the case that some persons who are mentally infirm have already participated in research and so should not be asked to participate again. If all persons have a duty of beneficence to help others, then it is morally relevant to know which individuals may have already fulfilled this duty.

1 RESEARCH INVOLVING PERSONS WITH MENTAL DISORDERS THAT MAY AFFECT DECISIONMAKING CAPACITY: REPORT AND RECOMMENDATIONS 18
NATIONAL BIOETHICS ADVISORY COMMISSION
(1998)

Plainly, . . . the capacity of the human subject to participate in th[e] process of informed decision making is a critical component, though not the total corpus, of the present system of public oversight of biomedical and behavioral research. Under a strict "protection model" those who lack the capacity to give informed consent, or whose capacity to do so is uncertain, may be excluded from participation as research subjects. Under the strict protection model such exclusion may seem appropriate since the underlying principle is that it is better to protect subjects from risks of harm, even at the cost of slowing the progress of scientific investigation, the development of new medical advances, and access to potentially beneficial but unproven therapies. In this model there would correspondingly be fewer opportunities to assess promising new clinical approaches to the diseases from which these potential subjects suffer. The obvious dilemma presented by such a strict protection standard is that research leading to therapies for those disorders would be slowed as a consequence of the limited capacity of those who suffer from such disorders to consent to participate in such research.

Conversely, under the "access model" a total barrier to research for persons with mental disorders is suspect precisely because it would prevent some people from obtaining the potential benefits that such research might offer them, either directly as a result of participating in the research or indirectly as a result of the improved understanding of their illness and of methods for treating it that may result from the research in question.

NOTES AND QUESTIONS

1. The National Commission's analysis was limited to individuals "institutionalized as mentally infirm." For two reasons, many prospective research subjects who lack decision-making capacity do not fall within this group. First, while individuals with psychiatric disorders were commonly institutionalized at the time the National Commission issued its report, involuntary institutionalization is now relatively rare. Second, psychiatric illness is not the only reason individuals may lose decision-making capacity:

> Empirical studies suggest that impaired decision-making capacity may be less common among psychiatric patients (it is estimated to be present in about 52 percent of hospitalized patients with schizophrenia) and more common among those with serious medical illnesses (about 12 percent) than previously believed. For example, a survey of patients with medical disorders found that 6 percent of those who believed they

had never participated in medical research had actually done so, and 7 percent of those who had participated in research did not understand that they had the right to withdraw from it.

Robert Michels, *Are Research Ethics Bad for Our Mental Health?* 340 NEW ENG. J. MED. 1427 (1999). Does the National Commission's analysis apply with equal force to mentally ill individuals who are not institutionalized? To individuals who lack decision-making capacity for reasons unrelated to mental illness?

2. The concept of beneficence plays an important role in the National Commission's analysis. Beneficence is a difficult concept to apply because it incorporates two often contradictory notions — the avoidance of harm and the provision of benefits. If a study offers a potential benefit to incapacitated subjects but also entails a certain amount of risk, can conducting the study be justified under the principle of beneficence? How should one decide whether it is appropriate to seek certain benefits despite the existence of risk? Does the National Commission adequately address this question?

3. As the National Commission notes, prohibiting the use of individuals who lack decision-making capacity in studies that do not offer a prospect of direct benefit to the subjects "might harm the class of mentally infirm persons as a whole by depriving them of benefits they could have received if the research had proceeded." Is this "class interest" argument a sufficient basis for enrolling decisionally impaired individuals in risky studies that will not benefit those individuals directly? Does the fact that these individuals probably have benefited from risks assumed by members of the "class" in previous generations create an obligation to assume comparable risks for the potential benefit of class members in the future?

4. The National Commission suggests that a policy preferring the use of noninstitutionalized individuals as research subjects whenever possible could be considered "a violation of [institutionalized patients'] right to pursue their moral obligations." Do you believe that individuals have a "right" to pursue their "moral obligations"? If so, does the existence of such a right provide a basis for enrolling mentally disabled individuals in research that does not hold out any prospect of direct benefit to the subjects?

5. What is at stake for society in the choice between the "strict protection" and "access" models described in the NBAC excerpt? What might incapacitated adults gain or lose by the choice between these two approaches? Who should decide which model is preferable — legislators, regulators, individual IRBs, or prospective subjects and their families? If you believe that the views of prospective subjects should be incorporated into the analysis, how can that be done? Would it be appropriate to require IRBs that regularly review protocols involving subjects with mental illnesses to include individuals who have such illnesses, and/or their family members? *See* NATIONAL ALLIANCE FOR THE MENTALLY ILL, POLICIES ON STRENGTHENED STANDARDS FOR PROTECTION OF INDIVIDUALS WITH SEVERE MENTAL ILLNESSES WHO PARTICIPATE AS HUMAN SUBJECTS IN RESEARCH (1995) (recommending such a policy).

§ 14.02 DETERMINING WHETHER SUBJECTS LACK DECISION-MAKING CAPACITY

[A] Defining Decision-Making Capacity

Assessing Decision-Making Capacity
Bernard Lo
18 L. Med. & Health Care 193 (1990)

Like the courts, philosophers have suggested that it usually makes more sense to speak of capacity to make specific decisions about medical care than capacity in some general or global sense. Therefore decision-making capacity should be assessed by directly testing the patient's ability to make a particular decision. The generally accepted standard is that the patient should have the ability to give informed consent (or refusal) to the proposed test or treatment. More specifically, a series of abilities is required:

(1) The patient appreciates that she has a choice. That is, the patient must realize that she has decision-making power, not the physician or family members.

(2) The patient appreciates the medical situation and prognosis, the nature of the recommended care, the alternatives, the risks and benefits of each, and the likely consequences.

(3) The patient's decision should be stable over time and consistent with her values and goals.

. . . Concerned that patients might be regarded as incapacitated merely because they make idiosyncratic decisions, some philosophers have recommended that assessments of decision-making capacity look only at the process by which the patient makes decisions, not at the content of the decision itself. . . . [M]any writers suggest a sliding scale for assessing decision-making capacity. The greater the risk posed by the patient's decision, the more exacting should be the standard of capacity that is applied.

Legal Judgments and Informed Consent
in Geriatric Research
Nancy Dubler
35 J. Am. Geriatrics Soc'y 545 (1987)

A decision concerning capacity contains elements relating to individual ability in the context of the specific risks and benefits of research. By extension, a patient could be somewhat demented and still understand the fact that the suggested intervention is research (and will not, or may not, provide a therapeutic benefit); the nature and consequence of the particular participation; and the fact that he or she may refuse, without jeopardizing the care and concern of health care providers.

If these three elements exist, the legal presumption of competence could remain in effect. The inclusion in research protocols of persons who can understand these elements may be acceptable depending on the complexity and risk of the protocol.

Capacity to consent involves the interaction of individual ability, in the context of the risks and benefits of a protocol in a specific site. The setting of research can thus affect this complex balance of factors; the more controlling and confining the setting, the more individual ability could arguably be required to avoid duress and coercion. Elderly mobile persons living in the community, if vigorous and independent, can accept or refuse with their feet. Elderly persons in institutional settings may have their abilities affected by needs for attention, fear of rejection, and what has been labeled as "learned helplessness." The setting weighs heavily in the individual balancing of the risks and benefits of any protocol.

1 RESEARCH INVOLVING PERSONS WITH MENTAL DISORDERS THAT MAY AFFECT DECISIONMAKING CAPACITY: REPORT AND RECOMMENDATIONS 18-21
NATIONAL BIOETHICS ADVISORY COMMISSION
(1998)

The use of the term "impaired decisionmaking capacity" implies a condition that varies from statistical or species-typical normalcy, especially in the context of discussions about the ethics of human subjects research. In this sense, for example, normal immaturity should not be regarded as a decisional "impairment" since the very young cannot be expected to have achieved the normative level of decisionmaking capacity. Conversely, normal aging need not involve impaired decision making, and assuming such an impairment is inappropriate. (Throughout this report the term "capacity" is used rather than the term "competence" — although the two are often used interchangeably — because the latter often refers to a legal determination made by a court, and the former refers to a clinical judgment.) Therefore, "decisional impairment" refers to a limitation or an incapacity that is not part of normal growth and development. For example, senile dementia and schizophrenia are conditions that deviate from regular developmental patterns (e.g., dementia is not part of the normal aging process) and are not captured under regulatory categories intended to address periods in the life cycle (e.g., fetuses and children) or certain defined groups (e.g., pregnant women or prisoners).

In practice, it is not usually difficult to determine whether a person lacks all ability to make decisions, so findings of incapacity in this global sense are not often subject to much disagreement. Much more challenging (and the subject of numerous "hard cases" in the law) is determining whether someone with limited decisional capacity has sufficient capacity to make a particular choice, thereby demonstrating a level of capacity that one, on moral principle, should honor.

Capacity refers to an ability, or set of abilities, which may be situation- or context-specific. There is a growing consensus that the standards for assessing decisionmaking capacity include the ability to evidence a choice, the ability to understand relevant information, the ability to appreciate the situation and its consequences, and the ability to manipulate information rationally. These standards were developed initially with a focus on the capacity to consent to treatment, not research. Recently, however, the American Psychiatric Association approved guidelines for assessing decisionmaking capacity in potential research subjects, which substantially rely on these same standards. Whether the context is treatment or research, the particular standard or combination of standards selected for assessing capacity will determine what counts as impaired decision making. For instance, when more stringent standards are used, the result could be over inclusive and thereby deprive a large number of people of their rights to make treatment or research decisions. Thus, what counts as decisional capacity is dependent on a subtle set of assumptions and evaluations.

When a standard of capacity has been chosen, one must set the threshold that distinguishes those who meet the standard from those who do not. Of course, different mental disorders may have an effect on decisionmaking capacity in different ways — some, not at all; some, intermittently; some, more persistently. The decision regarding where the threshold of capacity is set is influenced in part by a society's value system. In a liberal democratic society such as ours, in which the scope of state authority over individual lives is strictly limited and subject to careful scrutiny, this threshold tends to be low. But the selection of a threshold of decisional ability is not wholly a political one, as it must be justified by the individual's ability to satisfy certain benchmarks.

Another facet of decisional impairment that is often encountered in the clinical setting is the variable manifestation of such impairments. The gradual loss of capacity rarely follows a straight line, and in psychiatric illnesses such as bipolar disease, cycles of mania and depression sometimes follow substantial periods of lucidity.

Persistent Decisional Impairments

In a certain sense, all of us are decisionally impaired at various times in our lives. When we have been exposed to anesthetic agents, when we have had too little sleep, when a life event disrupts our equilibrium, or when we have overindulged in alcoholic beverages, our ability to process information and weigh alternatives in light of our values is likely to be reduced. These acute but temporary forms of decisional impairment are not usually matters of concern, because decisions about participation in a research project can normally wait until the impairment has passed. Rather, the impairments that raise the greatest concern are those that persist or can be expected to recur. Reference to a decisional impairment in this report relates principally, but not exclusively, to a relatively persistent condition, that is, a condition that is ongoing or that may periodically recur. There are other sources of decisional impairment that are normally more temporary, such as the transitory side effects of medical treatment, but that might also call for special planning if participation in a research protocol is being considered. Some of the discussion and recommendations in this report may be relevant to these other factors that may affect decision-making capacity but, again, the primary concern of this report is with the potential effect of neurologic or psychiatric conditions on the decisional capacity of potential research subjects. . . .

[I]t is neither ethically acceptable nor empirically accurate to presume that individuals with mental disorders are decisionally impaired. Less obviously, it is also inappropriate to suppose that those who exhibit some decisionmaking deficit cannot be helped to attain a level of functioning that would enable them to be part of a valid consent process. Once these facts are recognized, the special ethical obligations of scientific investigators and institutions sponsoring or carrying out research with persons who may be decisionally impaired become apparent.

Not only must psychological and medical factors affecting these potential research subjects be taken into account, but a full understanding of the nature of their impaired decision making is required. As previously noted, even those who would not normally be considered to be suffering from a decisional impairment may become disoriented if suddenly thrust into the role of a patient, with all of the attendant social inequities and feelings of vulnerability. Persons with a tendency toward impaired decision making due to a mental disorder may experience the consequences of institutionalization in an even more pronounced manner. Therefore, the conditions under which a consent process takes place, including how information is presented and who is responsible for obtaining consent, can be critical in influencing the quality and thus the ethical validity of the consent obtained. Appreciating these different perspectives may also provide practical insights that can improve the process, such as the use of peers (other persons with similar mental disorders who have already participated in the research) and/or their advocates in the consent encounter, or the use of written or visual aids to clarify the research details. It is imperative that all those who are engaged in the approval and conduct of research with persons with mental disorders enrich their appreciation of the importance of context in the consent process and thus set an appropriate foundation for ethically acceptable research involving persons from this population as subjects.

For all of these reasons, determining the proper standards and procedures to assess capacity poses a major challenge in formulating policy on research involving subjects with mental disorders that may affect decisionmaking capacity. Persons with such disorders vary widely in their ability to engage in independent decision making. They may retain such capacity, or possess it intermittently, or be permanently unable to make decisions for themselves.

Individuals with dementia, for example, frequently retain decisionmaking capacity early in the course of the illness, but with time they may become intermittently and then permanently unable to make their own decisions. Some individuals with cognitive disabilities are capable of making many choices for themselves; others completely lack such capacity.

Because of their moral consequences, incorrect capacity determinations can be inadvertently damaging — an assessment that a capable person is incapable of exercising autonomy is disrespectful, demeaning, and stigmatizing, and it may result in the unwarranted deprivation of an individual's civil liberties. Conversely, a judgment that an incapable person is capable leaves that individual unprotected and vulnerable to exploitation by others. In addition, the presence of many marginal cases among members of the relevant populations triggers concern about the ability to make those capacity assessments for many individuals.

It is also important to recognize that investigators seeking to enroll subjects face conflicting interests, and some may become too willing, perhaps unconsciously, to label prospective subjects capable when this will advance their research objectives. Investigators also must be alert to the possibility — and to its subsequent ramifications — that a research subject's decisionmaking status may change during the protocol. NBAC's view is that existing federal policy fails to provide adequate guidance to investigators and IRBs on the many complexities related to capacity determinations in research involving persons who are the subject of this report. Currently, individual IRBs determine (or at least approve) how investigators are to address these matters. Without adequate education and guidance, however, IRB members are likely to, albeit inadvertently, vary criteria too much and fail to institute adequate safeguards for such research. NBAC's review of protocols and consent documents failed to find evidence that researchers provide to IRBs an adequate description of how prospective subjects will be evaluated for their ability to consent. NBAC, along with some other commentators, supports more systematic and specific federal direction on capacity assessment, not only for defining decisional capacity in the research context but also for developing better procedures for assessing such capacity.

Probing Informed Consent in Schizophrenia Research
Joan Stephenson
281 JAMA 2273 (1999)

Many people with schizophrenia are capable of giving informed consent to participate in research after an educational process to help them understand a study's potential risks and other key issues, according to new findings reported here at the Eighth International Congress on Schizophrenia Research. . . .

Carpenter, Conley, and colleagues decided to test their hypothesis that an explicit educational effort would be a key factor in helping patients participate in the informed consent process in a study that assessed 30 patients' cognitive deficits, symptoms, and understanding of a hypothetical research protocol, compared with healthy controls. The investigators found that the patient group scored lower than the control group on an assessment of decisional capacity, but after the patients went through an educational process involving group and/or individual sessions reviewing information related to the hypothetical study, their scores were in the normal range.

"There was no longer a difference between the normal controls and these chronic, cognitively impaired schizophrenics on their decisional capacity scores," said Carpenter. "Severely ill patients with schizophrenia can often provide competent informed consent if educational procedures enhance the consent process."

The investigators also noted that while there was a modest correlation between how well patients performed on the decisional capacity test and psychotic symptoms, their performance was most strongly related to the cognitive impairments associated with schizophrenia.

Although there is limited information about how well potential research subjects with schizophrenia are able to retain such knowledge, the earlier study led by Conley found that when patients were tested for recall one and three months later, many appeared to retain enough information to pass a test with questions about the study's risks, how to withdraw as a participant, and other statements relevant to informed consent.

NOTES AND QUESTIONS

1. In what way are individuals harmed by erroneous judgments about their decision-making capacity? Consider both situations in which individuals are incorrectly found to *lack* decision-making capacity and situations in which individuals are incorrectly found to *have* decision-making capacity. Are the harms associated with each of these situations comparable? Does the answer to this question depend on why the determination is being made? For example, are the potential harms different when the determination is being made in the context of medical research as opposed to ordinary treatment? Might they vary depending on the type of research being conducted?

2. NBAC states that "it is neither ethically acceptable nor empirically accurate to presume that individuals with mental disorders are decisionally impaired." Do you agree? Why should we not begin with a presumption that individuals with mental disorders lack decision-making capacity, and then put the burden on the researcher to rebut that presumption after an investigation into the decision skills of the particular individual? What would be the advantages and drawbacks of such an approach, as compared to the approach suggested by NBAC? What about making such a presumption only in the case of certain mental disorders that are highly likely to affect decision-making capacity?

3. What does NBAC mean by a "threshold of decisional ability"? Consider NBAC's observation that the decision to select a particular threshold "is not wholly a political one." In what respects is the decision "political" in nature?

4. Lo suggests that individuals whose decisions are not "stable over time" may lack decision-making capacity. Do you agree that stability of decisions is an appropriate consideration? If so, in what circumstances might lack of stable decisions suggest decisional incapacity? Does the fact that someone changes her mind about the desirability of participating in research necessarily mean that she lacks the capacity to enroll in a study?

5. Does depression undermine a person's capacity to consent to medical research? The "conventional thinking" on this question, Carl Elliott argues, is that it usually does not:

> According to conventional thinking, depression is primarily about despair, guilt, and a loss of motivation, while competence is about the ability to reason, to deliberate, to compare, and to evaluate. Often these latter abilities are ones that depression leaves intact.

Carl Elliott, *Caring about Risks: Are Severely Depressed Patients Competent to Consent to Research?* 54 ARCH. GENERAL PSYCHIATRY 113 (1997). Elliot maintains that this conventional account is mistaken:

> There are 2 good arguments for the conclusion that some depressed patients are incompetent to consent to research, each of which is persuasive for a slightly different type of patient. The first might be called the argument from *authenticity*. When a person is caught in the grip of depression, his values, beliefs, desires, and dispositions are dramatically different from when he is healthy. In some cases, they are so different that we might ask whether his decisions are truly his. . . .
>
> Here is where the notion of competence as accountability is helpful. If a person were to behave badly while mentally ill — say, in a full-blown manic episode — we would very likely think it unfair to hold him fully responsible for what he has done. . . . Similarly for the depressed patient being asked to consent to research: his mental state is such that his behavior and choices do not seem to be truly his. If something untoward were to happen to him during the research, for instance, we could not in good conscience say that he bears the full responsibility for undergoing that risk. . . .
>
> [The second argument is] what might be called the argument from *self-interest*. Our ordinary relationships with other people are based on certain assumptions about their thoughts and behavior. One of these assumptions is that other persons have some minimal concern for their own welfare. For example, the assumption that other people ordinarily both have some minimal degree of self-interest and are best positioned

to judge their own interests lies at the heart of the institution of informed consent.

However, if we have reason to believe that severely depressed patients do not have this minimal degree of concern, then a fundamental assumption underlying informed consent is undermined.

Id. Do you agree with Elliott that authenticity and self-interest are necessary components of competent decision making? Do you think Lo would agree? What objections might be raised in response to Elliott's analysis?

[B] Assessing Decision-Making Capacity

1 RESEARCH INVOLVING PERSONS WITH MENTAL DISORDERS THAT MAY AFFECT DECISIONMAKING CAPACITY: REPORT AND RECOMMENDATIONS 21 NATIONAL BIOETHICS ADVISORY COMMISSION
(1998)

A capacity assessment process must adequately protect the interests of individuals with conditions that increase the risk of decisional impairment. To address this need a variety of approaches to capacity assessment are endorsed in the literature on research involving adults with cognitive impairment. Many commentators believe that IRBs should, at a minimum, require investigators to specify the method by which prospective subjects' decisional capacity will be evaluated and the criteria for identifying incapable subjects.

A complicating factor, however, is that any assessment tool measures capacity indirectly through manifest performance, and a person's performance does not always adequately reflect his or her capacity or potential. Many factors can inhibit performance, including anxiety or environmental conditions, the quality of the assessment instrument itself, and other characteristics of the assessment process. Everyone can attest to the variation on one occasion or another between actual performance — as on an examination or in a job interview — and actual capacity. The problem is aggravated in populations whose conditions are partly characterized by fluctuating capacity. The capacity-performance distinction suggests why the context in which the capacity assessment is made (under what conditions or by whom, for example) is so important.

There is divergence of opinion on whether capacity assessment and information disclosure should be conducted by an individual not otherwise connected with the research project. The National Commission recommended that, "where appropriate," IRBs should appoint a "consent auditor" for research involving those persons institutionalized as mentally infirm. IRBs would be authorized to determine whether a consent auditor is indicated and how much authority the consent auditor would have. For example, in research involving greater than minimal risk without the prospect of direct benefit to the subjects, the National Commission recommended that the auditor observe and verify the adequacy of the consent and assent process, and in appropriate cases observe the conduct of the study to ensure the subjects' continued willingness to participate. The Department of Health, Education and Welfare (DHEW) regulations proposed in 1978 contemplated mandating auditors for all projects involving this subject population, but opposition to this proposal reportedly was one reason the regulations never became final. . . .

[The material that follows is from earlier in this report, at page 10.]

At least four types of limitations in decisionmaking ability should be considered when planning and conducting research with this population. First, some individuals might have fluctuating capacity, what is often called waxing and waning ability to make decisions, as in schizophrenia, bi-polar disorders, depressive disorders, and some dementias. Second, decisionmaking deficits can be predicted in some individuals due to the course of their disease or the nature of their treatment. Although these individuals may be decisionally capable in the early stages of the disease progression, such as in Alzheimer's disease, they have prospective incapacity. Third, most persons with limited capacity are in some way still able to object or assent to research, as in the case of more advanced Alzheimer's disease. Fourth, persons who have permanently lost the ability to make nearly any decision that involves any significant degree of reflection are decisionally incapable, as in the later stages of Alzheimer's disease and profound dementia.

The situation is further complicated by the fact that two or more of these four categories often apply to the same individual over the course of a disease. Thus someone in the early stages of Alzheimer's disease may have prospective incapacity, then experience very subtle decisionmaking limitations or have fluctuating capacity, and, finally, progress to incapacity. It is therefore critical that researchers who work with this population be familiar with the ways that decisionmaking impairments manifest themselves, and that they design appropriate mechanisms to maximize the subject's ability to decide whether to enter or continue in a study. In addition, circumstantial factors often affect decisionmaking capacity. All persons feel more empowered and in control in some social situations than in others. Similarly, some persons with mental disorders may be more or less capable of making their own decisions depending on circumstances. For example, some individuals may feel more empowered in dealing with certain health care professionals or family members, and less so in dealing with others; or they may more effectively express their wishes at home than in an institution, or the reverse. Such insights can be critical in helping the individual achieve as high a degree of self-determination as possible.

Finally, a basic difficulty is central to deliberations on research involving those who may be decisionally impaired: our society has not decided what degree of impairment counts as a lack of decisionmaking capacity. Although there are certain clear cases of those who are fully capable and those who are wholly incapable, persons with fluctuating or limited capacity present serious challenges to assessment. When can those whose capacity is uncertain over periods of time be deemed capable of deciding about participating in research? In a society that treasures personal freedom and centers its political system on the integrity and value of each individual, this question goes to the very heart of our culture and must therefore be addressed with utmost caution.

NOTES AND QUESTIONS

1. Should researchers always be required to assess subjects' decision-making capacity, or should capacity assessments be required only in studies involving certain types of subjects? Should the researcher make the capacity assessment, or should it be made by someone not affiliated with the study?

2. Would you support a policy requiring the use of "consent auditors" to monitor capacity assessments? If so, in what type of studies should such auditors be required? What type of qualifications would you require for a consent auditor? What specific tasks should a consent auditor be assigned?

3. How should researchers and IRBs deal with the problem of "fluctuating capacity"? Is it appropriate to accept an individual's consent to participate in research as long as she has decision-making capacity at the time the consent is provided, even if there is reason to believe that she may repeatedly lose decision-making capacity during the course of the study? Conversely, is it appropriate to exclude an individual from research, or to rely on surrogate consent, if the person lacks decision-making capacity during her encounter with the researcher but there is reason to believe that she might have the capacity to make a decision if approached at another time?

4. In a 1991 report, the Working Party on Research on the Mentally Incapacitated of the British Medical Research Council made the following recommendation:

> Many people with mental impairment or disorder are able to consent to their inclusion in research provided care is taken to explain it to them. When there is doubt about an individual's mental capacity, we recommend that a judgment on his ability to consent should be sought from the physician responsible. When the individual is not under the care of a physician, or the physician is involved in the proposed research, a view should be sought from a relative, friend or other person acceptable to the [local research ethics committee].

WORKING PARTY ON RESEARCH ON THE MENTALLY INCAPACITATED, THE ETHICAL CONDUCT OF RESEARCH ON THE MENTALLY INCAPACITATED (1991), available at http://www.mrc.ac.uk/pdf-ethics-mental.pdf. What are the advantages and drawbacks of this approach?

5. A leading work on assessing decision-making capacity in the clinical setting is THOMAS GRISSO & PAUL S. APPELBAUM, ASSESSING COMPETENCE TO CONSENT TO TREATMENT: A GUIDE FOR PHYSICIANS AND OTHER HEALTH PROFESSIONALS (1998); *see also* American Psychiatric Association, *Guidelines for Assessing the Decisionmaking Capacity of Potential Research Subjects with Cognitive Impairments*, 155 AM. J. PSYCHIATRY 1649 (1998); Evan G. Renzo et al., *Assessment of Capacity to Give Consent to Research Participation: State-of-the-Art and Beyond*, 1 J. HEALTH CARE L. & POL'Y 66 (1998).

§ 14.03 INFORMED CONSENT

[A] Surrogate Decision Making

Under the federal regulations, informed consent to research must be provided by either the subject or the subject's "legally authorized representative." 45 C.F.R. § 46.116. A "legally authorized representative" is defined as "an individual or judicial or other body authorized under applicable law to consent on behalf of a prospective subject to the subject's participation in the procedure(s) involved in the research." 45 C.F.R. § 46.102(c).

In general, state law determines who can consent to health care on behalf of individuals who lack decision-making capacity. In most states, authority to make medical decisions for incapacitated patients derives from one of the following legal sources:

- *Guardianship proceedings* — A guardian is a person appointed by a court to make financial, medical, and/or other decisions on behalf of an individual who lacks decision-making capacity. All states have laws allowing courts to appoint guardians for individuals who lack capacity. In some states, guardians must obtain specific court authorization for decisions to enroll an incapacitated person in research. *See* NBAC, *supra*, at page 34.

- *Health care proxy statutes* — A health care proxy is a document in which a competent individual can designate another person (known as an "agent") to make health care decisions on the individual's behalf, in the event that person loses decision-making capacity. Health care proxy statutes generally require the agent to make decisions based on the patient's wishes or, if the patient's wishes cannot be determined, the patient's best interests. All states have health care proxy statutes. *See* Charles P. Sabatino, *The Legal and Functional Status of the Medical Proxy: Suggestions for Statutory Reform*, 27 J.L. MED. & ETHICS 52 (1999).

- *Surrogate decision-making statutes* — Many states have statutes that empower "surrogates" to make medical decisions on behalf of patients who lack decision-making capacity. These statutes typically include a priority list of surrogate decision-makers, beginning with the patient's spouse, moving down through other family members, and sometimes adding a category of "close friend" at the end of the list. Like health care proxy statutes, surrogate decision-making statutes typically require decisions to be based on the incapacitated patient's wishes or best interests. Some state statutes place restrictions on the type of decisions a surrogate can make, particularly with respect to decisions about life-sustaining treatment. Most — but not all — states have surrogate decision-making statutes. *See* AMERICAN BAR ASSOCIATION COMMISSION ON LAW AND AGING, HEALTH CARE SURROGATE DECISION-MAKING LEGISLATION, available at http://www.abanet.org/aging/ update.html; Jerry A. Menikoff et al., *Beyond Advance Directives: Health Care Surrogate Laws*, 327 NEW ENG. J. MED. 1165 (1992).

While a few states have laws that specifically address surrogate consent to medical research, most do not. Some states have laws expressly prohibiting surrogate consent to certain types of research with subjects who lack decision-making capacity. *See* NBAC, *supra*, at page 34.

In the absence of federal guidance on these issues, IRBs have taken a variety of approaches to determining who qualifies as a subject's "legally authorized representative." There is no consensus on whether, for example, a health care agent appointed through a health care proxy would qualify as a legally authorized representative, or if a family member empowered to make treatment decisions under a surrogate decision-making statute would qualify. There is also disagreement about the policy question of whether the regulations *should* permit these individuals to enroll incapacitated persons in research, particularly research from which the subjects are not expected to receive any direct benefits.

1 RESEARCH INVOLVING PERSONS WITH MENTAL DISORDERS THAT MAY AFFECT DECISIONMAKING CAPACITY
NATIONAL BIOETHICS ADVISORY COMMISSION
34-35, 62-63 (1998)

Should federal policy require formal legal guardianship for someone to be considered a suitable surrogate for decision making about research? The underlying question is whether such a requirement is necessary or sufficient to provide adequate protection against inappropriate involvement of a vulnerable population in research to advance the interests of others. The National Commission recommended that the permission of either a legal guardian or a judge be required to authorize the research participation of subjects institutionalized as mentally infirm in the following situations: the incapable subject objects to participation, or the subject is incapable of assent and the research presents greater than minimal risk.

Subsequent commentary by others questions whether formal legal proceedings are necessary to provide adequate protection for subjects who lack capacity, particularly those not residing in an institutional setting. As one writer notes, IRBs requiring legal guardianship, "to be on the safe side," could end up contributing to a deprivation of general decisionmaking rights of subjects. Moreover, the guardian appointment process ordinarily will not address research participation issues in any explicit way. In most cases, a judicial decision to confer guardianship status on a particular person is made without consideration of that person's suitability to make decisions regarding his or her ward's participation in research protocols.

Dissatisfaction with a requirement for legal guardianship has led to alternative proposals for granting authority to act as an incapable person's representative in research decision making. One option . . . is to allow decisionally capable persons to authorize in advance a specific individual to make decisions regarding their research participation during a future period of incapacity. [This option is discussed *infra*, at page 606.] . . .

A second potential source of authority is an existing health care power of attorney. It is doubtful that an individual's choice of a proxy to make treatment decisions in the event of incapacity can fairly be taken as an authorization for research decision making as well. Nevertheless, the choice does manifest a high degree of trust in the proxy, and that evidence of trust may entitle the health care proxy to a decisionmaking role in research. The NIH Clinical Center policy does allow previously chosen health care proxies to make some research decisions for subjects.

A third alternative is to regard state legislation authorizing family members (and, in a few states, friends) to make certain treatment decisions on behalf of relatives as conferring authority for research decisions as well. It might be argued that such legislation recognizes that important health-related decisions for persons lacking decisional capacity are properly assigned to appropriate relatives. Perhaps it would be reasonable to extend the law's application to a statutory proxy's decision regarding research offering potential health benefit to an incapable subject. Others believe that these laws should not be interpreted so expansively and that amendments or new legislation would be required to provide explicit statutory authority for delegating to relatives decisions about the subject's participation.

A final possible option is to assign such decisionmaking authority based on the simple status of being a close relative or a trusted individual. Support for this alternative, especially as regards relatives, comes from the long-held tradition in health care of relying on families to make decisions for incapable persons, as well as from the belief that relatives are most likely to make decisions in accord with the incapable person's values, preferences, and interests. This approach is easy to administer; moreover, it apparently has been and continues to be a common practice in many research settings.

Each of these options presents advantages and drawbacks. Requiring judicial involvement may cause unproductive delays, raise the costs of research, and may not always advance respect for and protection of incapable persons. Requiring explicit durable powers of attorney for research poses some practical difficulties, since relatively few persons have or can be expected to complete these documents, and it may not be possible to describe the future research protocol completely. Another question is whether the power of DPAs to consent to research risks for an incapable individual should be equal to the power of capable adult subjects to consent to such risks for themselves. New legislation authorizing a relative or a trusted friend to make research decisions for incapable persons would require action by the states; such legislation, however, might emerge slowly or, in some states, not at all.

All of these alternatives also raise questions about the accuracy with which incapable subjects' values and preferences as competent persons will be expressed by formal or informal representatives. There is also the problem of potential conflicts between subjects' interests and those of their representatives. Those most likely to act as representatives are family members, who may see the subject's research participation as an avenue "that may lighten the burden of care-giving or lead to treatment from which the family member may benefit." Two empirical studies found some family members willing to allow an incapable relative to be entered in a research study even though they thought the relative would refuse if competent. Some family members also stated they would allow an incapable relative to become a subject even though they would refuse to enroll in such a study themselves. At the same time, NBAC recognizes that these mechanisms might permit some important research to go forward. Moreover, NBAC is satisfied that the argument for encouraging the involvement of LARs is sound so long as there is a clear description of the role and authority of the LAR, and of the protections that must be in place in order for an IRB to assure itself that the LAR is appropriately acting on behalf of the incapable persons. In addition, there should be an ongoing evaluation of LARs in this context.

    . . . *Recommendation 14.* A LAR may give permission (within the limits set by the other recommendations) to enroll in a research protocol a person who lacks the capacity to decide whether to participate, provided that:

    (A) the LAR bases decisions about participation upon a best estimation of what the subject would have chosen if capable of making a decision; and

    (B) the LAR is available to monitor the subject's recruitment, participation, and withdrawal from the study; and

    (C) the LAR is a person chosen by the subject, or is a relative or friend of the subject. . . .

Expansion of the Category of Legally Authorized Representatives and of the Powers Granted under Statutes for Durable Powers of Attorney (DPA) for Health Care

Recommendation 15. In order to expand the category of LARs:

(A) an investigator should accept as an LAR, subject to the requirements in Recommendation 14, a relative or friend of the potential subject who is recognized as an LAR for purposes of clinical decision making under the law of the state where the research takes place.

(B) States should confirm, by statute or court decision, that:

(1) an LAR for purposes of clinical decision making may serve as an LAR for research; and

(2) friends as well as relatives may serve as both clinical and research LARs if they are actively involved in the care of a person who lacks decisionmaking capacity.

Recommendation 16. States should enact legislation, if necessary, to ensure that persons who choose to plan for future research participation are entitled to choose their LAR. . . .

Involving Subjects' Family and Friends

Recommendation 17. For research protocols involving subjects who have fluctuating or limited decisionmaking capacity or prospective incapacity, IRBs should ensure that investigators establish and maintain ongoing communication with involved caregivers, consistent with the subject's autonomy and with medical confidentiality.

NOTES AND QUESTIONS

1. The NBAC recommendations are just that — merely recommendations. Only a few states (such as California and Kansas) have enacted the type of legislation NBAC recommended. The California legislation is discussed *infra*, at page 608.

2. Note that the definition of "legally authorized representative" in the federal regulations states that the representative must have the authority to consent to "the subject's participation in the *procedure(s)* involved in the research." 45 C.F.R. § 46.102(c) (emphasis added). Does the wording of the definition imply that a family member who has authority to consent to a particular procedure when making "health care decisions" pursuant to a state surrogate decision-making statute would also be an appropriate "legally authorized representative" — even if the state statute does not specifically empower surrogates to make decisions about research? Does it depend on whether the research offers the subject a prospect of direct benefit?

3. Would your answer to the questions posed in the previous note change if the state statute specifically stated that the surrogate's authority extends only to "medical treatment" decisions? What if it went further and stated that the surrogate may not make decisions about research enrollment? In answering these questions, consider the implications of 45 C.F.R. § 101(f) (stating that the federal regulations do not preempt state laws that "provide additional protections for human subjects").

4. In 2002, OHRP sent determination letters (letters specifying OHRP's conclusions following an investigation) to a number of sites that had been participating in a controversial study in which subjects with severe lung injury were randomly assigned to have different volumes of air pumped into their lungs by a ventilator. In the case of Duke University, the university had previously told OHRP that North Carolina law permitted certain relatives to "provide informed consent to health care on behalf of a person who is not competent to consent." The university had further noted that it "interpreted" that North Carolina law as also authorizing such relatives to "consent on behalf of a subject to the subject's participation in the procedures involved in the research." In its letter to Duke, OHRP "acknowledged" this information and did not raise any further questions about this point. Letter from OHRP to Duke University Health System, dated February 1, 2002, available at http://www.hhs.gov/ohrp/ detrm_letrs/YR02/feb02a.pdf. If you were an attorney advising a medical center about when incapacitated subjects can be enrolled in studies, how would this determination letter affect your analysis, particularly with respect to the questions raised in note 2, *supra*? *See* Michele Russell-Einhorn & Thomas Puglisi, *Three Exceptions to the Requirement to Obtain Informed Consent in Research*, 1 MED. RES. L. POL'Y REP. (BNA) 514 (2002).

5. As noted above, state health care proxy statutes and surrogate decision-making statutes typically require the decision maker to follow the patient's wishes or, if the patient's wishes cannot be determined, the patient's best interests. If a legally authorized representative derives her authority from one of those statutes, would she be required to satisfy the wishes/best interests standard when making decisions about research participation? If the representative would remain bound by the state law's wishes/best interests standard, how should that standard be interpreted in the context of research? Does the fact that a study offers a prospect of direct benefit to subjects necessarily mean that enrolling in the study is in a particular individual's best interests? Or should an even stricter standard, such as the "good choice" standard that is articulated in 45 C.F.R. § 46.405 for some more-than-minimal-risk studies involving children, be employed? In what circumstances would an agent or surrogate be permitted to enroll an incapacitated subject in studies that do not offer any prospect of direct benefit to the subjects?

6. Even individuals who lack the capacity to consent to research may have sufficient capacity to designate another person to make decisions about research enrollment. A work group convened by the New York State Department of

Health recommended that individuals be permitted to designate "research agents" if they have

> the ability to understand the difference between medical treatment, conducted to benefit the physical or mental condition of the individual, and research conducted to advance scientific knowledge, which may or may not hold out a prospect of direct benefit to the individual. The person also must understand that he or she is choosing someone to make decisions about his or her participation in research, based on his or her advance instructions.

NEW YORK STATE DEPARTMENT OF HEALTH ADVISORY WORK GROUP ON HUMAN SUBJECT RESEARCH INVOLVING THE PROTECTED CLASSES, RECOMMENDATIONS ON THE OVERSIGHT OF HUMAN SUBJECT RESEARCH INVOLVING THE PROTECTED CLASSES (1998) [hereinafter NEW YORK STATE WORK GROUP], at 24.

7. Is it appropriate to presume that individuals with impaired decision-making capacity would want their family members to have the authority to make decisions about research? Might it depend on the reason the prospective subject lacks decision-making capacity? Consider the following:

> [P]sychiatric illness tends to strike much earlier in life [than Alzheimer's disease], leaving many persons with psychiatric illness unable to finish school, start or sustain careers, or establish their own families. Unlike Alzheimer's disease patients who have had a chance to contribute to society and raise a family, it is not uncommon for persons with psychiatric disease to have caused much burden and heartache for their families for many years. Much more so than in the Alzheimer's context, a split exists between persons with mental illness and their family members regarding research on this population and how it should be regulated. As might be expected, relatives of individuals with a psychiatric disease are largely supportive of regulations that allow for family consent to participation in research of a patient lacking decisional capacity. Some individuals with mental illness, however, fear that they might, all too quickly, be tagged as decisionally impaired and enrolled, by a member of their family, in a clinical trial in which they would not wish to participate. The division is analogous to the debate over the laws for civil commitment — family members of the mentally ill would like to see the laws loosened to allow more flexibility in committing mentally ill patients so that they can be treated; mentally ill patients prefer the narrow criteria of "dangerousness" to remain the commitment standard.

Diane E. Hoffmann et al., *Regulating Research with Decisionally Impaired Individuals: Are We Making Progress?* 3 DEPAUL J. HEALTH CARE L. 547 (2000). What are the implications of these observations for policies governing surrogate consent to research with mentally ill subjects?

CALIFORNIA HEALTH AND SAFETY CODE § 24178

(b) Subdivisions (c) and (f) shall apply only to medical experiments that relate to the cognitive impairment, lack of capacity, or serious or life-threatening diseases and conditions of research participants.

(c) For purposes of obtaining informed consent required for medical experiments in a nonemergency room environment, and pursuant to subdivision (a), if a person is unable to consent and does not express dissent or resistance to participation, surrogate informed consent may be obtained from a surrogate decisionmaker with reasonable knowledge of the subject, who shall include any of the following persons, in the following descending order of priority:

    (1) The person's agent pursuant to an advance health care directive.

    (2) The conservator or guardian of the person having the authority to make health care decisions for the person.

    (3) The spouse of the person.

    (4) An individual [who is a domestic partner of the person].

    (5) An adult son or daughter of the person.

    (6) A custodial parent of the person.

    (7) Any adult brother or sister of the person.

    (8) Any adult grandchild of the person.

    (9) An available adult relative with the closest degree of kinship to the person.

NOTES AND QUESTIONS

1. As noted earlier in this chapter, while many states have surrogate decision-making statutes that automatically appoint someone to make health care decisions for an incapacitated person, there are only a handful of states that have similarly broad laws specifically appointing surrogates to enroll people in research. California is one such state.

2. This provision of the California law was enacted in 2002, apparently in response to a request from the University of California system. Lawyers at the University of California at San Francisco had for years said that California law allowed the University to enroll incompetent people in research by getting the consent of their relatives. However, several other campuses of the University of California system had reached a quite different legal conclusion, determining that state law "forbids" such research. Thus, to remedy this situation, the University sought, and obtained, the change in the law. Oddly enough, while this

change was being debated by the legislature, the University of California at San Francisco was cited by OHRP for having violated the federal regulations by enrolling 105 incompetent patients in the national study on ventilators described on page 606. Many of the lawmakers apparently were not even aware of the UCSF controversy. *See* Bernadette Tansey, *UCSF Violated Patients' Rights: Doctors Improperly Got Consent for Study, Feds Say*, SAN FRANCISCO CHRONICLE, July 28, 2002, at A1.

3. California does not have a surrogate decision-making statute applicable to ordinary health care decisions (situations in which research is *not* taking place): it is only for research participation that there is a clear, statutorily authorized list of surrogate decision makers. From a policy perspective, what do you think of this circumstance?

4. Section (f) of this law, not reprinted above, provides a list of people who can give consent in an emergency room setting. It is the same as the list included in section (c), except it does not include items (8) and (9). Why do you think the legislators altered the list in that way?

5. What definition would you give to the term "medical experiment"? How, if at all, might this term differ from a medical research study?

6. What is the purpose of the limitations described in section (b)? If it were up to you, would you have included additional limitations, and if so, which ones? Or might you want to throw out some of the limitations listed in (b)?

[B] Research Living Wills

Mentally Disabled Research Subjects: The Enduring Policy Issues
Rebecca Dresser
276 JAMA 67 (1996)

The Role of Advance Consent

The prevailing view is that proxy decision makers should be guided by two considerations: any relevant values and preferences the decisionally incapable subject held during a prior period of competency, or, if such evidence is indeterminate or nonexistent, the incapable subject's best interests. To promote respect for the subject's former autonomous desires, some organizations and individuals have endorsed a device called the "advance directive for experimental intervention" or the "research living will." Through this device, a competent person expected to become temporarily or permanently incapable of autonomous choice may issue advance consent to research participation. Potential candidates include individuals in the earliest stages of progressive dementia and those experiencing intermittent incompetency due to mental disorder.

Advocates of this approach contend that it furthers respect for persons by creating a new opportunity for persons to exercise autonomous choice. Advance directives for research raise several ethical concerns, however. In many cases, the competent person considering a directive will lack adequate information to make an informed decision about a future research project; indeed, the project may not materialize until long after the directive was issued. Moreover, an important dimension of research autonomy is the freedom to withdraw consent if the burdens of participation become too heavy. Persons consenting in advance forgo the opportunity to withdraw if experimental burdens prove substantial. To protect such persons, a proxy decision maker must be appointed to exercise that choice on the subject's behalf. A further controversial issue is whether policy should permit competent persons to consent in advance to greater risks than are generally permitted for decisionally incapable subjects.

Research advance directives have serious practical shortcomings as well. A relatively small percentage of persons complete advance directives on future medical care. Because there is less public awareness of and interest in the advance directive for research, few persons are likely to complete these documents. A recent survey of healthy elderly persons found many to be uneasy about the concept, though some expressed interest in providing advance consent to research offering reasonable promise of direct benefit.

Advance consent alone cannot provide adequate protection to decisionally incapable individuals; conversely, mandating advance consent would drastically reduce the number of subjects eligible for research participation. Advance directives for research are best viewed as a potentially helpful, yet optional, supplement to the ordinary rule governing proxy decision making on behalf of incapable subjects.

1 RESEARCH INVOLVING PERSONS WITH MENTAL DISORDERS THAT MAY AFFECT DECISIONMAKING CAPACITY
NATIONAL BIOETHICS ADVISORY COMMISSION
61 (1998)

Recommendation 13. A person who has the capacity to make decisions about participation in research may give Prospective Authorization to a particular class of research if its risks, potential direct and indirect benefits, and other pertinent conditions have been explained. Based on the Prospective Authorization, an LAR may enroll the subject after the subject has lost the capacity to make decisions, provided the LAR is available to monitor the subject's recruitment, participation, and withdrawal. The greater the risks posed by the research protocol under consideration, the more specific the subject's Prospective Authorization should be to entitle the LAR to permit enrollment.

NOTES AND QUESTIONS

1. Dresser notes that a research living will should be an "optional" supplement to the usual ways in which we might enroll an incapable subject in a research study. However, as discussed later in this chapter, NBAC proposed that such documents might in some circumstances be *required* before someone could be enrolled in certain risky types of studies. Dresser addressed this issue in a later article she wrote after the NBAC recommendations had been released. *See* Rebecca Dresser, *Advance Directives in Dementia Research: Promoting Autonomy and Protecting Subjects*, 23 IRB, Jan.-Feb. 2001, at 1 (describing safeguards needed to make sure these documents do not result in subjects inappropriately being exposed to onerous procedures).

2. According to the American Society for Geriatrics:

Advance consent, including formal advance directives for research purposes, is an appropriate mechanism for allowing individuals with decision making capacity to express their preferences regarding research participation that should, in general, be respected when making decisions about research enrollment at points in the future when those individuals have lost decisional capacity.

At the same time, they argue that research advance directives should not take precedence over a surrogate's contemporaneous assessment of the subject's best interests. Thus, they recommend that:

Surrogates should be allowed to refuse to enroll potential subjects or to withdraw a subject from an ongoing trial on the basis that the surrogate believes that the research protocol is not in the best interests of the subject or is not what the subject intended, even if that decision would conflict with the subject's advance directive. . . . Instructions in advance directives for research are likely to be imperfect at best as they will be based on knowledge at one point in time, but will be applied perhaps several years in the future. The individual's condition, available treatments, and other factors may change in the intervening years, making it safer to allow surrogates to decline enrollment or withdraw the subject from a trial if the surrogate determines that enrollment would either not be in the subject's best interests or would not be consistent with what the subject intended.

AMERICAN GERIATRICS SOCIETY, POSITION STATEMENT: INFORMED CONSENT FOR RESEARCH ON HUMAN SUBJECTS WITH DEMENTIA (1998), available at www.americangeriatrics.org/products/ positionpapers/infconsentPF.html. Do you agree that surrogates should be permitted to deviate from subjects' advance directives based on the surrogate's own assessment of the subject's best interests or intent?

[C] Subject Assent and Refusal

REPORT AND RECOMMENDATIONS: RESEARCH INVOLVING
THOSE INSTITUTIONALIZED AS MENTALLY INFIRM
NATIONAL COMMISSION FOR THE PROTECTION
OF HUMAN SUBJECTS OF BIOMEDICAL AND
BEHAVIORAL RESEARCH
9-10 (1978)

If the subject, because of illness or institutionalization, is incapable of giving informed consent to participate in research presenting no more than minimal risk, the subject's "assent" should be sufficient to authorize participation, provided the research is relevant to the subject's condition.

The Commission has chosen the term "assent" to describe authorization by a person whose capacity to understand and judge is somewhat impaired by illness or institutionalization, but who remains functional. The standard for "assent" requires that the subject know what procedures will be performed in the research, choose freely to undergo those procedures, communicate this choice unambiguously, and be aware that subjects may withdraw from participation. This standard for assent is intended to require a lesser degree of comprehension by the subject than would generally support informed consent, and it is not related to judicial determination of incompetency or commitment status. Assent is not intended to serve as a substitute for informed consent, but rather as the applicable standard for agreement to participate where the subject is incapable of giving informed consent and certain other conditions are satisfied. . . . [T]hose conditions require that the research be relevant to the subject's condition and present no more than minimal risk. Additional circumstances under which assent may authorize participation in research are set forth in the [Commission's] recommendations.

Where the subject is incapable even of assenting, absence of objection should be sufficient to permit participation in research that is relevant to the subject's condition and presents no more than minimal risk.

NOTES AND QUESTIONS

1. Acccording to the American Geriatrics Society,

In general, the refusal of a (potential) subject, even if that subject has lost decision making capacity, should be followed. The only exception should be protocols that meet the following four conditions: (1) a very high potential benefit to risk ratio; (2) where access to this benefit is available only through the research study (e.g., a promising experimental drug for severe agitation in patients with dementia, being tried on subjects who have not benefited from standard treatments); (3) proxy consent is obtained; and (4) any additional safeguards selected by an IRB are in place.

AMERICAN GERIATRICS SOCIETY, POSITION STATEMENT: INFORMED CONSENT FOR RESEARCH ON HUMAN SUBJECTS WITH DEMENTIA (1998), available at http://www.americangeriatrics.org/products/positionpapers/infconsentPF.html.

By contrast, NBAC concluded that:

> Even when decisionmaking capacity appears to be severely impaired, respect for persons must prevail over any asserted duty to serve the public good as a research subject. Hence, a potential or actual subject's objection must be heeded, regardless of the level of risk or potential benefit, just as it would in the case of an individual who clearly retains decisional capacity. Respect for persons requires that we avoid forcing an individual to serve as a research subject, even when the research offers the possibility of direct medical benefit to the individual, when his or her decisional capacity is in doubt, or when the research poses no more than minimal risk. While objections must always be respected, situations may arise in which the investigator could legitimately return to the subject at a later point to ascertain whether the previous objection still stands.

NBAC, *supra*, at 58. Which position is more similar to the federal regulations governing research with children? *See* 45 C.F.R. § 408. Which do you find more persuasive in the context of research with decisionally impaired adults? If you agree with the American Geriatrics Society's position, would you impose any procedural constraints on researchers' ability to override individuals' objections to participating in research? For example, should the researcher be required to obtain IRB approval before enrolling an incapacitated subject in a study over his or her objection? Should judicial approval ever be required?

2. According to the National Alliance for the Mentally Ill, "Whenever consent is given by someone other than the research participant, the participant and involved family members must receive information on the same basis as the person actually giving consent." NATIONAL ALLIANCE FOR THE MENTALLY ILL, POLICIES ON STRENGTHENED STANDARDS FOR PROTECTION OF INDIVIDUALS WITH SEVERE MENTAL ILLNESSES WHO PARTICIPATE AS HUMAN SUBJECTS IN RESEARCH (1995). Do you agree that the subject and the "involved family members" should always receive the same information as "the person actually giving consent"? Can you envision circumstances in which it might be appropriate to limit the information given to the subject or her family members?

§ 14.04 LIMITATIONS ON PERMISSIBLE RISKS

As discussed in Chapter 13, the federal regulations governing pediatric research distinguish between studies involving minimal risk, a minor increase over minimal risk, and more than a minor increase over minimal risk. As the level of risk increases, the regulations impose greater limitations on the use of children as research subjects. *See* Chapter 13, at page 544. The following excerpts discuss whether such limits should also apply to research involving adults who lack decision-making capacity.

1 RESEARCH INVOLVING PERSONS WITH MENTAL DISORDERS THAT MAY AFFECT DECISIONMAKING CAPACITY NATIONAL BIOETHICS ADVISORY COMMISSION
46-48, 60-61 (1998)

Research Protocols Involving Minimal Risk

NBAC recognizes that there are both practical and philosophical difficulties with applying the concept of minimal risk. However, NBAC's view is that research protocols that involve minimal risk present fewer ethical issues for IRBs, researchers, and potential subjects than those protocols involving greater than minimal risk, where, in the latter case, the harms or discomforts may be expected to occur more often or are more serious. . . . [A]n IRB may approve protocols that present only minimal risk using several different routes for subject enrollment: when the potential subject gives informed consent (unless consent is waived); if the potential subject gives permission in advance . . . and a surrogate decision maker has given permission; or if a surrogate decision maker has given permission under certain conditions.

Research Protocols Involving Greater than Minimal Risk that Offer the Prospect of Direct Medical Benefit to Subjects

The general view is that it is permissible to include persons with mental disorders that may affect decisionmaking capacity in a research protocol that involves greater than minimal risk, but does not offer the prospect of direct medical benefit to subjects as long as the research presents a balance of risks and expected direct benefits similar to those available in the normal clinical setting. The ACP [American College of Physicians] guidelines allow surrogates to consent to research involving incapable subjects only "if the net additional risks of participation (including the risk of foregoing standard treatment, if any exists) are not substantially greater than the risks of standard treatment (or of no treatment, if none exists)." In addition, they suggest that there should be "scientific evidence to indicate that the proposed treatment is reasonably likely to provide substantially greater benefit than standard treatment (or no treatment, if none exists)." . . .

Research Protocols Involving Greater than Minimal Risk that Do Not Offer the Prospect of Direct Medical Benefit to Subjects

The ACP and other groups take the position that greater than minimal risk research offering incapable subjects no reasonable prospect of direct medical benefit should be permitted only when authorized by a research advance directive or after review and approval at the national level, through a process resembling that set forth in the current regulations governing research involving children. The National Commission also recommended a national review process for studies that could not be approved under its other recommendations on research involving persons institutionalized as mentally infirm. However, others see this position as either too liberal or too restrictive. In NBAC's view, the proposal of national review has considerable merit. . . .

On the one hand, based on the Nuremberg Code's and the Declaration of Helsinki's convictions that vulnerable unconsenting individuals should not be put at undue risk for the sake of patient groups or society, some favor an absolute prohibition on moderate- or high-risk research offering no benefit to subjects but great promise of benefit to others. Supporters of this position contend that when these documents were created, "[i]t was presumably well understood that a price of that prohibition would be that some important research could not proceed, some research answers would be delayed, and some promising therapies and preventive measures would, for the time being, remain untested and unavailable." Some explicitly label this stance the most ethically defensible position.

On the other hand, a position paper representing federally funded Alzheimer's disease centers adopts a somewhat different view: "Research that involves potential risks and no direct benefit to subjects may be justified if the anticipated knowledge is vital and the research protocol is likely to generate such knowledge." This group also believes that a national review process is not necessarily the best way to decide whether to permit research presenting no potential direct benefit and greater than minimal risk to incapable subjects. While acknowledging that "there may be some advantages" to national review, [it] contends that "immediate and direct monitoring of such research and on-site assurance of its humane ethical conduct are at least as important as the process of evaluation and approval of any proposed research."

Special Review Panel

The regulations governing research involving children subjects provide for a special review process to address studies that offer the subjects no prospect of direct benefit and that would pose greater than a minor increment over minimal risk. . . . [For a discussion of these regulations, see Chapter 13, at page 554.]

This type of process, *if modified,* offers an additional route for assessing some protocols involving persons with mental disorders. In NBAC's view, however, a more flexible and accessible process is required. It would be appropriate for the Secretary of DHHS to establish a Special Standing Panel (SSP) which would have the authority to review and approve particular protocols, involving greater than minimal risk and do not offer the prospect of direct medical benefit to potential subjects, that could not otherwise be approved by IRBs. These protocols would be forwarded to the SSP by the local IRB. The SSP . . . would also have the authority to establish guidelines over time for delegating to local IRBs the authority to approve certain types of protocols in this arena.

NBAC urges the Secretary of DHHS, when constituting the SSP, to be mindful of the reports NBAC has received from the research community asserting that a significant amount of important research may fall into this category and that medical progress for many suffering persons may very well depend upon the ability of IRBs to approve appropriate protocols in this area. In designing the SSP, the Secretary also should take into account the experience of the current panel mechanism identified in 45 CFR 46.407(b). In particular, NBAC believes that it is essential for the SSP to conduct its work in a timely and efficient manner. Although the mechanism for special cases in research with children has been used only twice, NBAC believes that a similar but modified mechanism could fulfill its intended purpose in research involving persons with mental disorders that may affect decisionmaking capacity.

Therefore, NBAC strongly encourages the Secretary to ensure sufficient administrative support of, and financing for, the SSP and to adopt procedures for the operation of the panel such that will: (a) make case-by-case decisions using a process that is easily accessible to IRBs; and (b) develop as appropriate, and issue, guidelines for categories of research that then can be used by IRBs without having to utilize the SSP. In addition, the process should include public participation and a public written decision that explains the SSP's rationale for each of its decisions. The system of review recommended here will serve several important functions. Most important to NBAC is that it will increase protections for a subject population believed to have been historically underprotected. Second, it will permit research to go forward that has passed uniform expert and public review of risks and benefits.

. . . *Recommendation 10.* An IRB may approve a protocol that presents only minimal risk, provided that:

    A. consent has been waived by an IRB, pursuant to federal regulations; or

    B. the potential subject gives informed consent; or

    C. the potential subject has given Prospective Authorization [see *Recommendation 13*, reprinted at page 610 of this chapter] . . . and the potential subject's LAR gives permission . . . ; or

    D. the potential subject's LAR gives permission . . .

Recommendation 11. An IRB may approve a protocol that presents greater than minimal risk but offers the prospect of direct medical benefit to the subject, provided that:

    A. the potential subject gives informed consent; or

    B. the potential subject has given Prospective Authorization . . . and the potential subject's LAR gives permission . . .; or

C. the potential subject's LAR gives permission . . .

Recommendation 12. An IRB may approve a protocol that presents greater than minimal risk but does not offer the prospect of direct medical benefit to the subject, provided that:

A. the potential subject gives informed consent; or

B. the potential subject has given Prospective Authorization . . . and the potential subject's LAR gives permission, consistent with Recommendation 14; or

C. the protocol is approved on the condition of its approval by [a special standing panel to be convened by the Secretary of the Department of Health and Human Services] or falls within the guidelines developed by the panel, and the potential subject's LAR gives permission. . . .

Regulating Research with Decisionally Impaired Individuals: Are We Making Progress?
Diane E. Hoffmann, Jack Schwartz & Evan G. DeRenzo
3 DePaul J. Health Care L. 547 (2000)

[The following excerpt discusses a report by the Maryland Commission on Research with Decisionally Impaired Individuals, which was convened by the Maryland Attorney General to recommend state legislation on research with decisionally impaired subjects. The Commission's recommendations have not been enacted into law.]

The Commission's report included an influential analysis of the relationship among the risk-benefit profile of the research, subject assent, and third-party consent. If the research in question involved no more than minimal risk and the subject was incapable of consenting, the Commission stated that the research must be "relevant to the subject's condition." In addition, the Commission recommended that the subject "assent" or, at least not object to participation. . . .

If the research under consideration involved greater than minimal risk, the Commission recommended that the research not be performed on this population unless it included an intervention that held out the prospect of direct benefit to the subject or included a monitoring procedure "necessary to maintain the well-being of those subjects." . . .

The Commission also addressed research that posed greater than a minimal risk with no possibility of direct benefit to the subject population. Under these circumstances, the research could be conducted only if the anticipated risk of participation in the research was a "minor increase over minimal risk," the knowledge expected from the research was "of vital importance for the understanding or amelioration of the type of disorder or condition of the subjects" or could "reasonably be expected to benefit the subjects in the future." . . .

This recommendation was particularly controversial even among Commission members. One commissioner, in fact, submitted a dissenting statement focusing on this recommendation, in which he argued as follows:

> Since it is accepted that normal persons should not be enrolled in nontherapeutic research with more than minimal risk unless they can give informed and meaningful consent, it is doubly unreasonable that the institutionalized mentally infirm should be so enrolled when society has had so much recent concern for their greater protection, and when they live in environments which seriously discourage any kind of decision making and the nature of their illnesses weakens their abilities to choose responsibly in most of life's usual situations.

Lastly, the Commission addressed research that involved greater than a minor increase above minimal risk and did not hold out the prospect of direct benefit to the subject. Under these circumstances, the research could only be performed if:

. . . The research presented an opportunity to understand, prevent or alleviate a serious problem affecting the health or welfare of persons institutionalized as mentally infirm; and

. . . A national ethical advisory board and, following opportunity for public review and comment, the head of the responsible Federal department or agency have determined that:

(I)   the conduct of the research will be in accord with the basic ethical principles that should underlie the conduct of research involving human subjects; and

(II) adequate provisions are made for obtaining consent or assent of each subject or permission from a guardian of the person.

The Commission stated explicitly that "because of the importance of the ethical issues at stake, debate [on this type of research] should be in a public forum, and conduct of the research should be delayed pending Congressional notification and a reasonable opportunity for Congress to take action regarding the proposed research."

NOTES AND QUESTIONS

1. NBAC also recommended that IRBs "should not approve research protocols targeting persons with mental disorders as subjects when such research can be done with other subjects." NATIONAL BIOETHICS ADVISORY COMMISSION, *supra*. Which of the following situations would be approvable under the NBAC recommendations (in each case assuming a surrogate decision-maker gives consent)?

(a) Researchers conduct a minimal risk study comparing two over-the-counter antacid drugs on a group of patients with moderate Alzheimer's disease.

(b) A genetic defect causes both severe mental retardation and a unique type of pancreatic dysfunction. Persons with this defect are to be enrolled in a more-than-minimal risk study that compares two methods for treating the pancreatic dysfunction.

(c) A study designed to find out more information about the causes of Alzheimer's disease involves hospitalizing persons with that condition for two days and giving them various intravenous compounds. It does not offer any possibility of benefit to the subjects, and involves a minor increase over minimal risk.

(d) A person with severe Alzheimer's disease is suffering from pancreatic cancer, for which there are few good treatments. There is a study that randomizes subjects between standard chemotherapy and a new drug that has not yet been FDA approved. The study's eligibility criteria permit anyone with pancreatic cancer to be enrolled.

2. How do NBAC's recommendations about the scope of surrogates' authority to consent to greater-than-minimal risk research differ from the regulations governing research with children? How do they differ from the Maryland Commission's recommendations? Which approach do you consider more appropriate?

3. Should policies governing surrogate consent to research with incapacitated adults be similar to those governing parental consent to research with children? Or are there reasons to give surrogates either broader or narrower decision-making authority than parents?

4. The New York State work group discussed above issued recommendations similar to those of the Maryland commission. See NEW YORK STATE WORK GROUP, *supra*. Shortly after the recommendations were announced, John Cardinal O'Connor, the Archbishop of New York, strongly criticized the proposal to allow surrogate consent to research involving a minor increase over minimal risk and no prospect of direct benefit to subjects:

> "It is in no way even remotely to impute bad faith or evil intentions to any of these researchers in our state, to anyone in the Department of Health in our state," he said at St. Patrick's Cathedral. "But every one of us perhaps could profit by a periodic reminder that much of what was done under the Nazi regime under Hitler began long before with the experiments of psychiatrists and other medical persons on people who were psychologically incapacitated or otherwise vulnerable."

Naomi Toy & Gregg Birnbaum, *O'Connor: No-Consent Testing Recalls Nazis*, N.Y. POST, Jan. 18, 1999, at 5. What do you think of the Cardinal's reference to the Nazis in this context?

5. None of the three proposals discussed above — NBAC, the Maryland Commission, or the New York State work group — has been enacted into law. Why do you think that is the case?

6. Imagine that you are in a state such as Kentucky, which has a surrogate decision-making statute that appoints relatives to make "health care decisions" for a person who lacks capacity (KY. REV. STAT. ANN. § 311.631), and no other relevant laws. In that state, could such a surrogate consent to enroll a person into (a) a minimal-risk study; (b) a study that involves a minor increase over minimal risk but no prospect of direct medical benefit to the subject; (c) a study that involves more than a minor increase over minimal risk, but offers no prospect of direct medical benefit to the subject; or (d) a study that meets the test of 45 C.F.R § 46.405 (relating to research on children, but in this instance applied to adults)? If you were a member of an IRB in that state, which of these studies would you find to be approvable? Based on what reasoning?

7. Answer the questions posed in note 6, but assume you are in California, and thus subject to California Health and Safety Code § 24178 (reprinted earlier in this chapter at page 608).

8. Missouri has a statute specifically dealing with enrolling subjects in research. It states that when "an adult person, because of a medical condition, is treated by a teaching hospital for [an accredited] medical school . . . and such person is incapable of giving informed consent for an experimental treatment, test or drug, then such treatment, test or drug may proceed upon obtaining consent of" certain surrogate decision-makers. MO. REV. STAT. § 431.064. Answer the questions posed in note 6, assuming that you are in Missouri.

9. Might the fact that a subject lacks decision-making capacity be relevant to the determination of whether a particular intervention involves more than a minimal risk? For example, is the possibility of short-term pain a more significant risk in a study involving a 92-year-old demented patient than in a study involving healthy middle-aged adults?

10. For additional discussions of the Maryland commission's proposal (including its full text) and similar issues, see volume 1 of the *Journal of Health Care Law & Policy* (1998), which is devoted to a symposium on research with decisionally impaired subjects.

§ 14.05 CONSTITUTIONAL CONSIDERATIONS

T.D. v. NEW YORK STATE OFFICE OF MENTAL HEALTH
Appellate Division of the Supreme Court of New York,
650 N.Y.S.2d 173 (1996)

The issues presented for determination in this matter concern the validity of regulations promulgated by the defendant New York State Office of Mental Health (OMH). The regulations, promulgated on November 7, 1990, state that their purpose is to "seek to ensure the protection of patients who participate in research while, at the same time, facilitating research into the very disorders from which they suffer and which underlie their impairment." Contained in the regulations are provisions which set out procedures for, and thereby sanction, the participation of adults and children, who are patients or residents of OMH operated and licensed facilities deemed incapable of giving consent, in so-called "more than minimal risk" nontherapeutic and possibly therapeutic experiments. These studies involve, *inter alia,* the administration of both Food and Drug Administration (FDA) approved and experimental antipsychotic and psychotropic drugs, which are capable of causing permanent harmful or even fatal side effects and/or highly invasive painful testing procedures on subjects with no benefit or only the possibility of a beneficial effect expected from their participation. Moreover, several of the studies involve a medication-free or placebo phase in which subjects, who are being successfully treated with approved drugs, are taken off the medication for a period of time before the experimental medication is introduced, during which time they may relapse and suffer the adverse symptoms of their particular illnesses or disorders.

The challenged regulations attempt to adequately provide, *inter alia,* for prescreening of potential subjects to ensure that participation in a particular study "does not come into substantial conflict with their individual service plans," and for obtaining consent or assent from the potential subject or, in the case of individuals who are deemed incapable of giving consent under the regulations, from one of a number of other individuals identified in the regulations as possible surrogates for the purpose of providing consent or from a court of competent jurisdiction. However, upon our review, we conclude that the challenged regulations do not adequately safeguard and therefore violate the State and Federal constitutional rights to due process, as well as the common-law right to personal autonomy, of the patients and residents in OMH licensed or operated facilities who are, or potentially may be, subjects for the experimentation at issue. In addition, we agree with the hearing court that the Commissioner of the OMH lacked the authority to promulgate the challenged regulations governing human subject research as such authority is given exclusively to the Commissioner of the Department of Health pursuant to article 24-A of the Public Health Law. . . .

It may very well be that for some categories of greater than minimal risk non-therapeutic experiments, devised to achieve a future benefit, there is at present no constitutionally acceptable protocol for obtaining the participation of inca-pable individuals who have not, when previously competent, either given spe-cific consent or designated a suitable surrogate from whom such consent may be obtained. The alternative of allowing such experiments to continue, without proper consent and in violation of the rights of the incapable individuals who participate, is clearly unacceptable. . . .

Plaintiffs herein are six individuals who are involuntarily hospitalized . . . at OMH supervised psychiatric facilities, and who have been adjudicated mentally incapable of giving or withholding informed consent. Each has been medicated over his or her objections and therefore fears being considered "incapable" pur-suant to the challenged regulations and forced to participate in the types of experimentation specifically challenged in the complaint.

[In a portion of the opinion not excerpted here, the court concluded that the reg-ulations were invalid because the Legislature granted the Commissioner of Health, not the Commissioner of Mental Health, the authority to enact regu-lations for the protection of human research subjects.]

It is evident that, even though the subject regulations have been declared invalid and unenforceable, defendants will seek to continue to carry out the human subject research at issue herein in the future. Therefore, analysis of the plaintiffs' constitutional and common-law claims is appropriate. . . .

The record demonstrates that defendants' experiments involving more than minimal risk expose the subjects to, *inter alia,* invasive and painful procedures and/or the administration of psychotropic drugs, antipsychotic drugs and other medications, which have harmful side effects as severe or even worse than sim-ilar medications and procedures currently used for treatment. Therefore, defen-dants' practices for assessing capacity and obtaining consent for such experimentation must, at the very least, provide the same safeguards to the con-stitutional and common-law rights of the incapable patients, who may be poten-tial subjects of these experiments, as provided to patients over whose objection treating physicians seek to administer, solely for therapeutic purposes, med-ications, that can cause similar side effects. It must be kept in mind throughout this discussion, that we are dealing herein with research that offers no benefit or only minimal benefit to the subject, as opposed to treatment where the sole motivation is a beneficial therapeutic effect on the patient with minimal adverse side effects. . . .

[T]he focus herein is upon the provisions applicable to children and adults deemed incapable of giving or withholding consent for participation in experi-ments involving more than minimal risk. Such individuals are in a position analogous to that of involuntarily committed individuals, who, in the context of treatment, may be subject to administration of medication without their consent and/or over their objection.

In *Rivers v Katz*, the leading case in this State on the subject, the Court of Appeals reaffirmed the principle of personal autonomy in this State's common law and explicitly held that "the due process clause of the New York State Constitution affords involuntarily committed mental patients a fundamental right to refuse antipsychotic medication." Plaintiffs in *Rivers* were involuntarily committed patients in State institutions whose refusals to be medicated with antipsychotic drugs were overruled following the administrative review procedures then in effect.

While the Court rejected any arguments that either mental illness or involuntary commitment, in and of itself, in any way diminishes the mentally ill individual's fundamental liberty interest in avoiding unwanted administration of antipsychotic medication, it recognized that the right to reject treatment with such medication is not absolute, and that in certain emergency situations, such as where the individual presents an imminent danger to himself or those in immediate proximity to him, that right may yield to compelling State interests. However, the Court expressly rejected any implication that State interests unrelated to the patient's well-being or those in close proximity to the patient can outweigh the individual's fundamental autonomy interest.

The Court held that in situations where the State's police power is not implicated, and the patient refuses to consent to the administration of antipsychotic drugs, there must be a judicial determination of whether the patient has the capacity to make a reasoned decision with respect to the proposed treatment before the drugs may be administered pursuant to the State's *parens patriae* power. . . .

Plaintiffs herein also have the benefit of the protection of the Due Process Clause of the Fourteenth Amendment of the United States Constitution. . . .

Therefore, in order to be sustained as constitutional and otherwise viable, the regulations here at issue must, at the very least, contain appropriate and specific provisions for notice to the potential subject that his or her capacity is being evaluated and for appropriate administrative and judicial review of a determination regarding capacity.

The regulations generally provide that no capable patient shall become involved or remain in research over his or her objection and that such patients have the right to withdraw consent to participate after the commencement of the research. However, once a patient is deemed incapable, his or her ability to have an objection to participation or continued participation honored is severely, and as we find below, in some instances impermissibly, curtailed by provisions allowing for override of the objection and for surrogate consent by individuals other than legal guardians and/or individuals designated pursuant to a durable power of attorney. Thus, the determination of capacity or lack thereof is the key determination under the regulations. . . .

The general principle under which the regulations operate with respect to the participation of incapable patients is stated at 14 NYCRR 527.10(d)(6). There, it is provided that research that involves patients who lack the capacity to consent may not be approved unless the IRB has determined and documented that the study cannot be conducted without the involvement of incapable subjects. The section provides further that research that involves more than minimal risk and/or invasive procedures may only involve incapable subjects if the IRB determines and documents that the project is likely to produce knowledge that has overriding therapeutic importance for the understanding or treatment of a condition that is presented by the patient. However, paragraph (7) of section 527.10(d) provides that an IRB may waive the conditions established in the above-stated paragraph (6) for a patient who lacks the capacity to consent, if the IRB determines and documents that the research holds out a prospect of direct benefit that is important to the general health or well-being of the patient and is available only in the context of the research. The term "benefit" is left undefined, and therefore could be viewed as any benefit important to the general health and well-being of the patient whether or not related to the patient's condition. Moreover, it is apparent that "a prospect of direct benefit" important to the general health or well-being of the subjects is something significantly less than what is expected or intended in a treatment context. Thus, it is apparent that, under the general principles of the regulations, if a research project holds out any prospect for a direct benefit that may or may not relate to the specific condition presented by the incapable patients, the limiting conditions of 14 NYCRR 527.10(d)(6) may be waived and researchers may involve incapable patients in greater than minimal risk studies, which could be carried out using capable patients, but to which no capable individual would submit. This option provided to researchers is cause for alarm, given the inadequacies of the regulations discussed below. . . .

The provisions concerning the assessment of a potential subject's capacity do not adequately protect the common-law privacy and due process rights of potential subjects. The regulations do not identify or set out specific or even minimum qualifications for the individual or individuals who initially assess a potential subject's capacity, and do not contain a specific protocol for how the assessment is to be carried out. Further, there are no provisions requiring any notice to the patient that his or her capacity to provide or withhold consent for a particular study is being questioned. Consequently, there is no provision for review of a determination of lack of capacity at the patient's request. . . .

It is apparent therefore that the regulations were drafted to provide maximum flexibility in the assessment of capacity with the primary consideration being the researchers' need to determine an individual patient's suitability for the specific study involved. To that end, the IRB has complete discretion in designating the individual or individuals who will make the assessment and who will thereafter review the researcher's initial assessment; no other requirements are stated. While the regulations provide the IRB with the authority to have persons not affiliated with the research evaluate capacity, in practice, it is often the researchers or others affiliated with them who conduct interviews and make the initial determination. . . .

This practice is unacceptable given the significance of a determination of lack of capacity and the absence of any provision for patient-requested review of the determination of capacity, and in light of the provision for surrogate consent. Subdivision (e)(2)(iv) of the regulations allows for any one of a number of individuals, other than a legal guardian or a committee of the person, to be accepted as a surrogate for the purposes of obtaining informed consent. While these individuals may be related to the patient, or, in the case of a "close friend" as defined in the regulations, swear in an affidavit that they have sufficient contact and concern for the patient to be allowed to give consent, in neither case is the individual appointed as guardian pursuant to a finding of legal incapacity . . . or in any way guaranteed to act in the patient's best interests. . . . [I]t is possible that, under regulations, an otherwise capable person may be determined to be incapable for defendants' purposes because he or she is found to lack the ability to understand and make a decision about whether or not to participate in a specific study. In that event, neither the determination of lack of capacity itself nor the decisions of the surrogate are reviewable at the patient's request. Indeed, given the lack of a notice requirement, the patient may not even be informed of either determination and may not even be aware he or she is involved in research. Therefore, we hold that the provisions for determining a potential subject's capacity under the challenged regulations fail to adequately protect the individual's due process rights guaranteed under both the New York State and United States Constitutions and declare them unconstitutional for that reason.

The law with respect to surrogate decision-making in health care has been developed mainly in the context of the termination or withholding of treatment. The basic rule in New York is that in the absence of specific legislation, and where there is no evidence of personal intent, a surrogate has no recognized right to decide that a patient's quality of life has declined to a point where treatment should be withheld and the patient allowed to die.

Defendants contend that the reasoning of the case law in this State concerning surrogate decision-making resulting in the withholding of life-sustaining treatment, "suggests that surrogate decision-making that does not involve the withholding of treatment so as to lead to the patient's death is permissible under the common law of this State." Defendants argue therefore that surrogate consent for participation in research, being "quite a different matter" from a decision to withhold treatment, should be allowed. Defendants' argument is unpersuasive with regard to the greater than minimal risk nontherapeutic studies with which we are concerned herein. It is not disputed that participation in studies involving greater than minimal risk exposes the subjects to possible harmful, and even fatal, side effects. Thus, similar substantive and procedural safeguards should be provided to these potential research subjects as are provided to patients in life-sustaining treatment settings.

Defendants also rely on the argument that the Legislature has provided for surrogate decision-making in various other health care treatment situations and maintain that the provisions of their regulations regarding surrogate consent are derived from these statutes. As examples defendants cite Public Health Law articles 29-b (the "do-not-resuscitate law") and 29-C (the "health care proxy law"), and Mental Hygiene Law articles 80 (surrogate decision-making committees and panels for major medical treatment of mentally disabled persons) and 81 (appointment of a guardian for personal needs and property management). However, unlike defendant's regulations, each of these statutory schemes contains provisions for notice to the individual patient and/or exhaustive administrative and judicial review procedures. . . .

Defendants contend, however, that Mental Hygiene Law articles 80 and 81 are not appropriate vehicles for obtaining surrogate consent to participation in research because "a person can be capable of providing consent for his or her health care needs in general, and thus ineligible for surrogate decision making pursuant to these statutes, but at the same time be incapable of understanding the issues necessary to provide informed consent to participation in research." Given the absence of notice and review provisions, this contention of defendants states precisely the reason why their practices are unacceptable with respect to greater than minimal risk nontherapeutic experiments. A person otherwise competent to make health care choices may, by defendants' standards, be found incapable to understand the issues necessary to provide consent for research and then be enrolled in a study involving greater than minimal risk based on the consent of a surrogate, without ever being informed. Such a practice is unacceptable for treatment purposes, let alone for research, involving significant risk of harm and offering no benefit. . . .

Lastly, we examine the portion of the regulations that allow for the objection of an incapable patient to be overridden. While the regulations provide generally that no incapable patient shall become or remain a research subject over his or her objection or over the objection of any of the persons authorized to consent on the patient's behalf, that objection can be overridden by "a psychiatrist who is not associated with the research" who "finds and documents that the intervention or procedure involved in the research holds out a prospect of direct benefit that is important to the health or well-being of the patient and is available only in the context of the research and a court of competent jurisdiction specifically authorizes overruling the objection." . . .

The provisions allowing for override of a patient's objection do not require notice to the patient or patient's representative. . . . Therefore, the patient has no opportunity to seek administrative or judicial review of the psychiatrist's determination. . . . Both sections dealing with participation over the objection of the research subject base the override on the finding of a psychiatrist that the intervention or procedure involved holds out "a prospect of direct benefit." [T]he nature of the benefit is left undefined. Thus, the benefit while required to be important to the health or well-being of the adult or minor patient, is not required to be a product of the research procedures or even related to the psychiatric condition presented by the patient.

We take notice of the fact that a new generation of more powerful, faster acting psychiatric drugs predicted to be "10 times better than those we have now," with fewer unwanted effects, is forthcoming from the pharmaceutical industry, and that "the race to market is on" with several of the new drugs "close to or already undergoing the first phase of clinical trials, tests for toxicity and side effects in humans." It has also been reported that "[m]ost major pharmaceutical companies report a surge in research on new psychiatric drugs." It is evident that, given the motivation to test these medications and quickly bring them to market, industry-sponsored studies, which will not rely on Federal funds and therefore will not be strictly subject to Federal guidelines and oversight, will proliferate. These developments serve to highlight the importance of safeguarding the rights of incapable adults and minors, who may be potential subjects of greater than minimal risk studies involving psychiatric medications, through constitutionally acceptable protocols and guidelines promulgated by the appropriate agency.

NOTES AND QUESTIONS

1. In portions of the opinion not reprinted here, the court reached similar conclusions about research involving minors.

2. In the last paragraph of the opinion, the Court states that industry-sponsored studies that do not rely on federal funds "therefore will not be strictly subject to federal guidelines and oversight." Is that statement correct?

3. The court was particularly concerned about the regulatory provisions governing capacity determinations, notice to patients, and objections by patients. What aspects of those provisions posed due process problems, according to the court? Could the regulations be changed to avoid those problems? If so, how?

4. Much of the court's opinion is concerned with the need for greater procedural protections for determining whether a person has the capacity to make his or her own decisions. Do you think the court would find Recommendation 8 from the NBAC Report acceptable?

> For research protocols that present greater than minimal risk, an IRB should require that an independent, qualified professional assess the potential subject's capacity to consent. The protocol should describe who will conduct the assessment and the nature of the assessment. An IRB should permit investigators to use less formal procedures to assess potential subjects' capacity if there are good reasons for doing so.

Would it be a good thing to implement such a proposal? What modifications might you suggest?

5. Perhaps the most controversial part of this opinion was the court's observation that it "may very well be that for some categories of greater than minimal risk nontherapeutic experiments, devised to achieve a future benefit, there

is at present no constitutionally acceptable protocol for obtaining the participation of incapable individuals who have not, when previously competent, either given specific consent or designated a suitable surrogate from whom such consent may be obtained." Having read the rest of the opinion, can you better define which types of "greater than minimal risk nontherapeutic experiments" the court would probably put into that category? If you accept the court's conclusions, to what extent do you think this would prevent important types of research from being conducted?

6. Assuming that there were adequate procedures in place to review the decisions made by surrogate decision makers, what do you think this court would say about each of the following standards for enrolling subjects: (a) NBAC's Recommendation 11 (see supra, page 616); (b) NBAC's Recommendation 12 (see supra, page 617); (c) 45 C.F.R. § 46.405 (if applied to studies involving adults who lack decision-making capacity); and (d) 45 C.F.R. § 46.406 (again, if applied to adults who lack decision-making capacity)?

7. The decision excerpted above was issued by the Appellate Division of the New York State Supreme Court, which is the court that hears appeals from the state's trial courts. The plaintiffs subsequently appealed that decision to the New York Court of Appeals, the highest court in the state. Although they were satisfied with the Appellate Division's constitutional analysis, they argued that the court erred in limiting its holding to non-federally funded research; the appeal sought to extend the ruling to all research conducted by OMH, regardless of its source of funding. The Court of Appeals concluded that, because the Appellate Division had struck down the challenged regulations, the plaintiffs had "received the complete relief sought in this litigation" and therefore had "no grounds for appeal." It further observed that:

> once the Appellate Division in its decision below had concluded that the challenged regulations were invalid because OMH lacked statutory authority to promulgate them, it was unnecessary under the circumstances here presented to prospectively declare the regulations invalid on additional common-law, statutory, and constitutional grounds. In doing so, the Appellate Division issued an inappropriate advisory opinion.

T.D. v. New York State Office of Mental Health, 91 N.Y.2d 860 (1997). Thus, most of the legal analysis you just read in the excerpt from the Appellate Division opinion has no binding legal effect, because that court was not supposed to be discussing these issues.

8. For additional discussion of the *T.D.* case, see, e.g., Stephan Haimowitz et al., *Uninformed Decisionmaking: The Case of Surrogate Research Consent*, 27 HASTINGS CENTER REP., Nov.-Dec. 1997, at 9 (a criticism of the Appellate Division opinion by officials of the New York State Office of Mental Health, a defendant in that case); Paula Walter, *The Mentally Incompetent and Medical/Drug Research Experimentation: New York Saves the Day for the Underdog*, 6 HEALTH L.J. 149 (1998).

Chapter 15

RESEARCH WITH PRISONERS

The classic "captive population," prisoners are an especially vulnerable class of potential research subjects. Historically, researchers viewed prisoners as an easy source of research subjects. (When prisoners were not available, orphans and residents of the poor house were frequently used as a convenient substitute.) Today, federal regulations and state laws significantly limit the extent to which prisoners can be used as research subjects, to the point that some prison advocates now claim that prisoners are being unfairly excluded from the potential benefits of research participation. As you read this chapter, keep in mind the challenge of protecting prisoners from exploitation by researchers without unduly restricting prisoners' access to potentially beneficial research. Consider whether existing federal and state policies appropriately balance the twin goals of protection and access to research in the prison setting.

§ 15.01 GENERAL CONSIDERATIONS

[A] Health Status and Health Care in Prisons

On Research on HIV Infection and AIDS in Correctional Institutions
Nancy Dubler & Victor Sidel
67 MILBANK Q. 171, 177-78 (1989)

Rudimentary health care has been provided to confined inmates since the mid-nineteenth century. In England in 1784, social reformer Sir George Onesiphorus Paul instituted basic procedures for hygiene, not for the benefit of the prisoners, but rather to increase the "salutory humiliation" of prison life and to prevent the spread of epidemic disease beyond the prison walls to the general citizenry. The object was clear: "The daily cleanups and hygienic inspections were intended not only to guard against disease, but also to express the State's power to order every feature of the institutional environment, no matter how minor."

Health care in most correctional settings was woefully inadequate through the late 1960s when, following the revolt at Attica and the reports of civil rights advocates who had experienced incarceration, citizen groups, civil liberties organizations, and newly funded prisoners' rights attorneys began to investigate conditions of confinement. The descriptions presented to the federal courts were shocking: prisoners performing surgery on fellow inmates; inmates left to die with wounds covered with maggots and encased in their own filth; and systems that separated sick and disabled inmates from medical care givers by two locked sets of doors and no means of communication across them. A survey by the American Medical Association in 1973 to determine the health care capacity of jails found that among over 3,000 jails surveyed, 82 percent had no formal arrangement for any medical care; 18 percent said they called a doctor when needed; 65 percent had only first aid available on site; and 16.7 percent had no medical facility, not even a first-aid kit. . . . Since then federal court decisions have documented continuing and severe health deprivations in many states.

2 THE HEALTH STATUS OF SOON-TO-BE-RELEASED INMATES: EXECUTIVE SUMMARY VIII-IX NATIONAL COMMISSION ON CORRECTIONAL HEALTH CARE
(2002)
http://www.ncchc.org/stbr/Volume2/ExecutiveSummary.pdf

The estimated prevalence of selected communicable diseases in prisons and jails is as follows:

- An estimated 34,800 to 46,000 inmates in 1997 were infected with HIV. An estimated 98,500 to 145,500 HIV-positive inmates were released from prisons and jails in 1996.

- Included among the HIV-positive inmates in 1997 were an estimated 8,900 inmates with AIDS. An estimated 38,500 inmates with AIDS were released from prisons and jails in 1996.

- There were an estimated 107,000 to 137,000 cases of STDs among inmates in 1997 and at least 465,000 STD cases among releasees: 36,000 inmates in 1997 and 155,000 releasees in 1996 had current or chronic hepatitis B infection; between 303,000 and 332,000 prison and jail inmates were infected with hepatitis C in 1997; and between 1.3 and 1.4 million inmates released from prison or jail in 1996 were infected with hepatitis C.

- About 12,000 people who had active TB disease during 1996 served time in a correctional facility during that year. More than 130,000 inmates tested positive for latent TB infection in 1997. An estimated 566,000 inmates with latent TB infection were released in 1996.

Thus, a highly disproportionate number of inmates suffer from infectious disease compared with the rest of the Nation's population. During 1996, about 3 percent of the U.S. population spent time in a prison or jail; however, between 12 and 35 percent of the total number of people with selected communicable diseases in the Nation passed through a correctional facility during that same year.

- Seventeen percent of the estimated 229,000 persons living with AIDS in the United States in 1996 passed through a correctional facility that year. The prevalence of AIDS among inmates is five times higher than among the general U.S. population.

- The estimated 98,000 to more than 145,000 prison and jail releasees with HIV infection in 1997 represented 13 to 19 percent of all HIV-positive individuals in the United States.

- The estimated 155,000 releasees with current or chronic hepatitis B infection in 1996 indicate that between 12 and 15 percent of all individuals in the United States with chronic or current hepatitis B infection in 1996 spent time in a correctional facility that year.

- The estimated 1.3–1.4 million releasees infected with hepatitis C in 1996 suggest that an extremely high 29–32 percent of the estimated 4.5 million people infected with hepatitis C in the United States served time in a correctional facility that year. The 17.0–18.6 percent prevalence range of hepatitis C among inmates — probably an underestimate — is 9–10 times higher than the estimated hepatitis C prevalence in the Nation's population as a whole.

- Of all people in the Nation with active TB disease in 1996, an estimated 35 percent (12,200) served time in a correctional facility that year. The prevalence of active TB among inmates is between 4 and 17 times greater than among the total U.S. population.

Prevention and Control of Infection with Hepatitis Viruses in Correctional Settings
Cindy Weinbaum et al.
52 MORBIDITY & MORTALITY WEEKLY REP. 1, 5 (January 24, 2003)
http://www.cdc.gov/mmwr/PDF/RR/RR5201.pdf

Upon incarceration, all adults and the majority of juveniles lose access to the usual public and private health-care and disease-prevention services. Their health care becomes the sole responsibility of either the correctional system (federal, tribal, state, or local), or less frequently, the public health system.

For the majority of persons, entry into the correctional system provides an opportunity to access health care. In one series, approximately 78% of newly incarcerated females had abnormal Papanicolaou smears, and >50% had vaginal infections or STDs. However, the rapid turnover of the incarcerated population, especially in jails, and the suboptimal funding of correctional health and prevention services, often limits the correctional system in providing both curative and preventive care.

Infectious diseases — including acquired immune deficiency syndrome (AIDS), STDs, TB, and viral hepatitis — are more prevalent among correctional inmates than the general population. In 1997, an estimated 46,000–76,000 prison and jail inmates had serologic evidence of syphilis; 8,900 had AIDS (4% of the U.S. AIDS burden); and 1,400 had active TB (4% of the U.S. TB burden).

Among incarcerated persons, shared risk factors (e.g., injection-drug use) can result in populations coinfected with HBV, HCV, or HIV. Coinfections can make treatment of chronic viral hepatitis, AIDS, and TB more difficult because of the need to use multiple drugs, which increases the chance of hepatotoxicity and other adverse events. In addition, both TB chemoprophylaxis and HIV postexposure prophylaxis can be complicated by the presence of chronic liver disease.

United States: *Mentally Ill Mistreated in Prison: More Mentally Ill in Prison Than in Hospitals*
Press Release, Human Rights Watch
(October 22, 2003)
http://www.hrw.org/press/2003/10/us102203.htm

According to the 215-page report, *Ill-Equipped: U.S. Prisons and Offenders with Mental Illness*, prisons are dangerous and damaging places for mentally ill people. Other prisoners victimize and exploit them. Prison staff often punish mentally ill offenders for symptoms of their illness — such as being noisy or refusing orders, or even self-mutilation and attempted suicide. Mentally ill prisoners are more likely than others to end up housed in especially harsh conditions, such as isolation, that can push them over the edge into acute psychosis.

"Prisons have become the nation's primary mental health facilities," said Jamie Fellner, director of Human Rights Watch's U.S. Program and a co-author of the report. "But for those with serious illnesses, prison can be the worst place to be."

Woefully deficient mental health services in many prisons leave prisoners undertreated — or not treated at all. Across the country, prisoners cannot get appropriate care because of a shortage of qualified staff, lack of facilities, and prison rules that interfere with treatment.

According to Human Rights Watch, the high rate of incarceration of the mentally ill is a consequence of underfunded, disorganized, and fragmented community mental health services. State and local governments have shut down mental health hospitals across the United States, but failed to provide adequate alternatives. Many people with mental illness — particularly those who are poor, homeless, or struggling with substance abuse problems — cannot get mental health treatment. If they commit a crime, even low-level nonviolent offenses, punitive sentencing laws mandate imprisonment. . . .

[The Human Rights Watch report] describes prisoners who, because of their illness, rant and rave, babble incoherently, or huddle silently in their cells.

They talk to invisible companions, living in worlds constructed of hallucinations. They lash out without provocation, beat their heads against cell walls, cover themselves with feces, mutilate themselves until their bodies are riddled with scars, and attempt suicide.

The Human Rights Watch report documents how prisoners with mental illness are likely to be picked on, physically or sexually abused, and manipulated by other inmates, who call them "bugs." For example, a prisoner in Georgia, who is both mentally ill and mildly retarded, has been raped repeatedly and exchanges sex for commissary items such as cigarettes and coffee.

Mentally ill prisoners can find it difficult if not impossible to comply with prison rules, and end up with higher than average rates of disciplinary infractions. Security staff — who usually lack training in mental illness — do not distinguish between the prisoner who is disruptive or fails to obey an order because of illness and a prisoner who causes problems for other reasons.

NOTES AND QUESTIONS

1. The Bureau of Justice Statistics releases an annual study of the number of people incarcerated in the United States. It reported that, at the end of 2002, there were 2,166,260 Americans in local jails, state and federal prisons, and juvenile detention facilities. In particular, 442,300 of those prisoners were black men from age 25 to 29, which amounts to 10.4 percent of all black men in the U.S. from that age group. By comparison, 2.4 percent of Hispanic men and 1.2 percent of white men in the same age group were in prison. That report also documented that fifty-seven percent of jail inmates reported they were under the influence of alcohol or drugs at the time they committed their offense. *See* Fox Butterfield, *Study Finds 2.6% Increase in U.S. Prison Population*, N.Y. TIMES, July 28, 2003, at A12. How might these characteristics of the prison population be relevant to the development of public policies on prison research?

2. As reported in the *New York Times* in 2003, "jails and prisons have become giant incubators for some of the worst infectious diseases." Experts commented that "the high rate of communicable diseases among inmates is a critical issue for two reasons: the danger inmates pose of infecting others when they are released, and the opportunity to treat them that is largely being wasted." Fox Butterfield, *Infections in Newly Freed Inmates Are a Rising Concern*, N.Y. TIMES, Jan. 28, 2003, at A14.

3. The Eighth Amendment to the U.S. Constitution forbids the government from inflicting "cruel and unusual punishments." In *Estelle v. Gamble*, 429 U.S. 97 (1976), the United States Supreme Court ruled that "deliberate indifference to serious medical needs of prisoners constitutes the unnecessary and wanton infliction of pain proscribed by" that Amendment. *Id.* at 104. The Court reasoned that, to put inmates in a setting where they could not arrange for their own care,

and then not to provide that care, amounted to precisely the sort of torture that the Eighth Amendment was designed to prohibit.

4. Despite the holding in *Estelle*, the data presented above demonstrate that prisoners often do not receive adequate health care. What implications do these data have for policies on prison research? Do they provide a public health justification for increased research related to the health problems of prisoners? Do the limited health care options available to prisoners affect prisoners' ability to provide informed consent to participate in research?

5. It is often impossible to distinguish between a refusal of care and a denial of care in a correctional setting. For example, if an inmate does not appear for a scheduled intervention or procedure, it is possible that he has: (1) decided not to come; (2) been barred from coming by a guard; (3) been taken to the court for an unscheduled appearance; or (4) received an unscheduled visitor. Can you think of any way for researchers and IRBs to deal with this problem?

6. Maintaining confidentiality is virtually impossible in prisons or jails. All of the walls are open. Everyone sees who moves where in the institutions and can speculate on what that movement means. Thus, a trip to a research unit that is directing its attention to research on AIDS or Hepatitis C makes quite clear what the inmate's visit portends. How might researchers design studies so that exposure of inmates' health status is kept to a minimum?

8. In thinking about the consequences of introducing research into prisons, keep in mind the power dynamics inherent in the prison setting. The following excerpt from a prison inmate magazine is particularly sobering:

> Louisiana pays its prisoners from two to five cents an hour for their labors, an amount grossly inadequate to meet their needs. To augment that income, many inmates sell their "plasma" twice weekly to the privately-owned plasma company located in the Main Prison, getting $9.50 each time. The process involves the plasma firm drawing a pint of blood from the inmate, extracting the plasma, then returning the "red blood" back to the inmate. Whenever the bag containing the donor's blood accidentally bursts, preventing the return of the blood into the inmate, the firm's policy is to suspend the inmate from the plasma program for six weeks to allow sufficient time for his blood cells to build back up. Such a suspension entails a total loss of $114 income for the inmate, money he would have earned during that six-week period.

> But, as it turns out, the bursting of the blood bags of some donors weren't (sic) always caused by accidents. According to information from inmates and security personnel, a number of inmate-employees of the plasma firm were threatening to deliberately bust the bags of homosexuals and inmates in protective custody units if the inmate-victim did not agree to "belong" to them. It was reported that such threats were also utilized to extort sex from them.

According to an informed source, some of the inmate-victims complained to the Warden's office, providing names of those allegedly involved in the homosexual extortion scheme. And, in a move that caught the entire Main Prison by surprise, the Warden's Office ordered the immediate transfer of nine inmate plasma workers out of the Main Prison to out-camps, all those believed to be involved. "I've been in this business for a long time, and I thought I knew all the prison games," the source told The Angolite, shaking his head, "but this is a new one on me . . . 'starving them out,' they called it."

Office for Protection from Research Risks, IRB GUIDEBOOK, available at http://www.hhs.gov/ohrp/irb/irb_chapter6ii.htm#g6. Can IRBs do anything to ensure that this sort of behavior will not occur?

9. If you were on an IRB reviewing a protocol for prison research, what would you want to know about the prison, its population, and the health care options available to inmates? What sorts of ongoing oversight mechanisms might you want to require to help ensure the integrity of the research?

[B] History of Medical Research in Prisons

Beneficial and Unusual Punishment:
An Argument in Support of Prisoner Participation
in Clinical Trials
Sharona Hoffman
33 IND. L. REV. 475 (2000)

Throughout history many different cultures used prisoners for biomedical experimentation. In ancient Persia physicians were permitted to utilize incarcerated individuals as research subjects. The Roman empire subjected prisoners to the testing of poisons. Eighteenth century European physicians exposed prisoners to venereal disease, cancers, typhoid, and scarlet fever in order to conduct medical research.

In the United States the earliest known experimentation involving prisoners dates back to 1914, when white male convicts in Mississippi were used in pellagra studies. Pellagra is a disease that causes dermatitis, diarrhea, dementia, and, at times, death. The purpose of the experiment was to induce pellagra in twelve volunteers and to study the effects of diet on the disease. All twelve received pardons and survived, but they were not permitted to leave the clinical trial, even after suffering severe symptoms and begging to be released from it.

In California, between 1919 and 1922, hundreds of prisoners took part in a testicular transplant experiment, designed to test whether lost male potency could be reinvigorated. During World War II great enthusiasm developed for prisoner experimentation, and prisoners signed up for research trials in large numbers in order to show their patriotism. In New York scores of inmates volunteered for daily doses of various drugs to assist the Army in determining whether soldiers could carry full workloads under the drugs' influence. New Jersey supplied the Army with willing participants for research regarding sleeping sickness, sand-fly fever, and dengue fever. In the Stateville Penitentiary in Illinois, more than 400 prisoners were included in a two-year-long study aimed at finding a cure for malaria, and at the U.S. Penitentiary in Atlanta 600 inmates participated in other malaria research. As these experiments were developed, researchers began utilizing informed consent forms to provide test subjects with information regarding the trials so that investigators could claim that participants understood the studies in which they enrolled and so that authorities could be absolved from legal repercussions. A considerable portion of participants in the malaria studies received pardons as a reward for their bravery. . . .

The Ohio prison system was involved in some of the most dangerous and controversial experiments of the mid-1950s. The research was conducted in conjunction with the Sloan-Kettering Institute for Cancer Research and Ohio State University's medical research department. Inmates volunteered to be injected with live cancer cells in both forearms. Two weeks after the injection, the affected area of one forearm would be surgically removed for study, while the malignant cells remained in the other forearm for an indefinite period of time.

Medical experimentation in the 1950s was not limited to physical ailments. At the Ionia State Hospital in Michigan, at least 142 inmates participated in secret mind-control experiments for the CIA. The CIA gave numerous "sexual psychopaths" LSD and marijuana in order to "test the effectiveness of certain medications in causing individuals to release guarded information under interrogation."

Biomedical experimentation on prisoners could be extremely lucrative for doctors. Dr. Austin R. Stough, an Oklahoma physician, is estimated to have earned approximately $1 million a year by selling blood plasma extracted from volunteer prisoners in Oklahoma, Arkansas, and Alabama and by using the prisoners for drug testing. His customers included Bristol-Myers, Merck, Sharp & Dohme, Upjohn, Lederle, and American Home Products.

Throughout the 1960s, in fact, drug companies competed for access to prison populations. In 1964, Upjohn and Parke-Davis contributed over a half million dollars to build a state of the art laboratory inside the State Prison of Southern Michigan at Jackson, which was the largest walled penitentiary in the world and housed 4,100 inmates. Inmates were trained to run the tests in prison labs themselves and were paid between $.35 and $1.25 per day, a small fraction of what employees doing such work would earn in a non-prison environment.

Medical experimentation in prisons continued throughout the 1960s and early 1970s. In 1969 eighty-five percent of all new drugs were tested on prisoners in forty-two prisons. As late as 1975 at least 3,600 prisoners in the United

States were used by drug companies as the first humans on whom the safety of new medication was tested. The federal government, through the Atomic Energy Commission, funded a decade-long radiation study on inmates in Oregon and Washington State prisons. The experiments were designed to determine how much radiation U.S. astronauts could tolerate during space flights. Prisoners volunteered for the testing and received small monetary payments, but were required to undergo radiation exposure to their testicles at rates equivalent to approximately twenty diagnostic x-rays. Test subjects suffered painful, lasting effects, and, according to some estimates, almost half of them have since died. From 1970 to 1975 five agencies of the federal government utilized prison inmates in 125 biomedical experiments and nineteen behavioral research studies.

In Petersburg, Virginia, Dr. John L. Sever of the National Institutes of Health conducted a rubella project, exposing prisoners to the disease for sixteen weeks at a time. Inmates earned twenty dollars for their participation. In California and Arizona prisoners were involved in weightlessness experiments for the National Aeronautics and Space Administration. Prisoners were required to remain in bed at all times, some for over six months. In addition, some were placed in compression suits and were forced to endure repeated blood and calcium tests and radioactive isotope injections. Subjects were paid fifty dollars per month and an additional fifty dollars for completing the study. They also signed informed consent forms, and these, unlike their predecessors, provided inmates with some degree of protection by stating that the consent forms "shall not be construed as a release of NASA from any future liability."

BAILEY v. LALLY

United States District Court for the District of Maryland,
481 F. Supp. 203 (D. Md. 1979)

Plaintiffs, . . . current and former state prisoners, initiated this class action . . . on behalf of all prisoners who were incarcerated at the Maryland House of Correction (MHC), a medium security penal institution, on or after December 7, 1973, and who participated in any medical research tests in the Medical Research Unit (MRU) of the MHC. Defendants are prison administrators, officials of the University of Maryland and the University of Maryland School of Medicine under whose auspices the medical research was sponsored, and doctors on the faculty of the University of Maryland School of Medicine who were responsible for conducting the research studies at the MRU. Presented herein, in a non-jury trial, after the disposition of other issues, is the issue of whether conditions of incarceration at the MHC were so bad and the inducements to participate in the MRU so great that the prisoners' participation in the medical research program was not voluntary and therefore in violation of constitutional rights to due process, privacy and protection against cruel and unusual punishment. Many of the facts were stipulated. Others are determined herein following trial.

The MHC was opened in 1879. Various additions and new facilities have been since incorporated. Conditions at the institution often have been the subject of controversy; certain of those conditions related to overcrowding have been declared unconstitutional.

The design capacity of the MHC is approximately 1100. The population of the MHC on January 1 during the years 1971 to 1975 ranged from 1498 to 1617. Approximately 978 prisoners were housed two men to a cell at any one time from 1971 through 1975. The cells which housed two men measured about 40 square feet and were designed for one person. There were sometimes time-consuming problems in finding compatible cellmates. Prior to 1976 there was no hot water in the cells at the MHC. Heat in the winter was inadequate and the institution was very hot in the summer. The building suffered from lack of repairs; the environment has been described as dreary and some have characterized the living conditions as barbaric. Overcrowding resulted in an excessive noise level, sanitation problems, and adverse psychological effects, including increased stress, anxiety and fear. . . .

[The court describes the conditions of employment at the prison. Unemployment was chronic, ranging from 16 to 37 percent. The $2 per /day for the MRU was excellent, steady pay, which many prisoners desired.]

The MRU live-in section contained 34 beds, which were generally 70-75 percent occupied. The unit was air conditioned, adequately heated, and quiet. It had hot water at all relevant times, color television, and three separate bathroom facilities. The new MRU facilities were opened in 1972 and complied with all relevant public health regulations. Prisoners participating on in-patient studies and confined to the MRU had certain advantages: "[T]he physical set-up . . . is considered superior in many ways to the normal correctional situation. Not only is the volunteer free to do as he wishes, but he associates with persons who are not inmates nor guards and has a definite break in routine."

Prisoners found out about the MRU through several methods, including word of mouth. Participation by prisoners in the MRU was initiated by application. Application forms were published in the prison newspaper and, during some periods, those forms were given to prisoners when they entered the MHC. There was no other solicitation of volunteers. The defendant doctors testified that there was always a shortage of volunteers and that some studies had to be aborted because of insufficient volunteers. On the other hand, those who did volunteer seemed generally willing to participate again, usually, apparently, because the prisoner who volunteered wanted to make the extra money.

[The opinion discussed the informed consent process and focused on the fact that the prisoners could drop out from the study at any time.]

[The opinion detailed studies involving non-therapeutic interventions addressing various infectious diseases, including malaria, cholera, shigella, viral diarrhea, influenza, typhoid, E. Coli and rhubivirus. The court concluded that the inmates agreed to stay in the studies for the money paid to them.]

For various reasons some volunteers would not be accepted for a particular study. Those accepted were again told what they should expect while on the study and were again asked if they wanted to be on the study and told that they could withdraw without any adverse consequence if they so desired. Many did withdraw for various reasons and at various stages both before and during a study. One doctor (Dr. Gilman) characterized attrition as "out-of-sight."

[The court then describes the rigorous nature of the review of the proposals by various federal agencies and by the Human Volunteers Research Committee (HVRC) of the University of Maryland School of Medicine, which functioned as the University's IRB.]

While there is no legal or moral objection to the participation of normal volunteers in research, there are problems surrounding the participation of volunteers who are confined in an institution. Many aspects of institutional life may influence a decision to participate; the extent of that influence might amount to coercion, whether it is intended or not. Where there are no opportunities for productive activity, research projects might offer relief from boredom. Where there are no opportunities for earning money, research projects offer a source of income. Where living conditions are unsatisfactory, research projects might offer a respite in the form of good food, comfortable bedding, and medical attention. While this is not necessarily wrong, the inducement (compared to the deprivation) might cause prisoners to offer to participate in research which would expose them to risks of pain or incapacity which, under normal circumstances, they would refuse. In addition, there is always the possibility that the prisoner will expect participation in research to be viewed favorably, and to his advantage, by prison authorities (on whom his other few privileges depend) and by the parole board (on whom his eventual release depends). This is especially true when the research involves behavior modification and may be termed "therapeutic" with respect to the prisoner. In such instances, participation inevitably carries with it the hope that a successful result will increase the subject's chances for parole. Thus, the inducement involved in therapeutic research might be extremely difficult to resist; and for this reason, special protection is necessary for prisoners participating in research whether or not the research is therapeutic.

[The court discussed the draft federal regulations on prison research, what is now Subpart C of 45 C.F.R. part 46.]

While this debate was taking place, numerous articles concerning the medical research at the MHC were accepted and published in medical journals. Over 100 articles concerning that research have been published since 1971, 45 since 1974. The articles appeared in such highly regarded journals as the *New England Journal of Medicine* and the *Journal of Infectious Diseases*. The acceptance of an article for publication apparently implies that the study discussed by the article is viewed as having been conducted in accordance with medically ethical standards. No article concerning a study at the MHC was ever refused because the study had been conducted in an unethical manner. . . .

Constitutional Issues

A. Cruel and Unusual Punishment

Plaintiffs contend that the poor prison conditions, idleness, and high level of pay relative to other prison jobs render the prisoners' participation in the studies conducted in the MRU coerced and in violation of their Eighth and Fourteenth Amendment rights.

The tests as to whether defendants' conduct subjected plaintiffs to cruel and unusual punishment or deprived plaintiffs of substantive due process are well established. In *Estelle v. Gamble,* 429 U.S. 97 (1976), Mr. Justice Marshall wrote concerning cruel and unusual punishment:

> The history of the constitutional prohibition of "cruel and unusual punishments" has been recounted at length in prior opinions of the Court and need not be repeated here. It suffices to note that the primary concern of the drafters was to proscribe "torture(s)" and other "barbar(ous)" methods of punishment. Accordingly, this Court first applied the Eighth Amendment by comparing challenged methods of execution to concededly inhuman techniques of punishment.
>
> Our more recent cases, however, have held that the Amendment proscribes more than physically barbarous punishments. The Amendment embodies "broad and idealistic concepts of dignity, civilized standards, humanity, and decency . . . ," against which we must evaluate penal measures. Thus, we have held repugnant to the Eighth Amendment punishments which are incompatible with "the evolving standards of decency that mark the progress of a maturing society," or which "involve the unnecessary and wanton infliction of pain."

A violation of substantive due process occurs when the acts of the defendants "shock the conscience" of mankind. . . .

Medical research studies offered at least a partial escape from [the poor prison conditions] since the MRU provided a clean, less-restrictive environment, and those who took part in its experiments were paid more than were prisoners generally except in a few other prison jobs. Additionally, some volunteers who did not live in the MRU and who had other jobs were able to earn money from both endeavors. The prisoners testified (and the doctors did not contest) that prisoners volunteered principally because of the money inducement and because they also hoped that their participation in the MRU would influence their chances for parole. While prisoner volunteers were told, either as a matter of course or upon a question being raised, that participation in the MRU program would have no impact on parole, "hope springs eternal in the human breast" and almost surely so did in the breast of each volunteer at the MRU. Nevertheless, it is to be noted that while some of the plaintiffs have stated that parole was never raised as a subject and that they were not told that participation would not affect parole, no prisoner has stated that parole was ever promised to any volunteer or that any volunteer was ever told that his parole would be facilitated through participation in the MRU. Additionally, the testimony of the prisoners indicates that they understood that they were free to withdraw from the studies at any time and that indeed some of them did withdraw for various reasons. Some prisoners participated only in out-patient studies and withdrew upon learning that a study would be in-patient. . . .

The doctors made diligent, continuing efforts orally to inform the prisoner volunteers concerning the various studies. They did not simply rely on a written consent form. They also made it clear to the inmates that the latter were free to withdraw at any time. Prisoners participating in studies were regularly and carefully examined and any volunteer who became ill received prompt, high-grade medical attention.

Accordingly, nothing in defendants' conduct of these studies is "incompatible with evolving standards of decency" nor "shocks the conscience" of mankind. That does not mean that there is not strong reason to question or disapprove of the use of prison inmates for research purposes. The issue of informed consent is a most thorny one. Informed consent consists of two elements: information and voluntariness. There is no question that the prisoner volunteers were informed. Each doctor who testified detailed the procedures already described to provide information to the applicants. Plaintiffs' allegation of coercion thus hinges on lack of voluntariness growing out of unconstitutional conditions such as overcrowding and other undesirable aspects of regular institutional life at the MHC. Those conditions may well have caused inmates to value even a few additional hours outside of their cells as worth the risk of participation in the MRU. That plus the high level of pay may have made such participation very attractive to certain inmates. Yet, while the level of pay was an inducement, some prisoners did not find it sufficiently attractive so as to be worth the risk of losing the right to return to their cells or their jobs. Further, there was always a shortage of volunteers. Only some 14 percent of all prisoners who went through the MHC during the years here involved participated in the medical studies. Thus, the program was hardly universally or overwhelmingly attractive to most inmates. . . .

Prisoners at the MHC were not subject to physical abuse, or confined in segregated cells, or restricted to meager diets, until they consented to participate in MRU studies. Prisoners were not pressured to participate. To the contrary, prisoners had a viable choice and, even after choosing to participate, had the option to withdraw from the medical studies. The defendant doctors, closely watched by the HVRC and other review committees, took the necessary measures to assure that the prisoners were exercising their free choice. . . .

In sum, though the MRU may have appeared attractive to some prisoners, the totality of the record fails to disclose any violation of the fundamental right of every person, including each inmate, to be free from undue coercion.

NOTES AND QUESTIONS

1. Do you agree with the reasoning of the court?

2. In one of the studies at issue in *Bailey*, the informed consent form disclosed the following risks:

> You may develop acute "viral diarrhea." You may have fever, abdominal pain, diarrhea and vomiting. If you agree we would like to obtain a small piece of small or large intestine. On rare occasions following such a procedure small amounts of intestinal bleeding might result and even more rare is the occurrence of intestinal perforation which might require blood transfusions and surgery.

Are these the type of risks to which prisoners should be asked to consent?

3. Consider the following guidance statement from the Office for Human Research Protections (OHRP):

> In addition to problems of coercion and undue inducement, the involvement of prisoners in research raises questions of burden and benefit. Prisoners should neither bear an unfair share of the burden of participating in research, nor should they be excluded from its benefits, to the extent that voluntary participation is possible. Prisoners' rights to self-determination (autonomy) should not be circumscribed more than required by applicable regulations. IRBs should refrain from assuming, without cause, that prospective prisoner-subjects will lack the ability to make autonomous decisions about participation in research. To the extent that prisoner-subjects are found able to voluntarily consent to participation, and to the extent allowable under applicable regulations, prisoners should be allowed the opportunity to participate in potentially beneficial research.

OHRP GUIDANCE ON THE INVOLVEMENT OF PRISONERS IN RESEARCH (May 23, 2003), available at http://www.hhs.gov/ohrp/humansubjects/guidance/prisoner.htm. Does this statement support the court's reasoning?

§ 15.02 FEDERAL REGULATION OF PRISON RESEARCH

[A] Overview of Subpart C

45 C.F.R. PART 46, SUBPART C (§§ 46.301-46.306): ADDITIONAL PROTECTIONS PERTAINING TO BIOMEDICAL AND BEHAVIORAL RESEARCH INVOLVING PRISONERS AS SUBJECTS

These provisions are reproduced in Appendix A, at page A-23. Please review them before proceeding.

NOTES AND QUESTIONS

1. What type of person should IRBs look for in appointing a "prisoner representative"? Should he or she be a person of color or someone with training in cultural sensitivity? Would an advocate from the local Legal Aid Society suffice? What about a former correctional officer or a warden, or the local prison or jail chaplain?

2. Assume that you are a member of an IRB that is considering research similar to the studies at issue in *Bailey v. Lally*. The prisoner representative on the IRB is a former inmate, and he sympathizes with the desire of inmates to maximize their income while in prison. If that person votes to approve the protocol, what weight would you give his decision? On questions related to the appropriateness of prison research, are the views of the prisoner representative entitled to greater deference than those of the other IRB members?

3. Does Section 305 provide adequate direction to the IRB for reviewing prison research? Are there issues not covered in that section that IRBs should be required to address?

4. What is the rationale for prohibiting parole boards from taking into account a prisoner's participation in research in making decisions regarding parole? Do you agree that a prisoner's willingness to participate in research should never be used in parole determinations?

5. Consider the types of permissible research detailed in Section 306(a)(2). Is it clear what is being designated under each subsection? Can you think of examples of research that might be approvable under the first two subsections?

6. Note that the first two subsections under Section 306(a)(2) require the IRB to determine that the risks to prisoners are "minimal." The definition of "minimal risk" under Subpart C (§ 46.303(d)) is different from the definition applicable to other parts of the regulations (§ 102(i)). What are the specific differences between the two definitions? What are the implications of those differences for prison research?

7. Given the prevalence of hepatitis C in prisons and the serious nature of the disease, would it be appropriate to conduct a clinical trial in a prison comparing a new treatment for the disease against standard treatment? Under Section 306(a)(2)(D), would the Secretary have to consult with experts and publish notice to the public before approving such a study? What if the subjects in the control group were given a placebo? Is it appropriate to condition the requirement for expert consultation and public notice on whether the "control groups" will "benefit from the research?" Does such a requirement implicitly assume that subjects receiving the investigational intervention will necessarily benefit?

8. Compare the requirements of Section 306(a)(2)(D) with those of Section 405, which applies to research with children that offers "a prospect of direct ben-

efit to the individual subjects." Under the children's regulations, it is not enough for the IRB to find that an intervention or procedure offers a possibility of benefiting the subjects; it must also find that "the relation of the anticipated benefit to the risk is at least as favorable to the subjects as that presented by available alternative approaches." 45 C.F.R. § 46.405(b). Under the prisoners' regulations, by contrast, the IRB need only find that practices being studied have "the intent and reasonable probability of improving the health or well-being of the subject." 45 C.F.R. § 46.306(a)(2)(D). In what type of studies might the difference between these two provisions be relevant? What do you think accounts for the difference?

9. The regulations do not address the challenges facing research staff when they are working in correctional settings. For example, if there is a research protocol studying sexually transmitted diseases, and the researcher finds that a particular prisoner has been raped by a fellow inmate, what is she to do? How should she balance the obligation to protect the subject's confidentiality against the prison's interest in deterring and punishing prison violence? Should the IRB require investigators to anticipate and develop plans for addressing these sorts of issues?

10. DHHS has waived the applicability of §§ 46.305(a)(1) and (a)(2) for epidemiological research conducted or supported by DHHS that meet the following criteria:

(1) In which the sole purposes are

  (i) To describe the prevalence or incidence of a disease by identifying all cases, or

  (ii) To study potential risk factor associations for a disease, and

(2) Where the institution responsible for the conduct of the research certifies to the Office for Human Research Protections, DHHS, acting on behalf of the Secretary, that the IRB approved the research and fulfilled its duties under 45 C.F.R. § 46.305 (a)(2)-(7) and determined and documented that

  (i) The research presents no more than minimal risk and no more than inconvenience to the prisoner-subjects, and

  (ii) Prisoners are not a particular focus of the research.

Department of Health and Human Services, *Waiver of the Applicability of Certain Provisions of Department of Health and Human Services Regulations for Protection of Human Research Subjects for Department of Health and Human Services Conducted or Supported Epidemiological Research Involving Prisoners as Subjects*, 68 FED. REG. 36929 (2003). Does this waiver seem reasonable in light of what you have read about prisons and jails and in light of the overall regulatory structure?

11. The federal regulations are not the only source of limitations on prison research. Many states have their own prison research laws, which are often much more restrictive than the federal regulations. Twenty-two states have laws prohibiting all biomedical research involving prisoners. *See* Hoffman, *supra*, at 492.

[B] OHRP Questions to NHRPAC on the Interpretation of Subpart C

The National Human Research Participant Advisory Committee [NHRPAC] was established as an advisory committee to OHRP in 2000. The Secretary's Advisory Committee on Human Research Protections (SACRHP) has since replaced this committee and has similar functions, as was discussed in Chapter 2. One of the tasks these committees were asked to undertake was an analysis of the continuing appropriateness of Subpart C.

LETTER FROM DR. GREG KOSKI, DIRECTOR OF OHRP, TO MARY FAITH MARSHALL, CHAIRPERSON OF NHRPAC
(APRIL 9, 2002)

Dear Dr. Marshall:

As you know, the National Human Research Protections Advisory Committee (NHRPAC) has responsibility for providing expert advice and recommendations to the Department of Health and Human Services, through the Director of the Office for Human Research Protections (OHRP). As Director of OHRP, I request that NHRPAC provide to the Department advice and recommendations on current requirements for research involving prisoners as subjects in Subpart C of Title 45 C.F.R. Part 46. Specifically, I am asking NHRPAC to: (1) provide recommendations for guidance on the current Subpart C; and (2) consider whether or not Subpart C is adequate; if not, provide recommendations on how Subpart C should be revised. More details are provided below.

Provide recommendations for guidance on the current Subpart C for the following:

- § 46.301(a): Should Subpart C apply to research involving a subject who is not a prisoner when he or she enrolls in a study but becomes a prisoner later during the study?

- § 46.303(c): What should the term "prisoner" encompass under the definition provided in the regulations? For example, should the term "prisoner" include someone civilly committed to a mental institution based on a "not guilty by reason of insanity" defense; or, to someone under house arrest?

- § 46.304(b): What would constitute appropriate background and expertise for an individual to serve as a "prisoner representative"?

- § 46.305(a)(7): What would constitute "adequate provision" for follow-up examination or care of participants *after* their participation has ended (OHRP notes that *after participation* can extend beyond the period of incarceration)?

- § 46.306(a)(2)(iv): How should "research on practices . . . which have the intent and reasonable probability of improving the health or well-being of the subject" be interpreted?

- § 46.306(a)(2)(iv): How should "control groups which may not benefit from the research" be interpreted? For example, should a control group where subjects receive only standard medical interventions for a particular disorder be considered as benefiting or not benefiting from the research?

2. Consider whether or not Subpart C is adequate; if not, provide recommendations on how it should be revised. For example:

- Is the current Subpart C adequate to ensure appropriate inclusion and avoid inappropriate exclusion of prisoners in research?

- Should the requirement for institutions to certify to the Secretary that the Institutional Review Board (IRB) has fulfilled its duties under Subpart C be retained (*see* 45 C.F.R. § 46.305(b))?

- Should the requirement that the Secretary judge that the research involves solely one of the four categories of research stipulated under 45 C.F.R. § 46.306(a)(2) be retained?

- Are the current four categories in 45 C.F.R. § 46.306(a)(2) sufficient? Should more categories be added?

NOTES AND QUESTIONS

1. Under current OHRP policy, an investigator who discovers that a subject has become a prisoner after enrollment in the study must report this fact to the IRB, and all interventions involving the subject must cease until the IRB is satisfied that the requirements of Subpart C have been satisfied. *See* OHRP GUID-ANCE ON THE INVOLVEMENT OF PRISONERS IN RESEARCH (May 23, 2003), available at http://www.hhs.gov/ohrp/humansubjects/guidance/prisoner.htm. What is the rationale for imposing the Subpart C requirements with regard to someone who chose to participate in a study before he became a prisoner? Assume you are a member of an IRB that learns that a subject in a Phase 3 study of a new cancer drug has been imprisoned. What facts would you want to know about the prison conditions and the level of care the individual can expect in the prison

before deciding whether it would be appropriate to allow the individual to continue in the study?

2. What should the IRB do when it can reasonably be anticipated that some of the subjects in a protocol might be incarcerated during the course of the research, such as in a protocol involving intravenous drug users with histories of prior incarceration?

3. The SACHRP Subcommittee on Subpart C suggested that the definition of "prisoner" under the federal regulations be changed to read:

> any individual involuntarily confined or detained (1) in a penal institution, medical or mental health facility, work release facility, halfway house, or prerelease facility, as a result of a criminal proceeding, or (2) in a penal institution due to a commitment pursuant to a civil statute, including those confined for civil or criminal contempt or as a material witness. This should include persons confined in medical or mental health facilities by virtue of statutes or commitment procedures that provide alternatives to criminal prosecution or incarceration in a penal institution or individuals detained in such facilities pending arraignment, trial, or sentencing.

See SUBCOMMITTEE ON 45 C.F.R. § 46, SUBPART C, REPORT TO SACHRP (July 26, 2004), available at http://www.hhs.gov/ohrp/sachrp/mtgings/mtg07-04/present/subpartc_files/frame.htm. How does this proposal differ from the existing definition? Which definition is preferable?

4. One could argue that application of Subpart C should depend on whether there is a substantial curtailment of the person's liberty such that the person cannot do, go, or act as she pleases. If that nexus to deprivation of liberty is not sufficiently close to trigger a formal application of Subpart C, the IRB could still require additional protections for subjects by treating them as a "vulnerable population" under Subpart A of the regulations. *See* 45 C.F.R. § 46.111(a)(3). How would this approach apply to a newly released prisoner in a halfway house who is subject to reincarceration for any infraction of the rules? If this person is not considered a "prisoner" under Subpart C, would treating him as a member of a "vulnerable population" under Subpart A provide adequate protection?

§ 15.03 THE SHIFT FROM PROTECTION TO ACCESS

Should we presume that prisoners necessarily want to be "protected" from research? Consider the following:

> When the National Commission visited the Jackson State Prison in Michigan on November 14, 1975, they met with a group of highly articulate prisoners. The leader of the group greeted them with the following opening statement: "Ladies and gentlemen: You are in a place where death at random is a way of life. We have noticed that the only place in

this prison that people don't die is in the research unit. Just what is it that you think you are protecting us from?

Nancy Dubler & Victor Sidel, *On Research on HIV Infection and AIDS*, 67 MIL-BANK Q. 171, 185-86 (1989) (quoting Alan Bronstein). In the intervening thirty years, criticism of the protectionist stance of prison research policies has increased.

On Research on HIV Infection and AIDS in Correctional Institutions
Nancy Dubler & Victor Sidel
67 MILBANK Q. 171, 171-72 (1989)

The AIDS epidemic challenges traditional analyses of public health responsibilities and civil liberty protections. Urgent demands for prevention and treatment also require us to rethink many of our regulations and practices, including the elaborate regulatory provisions and professional proscriptions that have been developed to protect research subjects from the risks of innovative but untested therapies. Since there are specially identified problems in conducting research on prisoners, for whom federal regulations governing research on human subjects specifically provide additional protection, and since a disproportionate number of prisoners suffer from HIV infection, the AIDS epidemic poses unique problems and unique opportunities in jails and prisons for epidemiological research on HIV infection and AIDS and for the conduct of clinical trials of new treatments.

Indeed, the AIDS epidemic may be reversing the ways in which the public, in general, and regulatory agencies, in particular, think about risk and innovation in human experimentation and drug development. As is often the case, two perspectives competed for ascendancy — one intent on minimizing risk, the other eager to foster useful innovation. Until very recently most regulatory bodies, including the wide variety of institutional review boards for the protection of human subjects (IRB) and the United States Food and Drug Administration (FDA), defined the essence of their mission in terms of protection: the protection of the human subject from the excesses of researchers. The presumption that most often guided policy was the risk-minimizing one: unless researchers and drug companies were carefully regulated, abuse was likely to follow. The public seemed to concur in these policies, ready to support the presumption that researchers left on their own would allow scientific curiosity, eagerness to conquer disease, and possibly desire for fame and personal gain to take precedence over all other considerations, including the immediate well-being or the autonomy of the human subjects of their research.

The pressures generated by the AIDS epidemic may be transforming this orientation and definition of purpose. It is this prospect that forces the rethinking of policy on epidemiological and therapeutic research on prisoners. Challengers to the FDA process are demanding bureaucratic and regulatory change to permit early approval and subsequent wide distribution of promising therapeutic interventions. The equilibrium is tilting, particularly in clinical trials, from restricting access to experimental protocols to enrolling as many subjects as possible. IRBs and federal regulators must consider whether these new perspectives should be allowed to alter policies and practices on experimentation in jails and prisons. With special reference to treatment, these bodies must decide whether the clinical situation of HIV disease demands a reevaluation of the previously constructed balance between protection from abuse and access to possibly beneficial treatments.

NOTES AND QUESTIONS

1. As noted above, the Supreme Court has held that "deliberate indifference to serious medical needs of prisoners" violates the Eighth Amendment to the Constitution. *See supra*, page 633. One commentator argues that, under this logic, it is a violation of the Eighth Amendment for prison officials to deny a seriously ill prisoner access to a clinical trial if the trial offers the possibility of benefiting the prisoner. *See* Hoffman, *supra*. Hoffman similarly argues that state laws restricting prison research are constitutionally invalid to the extent they deny seriously ill prisoners "promising treatment for a particular disease." *Id.* at 502. Do you find these arguments persuasive? Do you agree that clinical trials should be considered a form of medical treatment for purposes of the Eighth Amendment?

2. If sponsors of research choose to rely on prisons as a source of potential subjects, should they be required to ensure that there are adequate alternatives to research participation available in the prison? Hoffman notes that some research institutions provide ordinary medical treatment to prisoners in addition to the opportunity to participate in clinical trials. *See* Hoffman, *supra*, at 510-11. Should such arrangements be encouraged? Are there potential dangers in having a single institution both provide ordinary medical care and conduct research in prisons?

3. Rather than making it easier for prisoners to enroll in clinical trials, would it be better to give prisoners the opportunity to receive investigational interventions outside of a study, through the expanded use of "compassionate use" exemptions? (For a discussion of compassionate use exemptions, see Chapter 3, at page 147.) What are the potential advantages and drawbacks of such an approach?

4. In addition to access to experimental interventions, research may offer intangible benefits to inmates. For example, being a research subject gives prisoners access to the medical facility and its staff, who are likely to be more supportive and available than the correctional staff. In addition, "[b]iomedical research may also provide inmates with the moral satisfaction of contributing to the advancement of . . . research and with the opportunity 'to give something

back to society, to redeem, atone, and reconcile.' " Hoffman, *supra*, at 499. Should these intangible benefits be taken into account in the development of policies on prison research?

5. In addition to individual prisoners' interest in obtaining access to particular protocols, prisoners also have a stake in the *types* of research that investigators choose to conduct, and that funders choose to support. Does society have an obligation to support research relevant to the unique health problems of prisoners as a group? In determining how to spend its limited resources, how should the NIH prioritize research related to reducing the incidence of Hepatitis C in prisons, as compared to research related to health problems that do not disproportionately affect prisoners?

§ 15.04 RESEARCH WITH INCARCERATED CHILDREN

Prevention and Control of Infections with Hepatitis Viruses in Correctional Settings
Cindy Weinbaum et al.
52 MORBIDITY & MORTALITY WEEKLY REP. 1, 2 (January 24, 2003)
http://www.cdc. gov/mmwr/PDF/ RR/RR5201.pdf

In 1997, approximately 12% of persons aged 16 years reported at least one arrest in their lifetimes. In 1999, a reported 108,965 juvenile offenders were held in residential placement facilities. In 1994, the average length of stay in public facilities for juvenile releasees was 2 weeks for those detained and 5 months for those committed; the stay in private facilities (primarily a committed population) averaged 3.5 months. Of arrested juveniles not incarcerated, the majority are diverted to alternative programs (e.g., teen courts or restorative justice) where they remain under supervision of the juvenile justice system. Approximately 74% of incarcerated juvenile offenders are held in public facilities, and the rest in facilities operated by private contractors. Adult jails hold >7,600 juveniles, and approximately 3,100 are held in adult prisons. Females account for 27% of juveniles arrested and 13% of those in residential placement. Of juveniles arrested in 1999, approximately 72% were white, 25% black, and 3% of other races. However, a disproportionate number of racial and ethnic minorities were detained in residential placement (40% black and 18% Hispanic).

Biomedical and Behavioral Research on Juvenile Inmates:
Uninformed Choices and Coerced Participation
Brian Wyman
15 J.L. & HEALTH 77 (2000)

There are many reasons why juvenile inmates are an especially beneficial population of research subjects to target for conducting biomedical and behavioral research. The most prominent of those reasons is that the benefits of researching on children and prisoners are combined. Juvenile inmates for the most part consist of poor urban males. Many of the juveniles who are detained are uneducated and have a great number of medical problems upon admission to the detention facility, ranging from sexually transmitted diseases to mental illnesses. These diseases give researchers an opportunity to research and test possible cures and treatments. Something else that works to the benefit of researchers is the fact that, when admitted to the detention facility, most juvenile inmates need medical treatment and cannot afford to obtain such treatment. Juvenile inmates in such a situation will likely be willing to undergo experimental treatment if they are led to believe it will help them. Researchers can test their promising drugs and cures on these children without having to spend money coercing them, and without obtaining "assent" (consent) to the research since it directly benefits the welfare of the child. [For a discussion of the "assent" requirement in pediatric research, see Chapter 13, at page 538.]

There are also a number of behavioral problems among juvenile inmates that might lead researchers to conduct experiments on this group. Behavioral problems, depression and even learning disabilities are higher in juvenile inmates than other children. Antisocial personality disorder, borderline personality disorder, paranoid disorder, and passive-aggressive disorder are the most common personality disorders found among juvenile inmates. These are heavily researched areas of psychology, and therefore, juvenile inmates are one of the best sources for that research. . . .

One important issue that relates to juvenile inmates seeking remedies for any injury caused by research is the statute of limitations. This issue arises when side effects due to the research show up years after the actual experiment. These side effects are the injury resulting from the participation in the research while in prison. By the time the side effects are known by the former juvenile inmate, possibly now an adult, the statute of limitations may have run, which bars any claims the injured individual might otherwise be able to bring. What is referred to as the discovery rule is often the determining factor in these cases. Under the discovery rule, once the injured person discovers the injury the statute of limitations starts to run, but diligence must be used in discovering the critical facts of the injury. . . .

Coercion is a much more difficult problem among juvenile inmates than any other class or group of individuals who participate in biomedical and behavioral research. The same modes of coercion or influence that may be tolerated in research on adult prisoners would be very problematic in the experimentation on juvenile prisoners. The inducement needed to obtain consent in a vulnerable class of individuals is easier than that required for obtaining consent from average individuals. The more disadvantaged a class of individuals is, the less inducement or coercive external force is needed. The combination of prison life and maturity level of children, often with behavioral problems, makes for a very disadvantaged population. . . .

This leads to another major problem with juvenile inmates, which is that they usually have no legal representation and often fail to recognize when legal representation is needed. Juvenile prisoners can hardly seek to recover under any of the possible claims when they cannot receive legal advice. One suggestion is that the researchers and institutions that seek to conduct experiments on this particularly vulnerable population provide legal representation for the individual subjects. However, this presents a conflict of interest where the attorney would be hired by the researcher, yet at the same time represent the inmate. Again, there is a risk that the juveniles will not be able to comprehend what it is that the attorney is advising.

NOTES AND QUESTIONS

1. The OHRP guidance statement on research with prisoners includes the following question and response:

> Is an adolescent (e.g., age 14) detained in a juvenile detention facility a prisoner?

> Answer: Yes. In addition to subpart C, most likely subpart D would also apply.

OHRP Guidance on the Involvement of Prisoners in Research, available at http://www.hhs.gov/ohrp/humansubjects/guidance/prisoner.htm

Why do you think OHRP qualifies its answer by saying that Subpart D "most likely" would apply? Can you conceive of a situation in which Subpart D would not apply?

2. What sorts of research would be appropriate with incarcerated children? As discussed in Chapter 13, research with children normally requires the "permission" of the children's parents, but IRBs can waive this requirement if they determine that a study "is designed for conditions or for a subject population for which parental or guardian permission is not a reasonable requirement to protect the subjects," and an "appropriate mechanism for protecting the children who will participate as subjects in the research is substituted." *See* Chapter 13, at page 537. Could such waivers ever be appropriate in prison settings? For example, would it be appropriate to waive the permission requirement in a

study investigating risk factors for illness, disease, or bad social outcomes among incarcerated children?

3. Because many incarcerated children are in situations in which it is difficult to contact and involve parents or guardians, would it be appropriate to set up some sort of advocate team to supervise the research and give permission for the inmate children to participate? Note that this is the approach used for research with children who are wards of the state. *See* 45 C.F.R. § 46.409.

Chapter 16

FETUSES AND EMBRYOS

In a society polarized by the issue of abortion, it should come as no surprise that research involving embryos and fetuses is especially controversial. For those who believe human personhood begins at conception, embryos and fetuses are the ultimate vulnerable population — obviously incapable of consenting to research on their own behalf, and subject to abuse by a society that fails to respect their inherent rights. Other people, by contrast, believe that efforts to restrict embryo and fetal research place undue weight on the interests of those entities at the expense of patients who might benefit from such research. In studying this chapter, consider whether it is possible to be opposed to abortion while favoring at least some forms of embryo and fetal research, or to be pro-choice on abortion but against research in which a fetus or embryo might be harmed.

§ 16.01 FETAL RESEARCH

Current federal regulations on human subject protection owe their existence at least partly to the controversy about fetal research that erupted in the early 1970s, after a National Institutes of Health (NIH) advisory panel announced recommendations "encourag[ing] the use of newly delivered live fetuses for medical research before they died." ALBERT R. JONSEN, THE BIRTH OF BIOETHICS 94 (1998). These recommendations, which were released shortly after the Supreme Court's recognition of a constitutional right to abortion in *Roe v. Wade*, 410 U.S. 113 (1973), were one of the main factors that led to congressional interest in regulating research with human subjects. *See* JONSEN, *supra*, at 98. When the National Research Act was passed in 1974, it included a moratorium on federal funding of research involving fetuses "before or after abortion," but the moratorium was lifted the following year when federal regulations on research with fetuses were adopted. *See* Heather Boonstra, *Human Embryo and Fetal Research: Medical Support and Political Controversy*, GUTTMACHER REP. PUB. POL'Y, Feb. 2001, at 3.

[A] Research on Fetuses in Utero

In utero fetuses (i.e., fetuses inside a woman's uterus) can be used as research subjects for a variety of purposes, ranging from studies investigating new forms of fetal monitoring to tests of new types of surgical techniques. For obvious reasons, research on fetuses in utero necessarily entails using pregnant women as research subjects. For further discussion of research with pregnant women, see Chapter 9, at page 415.

45 C.F.R. § 46.204: RESEARCH INVOLVING PREGNANT WOMEN OR FETUSES

This provision is reproduced in Appendix A, at page A-19. Please review it before proceeding.

NOTES AND QUESTIONS

1. Under 45 C.F.R. § 46.204(b), research that does not hold out a prospect of direct benefit for either the woman or the fetus may not be approved if it poses more than a minimal risk to the fetus. What type of studies might this subdivision preclude? Contrast the limits on risk in subdivision (b) with the regulations on research with children, which in some circumstances permit greater-than-minimal risks even without a prospect of direct benefit to the children in the study. *See* 45 C.F.R. §§ 46.406, 46.407; *see also* Chapter 13, at page 548. What do you think explains the greater restrictions on risks to fetuses than on risks to children?

2. One of the most controversial aspects of § 46.204 is the requirement for the consent of the fetus's father in certain circumstances. Is it appropriate to require paternal consent to research on fetuses? Can such a requirement be reconciled with the Supreme Court's holding in *Planned Parenthood v. Casey*, 505 U.S. 833 (1992), which struck down a state law requiring women to notify their spouses before obtaining an abortion? Note that paternal consent is required only if the research "holds out the prospect of direct benefit solely to the fetus." Assuming paternal consent is appropriate because of the father's interest in the fetus's welfare, should it also be required when the research does *not* hold out a prospect of direct benefit to the fetus?

3. A new rule issued in the final days of the Clinton administration would have eliminated the paternal consent requirement for fetal research, but the Bush administration withdrew the changed rule before it went into effect. *See Bush Replaces Clinton Rule, Requires Paternal Nod for Some Studies on Fetuses*, HEALTH CARE DAILY REP. (BNA), Nov. 14, 2001. For further discussion of the paternal consent requirement, see Karen H. Rothenberg, *Gender Matters: Implications for Clinical Research and Women's Health Care*, 32 HOUS. L. REV. 1201 (1996).

4. Under the regulations, research on newborns of uncertain viability must either pose "no added risk to the neonate" or hold out the prospect of enhancing the neonate's survival. 45 C.F.R. § 46.205(b)(1). What is the difference between this "no added risk" standard and the minimal risk standard used in

the provisions governing fetuses (§ 46.204(b)) and children (§46.404)? What do you think explains the use of a different standard for research with neonates?

[B] Research on Tissue from Aborted Fetuses

Researchers have long used tissue from aborted fetuses to develop medical treatments. For example, the recipients of the 1954 Nobel Prize for Medicine used fetal tissue in their research on the polio virus, and in 1968 researchers successfully transferred fetal liver cells into patients with DiGeorge Syndrome, a genetic disorder. *See* Note, *Down for the Count? State Regulation of Aborted Fetal Tissue Research*, 37 WAKE FOREST L. REV. 217, 223 (2002). More recently, researchers used fetal tissue transplants in a highly publicized study designed to develop new treatments for Parkinson's disease. At the time of the study, many scientists expected that fetal tissue transplants would offer considerable benefits to Parkinson's patients. However, not only did those benefits fail to materialize, but many subjects who received the fetal tissue transplants ended up suffering from "disastrous" side effects. *See* Gina Kolata, *Parkinson's Research Is Set Back by Failure of Fetal Cell Implants*, N.Y. TIMES, March 8, 2001, at A1.

Opponents of fetal tissue research believe that the process "involves a 'trafficking of fetal body parts [that] not only violates basic human rights but is essentially legalized murder.'" *Down for the Count? supra* at 225. Others, however, ask "what compassionate, loving and caring person wants to mandate that fetal tissue, obtained in strict compliance with the law, be discarded when it can be used to help so many?" *Id.*

[1] Federal Law

45 C.F.R. § 46.206: RESEARCH INVOLVING, AFTER DELIVERY, THE PLACENTA, THE DEAD FETUS, OR FETAL MATERIAL

This provision is reproduced in Appendix A, at page A-21. Please review it before proceeding.

NOTES AND QUESTIONS

1. Would IRB approval be required for research with tissue from aborted fetuses in which no identifying information about living individuals will be recorded? *See* 45 C.F.R. § 101(b)(4).

2. In 1988, the Reagan administration imposed a moratorium on federal funding for research with fetal tissue from induced abortions. President Clinton issued an executive order lifting the moratorium in 1993. *See* Boonstra, *supra*, at 3-4. Later that year, Congress enacted the National Institutes of Health

Revitalization Act, which expressly authorized the Secretary of Health and Human Services to support research on the transplantation of human fetal tissue "regardless of whether the tissue is obtained pursuant to a spontaneous or induced abortion or pursuant to a stillbirth." 42 U.S.C. § 289g-1(a)(2). The Act requires the written consent of the woman donating the tissue and, if the tissue is obtained pursuant to an induced abortion, assurances that the woman's consent to the abortion was obtained before a request for donation of the tissue was made. The woman may not place restrictions on the recipients of the tissue, and she must affirm that she has not been informed of the identity of the recipients. *Id.*, § 289g-1(b). The legislation also requires the informed consent of both the researchers and any recipients of the tissue, to ensure that these individuals are aware that they are working with or receiving human fetal tissue. *Id.*, § 289g-1(c). What do you think is the rationale for each of these requirements?

3. Note that the NIH Revitalization Act does not require the consent of the father of the fetus. Given that paternal consent is required for some types of *in utero* fetal research, should it also be required for research involving tissue from fetuses that have been aborted?

4. Both the NIH Revitalization Act and the National Organ Transplant Act of 1984 prohibit the sale of fetal tissue for transplantation. *See* 42 U.S.C. §§ 289g-2, 274e. However, "both federal statutes could be interpreted to apply only to sales for transplant or therapeutic purposes, not laboratory research." NATIONAL BIOETHICS ADVISORY COMMISSION, 1 ETHICAL ISSUES IN HUMAN STEM CELL RESEARCH 33 (1999) [hereinafter NBAC, STEM CELL RESEARCH].

[2] State Law

Although research on fetal tissue is permissible under federal law, some states have laws limiting or prohibiting such research. The following case involves a constitutional challenge to one such law.

FORBES v. NAPOLITANO
United States Court of Appeals for the Ninth Circuit,
236 F.3d 1009 (9th Cir. 2000)

Plaintiffs challenge the constitutionality of an Arizona statute that criminalizes any medical "experimentation" or "investigation" involving fetal tissue from induced abortions unless necessary to perform a "routine pathological examination" or to diagnose a maternal or fetal condition that prompted the abortion. The plaintiffs include individuals suffering from Parkinson's disease who because of the statute are unable in Arizona to receive transplants of fetal brain tissue that many medical experts believe hold out promise for eventual amelioration or treatment of the disease. Plaintiffs also include doctors in Arizona who fear possible criminal prosecution if they provide services to their patients that the doctors would like to provide. . . .

Fetal tissue is also useful in diagnosing and testing for fertility problems. One of the plaintiff physicians who specializes in fertility treatments, Dr. Tamis, was the target of a potentially criminal investigation some years ago when he endeavored to study the effects on the fetus of a drug ingested by pregnant women before an induced abortion was performed. The study was to determine whether the drug passed through the placental wall. Although the state eventually dismissed the grand jury subpoenas issued to Dr. Tamis, he is still uncertain about the proper interpretation of the statute.

Other physicians and expert witnesses explain that many established treatments for illness have developed from fetal research and experimentation, including the polio vaccine. They point out the difficulties of knowing at what stage or point in time "experiments" become recognized as "treatment." They also point out that the terms "investigation" and "routine examination" are fundamentally ambiguous. In particular, the experts highlight doctors' lack of consensus about what procedures are purely experimental. In the view of one expert submitted to the district court, virtually every procedure with a therapeutic objective is experimental to some extent.

The due process clause of the Fourteenth Amendment guarantees individuals the right to fair notice of whether their conduct is prohibited by law. Although only constructive rather than actual notice is required, individuals must be given a reasonable opportunity to discern whether their conduct is proscribed so they can choose whether or not to comply with the law. Statutes need not be written with "mathematical" precision, nor can they be thus written. But they must be intelligible, defining a "core" of proscribed conduct that allows people to understand whether their actions will result in adverse consequences.

If a statute subjects transgressors to criminal penalties, as this one does, vagueness review is even more exacting. In addition to defining a core of proscribed behavior to give people constructive notice of the law, a criminal statute must provide standards to prevent arbitrary enforcement. Without such standards, a statute would be impermissibly vague even if it did not reach a substantial amount of constitutionally protected conduct, because it would subject people to the risk of arbitrary deprivation of their liberty. Regardless of what type of conduct the criminal statute targets, the arbitrary deprivation of liberty is itself offensive to the Constitution's due process guarantee. . . .

The district court concluded that these criminal statutes fail to establish any "core" of unquestionably prohibited activities. It explained this conclusion with reference to three of the statute's key terms: "experimentation," "investigation" and "routine," none of which the statute defines. With respect to "experimentation," the district court pointed out two difficulties. First, the term is ambiguous, lacking a precise definition to focus application of the statute. Second, the distinction between experimentation and treatment changes over time. The district court also found the term "investigation" to be ambiguous, since common definitions of the term can encompass pure research as well as more common, therapeutic medical techniques. In examining the statute's use of "routine pathological examinations" to carve out an exception to criminal liability, the district court determined that the term "routine" was also ambiguous. The statute itself does not define "routine," nor does the medical community provide any official standards to help. The district court was thus concerned that any examination of post-abortion fetal tissue beyond simply mounting fetal tissue on a slide could expose doctors to criminal liability. . . .

A criminal statute such as A.R.S. § 36-2302 that prohibits medical experimentation but provides no guidance as to where the state should draw the line between experiment and treatment gives doctors no constructive notice, and gives police, prosecutors, juries, and judges no standards to focus the statute's reach. The dearth of notice and standards for enforcement arising from the ambiguity of the words "experimentation," "investigation," and "routine" thus renders the statute unconstitutionally vague. . . .

The judgment of the district court is AFFIRMED.

SNEED, J., Circuit Judge, concurring:

Roe v. Wade held that the constitutional right to personal privacy encompasses a woman's decision whether or not to terminate her pregnancy. *Roe* and its progeny established that the pregnant woman has a right to be free from state interference with her choice to have an abortion. These cases do not hold that the State is under an affirmative obligation to ensure access to abortions for all who may desire them. Rather they require that the State refrain from wielding its power and influence in a manner that might burden the pregnant woman's freedom to choose whether to have an abortion.

A prohibition on aborted fetal tissue research could burden the rights of women and couples to make both present and future reproductive choices. Fetal tissue experimentation may aid in the development and continued improvement of techniques and procedures necessary to make such choices. Prohibiting research on aborted fetal tissue could prevent the advancement of important diagnostic techniques, the creation of safer abortion techniques, and the discovery of medical defects that would influence a woman's decision regarding future pregnancies.

Experimentation on aborted fetal tissue may foster the development of reproductive technology that is related to reproductive decisions. Governmental restrictions on reproductive decisions are only justifiable given compelling state interests. The Supreme Court has identified three state interests in regulating abortion: safeguarding the health of the woman; protecting the potential life of the fetus; and regulating the medical profession. None justify Arizona's prohibitions of fetal experimentation.

NOTES AND QUESTIONS

1. For other decisions invalidating state laws restricting fetal experimentation, see *Jane L. v. Bangerter*, 61 F.3d 1493 (10th Cir. 1995), *Margaret S. v. Edwards*, 794 F.2d 994 (5th Cir. 1986), and *Lifchez v. Hartigan*, 735 F. Supp. 1361 (N.D. Ill. 1990), *aff'd*, 914 F.2d 260 (7th Cir. 1990).

2. Does the majority's rationale suggest that states *must* permit fetal research? If not, how might the statute be rewritten to avoid the problems the court identified?

3. How does the concurring judge interpret the scope of the constitutional right recognized in *Roe v. Wade*? In what way does he believe the Arizona statute burdens that right? What other medical procedures might enjoy constitutional protection under the concurring judge's analysis? Is the concurring opinion consistent with the Supreme Court's decision in *Planned Parenthood v. Casey*, 505 U.S. 833 (1992), which held that states may place limits on abortion as long as those limits do not place an "undue burden" on the woman's ability to terminate her pregnancy?

4. A few states have statutes that expressly permit research on fetal remains, provided the woman who was pregnant with the fetus consents. *See* NBAC, STEM CELL RESEARCH, *supra*, at 32-33.

5. The 1987 revision of the Uniform Anatomical Gift Act (a model statute drafted by the National Conference of Commissioners on Uniform State Laws, which has been adopted in most states) prohibits the sale or purchase of any human body part, including fetal tissue. However, the law allows the payment of reasonable expenses associated with the removal, processing, and transportation of the tissue. *See* UNIFORM ANATOMICAL GIFT ACT § 10 (1987).

§ 16.02 EMBRYO AND EMBRYONIC STEM CELL RESEARCH

The development of in vitro fertilization (IVF) has made it possible for scientists to conduct research on embryos that are just a few hours or days old. With IVF, embryos are created in a laboratory by combining sperm with eggs that have been surgically retrieved from a woman's body. While it is possible for researchers to use IVF in order to create embryos specifically for research purposes (see *infra*, page 671), IVF is more often used by individuals seeking to have children. Typically, these individuals create multiple embryos at one time, transferring some of them to the woman's uterus to establish a pregnancy and freezing the remainder for possible use in the future. If they have embryos left over after their treatment is completed, they may choose to donate some or all of them to scientists for medical research. *See generally* NEW YORK STATE TASK FORCE ON LIFE AND THE LAW, ASSISTED REPRODUCTIVE TECHNOLOGIES: ANALYSIS AND RECOMMENDATIONS FOR PUBLIC POLICY (1994).

While it is possible to conduct research on embryos intended to be transferred into a woman's uterus (for example, a study of different methods of culturing embryos in the laboratory prior to implantation), researchers typically conduct research with embryos that would otherwise be discarded. This research will not benefit the embryos that are the subject of the experimentation. On the contrary, research on embryos not intended to be used to establish a pregnancy inevitably results in the destruction of the embryos.

Embryo research gained national attention in 1998, when scientists announced that they had learned how to isolate human embryonic stem cells and grow them in the laboratory. Embryonic stem cells are a small group of unspecialized cells that ultimately develop into all of the specialized cells that make up an adult organism. Under certain conditions, these cells "can be induced to become cells with special functions such as the beating cells of the heart muscle or the insulin-producing cells of the pancreas." NATIONAL INSTITUTES OF HEALTH, STEM CELL BASICS, available at http://stemcells.nih.gov/info/basics/. Scientists believe that, if they can direct embryonic stem cells to become specific cell types, they may be able to use the resulting cells to treat a variety of serious conditions, including Parkinson's disease, diabetes, traumatic spinal cord injury, heart disease, and vision and hearing loss. *See id.*

[A] Perspectives on Embryo and Embryonic Stem Cell Research

Testimony on Behalf of the Juvenile Diabetes Research Foundation International Regarding Federal Support of Juvenile Diabetes Research
Before the Senate Permanent Subcommittee on Investigations
Mary Tyler Moore
June 26, 2001

[Mary Tyler Moore, who was diagnosed with juvenile diabetes as a young adult, is the International Chairman of the Juvenile Diabetes Research Foundation.]

The only current source for islets [of Langerhans, the clusters of pancreatic cells that produce insulin and whose destruction causes juvenile diabetes] suitable for human transplant are cadaver pancreases. And in the U.S. less than 2000 such pancreases become available for transplant each year. If tomorrow we had the perfect solution to immune tolerance, we would still only be able to offer islet transplantation to a tiny fraction of the millions of people with diabetes who might benefit. There is hope, though, that an alternative, inexhaustible supply of islet cells can be created. Hope that very much depends on actions you, your colleagues, and the Administration choose to take. The hope I refer to resides in the potential of embryonic stem cells to be coaxed to develop into any cell in the body, including islet cells. This would solve the islet cell supply problem. Of course the promise of stem cell research is not exclusive to islet transplantation, or to patients with diabetes. Stem cells could, potentially, help restore vision for those with macular degeneration, prevent Alzheimers, or reverse Parkinson's disease eventually helping as many as 100 million Americans who suffer from chronic illnesses. Stem cells could improve heart muscle function after heart attack, allow spinal injury patients to walk again, or replace bone marrow in cancer patients. As a greater authority than I, Dr. Harold Varmus, former director of NIH, has stated: "it is not unrealistic to say that [stem cell] research has the potential to revolutionize the practice of medicine and improve the quality and length of life." To make our hope a reality, embryonic stem cell research requires federal support. . . .

I understand that support for this research raises concerns among people of good will, each trying to do what's right based on their very personal religious and moral beliefs. I have not shied from that personal soul searching, nor has JDRF in its policy making, nor should anyone. I have found comfort in my heartfelt view that embryonic stem cell research is truly life affirming. It is a direct outcome of a young family making a choice, without coercion or compensation, to donate a fertilized egg not used for in vitro fertilization, for research. An egg that otherwise would have been discarded or frozen forever. Because of the great potential of stem cell research, donating unused fertilized eggs is much like the life-giving choice a mother whose child has died tragically in an automobile accident makes when donating his organs to save another mother's child. It is the true pinnacle of charity to give so totally, so freely, of ones self, to give life to another. Federal support for stem cell research is, therefore, an extension of this affirmation of life and is the best way to insure it is undertaken with the highest of ethical standards.

Instruction on Respect for Human Life in Its Origins and on the Dignity of Procreation Congregation for the Doctrine of the Faith
16 Origins 702 (1987)

At the Second Vatican Council, the church for her part presented once again to modern man her constant and certain doctrine according to which: "Life once conceived, must be protected with the utmost care; abortion and infanticide are abominable crimes." More recently, the Charter of the Rights of the Family, published by the Holy See, confirmed that "human life must be absolutely respected and protected from the moment of conception." . . .

The congregation recalls the teachings found in the Declaration on Procured Abortion:

From the time that the ovum is fertilized, a new life is begun which is neither that of the father nor of the mother; it is rather the life of a new human being with his own growth. It would never be made human if it were not human already. To this perpetual evidence . . . modern genetic science brings valuable confirmation. It has demonstrated that, from the first instant, the program is fixed as to what this living being will be: a man, this individual man with his characteristic aspects already well determined. Right from fertilization is begun the adventure of a human life, and each of its great capacities requires time . . . to find its place and to be in a position to act.

This teaching remains valid and is further confirmed, if confirmation were needed, by recent findings of human biological science which recognize that in the zygote (the cell produced when the nuclei of the two gametes have fused) resulting from fertilization the biological identity of a new human individual is already constituted.

Certainly no experimental datum can be in itself sufficient to bring us to the recognition of a spiritual soul; nevertheless, the conclusions of science regarding the human embryo provide a valuable indication for discerning by the use of reason a personal presence at the moment of this first appearance of a human life: How could a human individual not be a human person? The magisterium has not expressly committed itself to an affirmation of a philosophical nature, but it constantly reaffirms the moral condemnation of any kind of procured abortion. This teaching has not been changed and is unchangeable.

Thus the fruit of human generation from the first moment of its existence, that is to say, from the moment the zygote has formed, demands the unconditional respect that is morally due to the human being in his bodily and spiritual totality. The human being is to be respected and treated as a person from the moment of conception and therefore from that same moment his rights as a person must be recognized, among which in the first place is the inviolable right of every innocent human being to life.

This doctrinal reminder provides the fundamental criterion for the solution of the various problems posed by the development of the biomedical sciences in this field: Since the embryo must be treated as a person, it must also be defended in its integrity, tended and cared for, to the extent possible, in the same way as any other human being as far as medical assistance is concerned.

The two excerpts set forth above put the controversy over embryo research in stark relief. On the one hand, supporters of such research believe that its has the potential to lead to medical breakthroughs that will save the lives of many people. On the other hand, opponents of such research believe that it amounts to murder. What are the chances of finding a compromise that would satisfy those on both sides of this debate?

The following excerpt is taken from the report of an NIH committee charged with developing federal policy on embryo research. (The committee's work is discussed further *infra*, at page 673.) As you read the excerpt, consider how individuals with strong positions for or against legalized abortion probably reacted to the report.

REPORT OF THE HUMAN EMBRYO RESEARCH PANEL
NATIONAL INSTITUTES OF HEALTH
(1994)

Single Criterion Views

A single criterion approach to analyzing the moral status of the human embryo can lead to widely different conclusions. One view holds that the embryo is a person, a being meriting full and equal moral respect, from the moment of conception or fertilization because at this moment a unique diploid genotype comes into being. For those who hold this view, humanness, in a moral sense, is the possession of a distinctive human genetic identity.

Others arrive at this same conclusion by emphasizing the significant increase in potential for development that accompanies the transition from gametes to embryo. . . .

For all who believe that moral personhood begins at conception the embryo ought to have the same moral rights as any other human research subject. No experimentation on the human embryo is permissible that would not also be allowed on the fetus in utero or on a newborn child.

Moral positions emphasizing genetic identity or developmental potential offer a definitive standpoint on the status of the embryo, but they create paradoxes in logic and run counter to many widely accepted practices, including use of the intrauterine device and other contraceptive methods that work by preventing implantation. The equation of genetic diploidy with personhood leads to a logical paradox because twinning and the aggregation of two or more morula-stage embryos (sometimes inaccurately called "recombination") can occur well after fertilization. The emphasis on potential for development raises, but does not answer, the question of just *how much* potential is needed for moral respect. It also ignores the fact that even though developmental potential increases at conception, it remains relatively low at least until implantation. For example, it is estimated that approximately 60 percent of conceptuses are spontaneously aborted in the first days and weeks of pregnancy. As the British Royal College of Obstetricians and Gynaecologists observes, "it is morally unconvincing to claim absolute inviolability for an organism with which nature itself is so prodigal."

Among other single-criterion approaches to personhood, several positions exist that come to a very different moral conclusion about the status of the preimplantation embryo. One position bases full moral personhood on sentience

— the ability to feel or to experience pain. A second view emphasizes the beginning of brain activity or brain function. This view derives from the belief that the brain is the essential organ underlying our specifically human capacities. It is also an effort to render an account of the beginning of life that is consistent with the criterion of whole-brain death as the end of life. A third position takes as the marker for the beginning of personhood certain well-developed cognitive abilities such as consciousness, reasoning ability, or the possession of self-concept.

While these views can lead to different conclusions as to when personhood begins, all support the conclusion that the preimplantation embryo does not merit the same degree of moral protection given to children or adult human beings. The absence of a nervous system until after gastrulation or neurulation makes it certain that the preimplantation embryo cannot experience pain, has no brain activity, and is not conscious or self-aware.

But these views also face conceptual and practical difficulties. Insistence on sentience as the criterion of personhood, for example, might require extending equal moral respect to animals. Some who hold this position welcome this extension, but others see it as running counter to our practices of using animals as a source of food or in scientific research. Equating personhood with an earlier stage such as the commencement of brain activity raises the same parallel with animal rights and a further question of what is meant by brain activity in this context. There are a variety of stages of early neural development to choose from, ranging from 6.5 weeks (time of earliest brain waves) to 24 to 28 weeks (when almost all sequences of nervous system development have begun). Finally, a view based on consciousness, reasoning, or the possession of self-concept might lead to the exclusion of newborns from the class of protected subjects.

A Pluralistic Approach

A second broad approach to understanding how personhood and moral protectability are established is pluralistic. It does not focus on a single criterion of personhood (such as genetic diploidy or self-concept) but emphasizes a variety of distinct, intersecting, and mutually supporting considerations. According to this view, the commencement of protectability is not an all-or-nothing matter but results from a being's increasing possession of qualities that make respecting it (and hence limiting others' liberty in relation to it) more compelling.

Among the qualities considered under a pluralistic approach are those mentioned in single-criterion views: genetic uniqueness, potentiality for full development, sentience, brain activity, and degree of cognitive development. Other qualities often mentioned are human form, capacity for survival outside the mother's womb, and degree of relational presence (whether to the mother herself or to others). Although none of these qualities is by itself sufficient to establish personhood, their developing presence in an entity increases its moral status until, at some point, full and equal protectability is required.

According to this view, the increased potentiality for development that marks the transition from gametes to zygote — and the establishment at this stage of at least the beginnings of biological uniqueness counsel giving the preimplantation embryo a measure of respect that is not due the sperm or egg. However, the absence at this stage of almost all other qualities evoking respect makes it unreasonable to think of personhood as beginning here and places limits on the degree of respect accorded. . . .

Formation of the primitive streak at 14 days of development and the beginning of cellular differentiation and organization of a single body axis marks yet another stage of development that merits an enhanced degree of protectability. As gestation continues the further development of human form, the onset of a heartbeat, the development of the nervous system leading to brain activity and with this at least some of the physical basis for future sentience, relational presence to the mother, and capacity for independent existence all counsel toward according an increasing degree of protectability. This line of thinking culminates at birth, where substantial development and independent existence outside the mother's womb provide the moral basis for full and equal personhood.

NOTES AND QUESTIONS

1. How do you think the authors of the Vatican statement, *supra* page 663, would respond to the panel's assertion that "[m]oral positions based on genetic identity . . . create paradoxes in logic and run counter to many widely accepted practices"?

2. Consider the panel's comments about the relationship between the moral status of embryos and the moral status of animals. In your view, is it justifiable to use animals in research that would not be permitted with human subjects?

3. The panel suggests that, under a "pluralistic approach," the embryo "merits an enhanced degree of protectability" as gestation proceeds. Does this approach suggest when research resulting in the embryo's destruction should no longer be permitted? What are the implications of the approach for the restrictions on *in utero* fetal research discussed above, at page 656?

4. The Supreme Court has held that a fetus is not a "person" under the Fourteenth Amendment to the Constitution. *See Roe v. Wade*, 410 U.S. 113, 157 (1973). As a result, states do not have a constitutional obligation to afford fetuses "due process of law" or the "equal protection of the laws." However, states are free to enact laws protecting fetal interests if they choose to do so, as long as those laws do not infringe on pregnant women's constitutional rights. In *Planned Parenthood v. Casey*, the Court concluded that states may enact laws designed to protect a nonviable fetus's interest in potential life as long as those laws do not impose an "undue burden" on the woman's constitutionally protected right to obtain an abortion. *Planned Parenthood v. Casey*, 505 U.S. 833, 876

(1992) (plurality opinion). After viability, states may prohibit abortion outright, as long as they make exceptions for pregnancies that endanger the pregnant woman's life or health. *See id.* at 846.

5. Many commentators agree with the position articulated in 1994 by the American Fertility Society (now known as the American Society for Reproductive Medicine), which states that embryos are not persons but that they should be accorded a "special respect" not afforded other human tissue. *See* Ethics Committee of the American Fertility Society, *Ethical Considerations of Assisted Reproductive Technologies*, 62 FERTILITY & STERILITY 33S (Supp. 1 1994). This "special respect" position is generally interpreted as consistent with at least some forms of embryo research. *See id.; see also* Geron Ethics Advisory Board, *Research with Human Embryonic Stem Cells: Ethical Considerations*, HASTINGS CENTER REP., March-April 1999, at 31, 33 (concluding that research with early embryos is consistent with the special respect position if the embryos are "used with care only in research that incorporates substantive values such as reduction of human suffering"). Is it coherent to maintain that embryos deserve special respect while authorizing research that will result in their destruction? That question is the focus of the next excerpt.

Respecting What We Destroy: Reflections on Human Embryo Research
Michael J. Meyer & Lawrence J. Nelson
31 HASTINGS CENTER REP., Jan.-Feb. 2001, at 16-23

How can one have moral respect for something that one intentionally destroys? . . . The puzzle raises two questions: Does not having an attitude of respect for something rule out its ultimate destruction? Second, even if this is not so, is not the research use and destruction of embryos "more honestly done by simply stripping [these] embryos of any value at all?"

Our answer to both questions is no. What respect requires can be an alternative both to a prohibition on destruction and to a moral license to kill. . . .

We employ the method of ascertaining moral status recently elaborated by Mary Anne Warren, who has argued convincingly that no one criterion can determine moral status. In fact, for Warren, a judgment about an entity's moral status involves seven different principles, which include both intrinsic and relational properties of the entity in question. In abbreviated form, Warren's seven principles are: (1) respect for life: living organisms may not be killed or harmed without good reasons; (2) anti-cruelty: sentient beings ought not to be killed or subjected to pain unless there is no other way of furthering goals that are both consistent with the other principles and important to entities that have higher moral status than can be based on sentience alone; (3) agent's rights: moral agents have full and equal moral rights, including rights to life and liberty; (4) human rights: within the limits of their capacities, human beings capable of sentience but not moral agency have the same moral rights as moral agents; (5) ecological importance: ecologically important entities (living and nonliving) may have a stronger moral status than they would independent of their relationship to the ecosystem; (6) interspecific communities: animals that are part of a human community may have stronger moral status than they would standing alone; (7) transitivity of respect: within the limits of the above principles and to the extent that is reasonable, moral agents should respect one another's attributions of moral status.

... In this account, moral agents have the highest moral status and possess full and equal basic moral rights. An individual who displays only minimal consciousness has the same basic moral rights and status as an agent, even though he lacks those rights his diminished capacities render irrelevant. Nonhuman but sentient creatures possess a moral status that is significant but typically less than that of humans. Other, nonsentient living entities have even lower status but still merit some, even if in most cases quite minimal, moral respect.

If Warren's account is right, human embryos have a weak moral status and deserve a weak but genuine moral respect. The moral status of embryos does not, contrary to the suggestion of some, rest exclusively on their being the result of reproductive activity. Rather, the human embryo has a claim to some moral status both in virtue of being alive and in virtue of Warren's rule of the "transitivity of respect." Although frozen embryos are in a state of suspended animation, they are still living entities, and purely gratuitous harm to or destruction of a living thing is, many would say, clearly morally problematic. When a living thing is harmed or destroyed there must be some reasonable justification for doing so. Thus while the claim that life itself is worthy of moral respect is surely controversial, it is hardly unusual, and indeed seems rather plausible if moral respect is held to admit of different levels.

The moral status of embryos also turns on the fact that, in addition to being alive, they are valued, in some cases very highly, by many people. The value ascribed to an embryo covers a wide range, of course; it is sometimes essentially given the full worth and status of a moral agent, sometimes a very high status but not at every stage the equal of a moral agent, and sometimes only very modest moral status. Some hold that an extracorporeal human embryo naturally engenders a sense of wonder, or that it is a thing of beauty. What gives rise to these reactions provides a reason to hold that the extracorporeal embryo has some modest moral status. One might, for instance, have a sense of wonder about embryos because of the simple realization that an embryo is, in some rough sense, "the stuff of life." Its beauty alone is also a distinct reason to accord it some moral status.

The transitivity principle does not depend on a defense of any particular view an agent might hold about the embryo's moral status. The whole point of the transitivity principle is that the actual valuations of other agents merit respect even when one does not share their valuations. ...

Surely, then, there is good reason to say that the extracorporeal embryo has some moral status and is worthy of some moral respect. More specifically, our interpretation of Warren's account leads us to conclude that its status is weak or modest. The only intrinsic property that provides a reason to grant it moral status is its being alive. The embryo is neither an agent, a human being capable of sentience but not agency, a nonhuman sentient creature, nor an entity of ecological significance. Nor is an embryo a person, or an early stage of a person, in the typical understandings, both metaphysical and moral, of the muddied term "person." One oft-noted reason it isn't is that an embryo prior to the formation of the "primitive streak" (which usually appears around fourteen days of development) is not clearly even an individual, as it can still be divided into twins. Personhood is usually taken to imply individuality. Another reason is that, if an embryo is maintained outside a woman's body and those who provided the gametes for it have not decided to permit its development in a womb, it is not effectively a stage in the early development of a person. Put differently, an extracorporeal embryo — whether used in research, discarded, or kept frozen — is simply not a precursor to any ongoing personal narrative. An embryo properly starts on that trajectory only when the gamete sources intentionally have it placed in a womb. . . .

The moral respect an agent has for something or someone is demonstrated in two fundamental ways: in what the agent does or refuses to do with the object of respect, and in the attitudes the agent adopts in relation to that which he or she respects. Behavior must be consistent with attitude; someone cannot legitimately claim she holds a respectful attitude about something while her behavior clearly manifests indifference, disregard, or contempt. Morally respectful behavior can assume a variety of forms: addressing the respected entity in a certain manner, protecting and preserving it from destruction or degradation, thinking of it or talking about it in terms that accurately reflect its value, and encouraging or requiring others to behave respectfully. The precise forms of respectful behavior adopted by an agent should also be congruent with the degree of respect owed to the particular object in question. To solve the puzzle of how we can show respect for what we destroy, we must recognize the moral weight of both the sincerely respectful attitude of the destroying agent toward the destroyed object, as well as the purposefully adopted behavioral manifestations of this attitude.

Sometimes people destroy something because they respect it, as when a sacred artifact is destroyed to prevent its being treated in a profane way. In contrast, embryos are destroyed in the course of research in spite of the respect they deserve. Destroying an object in spite of the respect it is owed raises the tension we seek to resolve. To illustrate how the tension might be resolved, we offer some actual examples of people who have destroyed what they truly respect. . . .

[The authors discuss Native American practices designed to show respect for animals killed for food, the Japanese practice of mizuko kuyo, a set of spiritual rituals performed by women as memorial services for their aborted fetuses, and medical schools' efforts to show respect for human cadavers used for teaching.] [These examples] suggest that respecting what one destroys should include an attitude of regret, and some sense of loss, conjoined with a display of that respect. Respecting what is destroyed should include an attitude of regret and loss because the thing one has intentionally destroyed does in fact have moral value. Even the gains reaped through its destruction do not preclude honest and open acknowledgment of the regret and loss one should feel about it. . . .

Examples of restrictions on the treatment of embryos that would show respect for them (which are independent of justifications for their destruction) would include the following: (1) human extracorporeal embryos should be used in research only if the research goals cannot be obtained with other methods; (2) the use of extracorporeal embryos more than fourteen days old should be avoided or diminished, since this point is regarded by some as the morally significant onset of embryonic individuation; (3) researchers should avoid considering extracorporeal embryos as property and in particular should avoid buying and selling them; (4) researchers should recognize that the destruction of extracorporeal embryos provides a reason for them to have and demonstrate some sense of regret or loss. Further, handling extracorporeal embryos with respect in the lab should never be an empty or insincere gesture but might include both acquiring only the minimum number of embryos required to achieve the research goals and disposing of the remains of used embryos in a way respectful of their status (for example, the remains might be treated as if they were corpses and be buried or cremated).

NOTES AND QUESTIONS

1. Some supporters of embryo research believe that only leftover embryos originally created by individuals undergoing infertility treatment should be used in research. *See*, e.g., George J. Annas et al., *The Politics of Human-Embryo Research — Avoiding Ethical Gridlock*, 334 NEW ENG. J. MED. 1329, 1331 (1996) (arguing that "it is the intention to create a child that makes the creation of an embryo a moral act"). Others maintain that "it should not matter whether researchers use embryos left over from IVF or embryos created solely for research. In both cases the embryos are at the same stage of development." BONNIE STEINBOCK, LIFE BEFORE BIRTH: THE MORAL AND LEGAL STATUS OF EMBRYOS AND FETUSES 211 (1992); *cf.* William FitzPatrick, *Surplus Embryos, Nonreproductive Cloning, and the Intend/Foresee Distinction*, 33 HASTINGS CENTER REP., May-June 2003, at 29, 34 (arguing that creating embryos specifically for research "appears to be exploitative and disrespectful in a way that the other practices are not," but that creating embryos for research is nonetheless ethically acceptable, given the embryo's low moral status). How would you react to a researcher's plan to recruit women to provide eggs to be fertilized solely for use in a scientific study? Would your reaction depend on the medical risks asso-

ciated with egg donation? The amount of money paid to the women? The scientific merit of the proposed research? Some other factor?

2. Recall the Nazis' efforts to defend their medical experimentation by pointing to examples of nonconsensual research with military personnel in the United States. *See* Chapter 1, at page 25. However, a key difference between the Nazi and American experiments was that, in the former, all of the subjects were meant to be destroyed, many in the course of carrying out the experiments. In response to the Nazis' intentional destruction of human research subjects, the Nuremberg Code contains a specific prohibition on research in which "there is an a priori reason to believe that death or disabling injury will occur." NUREMBERG CODE, ¶ 5. Is this provision of the Nuremberg Code relevant to research with embryos?

3. One commentator argues that the most common objections to embryo research do not apply to research on "nonviable" embryos, defined as embryos that, "[i]n a healthy and physiologically receptive uterus . . . would either fail to implant or would implant and then spontaneously abort." Françoise E. Baylis, *The Ethics of* Ex Utero *Research on Spare 'Non-Viable' IVF Human Embryos*, 4 BIOETHICS 311, 318 (1990). How do you think the Vatican would respond to a proposal to use nonviable embryos in scientific research?

[B] Federal Law and Policy

[1] General Federal Policy on Embryo Research

ASSISTED REPRODUCTIVE TECHNOLOGIES: ANALYSIS AND RECOMMENDATIONS FOR PUBLIC POLICY
NEW YORK STATE TASK FORCE ON LIFE AND THE LAW
382-385 (1998)

In 1974, Congress imposed a temporary ban on [federal funding of] human fetal and human IVF research pending adoption of regulations on the subject. In August 1975, the Department of Health, Education and Welfare (now the Department of Health and Human Services, or DHHS) promulgated regulations that lifted the ban. The regulations allowed federal funding of human fetal or human IVF research subject to the approval of an ethics advisory board (EAB). The Secretary of Health, Education and Welfare did not instruct the EAB to review a request for federal funding until September 1978. A research proposal was then submitted to the EAB, which issued a report in March 1979.

The EAB's report concluded that the federal government should support human embryo research, including research on embryos not intended to be transferred for implantation. According to the report, research not involving embryo transfer must comply with existing regulations governing research on human subjects, must be designed to establish the safety and efficacy of embryo transfer and to obtain scientific information not reasonably attainable by other means, and must stop fourteen days after fertilization. The report also urged researchers to obtain specific informed consent for the use of gametes in research and to inform the public of possible risks associated with the practice of IVF. No action was ever taken by the Secretary of Health and Human Services on the board's report and the board was allowed to expire in 1980. Because the regulations required the board's approval of all embryo research proposals, without a board in place no federal funding of embryo research could be authorized.

In 1993, Congress passed the National Institutes of Health Revitalization Act, which removed the requirement that an EAB approve all embryo research proposals. Subsequently, the DHHS rescinded the regulatory provision requiring EAB approval of proposals for IVF-related research. In response, the National Institutes of Health (NIH) established a Human Embryo Research Panel to develop guidelines for the use of human embryos in federally funded research. The panel issued its report in September 1994.

The Human Embryo Research Panel was nearly unanimous in its recommendations concerning the conditions under which embryo research should be eligible for federal funding. For embryos intended to be transferred for implantation, the panel concluded that research should be permitted only if it will provide knowledge important to the health and well-being of the developing embryo, is related to establishing a normal pregnancy, or will otherwise provide a direct benefit to the embryo transferred. According to the panel, research on embryos intended for transfer should not pose any additional harm to the embryos and must be based on animal and human research with non-transferred embryos confirming the safety of the procedures.

The panel also developed a list of acceptable areas of research for embryos not intended to be used to initiate a pregnancy. The list included research on freezing or maturing oocytes, fertilization, the relative roles of maternal and paternal genes in embryo development, the development of undifferentiated embryonic cells, gene therapy, and research intended to increase the likelihood of successful pregnancy outcomes. The panel also listed other types of research that might be permissible upon additional review, as well as types of research considered unacceptable for federal funding. The unacceptable list included research on cloning (defined as studies designed to duplicate a genome or increase the number of embryos with the same genotype), research beyond the onset of closure of the neural tube, and research on cross-species fertilization and cross-species gestation.

The panel determined that research on embryos should not be conducted without the informed consent of the embryo donors as well as the donors of the gametes making up the embryos, if they are not the same. In addition, the rearing parents of any children created from related embryos must also consent. Whenever possible, donors should be told what type of research is to be undertaken on their gametes or embryos. The panel noted that some donors may want their gametes or embryos used only for specific types of research.

The panel also determined that no research should be performed on embryos after fourteen days. According to the panel, the appearance of the primitive streak at fourteen days makes the embryo "a distinct developing individual," and some "enhanced degree of protectability" is warranted because the nervous system is beginning to develop, twinning or aggregation is no longer possible, and cell differentiation is occurring. In the course of their deliberations, some panel members suggested other developmental markers as the point at which all research should be terminated, such as the occurrence of a heartbeat on the twenty-second day or some point beyond fourteen days at which sentience could be said to begin. In its conclusion, however, the panel determined that it was critical for public policy purposes to set an absolute time limit and that fourteen days was an appropriate point. The panel noted, however, that if further research shows that the primitive streak takes more than fourteen days to appear in vitro, research should be permitted up to the point at which the primitive streak actually appears.

The panel's most controversial conclusion was its support of federal funding for the creation of embryos expressly for research, as opposed to using only embryos donated by couples who originally created them to initiate a pregnancy. There was some disagreement about the types of research that would justify creating embryos. The majority of the panel concluded that it would be appropriate to fertilize oocytes specifically for research under two conditions: when the research cannot by its nature be conducted otherwise, as with research on oocytes prior to fertilization or on the process of fertilization itself, and when a representative group of embryos is needed to validate a study "of outstanding scientific and therapeutic value" and some of those embryos are not available through donations. The panel specifically stated that oocytes should not be fertilized for research merely because of a scarcity of embryos resulting from infertility treatment.

The panel suggested a number of possible sources of oocytes for projects requiring the creation of embryos, including women undergoing infertility treatment, women undergoing scheduled pelvic surgery, and women and girls who have died, if they gave specific consent prior to their death or their next of kin gives specific consent at the time of death with the understanding that the oocytes may be fertilized but will not be transferred for implantation. The panel concluded that it was not appropriate to fertilize oocytes from aborted fetuses for use in research.

The panel's report has received both praise for its "careful analysis of the moral status of the embryo," and criticism for failing "to come even close to making a persuasive case for pre-implantation embryo research." Critics maintain that the report does not adequately explain how research is consistent with the special respect that embryos are owed, that the "justifications for this research on health grounds are grossly overstated and mask important questions regarding the social origins of infertility," and that the scientific necessity and significance of embryo research is not sufficiently established.

NOTES AND QUESTIONS

1. Despite the NIH panel's recommendations, Congress has continued to pass annual resolutions barring the use of federal funds for research in which human embryos will be destroyed.

2. In the absence of federal funding for embryo research, many new infertility techniques are never tested in formal research protocols before they are introduced into clinical practice. Instead, they are tested on patients through trial and error, with successful techniques eventually becoming the standard of care. *See* Rebecca L. Skloot, *The Other Baby Experiment*, N.Y. TIMES, Feb. 22, 2003, at A17 (arguing that withholding federal support for embryo research "means experimenting on infertile women and their offspring instead"). Criticizing this practice, the New York State Task Force on Life and the Law concluded that, "when there is no evidence in the medical literature of a procedure's safety and efficacy, generally it should be introduced under a formal research protocol," and that "[s]uch procedures should not be advertised or promoted as accepted treatments." NEW YORK STATE TASK FORCE ON LIFE AND THE LAW, *supra*, at 174. What measures might be taken to enforce such a policy? *See* Chapter 3, at page 113; *see also* Chapter 7, at page 304 (discussing informed consent issues that arise when innovative therapies are offered outside of formal research protocols).

3. Institutions that receive federal research funding generally agree to comply with the federal regulations in all of their human subject research, including research supported entirely with private funds. *See* Chapter 3, at page 107. Under what circumstances would these institutions have to apply the federal regulations to privately funded embryo research? Consider both the definition of "human subject" in 45 C.F.R. § 102(f) and the exemptions set forth in 45 C.F.R. § 101(b)(4). How might these provisions apply to a study in which researchers recruit women to donate their eggs so that they can be fertilized with sperm from a sperm bank? A study involving "leftover" embryos donated by infertility patients whose identities are known to the researchers? A study that uses embryos from an embryo bank that have been stripped of all identifying information?

4. In an October 2002 charge to the Secretary's Advisory Council on Human Research Protections, DHHS Secretary Tommy G. Thompson directed the council to develop recommendations on "the responsible conduct of research involving human subjects with particular emphasis on . . . embryos and fetuses." M. Alexander Otto, *New HHS Science Committee to Consider Embryos, Fetuses Human Research Subjects*, 1 MED. RESEARCH L. & POL'Y REP. (BNA) 485 (2002). Secretary Thompson's characterization of embryos as "human subjects" generated significant media attention. *See, e.g.*, Rick Weiss, *New Status for Embryos in Research*, WASHINGTON POST, Oct. 30, 2002, at A1. What would be the implications for embryo research if the federal research regulations were changed to provide that embryos are to be considered human subjects?

[2] Application of Federal Embryo Research Policies to Research on Embryonic Stem Cells

After human embryonic stem cells were first isolated in 1998, the Clinton administration determined that research with these cells would be eligible for federal funding as long as no federal funds were expended on the process of deriving the stem cells from an embryo. *See* NATIONAL INSTITUTES OF HEALTH GUIDELINES FOR RESEARCH USING HUMAN PLURIPOTENT STEM CELLS, available at http://stemcells.nih.gov/news/newsArchives/stemcellguidelines.asp. The rationale was that only the derivation of embryonic stem cells — not the use of those cells once they have been isolated — would implicate the congressional ban on federal funding of embryo research, because it is only during the process of derivation that any embryos are destroyed. As a matter of statutory construction, what are the arguments for and against this interpretation? Even if the distinction between derivation and use is consistent with the letter of the federal prohibition on funding embryo research, does it violate the law's underlying spirit, which is to withhold federal support from activities that Congress has deemed objectionable? *See* John A. Robertson, *Ethics and Policy in Embryonic Stem Cell Research*, 9 KENNEDY INST. ETHICS J. 109, 113-114 (1999) (analyzing the ethical premises underlying the Clinton administration's policy). The National Bioethics Advisory Commission, while recognizing the logic of the Clinton administration's distinction as a legal matter, recommended that federal policy be changed to support both the derivation and use of embryonic stem cells, on the ground that relying solely on cell lines derived by privately funded researchers "could severely limit scientific and clinical progress." NBAC, STEM CELL RESEARCH, *supra*, at 70-71.

Embryonic stem cell research became a major issue during the 2000 presidential election campaign, with some conservative Republicans calling for a total ban on federal funding of such research. *See 7 Senators Protest Cell Research*, N.Y. TIMES, Feb. 20, 1999, at A11. Before President Bush announced his administration's policy on stem cell research in August 2001, researchers were concerned that they would lose all federal support for embryonic stem cell research. As the next excerpt shows, that did not happen.

George W. Bush
Remarks by the President on Stem Cell Research
The White House, Office of the Press Secretary
Aug. 9, 2001

The issue of research involving stem cells derived from human embryos is increasingly the subject of a national debate and dinner table discussions. The issue is confronted every day in laboratories as scientists ponder the ethical ramifications of their work. It is agonized over by parents and many couples as they try to have children, or to save children already born.

The issue is debated within the church, with people of different faiths, even many of the same faith coming to different conclusions. Many people are finding that the more they know about stem cell research, the less certain they are about the right ethical and moral conclusions.

My administration must decide whether to allow federal funds, your tax dollars, to be used for scientific research on stem cells derived from human embryos. . . .

Based on preliminary work that has been privately funded, scientists believe further research using stem cells offers great promise that could help improve the lives of those who suffer from many terrible diseases — from juvenile diabetes to Alzheimer's, from Parkinson's to spinal cord injuries. And while scientists admit they are not yet certain, they believe stem cells derived from embryos have unique potential.

You should also know that stem cells can be derived from sources other than embryos — from adult cells, from umbilical cords that are discarded after babies are born, from human placenta. And many scientists feel research on these types of stem cells is also promising. Many patients suffering from a range of diseases are already being helped with treatments developed from adult stem cells.

However, most scientists, at least today, believe that research on embryonic stem cells offer the most promise because these cells have the potential to develop in all of the tissues in the body.

Scientists further believe that rapid progress in this research will come only with federal funds. Federal dollars help attract the best and brightest scientists. They ensure new discoveries are widely shared at the largest number of research facilities and that the research is directed toward the greatest public good.

The United States has a long and proud record of leading the world toward advances in science and medicine that improve human life. And the United States has a long and proud record of upholding the highest standards of ethics as we expand the limits of science and knowledge. Research on embryonic stem cells raises profound ethical questions, because extracting the stem cell destroys the embryo, and thus destroys its potential for life. Like a snowflake, each of these embryos is unique, with the unique genetic potential of an individual human being.

As I thought through this issue, I kept returning to two fundamental questions: First, are these frozen embryos human life, and therefore, something precious to be protected? And second, if they're going to be destroyed anyway, shouldn't they be used for a greater good, for research that has the potential to save and improve other lives?

I've asked those questions and others of scientists, scholars, bioethicists, religious leaders, doctors, researchers, members of Congress, my Cabinet, and my friends. I have read heartfelt letters from many Americans. I have given this issue a great deal of thought, prayer and considerable reflection. And I have found widespread disagreement.

On the first issue, are these embryos human life — well, one researcher told me he believes this five-day-old cluster of cells is not an embryo, not yet an individual, but a pre-embryo. He argued that it has the potential for life, but it is not a life because it cannot develop on its own.

An ethicist dismissed that as a callous attempt at rationalization. Make no mistake, he told me, that cluster of cells is the same way you and I, and all the rest of us, started our lives. One goes with a heavy heart if we use these, he said, because we are dealing with the seeds of the next generation.

And to the other crucial question, if these are going to be destroyed anyway, why not use them for good purpose — I also found different answers. Many argue these embryos are byproducts of a process that helps create life, and we should allow couples to donate them to science so they can be used for good purpose instead of wasting their potential. Others will argue there's no such thing as excess life, and the fact that a living being is going to die does not justify experimenting on it or exploiting it as a natural resource.

At its core, this issue forces us to confront fundamental questions about the beginnings of life and the ends of science. It lies at a difficult moral intersection, juxtaposing the need to protect life in all its phases with the prospect of saving and improving life in all its stages.

As the discoveries of modern science create tremendous hope, they also lay vast ethical mine fields. As the genius of science extends the horizons of what we can do, we increasingly confront complex questions about what we should do. We have arrived at that brave new world that seemed so distant in 1932, when Aldous Huxley wrote about human beings created in test tubes in what he called a "hatchery."

In recent weeks, we learned that scientists have created human embryos in test tubes solely to experiment on them. This is deeply troubling, and a warning sign that should prompt all of us to think through these issues very carefully.

Embryonic stem cell research is at the leading edge of a series of moral hazards. The initial stem cell researcher was at first reluctant to begin his research, fearing it might be used for human cloning. Scientists have already cloned a sheep. Researchers are telling us the next step could be to clone human beings to create individual designer stem cells, essentially to grow another you, to be available in case you need another heart or lung or liver.

I strongly oppose human cloning, as do most Americans. We recoil at the idea of growing human beings for spare body parts, or creating life for our convenience. And while we must devote enormous energy to conquering disease, it is equally important that we pay attention to the moral concerns raised by the new frontier of human embryo stem cell research. Even the most noble ends do not justify any means.

My position on these issues is shaped by deeply held beliefs. I'm a strong supporter of science and technology, and believe they have the potential for incredible good — to improve lives, to save life, to conquer disease. Research offers hope that millions of our loved ones may be cured of a disease and rid of their suffering. I have friends whose children suffer from juvenile diabetes. Nancy Reagan has written me about President Reagan's struggle with Alzheimer's. My own family has confronted the tragedy of childhood leukemia. And, like all Americans, I have great hope for cures.

I also believe human life is a sacred gift from our Creator. I worry about a culture that devalues life, and believe as your President I have an important obligation to foster and encourage respect for life in America and throughout the world. And while we're all hopeful about the potential of this research, no one can be certain that the science will live up to the hope it has generated.

Eight years ago, scientists believed fetal tissue research offered great hope for cures and treatments — yet, the progress to date has not lived up to its initial expectations. Embryonic stem cell research offers both great promise and great peril. So I have decided we must proceed with great care.

As a result of private research, more than 60 genetically diverse stem cell lines already exist. They were created from embryos that have already been destroyed, and they have the ability to regenerate themselves indefinitely, creating ongoing opportunities for research. I have concluded that we should allow federal funds to be used for research on these existing stem cell lines, where the life and death decision has already been made.

Leading scientists tell me research on these 60 lines has great promise that could lead to breakthrough therapies and cures. This allows us to explore the promise and potential of stem cell research without crossing a fundamental moral line, by providing taxpayer funding that would sanction or encourage further destruction of human embryos that have at least the potential for life.

I also believe that great scientific progress can be made through aggressive federal funding of research on umbilical cord placenta, adult and animal stem cells which do not involve the same moral dilemma. This year, your government will spend $250 million on this important research.

I will also name a President's council to monitor stem cell research, to recommend appropriate guidelines and regulations, and to consider all of the medical and ethical ramifications of biomedical innovation. This council will consist of leading scientists, doctors, ethicists, lawyers, theologians and others, and will be chaired by Dr. Leon Kass, a leading biomedical ethicist from the University of Chicago.

This council will keep us apprised of new developments and give our nation a forum to continue to discuss and evaluate these important issues. As we go forward, I hope we will always be guided by both intellect and heart, by both our capabilities and our conscience.

NOTES AND QUESTIONS

1. President Bush's willingness to support even limited federal funding for research with embryonic stem cells, despite his apparent opposition to the destruction of human embryos, suggests that he rejects the idea that "benefiting from another person's wrongdoing" is inherently wrong. *See* Robertson, *supra*, at 113-114 (arguing that such a theory, if taken seriously, would require one to "object to transplanting or receiving organs from murder victims," as well as to many other "common activities, practices, and social arrangements"). Why, then, is he willing to support only research involving embryonic stem cells that already exist, as opposed to research involving embryonic stem cells created in the future?

2. If it is indeed morally wrong to continue destroying embryos in order to generate stem cells, why did President Bush limit his statement to the issue of federal funding? Wouldn't his analysis also suggest that Congress should enact legislation prohibiting the destruction of embryos by any researcher, regardless of his or her funding source?

3. Opponents of federal funding for embryonic stem cell research argue that the federal government should instead fund research with stem cells derived from adults. *See* NBAC, STEM CELL RESEARCH, *supra*, at 57-58 (discussing, and ultimately rejecting, this argument). Yet, despite a few studies suggesting that adult stem cells have greater developmental potential than was previously recognized, supporters of embryonic stem cell research argue that "no credible biologist would accept the idea that embryonic and adult stem cells have the same intrinsic or native developmental potency." George Q. Daley, *Cloning and Stem Cells — Handicapping the Political and Scientific Debates*, 349 N. ENG. J. MED. 211, 212 (2003).

4. While President Bush's position was intended to strike a compromise between supporters and opponents of embryonic stem cell research, most researchers have not found the compromise acceptable. First, while the NIH originally identified a total of 78 embryonic stem cell lines eligible for use in federally funded research, many of these lines were discovered to be either unavailable or unsuitable for research. In fact, as of May 2004, only 19 stem cell lines were actually available for use. Second, some scientists believe that those stem cell lines are "useless for treating human diseases" because they were grown in culture that contained mice and fetal calf serum, which contaminated the stem cells with animal molecules. *See* Jeannie Baumann, *Study Says Contamination of Cell Lines Available in U.S. Affects Future Human Uses*, 4 MED. RESEARCH L. & POL'Y REP. (BNA) 101 (2005) (quoting one scientist's concern that using the

available stem cells in human transplants would entail "a significant chance of a 'deleterious immune reaction' and possible rejection of the transplanted cells").

5. The policy also does not appear to satisfy the concerns of the Catholic Church. According to a statement on stem cell research issued by the Vatican, even if embryonic stem cells were "supplied by other researchers or are commercially obtainable," the use of those stem cells would still be immoral because it "entails a proximate material cooperation in the production and manipulation of human embryos on the part of those producing or supplying them." PONTIFICAL ACADEMY FOR LIFE, DECLARATION ON THE PRODUCTION AND THE SCIENTIFIC AND THERAPEUTIC USE OF HUMAN EMBRYONIC STEM CELLS, Aug. 25, 2000, available at www.vatican.va/roman_curia/pontifical_academies/acdlife/documents/rc_pa_acdl ife_doc_20000824_cellule-staminali_en.html.

6. Federally funded researchers may use private funds to conduct research with embryonic stem cells that are not eligible for federal funding, but they must "separate allowable and unallowable activities in such a way that permits the costs incurred in the research to be allocated consistently to the appropriate funding source." Provided they allocate their funding properly, they also may use private funds to derive new stem cell lines from embryos. NATIONAL INSTITUTES OF HEALTH, STEM CELL INFORMATION: FREQUENTLY ASKED QUESTIONS, available at http://stemcells.nih.gov/info/faqs.asp.

7. Some commentators worry that restrictions on federal funding for embryonic stem cell research will lead scientists to leave the United States for countries like Great Britain, which supports such research with public funds. *See, e.g.,* Michael Lasalandra, *Stem Cell Group: Bill Should Fund and Support Work,* BOSTON HERALD, Dec. 5, 2002, at 37. Should such considerations be relevant to the allocation of federal research dollars?

[C] State Law and Policy

While federal policy precludes the use of federal funds in research in which embryos will be destroyed, it does not bar embryo research supported by private funds. Such research, however, may be subject to more stringent state laws.

LOUISIANA REVISED STATUTES ANNOTATED

§ 9:122: Uses of human embryo in vitro

The use of a human ovum fertilized in vitro is solely for the support and contribution of the complete development of human in utero implantation. No in vitro fertilized human ovum will be farmed or cultured solely for research purposes or any other purposes. The sale of a human ovum, fertilized human ovum, or human embryo is expressly prohibited.

§ 9:129: Destruction

A viable in vitro fertilized human ovum is a juridical person that shall not be intentionally destroyed by any natural or other juridical person or through the actions of any other such person. An in vitro fertilized human ovum that fails to develop further over a thirty-six hour period except when the embryo is in a state of cryopreservation, is considered non-viable and is not considered a juridical person.

CALIFORNIA HEALTH & SAFETY CODE

§ 125115. The policy of the State of California shall be as follows:

(a) That research involving the derivation and use of human embryonic stem cells, human embryonic germ cells, and human adult stem cells from any source, including somatic cell nuclear transplantation, shall be permitted and that full consideration of the ethical and medical implications of this research be given.

(b) That research involving the derivation and use of human embryonic stem cells, human embryonic germ cells, and human adult stem cells, including somatic cell nuclear transplantation, shall be reviewed by an approved institutional review board.

NOTES AND QUESTIONS

1. In *Lifchez v. Hartigan*, 735 F. Supp. 1361 (N.D. Ill.), *aff'd*, 914 F.2d 260 (7th Cir. 1990), a federal district court struck down Illinois' ban on embryo experimentation, based on reasoning similar to that of the concurring judge in *Forbes v. Napolitano*, *supra*. Do you think the Louisiana statute would survive a constitutional challenge?

2. Like California, several other states have passed statutes encouraging embryonic stem cell research. What is the legal significance of these statutes? Why do you think they were passed? Under § 125115(b) of the California statute, what factors should an IRB consider in determining whether to approve a particular study? Should each IRB make its own assessment of the moral status of embryos?

3. In November 2004, California voters approved a ballot initiative directing the state to spend $300 million per year for ten years to support stem cell research. The state will obtain the money by issuing $3 billion in general obligation bonds. *See* Dean E. Murphy, *Defying Bush Administration, Voters in California Back $3 Billion for Stem Cell Research*, N.Y. TIMES, Nov. 4, 2004, at P1.

[D] Consent to Embryo and Embryonic Stem Cell Research

Donating Spare Embryos for Embryonic Stem-cell Research
Ethics Committee of the American Society for Reproductive Medicine
8 FERTILITY & STERILITY 957 (2002)

Informed consent is a basic requirement for the ethical conduct of all human subjects research, including studies using human embryos. Couples who donate embryos for research should be told of the risks and benefits of donation. For example, a risk might arise if the couple were later to wish they still had the embryos available for their fertility efforts. A benefit might be the satisfaction of knowing they have contributed to research designed to advance medical therapies. Couples should also be told of the purpose and nature of the research and of whether the research is expected to have commercial value. They should be told that they may change their minds at any time until the experiment begins, that their status in the in fertility program will not be affected if they do not donate spare embryos, and that no embryos used in the study will be transferred for pregnancy.

In the case of donation for ES [embryonic stem] cell research, other considerations may also be relevant. Given the wide range of uses to which ES cells may be put, couples should be informed of the specific research project, if known, or at least of the category of anticipated research, such as reproductive research, development of therapies for disease, or product development. Couples should also know that ES cell research typically involves deriving cells from the inner cell mass of an embryo at the blastocyst stage, which leads to the embryo's destruction. Potential donors also should be informed that the cell might exist indefinitely. They should be told that stem cells from embryos may have commercial value for a wide range of research and clinical purposes and that they as donors will not share in the commercial value. The clinic should develop a policy on privacy and confidentiality of donations and present this as part of the consent process. If identifiers are attached to the cell lines, the donors must be informed of this and of steps taken to assure their anonymity. The male and female partners must agree on the disposition of their spare embryos. If they cannot jointly agree to donate embryos for research, the embryos should not be used for research.

When Consent Should be Obtained

It is important that couples decide to donate embryos for research only after they have decided not to continue storing their embryos. Making separate decisions about no longer using embryos and donating them for research guards against pressure placed on couples to donate embryos. When embryos are created, couples often stipulate what should be done with their frozen embryos in the event of future contingencies, such as death, divorce, or no contact with the clinic. These directives usually involve donating the embryos to another couple, donating them for research, or discarding them. If no death or divorce occurs, the couple makes a separate decision about what should be done with the unused embryos when their fertility needs are met or they end their reproductive efforts with these embryos. At this point, the investigator has the opportunity to discuss more thoroughly the option of donating embryos for research.

Using only frozen embryos for research ensures that time passes between the creation of embryos for conception and their donation for research. Still, it is reasonable to expect questions eventually to arise about the donation of fresh but supernumerary embryos. Donation of fresh embryos raises the possibility that a physician might induce a patient to allow insemination of extra eggs so that they may be donated for research. Moreover, this increases the chance that decisions will be made quickly and later regretted by couples. Without evidence that fresh embryos are significantly preferable to frozen embryos for ES cell use, it is appropriate to use only spare embryos that have been frozen. The number of embryos created and frozen should be determined by the clinical needs of the infertile couple.

In some situations, couples with stored embryos cannot be contacted despite efforts on the part of the clinic. The Ethics Committee has previously concluded that programs may consider embryos abandoned if clinics have taken diligent steps to contact the couple, no written instructions exist, and more than 5 years have elapsed without contact with the couple. Abandoned embryos may be discarded, but they should not be used for research or donated to another couple without prior consent. In some cases, however, couples may have given consent to use spare embryos for research but were not informed of the possibility of ES cell research. The singular features of ES cell research make it advisable not to use such embryos for ES cell research unless couples have given specific advance consent for this purpose, in case they cannot later be reached for a decision. Advance permission to use abandoned embryos for research may thus prevail for ES cell studies if the couple has been informed of the possibility of ES cell research.

Who Should Secure Consent

Several advisory bodies have recommended that a person other than the fertility specialist secure consent to donate embryos. The rationale is that this will ensure that the couple's reproductive needs are foremost and avoid conflicts of interest when the fertility specialist is also the investigator. In some circumstances, however, this guideline may be difficult to follow. It is possible, for example, that the fertility specialist who knows the couple and is trusted by them may be better able to have a frank discussion with the couple about donation for research and may secure more informed consent.

Moreover, using a separate person to secure consent may be difficult if the physician is part of the research team. The possibility of undue influence by the physician will be lessened if the request for a donation is made after the couple decides to dispose of their embryos. Still, the fact that the physician is also a researcher is relevant information and should be conveyed to the couple along with a statement about financial incentives, if any, the physician has in the research. The rule that the number of embryos created and frozen must be determined by the clinical needs of the couple and not by research goals is especially pertinent when the physician is both the fertility specialist and investigator.

CALIFORNIA HEALTH & SAFETY CODE

§ 125116. Information regarding choice of disposition of human embryos to be provided to individuals undergoing fertility treatment

(a) A physician, surgeon, or other health care provider delivering fertility treatment shall provide his or her patient with timely, relevant, and appropriate information to allow the individual to make an informed and voluntary choice regarding the disposition of any human embryos remaining following the fertility treatment.

(b) Any individual to whom information is provided pursuant to subdivision (a) shall be presented with the option of storing any unused embryos, donating them to another individual, discarding the embryos, or donating the remaining embryos for research.

(c) Any individual who elects to donate embryos remaining after fertility treatments for research shall provide written consent.

NOTES AND QUESTIONS

1. The American Society for Reproductive Medicine (ASRM) states that "[t]he singular features of ES cell research" make it inappropriate for stem cell researchers to rely on a couple's general consent to embryo research if the possibility of stem cell research was not specifically discussed with the couple. What are those "singular features"? Is it likely that couples who are willing to have their embryos used in scientific research would object to studies involving the derivation of embryonic stem cells?

2. The ASRM statement focuses on the interests of the couple that is donating the embryo. What if the embryo was created with gametes from one of the donating partners combined with gametes from an anonymous sperm or egg donor? What if a couple creates embryos entirely with donor gametes? Should sperm and egg donors have the right to insist that any embryos created with their gametes not be used for research purposes, or that they be used only for some types of research but not others?

3. Some courts have held that advance agreements regarding the disposition of frozen embryos are not enforceable if either party to the agreement changes his or her mind. *See In re The Marriage of Arthur Lee Witten III and Tamera Jean Witten*, 672 N.W.2d 768 (Iowa 2003); *J.B. v. M.B.*, 783 A.2d 707 (N.J. 2001); *A.Z. v. B.Z.*, 725 N.E.2d 1051 (Mass. 2000). These courts have pointed to statutes and court decisions refusing to enforce surrogate parenting contracts or agreements by pregnant women to give up their future children for adoption. These precedents, the courts reasoned, indicate that prior agreements are an insufficient basis for extinguishing an individual's right to decide whether to become a parent. *See generally* Carl H. Coleman, *Procreative Liberty and Contemporaneous Choice: An Inalienable Rights Approach to Frozen Embryo Disputes*, 84 MINN. L. REV. 55 (1999). What are the implications of these decisions for the ASRM's position?

4. How does the California statute differ from the ASRM's recommendations? Which approach do you find preferable?

§ 16.03 CLONING

Although the possibility of cloning human beings has long fascinated both scientists and the lay public, until recently it was assumed that human cloning would never be possible. That assumption changed in 1997, when scientists in Scotland announced the birth of a lamb named "Dolly," who developed from the somatic cell nuclear transfer procedure described below. With the birth of Dolly, "the science fiction scenario of copying or 'cloning' an adult mammal, including humans, became science fact." Janet Rossant, *The Science of Animal Cloning*, in NATIONAL BIOETHICS ADVISORY COMMISSION, 2 CLONING HUMAN BEINGS B-10 (1997) [hereinafter NBAC, CLONING]. While most public discussions about cloning have focused on the use of the technology to create a child, many scientists are more interested in using embryos created through cloning for biomedical research. The following materials discuss both of these potential applications of cloning technology.

[A] What Is Cloning?

FREQUENTLY ASKED QUESTIONS ABOUT HUMAN CLONING
AND THE COUNCIL'S REPORT, "HUMAN CLONING AND
HUMAN DIGNITY: AN ETHICAL INQUIRY"
PRESIDENT'S COUNCIL ON BIOETHICS
(2002)

1. What is cloning?

Cloning is a form of reproduction in which offspring result not from the chance union of egg and sperm (sexual reproduction) but from the deliberate replication of the genetic makeup of another single individual (asexual reproduction). Human cloning, therefore, is the asexual production of a new human organism that is, at all stages of development, genetically virtually identical to a currently existing or previously existing human being.

2. How is cloning related to somatic cell nuclear transfer?

Somatic cell nuclear transfer (SCNT) is the technique by which cloning is accomplished. It involves introducing the nuclear material of a human somatic cell (donor) into an oocyte (egg cell) whose own nucleus has been removed or inactivated, and then stimulating this new entity to begin dividing and growing, yielding a cloned embryo.

3. For what purposes would anyone want to perform human cloning?

Human cloning might be undertaken for two general purposes. One potential use would be to produce children who would be genetically virtually identical to pre-existing individuals. Another would be to produce cloned embryos for research or therapy. For example, a scientist might wish to create a cloned embryo which would then be taken apart to yield embryonic stem cells that could potentially be used in biomedical research or therapies. The Council has termed the first use "cloning-to-produce-children" and the second "cloning-for-biomedical-research."

NOTES AND QUESTIONS

1. Note that cloning via somatic cell nuclear transfer results in offspring whose genes are "virtually" identical to those of an existing or previously existing human being, not "completely" identical. The reason is that a small amount of DNA is contained in the portion of the egg that surrounds the nucleus (known as "mitochondrial DNA"). This DNA comes from the woman who provided the egg used in the procedure, not from the donor who provided the somatic cell.

2. The President's Council on Bioethics (PCB) adopted the term "cloning-to-produce children" to refer to what many people have characterized as "reproductive" cloning, and "cloning-for-biomedical research" to refer to what is often called "therapeutic" cloning. Why might the PCB's terminology be less controversial than the terms "reproductive" and "therapeutic" cloning?

[B] Perspectives on Cloning

Frequently Asked Questions about Human Cloning and the Council's Report, "Human Cloning and Human Dignity: An Ethical Inquiry" President's Council on Bioethics
(2002)

8. Why might anyone want to clone a child?

Cloning-to-produce-children might serve several purposes. It might allow infertile couples or others to have genetically related children; permit couples at risk of conceiving a child with a genetic disease to avoid having an afflicted child; allow the bearing of a child who could become an ideal transplant donor for a particular patient in need; enable a parent to keep a living connection with a dead or dying child or spouse; or even to try to "replicate" individuals of great talent or beauty. These purposes have been defended by appeals to the goods of freedom, existence (as opposed to nonexistence), and well-being.

9. What are the arguments against cloning a child?

The Council holds that cloning-to-produce-children would violate the principles of the ethics of human research. Given the high rates of morbidity and mortality in the cloning of other mammals, cloning-to-produce-children would be extremely unsafe, and, as such, attempts to produce a cloned child would be highly unethical. Even conducting experiments in an effort to make cloning-to-produce-children safer would itself be an unacceptable violation of the norms of research ethics, so there seems to be no ethical way to try to discover whether cloning-to-produce-children can become safe, now or in the future. Beyond those safety issues, the Council holds that cloning-to-produce-children would be a radically new form of human procreation that leads to concerns about: (1) problems of identity and individuality; (2) concerns regarding manufacture; (3) the prospect of a new eugenics; (4) troubled family relations; and (5) effects on the family.

10. Why might anyone want to produce cloned embryos for biomedical research?

Some scientists believe that stem cells derived from cloned human embryos, produced explicitly for such research, might prove uniquely useful for studying many genetic diseases and devising novel therapies.

12. What are the arguments for and against cloning for biomedical research?

The primary argument for proceeding with cloning-for-biomedical-research is that it might lead to advances in medical knowledge and toward treatments and cures. Those members of the Council who support cloning-for-biomedical-research believe that it may offer uniquely useful ways of investigating and possibly treating many chronic debilitating diseases and disabilities, providing aid and relief to millions who are suffering, and to their families and communities. They also believe that the moral objections to this research — some of which are taken quite seriously by some of these members — are outweighed by the great good that may come from it.

The case against proceeding with the research does not deny the possibility (albeit speculative) of medical progress from this work, but rests on the belief of those members of the Council who oppose the research that it is morally wrong to exploit and destroy developing human life, even for good reasons, and that it is unwise to open the door to the many undesirable consequences that are likely to result from this research. These members point to concerns about our obligations to nascent human life; the crossing of an important moral boundary through the creation of human life expressly and exclusively for the purpose of its use in research; and possible further moral harms to our society.

16. What are the Council's policy recommendations on human cloning?

A minority of the Council (seven members) recommended a ban on cloning-to-produce-children, with federal regulation of the use of cloned embryos for bio-medical research. Such a policy, they argue, would permanently ban cloning-to-produce-children, which nearly all Americans oppose, and would allow potentially important biomedical research to continue, thus offering hope to many who are suffering. These members believe that a regulatory system would be sufficient to protect against abuses and to prevent the implantation of cloned embryos to initiate a pregnancy. Above all, they believe that society should support and affirm the responsible effort to find treatments and cures for those who need them.

A majority of the Council (ten members) recommended a ban on cloning-to-produce-children combined with a four-year moratorium on cloning-for-bio-medical research, and also called for a federal review of current and projected practices of human embryo research, pre-implantation genetic diagnosis, genetic modification of human embryos and gametes, and related matters.

Such a policy, they argue, would most effectively ban cloning-to-produce-children, which nearly all Americans oppose, and would provide time for further democratic deliberation about cloning-for-biomedical research, a subject about which the nation is divided and where there remains great uncertainty.

A moratorium would allow time for moral persuasion; for further animal experiments and progress on alternative avenues of research (including adult stem cells, and other approaches to the immune rejection problem); and for development of possible future regulations by those who do not wish to see the moratorium made permanent.

It would show respect for the views of the large number of Americans who have serious ethical problems with this research, and it would promote a fuller and better-informed public debate. The moratorium, they argue, would also enable society to consider this activity in the larger context of research and technology in the areas of developmental biology, embryo research, and genetics.

Finally, a moratorium, rather than a lasting ban, signals a high regard for the value of biomedical research and an enduring concern for patients and families whose suffering such research may help alleviate. These members believe that on this important subject American society should take the time to make a judgment that is well-informed, respectful of strongly held views, and representative of the priorities and principles of the American people. They believe this proposal offers the best available way to a wise and prudent policy.

Cloning, Ethics, and Religion
Lee M. Silver
7 CAMBRIDGE Q. HEALTHCARE ETHICS 168 (1998)

Let us take a look at the safety argument first. Throughout the 20th century, medical scientists have sought to develop new protocols and drugs for treating disease and alleviating human suffering. The safety of all these new medical protocols was initially unknown. But through experimental testing on animals first, and then volunteer human subjects, safety could be ascertained and governmental agencies — such as the Food and Drug Administration in the United States — could make a decision as to whether the new protocol or drug should be approved for use in standard medical practice.

It would be ludicrous to suggest that legislatures should pass laws banning the application of each newly imagined medical protocol before its safety has been determined. Professional ethics committees, institutional review boards, and the individual ethics of each medical practitioner are relied upon to make sure that hundreds of new experimental protocols are tested and used in an appropriate manner each year. . . .

Opposition to cloning on the basis of safety alone is almost surely a losing proposition. Although the media have concocted fantasies of dozens of malformed monster lambs paving the way for the birth of Dolly, fantasy is all it was. Of the 277 fused cells created by Wilmut and his colleagues, only 29 developed into embryos. These 29 embryos were placed into 13 ewes, of which 1 became pregnant and gave birth to Dolly. If safety is measured by the percentage of lambs born in good health, then the record, so far, is 100% for nuclear transplantation from an adult cell (albeit with a sample size of 1).

In fact, there is no scientific basis for the belief that cloned children will be any more prone to genetic problems than naturally conceived children. The commonest type of birth defect results from the presence of an abnormal number of chromosomes in the fertilized egg. This birth defect arises during gamete production and, as such, its frequency should be greatly reduced in embryos formed by cloning. The second most common class of birth defects results from the inheritance of two mutant copies of a gene from two parents who are silent carriers. With cloning, any silent mutation in a donor will be silent in the newly formed embryo and child as well. Finally, much less frequently, birth defects can be caused by new mutations; these will occur with the same frequency in embryos derived through conception or cloning. (Although some scientists have suggested that chromosome shortening in the donor cell will cause cloned children to have a shorter lifespan, there is every reason to expect that chromosome repair in the embryo will eliminate this problem.) Surprisingly, what our current scientific understanding suggests is that birth defects in cloned children could occur less frequently than birth defects in naturally conceived ones.

Once safety has been eliminated as an objection to cloning, the next concern voiced is the psychological well-being of the child. Daniel Callahan, the former director of the Hastings Center, argues that "engineering someone's entire genetic makeup would compromise his or her right to a unique identity." But no such "right" has been granted by nature — identical twins are born every day as natural clones of each other. Dr. Callahan would have to concede this fact, but he might still argue that just because twins occur naturally does not mean we should create them on purpose.

Dr. Callahan might argue that a cloned child is harmed by knowledge of her future condition. He might say that it's unfair to go through childhood knowing what you will look like as an adult, or being forced to consider future medical ailments that might befall you. But even in the absence of cloning, many children have some sense of the future possibilities encoded in the genes they got from their parents. Furthermore, genetic screening already provides people with the ability to learn about hundreds of disease predispositions. And as genetic knowledge and technology become more and more sophisticated, it will become possible for any human being to learn even more about his or her genetic future than a cloned child could learn from his or her progenitor's past.

It might also be argued that a cloned child will be harmed by having to live up to unrealistic expectations placed on her by her parents. But there is no reason to believe that her parents will be any more unreasonable than many other parents who expect their children to accomplish in their lives what they were unable to accomplish in their own. No one would argue that parents with such tendencies should be prohibited from having children.

But let's grant that among the many cloned children brought into this world, some *will* feel badly about the fact that their genetic constitution is not unique. Is this alone a strong enough reason to ban the practice of cloning? Before answering this question, ask yourself another: Is a child having knowledge of an older twin worse off than a child born into poverty? If we ban the former, shouldn't we ban the latter? Why is it that so many politicians seem to care so much about cloning but so little about the welfare of children in general?

Finally, there are those who argue against cloning based on the perception that it will harm society at large in some way. The *New York Times* columnist William Safire expresses the opinion of many others when he says that "cloning's identicality would restrict evolution." This is bad, he argues, because "the continued interplay of genes . . . is central to humankind's progress." But Mr. Safire is wrong on both practical and theoretical grounds. On practical grounds, even if human cloning became efficient, legal, and popular among those in the moneyed classes (which is itself highly unlikely), it would still only account for a fraction of a percent of all the children born onto this earth. Furthermore, each of the children born by cloning to different families would be different from each other, so where does the identicality come from?

On theoretical grounds, Safire is wrong because humankind's progress has nothing to do with unfettered evolution, which is always unpredictable and not necessarily upward bound. H.G. Wells recognized this principle in his 1895 novel *The Time Machine*, which portrays the evolution of humankind into weak and dimwitted but cuddly little creatures. And Kurt Vonnegut follows this same theme in *Galapagos,* where he suggests that our "big brains" will be the cause of our downfall, and future humans with smaller brains and powerful flippers will be the only remnants of a once great species, a million years hence.

As is so often the case with new reproductive technologies, the real reason that people condemn cloning has nothing to do with technical feasibility, child psychology, societal well-being, or the preservation of the human species. The real reason derives from religious beliefs. It is the sense that cloning leaves God out of the process of human creation, and that man is venturing into places he does not belong. Of course, the "playing God" objection only makes sense in the context of one definition of God, as a supernatural being who plays a role in the birth of each new member of our species. And even if one holds this particular view of God, it does not necessarily follow that cloning is equivalent to playing God. Some who consider themselves to be religious have argued that if God didn't want man to clone, "he" wouldn't have made it possible.

Should public policy in a pluralist society be based on a narrow religious point of view? Most people would say no, which is why those who hold this point of view are grasping for secular reasons to support their call for an unconditional ban on the cloning of human beings. When the dust clears from the cloning debate, however, the secular reasons will almost certainly have disappeared. And then, only religious objections will remain.

NOTES AND QUESTIONS

1. The PCB's report is the second by a federal commission charged with recommending public policy on cloning. The first was issued in 1997 by NBAC, shortly after the announcement of the birth of Dolly the lamb. NBAC unanimously concluded that "at this time it is morally unacceptable for anyone . . . to attempt to create a child using somatic cell nuclear transfer cloning." NBAC's conclusion was based on the risks the procedure would pose to "the fetus and/or

potential child." NBAC, CLONING, *supra*, at iii. NBAC did not address the use of cloning to create embryos for use in biomedical research.

2. According to John Robertson, the assumption "that resulting children are harmed by cloning is open to challenge: but for the procedure in question, the child would not have been born." Even if cloning results in severe birth impairments, Robertson argues, a cloned child cannot be said to be harmed unless "the child's present life is so full of suffering that it would now prefer nonexistence." John A. Robertson, *Wrongful Life, Federalism, and Procreative Liberty: A Critique of the NBAC Cloning Report*, 38 JURIMETRICS 69, 75 (1997). Is it possible to claim that cloning poses unacceptable risks to future children even if those children, once alive, would not wish to be dead? *See* Carl H. Coleman, *Conceiving Harm: Disability Discrimination in Assisted Reproductive Technologies*, 50 UCLA L. REV. 17 (2002).

3. Is Silver correct that opposition to cloning-to-produce-children is based primarily on religious views? Even if he is, if a majority of Americans hold that position, should it matter that they do so in part because of religious beliefs?

4. Are the issues raised by cloning-for-biomedical research significantly different from those raised by the use of IVF to create embryos specifically for research purposes? *See supra*, page 671.

5. If the regulatory approach suggested by a minority of the PCB were adopted, what measures should be included in the system to "protect against abuses and to prevent the implantation of cloned embryos to initiate a pregnancy"?

[C] Federal Law

Despite widespread congressional support for some sort of legislation prohibiting human cloning, at the time this book went to press no such legislation had been enacted. The problem has been that some legislators want the law to apply only to cloning-to-produce-children, while others insist that it also should apply to cloning-for-biomedical-research. *See* CENTER FOR PUBLIC INTEGRITY, IN CONGRESS, A CLONING STALEMATE: EFFORTS TO BAN CLONING FALTER OVER SCOPE OF PROPOSED PROHIBITION (June 20, 2004), available at http://www.publicintegrity.org/genetics/report.aspx?aid=281&sid=200 (noting that lawmakers are about equally divided between the two positions).

NOTES AND QUESTIONS

1. Under what circumstances would the human subject protection regulations apply to cloning-for-biomedical-research? Recall the discussion of the applicability of these regulations to research with embryos created through IVF. *See supra*, page 675.

2. The Food and Drug Administration has taken the position that "[c]linical research using cloning technology to create a human being is subject to FDA regulation under the Public Health Service Act and the Federal Food, Drug, and Cosmetic Act," and that anyone intending to proceed with such research must therefore submit an investigational new drug application to the FDA. *See* "Dear Colleague" Letter from Stuart L. Nightingale, M.D., Associate Commissioner, to IRB Chairs, Oct. 26, 1998, available at http://www.fda.gov/oc/ohrt/irbs/ irbletr.html. The premise of the FDA's assertion of jurisdiction is that a cloned embryo falls within the statutory definitions of "drug" and/or "biological product." *See House Commerce Members Grill Official on FDA's Ability to Regulate Human Cloning*, HEALTH CARE DAILY REP. (BNA), March 29, 2001. The Food, Drug, and Cosmetic Act defines "drugs" as "articles intended for use in the diagnosis, cure, mitigation, treatment, or prevention of disease in man or other animals; and articles (other than food), intended to affect the structure or any function of the body of man or other animals." 21 U.S.C. § 321(g)(1). The Public Health Service Act defines "biological product" as a "virus, therapeutic serum, toxin, antitoxin, vaccine, blood, blood component or derivative, allergenic product, or analogous product . . . applicable to the prevention, treatment, or cure of a disease or condition of human beings." 42 U.S.C. § 262(i). Do you think that cloning-to-produce-children fits within either of these definitions? *See* Christine Willgoos, *FDA Regulation: An Answer to the Questions of Human Cloning and Germline Gene Therapy*, 27 AM. J.L. & MED. 101, 119-20 (2002) (noting that many legal scholars dispute the FDA's assertion of jurisdiction over cloning-to-produce-children).

3. Even if the FDA has jurisdiction to regulate cloning-to-produce-children, would such research be subject to the FDA's human subject protection regulations, or would the FDA have to regulate it through some other mechanism? How would the definitions of "research" and "human subject" apply to both the laboratory aspects of cloning-to-produce children and the process of transferring a cloned embryo into a woman's body? Which person or entity should one consider in applying the definition of "human subject" to these activities — the person who provides the somatic cell, the woman who provides the egg, the woman who carries the pregnancy, the cloned embryo, and/or the resulting child?

4. Does the Constitution require heightened scrutiny of legal restrictions on cloning-to-produce-children? According to John Robertson,

> Couples who suffer from gametic infertility, who are seeking to have children to rear to whom they are genetically or biologically-related, may plausibly argue that cloning one of the partners is part of their constitutional right to reproduce. If so, their choice to form a family by cloning should not be restricted unless the practice were highly likely to cause substantial harm to children or others.

John A. Robertson, *Two Models of Human Cloning*, 27 HOFSTRA L. REV. 609, 622 (1999). Cass Sunstein, by contrast, disputes the claim "that there is a presumptive right to do whatever might be done to increase the likelihood of having, or not having, a child." Cass R. Sunstein, *Conceiving a Code for Creation: The Legal Debate Surrounding Human Cloning: Is There a Constitutional Right to Clone?* 53 HASTINGS L.J. 987, 994 (2002). Sunstein argues that "[u]nless there is some problem in the process that led to the law under review, courts should be hesitant to interpose their own views, at least outside of the most egregious cases." *Id.* at 1004; *see also* Carl H. Coleman, *Assisted Reproductive Technologies and the Constitution*, 30 FORD. URB. L.J. 57 (2002). Sunstein also concludes that there is no constitutional right to engage in cloning-for-biomedical-research. *See* Sunstein at 1002 (arguing that Supreme Court precedents lend no support to the claim that individuals "have a right to a particular set of medical experiments that might ultimately benefit them"). Should the Supreme Court recognize a constitutional right to engage in cloning-for-biomedical research and/or cloning-to-produce-children? What would be the implications of such a right?

[D] State Law

MICHIGAN COMPILED LAWS

§ 333.16274

(1) A licensee or registrant shall not engage in or attempt to engage in human cloning.

(2) Subsection (1) does not prohibit scientific research or cell-based therapies not specifically prohibited by that subsection. . . .

(5) As used in this section: (a) "Human cloning" means the use of human somatic cell nuclear transfer technology to produce a human embryo. . . .

§ 333.16275

. . . (3) A licensee or registrant or other individual who violates [the prohibition of human cloning] is subject to a civil penalty of $10,000,000.00.

RHODE ISLAND GENERAL LAWS § 23-16.42

No person or entity shall utilize somatic cell nuclear transfer for the purpose of initiating or attempting to initiate a human pregnancy nor shall any person create genetically identical human beings by dividing a blastocyst, zygote, or embryo.

NOTES AND QUESTIONS

1. Note that the Michigan law prohibits all forms of cloning, while the Rhode Island law prohibits only cloning-to-produce-children. In some states, the laws are ambiguous. For example, Virginia's law expressly permits "technologies to

clone molecules, including DNA, cells or tissues," but it says nothing about embryos. While the National Conference of State Legislatures believes the law prohibits only cloning-to-produce-children, some opponents of cloning believe it extends cloning-for-biomedical-research as well. *See* Sheryl Gay Stolberg, *States Pursue Cloning Laws as Congress Debates*, N.Y. TIMES, May 26, 2002, at 1.

2. What is the effect of paragraph (2) of the Michigan statute?

Chapter 17

GENETICS RESEARCH

This chapter examines two categories of research involving human genetics: (1) research designed to learn about the genome,[1] including studies exploring the relationship between genes and personal characteristics or susceptibility to disease; and (2) research designed to change the genome, which involves inserting "normal" genes into individuals who have undesirable mutations. In reading these materials, consider whether genetics research raises issues that are distinct from those involved in other types of human subject research, and, if it does, whether the existing regulatory framework is capable of addressing those concerns.

§ 17.01 RESEARCH DESIGNED TO LEARN ABOUT THE GENOME

Scientists employ a variety of methods to learn about the genome. *Pedigree studies* involve interviews and/or medical records reviews of individuals from families in which one or more members have an inherited disease or characteristic, in order to trace the natural history of the condition under investigation. *Genetic sequencing studies* seek to determine the chemical makeup of the human genome — i.e., the sequence in which the molecules of DNA (the chemical building block of genes) are organized. *Linkage studies* seek to identify disease-causing genes by connecting them to genetic markers that are transmitted through a family. Other forms of genetics research include *gene expression studies*, which seek to understand which genes are "turned on" or "turned off" in healthy and diseased tissues; *proteomics research*, which investigates the relationship between genes and the production of particular proteins in the body; and *DNA diagnostic studies*, which are designed to develop methods for learning about the genetic make-up of particular individuals. *See generally* LORI B. ANDREWS ET AL., GENETICS: ETHICS, LAW AND POLICY 86-87 (2002); NEW YORK STATE TASK FORCE ON LIFE AND THE LAW, GENETIC TESTING AND SCREENING IN THE AGE OF GENOMIC MEDICINE 29-77 (2000).

Genetics research is proceeding at an astonishingly fast pace, due largely to the efforts of the Human Genome Project, an international program launched in 1990 to sequence the human genome and to "map" all of the human genes to the twenty-three pairs of chromosomes that exist in all cells except sperm and egg cells. The National Human Genome Research Institute of the National

---

[1] The term "genome" refers to the total array of genes in either humans generally (the "human genome") or a particular individual.

Institutes of Health and the United States Department of Energy are jointly responsible for administering the Human Genome Project's activities in the United States.

[A] What the Genome Can Tell Us: The Power and Perils of Genetic Information

Although all individuals have the same basic set of genes, alternative forms of many genes exist throughout the population. The alternative forms of a gene are known as "alleles." Except for identical twins, every person has a unique combination of alleles, making each individual's overall genetic make-up (or "genotype") distinct.

Most observable characteristics of an individual (known as that person's "phenotype") are due to a combination of genetic and environmental factors. Thus, while genetic variations between individuals will sometimes result in observable differences in appearance, behavior, or disease susceptibility, in other cases genotypic variations may produce no phenotypic consequences. The imprecise link between genotype and phenotype can make it difficult to assess the clinical implications of genetic information.

Is genetic information inherently different from other probabilistic health information? Consider the distinctions identified in the following excerpt.

GENETIC TESTING AND SCREENING IN THE AGE OF GENOMIC MEDICINE NEW YORK STATE TASK FORCE ON LIFE AND THE LAW 98-101 (2000)

Genetic testing and information differ from other health-related testing and information, in kind or in degree, by a number of different, sometimes overlapping qualities, outlined below. . . .

Predictive Power of Genetic Information

Many medical tests, including serum cholesterol and blood pressure measures, can predict future health risks. However, genetic testing has more far-reaching predictive powers. It can indicate an individual's risk probabilities for late-onset disorders many decades before the presence of clinical signs or symptoms; reproductive genetic testing can predict the same risks for an embryo, a fetus, or an individual's future offspring. . . .

Stability of DNA

The stability of DNA is a fundamental difference between DNA-based genetic testing and other medical testing. Information determined by genetic testing of inherited gene variants of a newborn infant will not change over that infant's lifetime while medical signs and symptoms detected by other medical tests may. Samples may be stored indefinitely, enabling testing of long-deceased individuals.

Limited Sample Requirement

Another unique aspect of DNA-based genetic testing is that it can be performed with tiny samples, as little as a single cell. This allows predictive testing of pre-implantation embryos and forensic testing with microscopic tissue samples. . . .

Precision of Genetic Information

Genetic testing, by detection of specific gene variants, has a very high capacity for precision. In some cases, for example DNA-based cystic fibrosis testing, detection of particular gene mutations may enable prediction not only of the disorder, but also of the type and severity of the disorder. For more complex disorders, testing for inherited susceptibility variants can provide precise information about innate risk, although it cannot predict that a person will develop a disorder. The level of precision of genetic tests is greater than that of most other medical tests.

Personal Nature of Genetic Information

Genetic testing of health-related or other DNA "markers" that vary among the population can theoretically produce a "unique identifier" profile for any person. This is the basis for DNA-based forensic testing, which can identify a single individual from millions of others. Some view this difference of genetic information as qualitatively different from other health data. One commentator, however, claims that some nongenetic data in a medical record, such as gross obesity and loss of limbs, also may serve to identify an individual. He also suggests that the "considerable work and expense" needed to compile an identifying genetic profile would act as a deterrent to the use of genetic information in this manner, but evolving technologies may eventually render this claim obsolete.

Familial Nature of Genetic Information

Genetic information, while personal, also is inherently familial. Identical twins share 100 percent of their genes, other siblings (and a parent and a child) share 50 percent, and more distant relatives share a lower but calculable percentage of genes. Genetic testing, including blood group antigen testing and tissue typing to match donors and recipients for tissue transplantation, also may reveal nongenetic relationships within families, such as nonpaternity.

While other medical information also may help identify shared family risks, for example, information about infectious disease, the level of precision of genetic testing places genetic information at a significantly different level. One example of the power of genetic testing to disclose family relationships: Genetic testing of living descendants of Thomas Jefferson and descendents of one of his slaves, Sally Hemings, established Jefferson, or one of his nephews, as the father of at least one of Hemings' sons 200 years earlier.

History of Misuse and Misunderstanding of Genetics

Some think that past misuse of genetic information to stigmatize and victimize people is another factor that sets genetic information apart from other medical information. One commentator states that claims for genetic exceptionalism are partly due to a cultural overemphasis on the power of genetic information. Another group counters that public misperceptions about the power of genes: may be a reason to treat genetic information differently from other medical information.

NOTES AND QUESTIONS

1. For further discussion, *see,* e.g., Thomas H. Murray, *Genetic Exceptionalism and "Future Diaries:" Is Genetic Information Different from Other Medical Information*, in GENETIC SECRETS: PROTECTING PRIVACY AND CONFIDENTIALITY IN THE GENETIC ERA 60 (Mark Rothstein ed. 1997) (summarizing arguments for and against treating genetic information differently from other personal medical information).

2. Many of the "misuses" of genetic information mentioned in the excerpt from the New York State Task Force on Life and the Law were a product of the eugenics movement, which flourished in the United States in the early part of the twentieth century. Eugenicists attributed virtually all human characteristics to genetic factors and sought to limit reproduction to individuals deemed genetically "fit." Eugenic theories led to the adoption of marriage and immigration restrictions, the forcible sterilization of individuals considered unfit for reproduction, and other coercive laws and policies at the state and federal levels. Eugenics policies in this country had a significant influence on the Nazis, who cited legislation in California and other states "not only as precedents but also as models." ALLEN BUCHANAN ET AL., FROM CHANCE TO CHOICE: GENETICS AND JUSTICE 38 (2000).

3. Concerns about potential abuses of genetic information have led many states to adopt laws that require written informed consent to genetic testing, protect the confidentiality of genetic test results, and/or prohibit the adverse use of genetic information in employment, insurance, and other decisions. *See* George J. Annas, *The Limits of State Laws to Protect Genetic Information*, 345 NEW ENG. J. MED. 385 (2001) (noting that state anti-discrimination laws often provide only partial protections). Most of these laws were adopted after the Human Genome Project began in 1990. Given that the eugenics movement had long been discredited by that time, what sort of abuses do you think lawmakers were most worried about? Why, for example, might lawmakers have worried that an individual's genetic predisposition to developing early-onset cancer might be used against her by employers?

4. The New York State Task Force on Life and the Law also refers to a history of "misunderstanding" about genetics, a problem that continues today. Despite the fact that most individual characteristics are the result of a complex interplay of genetic and environmental factors, many people are wedded to a highly deterministic view of the role of genes. In their 1995 book, THE DNA MYSTIQUE: THE GENE AS CULTURAL ICON, Dorothy Nelkin and M. Susan Lindee coined the term "genetic essentialism" to describe the common perception that "genetics is destiny." Genetic essentialism, combined with widespread misunderstanding about the meaning of probabilistic information, makes it difficult to counsel people about the value of genetic testing and the meaning of genetic test results. *See* NEW YORK STATE TASK FORCE ON LIFE AND THE LAW, *supra*, at 89-90.

5. What are the implications of each of the factors outlined in the excerpt from the New York State Task Force on Life and the Law for an IRB's review of genetics research?

[B] Sources of Biological Materials for Genetics Research

Some genetics research is performed by recruiting individuals to donate tissue samples, including blood, saliva, and other bodily fluids, and/or to provide information about their family medical history. In many cases, however, researchers conduct studies using preexisting samples originally obtained for other purposes, sometimes combined with an analysis of the sample source's medical records. The next excerpt discusses where researchers find these samples.

1 RESEARCH INVOLVING HUMAN BIOLOGICAL MATERIALS: ETHICAL ISSUES AND POLICY GUIDANCE NATIONAL BIOETHICS ADVISORY COMMISSION
2 (1999)

The most common sources of human biological materials are diagnostic or therapeutic interventions in which diseased tissue is removed or tissue or other material is obtained to determine the nature and extent of a disease. Even after the diagnosis or treatment is complete, a portion of the specimen routinely is retained for future clinical, research, or legal purposes. Specimens also are obtained during autopsies. In addition, volunteers donate organs, blood, or other tissue for transplantation or research, and some donate their bodies after death for transplantation of organs or anatomical studies. . . .

Just as a clinician chooses biological materials appropriate to the clinical situation at hand, a researcher's choice of such materials depends on the goals of the research project. The selected tissue can be used only once, or it can be used to generate a renewable source of material, such as by developing a cell line, a cloned gene, or a gene marker. In addition, proteins can be extracted, or DNA isolated, from particular specimens.

There is substantial research value both in unidentified material (i.e., material that is not linked to an individual) and in material linked to an identifiable person and his or her continuing medical record. In the former, the value to the researcher of the human biological material is in the tissue itself and often in the associated clinical information about that individual, without the need to know the identity of the person from whom it came. For example, investigators may be interested in identifying a biological marker in a specific type of tissue, such as cells from individuals with Alzheimer's disease or specific tumors from a cancer patient. In such cases, beyond knowing the diagnosis of the individual from whom the specimen was obtained, researchers may not require more detailed medical records, either past or ongoing.

Sometimes, however, it is necessary to identify the source of the research sample, because the research value of the material depends upon linking findings regarding the biology of the sample with updated information from medical or other records pertaining to its source. For example, in a longitudinal study to determine the validity of a genetic marker as a predictor of certain diseases, the researchers would need to be able to link each sample with the medical record of its source in order to ascertain whether those diseases developed. In one case, a recent study of late-onset Alzheimer's disease linked the presence of the disease with the apolipoprotein-E allele by studying the stored tissues of 58 families with a history of Alzheimer's disease and then examining autopsy records for evidence of the disease in those individuals whose tissue revealed the presence of that allele.

Already, research using biological materials has produced tests to diagnose a predisposition to conditions such as cancer and heart disease and to a variety of genetic diseases that affect millions of individuals. In some cases, prevention or treatment is available once a diagnosis is made; in those cases, knowing the identity of the specimen source would permit communication of relevant medical information to the source that may be of importance to his or her health. In other cases, when medical interventions are unavailable, having one's specimen linked with a disease predictor is likely to be of less clinical value to the individual and might even be troubling.

NOTES AND QUESTIONS

1. How much of your own tissue do you think is currently available to genetics researchers? Consider all of the circumstances in which you have authorized physicians to remove blood or other tissue from your body. Do you know where those materials eventually ended up? Do you care?

2. In what way does the manner in which researchers obtain tissue for genetics research affect the issues an IRB should consider in reviewing a particular protocol?

[C] Necessity of IRB Review of Genetic Testing Research

[1] Definition of "Human Subject"

IRB approval is not required for research that does not involve "human subjects." Under the federal regulations, a "human subject" is defined as "a living individual about whom an investigator . . . obtains (1) data through intervention or interaction with the individual; or (2) identifiable private information." 45 C.F.R. § 46.102(f). Information is considered "identifiable" if "the identity of the subject is or may readily be ascertained by the investigator or associated with the information." 45 C.F.R. § 46.102(f)(2).

When researchers recruit individuals to donate tissue specifically for use in genetics research, they are clearly conducting research with human subjects under subdivision (1) of this definition. Whether research involving pre-existing or discarded tissue samples constitutes human subject research depends on whether the researchers have access to "identifiable private information" about the sample source.

Tissue samples used in research are often categorized into four types, depending on the ease of learning the sample source's identity:

- *Anonymous* samples are provided to researchers from specimens that were collected without any individually identifying information.

- *Anonymized* samples are provided by researchers from specimens that were collected with individually identifying information, but that have had this information permanently removed by the storage facility.

- *Coded* samples are provided by researchers from individually identifiable specimens; however, before sending the specimens to the researchers, the storage facility replaces the identifying information with a code. Only the storage facility, which retains the key to the code, has the ability to link the research findings with the sample source's identity.

- *Identified* samples are samples sent to researchers with individually identifiable information.

National Bioethics Advisory Commission, *supra*, at 58.

Research with identified samples would constitute human subject research under 45 C.F.R. § 109(f) because the researcher has access to the subject's identity. The next excerpt discusses whether the definition also should apply to research with coded samples.

GUIDANCE ON RESEARCH INVOLVING CODED PRIVATE INFORMATION OR BIOLOGICAL SAMPLES
OFFICE FOR HUMAN RESEARCH PROTECTIONS
http://www.hhs.gov/ohrp/humansubjects/guidance/cdebiol.pdf

In general, OHRP considers private information or specimens to be individually identifiable as defined at 45 C.F.R. 46.102(f) when they can be linked to specific individuals by the investigator(s) either directly or indirectly through coding systems.

Conversely, OHRP considers private information or specimens not to be individually identifiable when they cannot be linked to specific individuals by the investigator(s) either directly or indirectly through coding systems. For example, OHRP does not consider research involving *only* coded private information or specimens to involve human subjects as defined under 45 C.F.R. 46.102(f) if the following conditions are both met:

(1) the private information or specimens were not collected specifically for the currently proposed research project through an interaction or intervention with living individuals; and

(2) the investigator(s) cannot readily ascertain the identity of the individual(s) to whom the coded private information or specimens pertain because, for example:

   (a) the key to decipher the code is destroyed before the research begins;

   (b) the investigators and the holder of the key enter into an agreement prohibiting the release of the key to the investigators under any circumstances, until the individuals are deceased (note that the HHS regulations do not require the IRB to review and approve the agreement);

   (c) there are IRB-approved written policies and operating procedures for a repository or data management center that prohibit the release of the key to the investigators under any circumstances, until the individuals are deceased; or

   (d) there are other legal requirements prohibiting the release of the key to the investigators, until the individuals are deceased.

This guidance applies to existing private information and specimens, as well as to private information and specimens to be collected in the future for purposes other than the currently proposed research.

NOTES AND QUESTIONS

1. A surgeon agrees to send a group of researchers all tissue obtained from surgical patients meeting specified clinical criteria over a period of six months. The surgeon will assign each sample a code number, keep the key to the code in a secure place, and release only the samples and the code numbers to the researchers. After the patients return for follow-up care, the surgeon will send updated medical information to the researchers, again identifying the sample sources only by their code number. Assuming the researchers and the surgeon enter into an agreement prohibiting the researchers access to the key to the code under any circumstances, would the researchers be conducting "human subject" research under the OHRP guidance statement? How would the HIPAA privacy regulations discussed in Chapter 10 apply to this situation? Would the surgeon be required to obtain an HIPAA authorization or waiver of the authorization requirement before releasing the samples or the updated medical records, assuming that no identifying information about the patients is released? Would the surgeon be under any obligation to inform her patients about her use of their samples and their medical information?

2. In contrast to OHRP, the National Bioethics Advisory Commission (NBAC) concluded that the definition of human subject should be interpreted to include research with both anonymized and coded samples. *See* NATIONAL BIOETHICS ADVISORY COMMISSION, *supra*, at 58-60. Why do you think they made this recommendation? Why do you think OHRP did not follow it?

3. Under 45 C.F.R. § 102(f), only living individuals count as human subjects. Because research with tissue samples obtained from deceased individuals can have significant ramifications for those individuals' living relatives, it has been suggested that "investigators reconceptualize 'the family' as the 'subject' requiring protection and regulatory oversight" in these situations, thereby triggering the obligation to seek IRB review of protocols involving tissue samples from deceased individuals. Evan G. DeRenzo et al., *Genetics and the Dead: Implications for Genetics Research with Samples from Deceased Persons*, 69 AM. J. MED. GENETICS 332 (1997). Note that, although the research regulations do not apply to dead people, the HIPAA privacy regulations do apply to those persons' medical information. *See* Chapter 10, at page 461. Therefore, while researchers can use deceased persons' tissue samples without obtaining IRB approval, researchers who are part of a "covered entity" under HIPAA may not use those persons' medical records without complying with the HIPAA privacy rules.

4. In 2000, federal authorities suspended most human subject research at Virginia Commonwealth University after finding deficiencies in the IRB's oversight of a study involving adult twins. As part of the study, adult twins were sent a survey that included questions about the health of their family members, including whether they "had ever suffered from depression or had abnormal genitalia." Jay Mathews, *Father's Complaints Shut Down Research; U.S. Agencies Act on Privacy Concerns*, WASHINGTON POST, Jan. 12, 2000, at B7. The Office of

Protection from Research Risks (OPRR, the predecessor of OHRP) found that the IRB "should have considered whether family members were human subjects in this research by virtue of their relationship to the respondent and the nature of the family information obtained from the respondent." Jeffrey R. Botkin, *Protecting the Privacy of Family Members in Survey and Pedigree Research*, 285 JAMA 207 (2001).

Assume that you are a member of an IRB charged with reviewing a survey similar to that used in the Virginia Commonwealth study. What facts would you want to know before you decided whether the family members of the survey respondents constituted "human subjects"? What would be the implications of deciding that the family members do constitute human subjects? *See* Botkin, *supra*; Jeffrey R. Botkin et al., *Privacy and Confidentiality in the Publication of Pedigrees: A Survey of Investigators and Biomedical Journals*, 279 JAMA 1808 (1998). For further discussion of the confidentiality issues in pedigree research, see Chapter 10, at page 451.

[2] Exempt Research

Even if a study constitutes research with "human subjects," it may still be exempt from IRB review under 45 C.F.R. § 46.101(b)(4) (exempting from IRB review "research involving the collection or study of existing . . . pathological specimens, or diagnostic specimens, if these sources are publicly available or if the information is recorded by the investigator in such a manner that subjects cannot be identified, directly or through identifiers linked to the subjects").

NOTES AND QUESTIONS

1. Note that an exemption under § 46.101(b)(4) is available only for samples that are "existing" — i.e., samples that were collected before the research was initiated. What is the rationale for that limitation?

2. One of the situations in which research with existing samples is exempt from IRB review is if the samples are "publicly available." What is the rationale for exempting such studies from the regulatory requirements? Should tissue samples contained in a government repository be considered "publicly available" when they are freely accessible to any scientist who requests them but not to members of the general public who are not researchers? *See* NATIONAL BIOETHICS ADVISORY COMMISSION, *supra*, at 59 (arguing that such samples should not be considered publicly available).

3. Research with existing tissue samples also is exempt from IRB review if the information will be "recorded by the investigator in such a manner that the subjects cannot be identified." Note that, under this provision, the availability of an exemption depends not on whether the investigator is able to obtain information about the identity of the tissue sources (the issue of concern in the def-

inition of "human subject"), but on the manner in which the investigator records the data. Thus, even if the investigator has access to identifying information regarding the source of the samples, the study would still be exempt if she merely refrains from recording that identifying information. Is it appropriate to permit researchers to sift through the sample source's medical information without being subject to IRB review — and without obtaining the sample source's consent — as long as they do not record any identifying information?

4. A researcher wants to examine tissue samples from families affected with a rare genetic disorder. Before beginning the study, she will strip all references to the family names from the samples and mark each sample by its position within the family group (e.g., "family #1 father," "family #2 sister," etc.). Is the research exempt from the human subject protection regulations under 45 C.F.R. § 101(b)(4)?

5. Under the HIPAA privacy regulations, would any of the arrangements described in the previous note require an authorization or waiver of authorization by an IRB or a Privacy Board? *See* Chapter 10, at page 459.

6. Are the categories of genetics research that may be conducted without IRB review too broad? Can you think of an example of a study that would escape IRB review despite the fact that it involves significant risks?

[D] Risk Assessment

[1] Risks to Subjects

INSTITUTIONAL REVIEW BOARD GUIDEBOOK
Chapter 5H
U.S. DEPT. OF HEALTH AND HUMAN SERVICES,
OFFICE FOR PROTECTION FROM RESEARCH RISKS
(1993)

Genetic studies that generate information about subjects' personal health risks can provoke anxiety and confusion, damage familial relationships, and compromise the subjects' insurability and employment opportunities. . . .

Psychological risk includes the risk of harm from learning genetic information about oneself (e.g., that one is affected by a genetic disorder that has not yet manifested itself). Complicating the communication of genetic information is that often the information is limited to probabilities. Furthermore, the development of genetic data carries with it a margin of error; some information communicated to subjects will, in the end, prove to be wrong. In either event, participants are subjected to the stress of receiving such information. For example, researchers involved in developing presymptomatic tests for Huntington Disease (HD) have been concerned that the emotional impact of learning the results may lead some subjects to attempt suicide. They have therefore asked whether prospective participants should be screened for emotional stability prior to acceptance into a research protocol.

Note that these same disclosures of information can also be beneficial. One of the primary benefits of participation in genetic research is that the receipt of genetic information, however imperfect, can reduce uncertainty about whether participants will likely develop a disease that runs in their family (and possibly whether they have passed the gene along to their children). Where subjects learn that they will likely develop or pass along the disease, they might better plan for the future.

To minimize the psychological harms presented by pedigree research, IRBs should make sure that investigators will provide for adequate counseling to subjects on the meaning of the genetic information they receive. Genetic counseling is not a simple matter and must be done by persons qualified and experienced in communicating the meaning of genetic information to persons participating in genetic research or persons who seek genetic testing.

Social risks include stigmatization, discrimination, labeling, and potential loss of or difficulty in obtaining employment or insurance. Changes in familial relationships are also social ramifications of genetic research. For example, an employer who knew that an employee had an 80 percent chance of developing HD in her 40s might deny her promotion opportunities on the calculation that their investment in training would be better spent on someone without this known likelihood. Of course, the company may be acting irrationally (the other candidate might be hit by a car the next day, or have some totally unknown predisposition to debilitating disease), but the risk for our subject of developing HD is real, nonetheless. One problem with allowing third parties access to genetic information is the likelihood that information, poorly understood, will be misused. Likewise, an insurer with access to genetic information may be likely to deny coverage to applicants when risk of disease is in an unfavorable balance. Insuring against uncertain risks is what insurance companies do; when the likelihood of disease becomes more certain, they may refuse to accept the applicant's "bet."

NOTES AND QUESTIONS

1. As the preceding excerpt notes, genetic information is often "limited to probabilities." Consider, for example, the genetic tests now available for mutations in the BRCA1 and BRCA2 genes that have been associated with an increased risk of developing breast and/or ovarian cancer. Studies suggest that women who have one of these gene mutations but do not also have an extensive family history of breast and/or ovarian cancer face a lifetime breast cancer risk of between 36 and 56 percent. *See* NEW YORK STATE TASK FORCE ON LIFE AND THE LAW, *supra*, at 65. If you were one of these women, what would you do with that

information? Would you consider prophylactic mastectomy or prophylactic hormonal therapy, both of which have significant risks of their own? More frequent mammograms? Would you prefer not to know of your increased risk, given the lack of clear preventive options?

2. For studies in which individuals will receive the results of genetic testing, how should an IRB assess the significance of the risks identified above? Should it depend on the severity of the condition associated with the genetic information? The degree of stigma attached to the particular condition? The predictive value of the information? Whether the information is likely to affect an individual's reproductive decision making?

3. As discussed below, at page 723, researchers do not always reveal the results of genetic testing to the individuals who provided the samples, even when the sample source's identity is known. What risks exist in studies involving identifiable samples when the results of genetic tests will not be disclosed to the sample sources?

4. What, if any, risks to subjects exist in studies involving pre-existing tissue samples that lack any identifying information about the sample sources (i.e., anonymous, anonymized, or coded samples)?

5. Can you envision any circumstances in which the risks of genetics research might be sufficiently serious for an IRB to reject a study? Or is the primary reason for assessing the risks of genetics research to identify issues to disclose to subjects during the informed consent process?

[2] Risks to Others

Information about one person's genetic make-up necessarily has implications for that person's blood relatives. For example, if researchers discover that an individual has a genetic mutation associated with an increased risk of developing a particular form of cancer, there is a good chance that the person's siblings also share the mutation. If those siblings are told of these findings, they may be burdened with information they would rather not know, and they generally will not have been given the opportunity to receive appropriate counseling about the implications of the information. Moreover, if the information is not kept confidential, it may be used against them in employment, insurance, or other contexts.

Genetic information also can have implications for individuals not related to the subject of testing. For example, many genetic studies have focused on Ashkenazi Jews — not because these individuals have higher rates of genetic disorders than any other group of people, but because "centuries of living and marrying within the confines of ghettoes have produced a relatively homogenous population in which tiny genetic alterations, or mutations, that cause disease are easy to find." Sheryl Gay Stolberg, *Concern Among Jews Is Heightened as Scientists Deepen Gene Studies*, N.Y. TIMES, April 22, 1998, at A24. As more and more studies reveal genetic mutations common among the Ashkenazi Jewish population, some people worry that Ashkenazi Jews are " 'getting a bad reputation.' " *Id.* (quoting Rabbi Moshe David Tendler, a professor of medical ethics at Yeshiva University in Manhattan). Some Native Americans have similarly expressed concerns about the stigmatizing potential of genetics research, including "the fear that looking for genetic contributions to diseases such as diabetes mellitus and alcoholism will shift the focus away from the social factors, such as diet, poverty, and stress, that influence these disorders." Ellen Wright Clayton, *The Complex Relationship of Genetics, Groups, and Health: What It Means for Public Health*, 30 J. L. MED. & ETHICS 290, 294 (2002).

As discussed in the following excerpt, one method that has been proposed to address the implications of genetics research for racial or ethnic populations is to involve those populations more directly in the design and/or review of such research.

Involving Study Populations in the Review of Genetic Research
Richard R. Sharp & Morris W. Foster
28 J. L. MED. & ETHICS 41 (2000)

Forms of community review

. . .

Community dialogue

This form of review includes both formal and informal discussion of a proposed study and its potential implications for a socially identifiable group. These discussions may be initiated by researchers or arise independently within a community after contact with researchers. Community dialogue is meant to identify collective concerns and consider ways of minimizing research-related risks, but does not provide a comprehensive review of the research in question and often will not engage a representative sample of community members.

Community consultation

In contrast to community dialogue, this type of review is more structured. Community consultation documents and records the concerns of a socially identifiable group by consulting a representative subset of its individual members and organizations. Other reviewers can then incorporate these perspectives in their assessments of the research. How these perspectives are documented will vary, ranging from structured community forums to the creation of an independent community review panel. These forums and review panels may choose to endorse or oppose the research in an explicit way, but with community consultation, these evaluations are not binding on researchers.

Formal community approval (disapproval)

An even more structured type of community review is the negotiation of a formal contractual agreement between researchers and a study population. This arrangement can be thought of as roughly analogous to obtaining informed consent from individual research participants. In this form of review, members of a study population (or recognized political representatives) are asked to give their collective permission for a research study. That collective decision, however, is not binding on individual community members, who still may choose to participate in the research (or not to participate).

Community partnership

The most structured way to involve members of a study population in the review process is to make them partners in the research. As partners, members of the study population are involved early in the design of the research project and "review" the study by helping to define its goals and methodology, and implement its experimental design. . . .

Tailoring review to the community

The form of community review that is most appropriate for a given community, or a particular study, depends upon several factors. Formal community approval, for instance, requires that there be authorities empowered to speak for the study population at large. Similarly, community consultation assumes the existence of shared communal interests and values. Culturally heterogeneous populations may not possess such shared interests, and thus may not be able to reach consensus about the most salient research-related risks. Other factors affecting the form that community review should take include: the size of the population, the extent of shared social and cultural structures, the frequency with which individual members interact with each other, the types of risks presented by the study, and the nature and scope of the proposed research. . . .

For example, if interactions between members of a study population are infrequent, and their distinctive beliefs few, then genetic research is unlikely to present risks that are unique to that population's particular sociocultural structures. In such populations, the primary risks presented by genetic research involve potential misuses of genetic information by others outside the community. These risks, what we might call "external" risks, include discrimination and stigmatization of members of the study population. Many of these external risks, however, are not unique to any particular group and often can be identified by individuals who are not themselves members of the population placed at-risk (though these external threats may be more readily identifiable by members of the study population). Hence, where the primary risks are presented by outsiders and are not linked to distinctive interactions between members of the study population, supplemental community review may not be necessary. Nonetheless, community dialogue or consultation can still be helpful in identifying research-related risks and assessing how members of the study population view the significance of these risks. For example, community review may reveal that members of the study population place a different weight on these risks than those assumed by outside reviewers. . . .

In contrast, where the frequency of social interaction between members of a study population is high, and a number of distinctive sociocultural beliefs help to distinguish members of the population from outsiders, genetic research can present additional risks. These two factors can heighten the external risks of a study because the study population's cultural discreteness may make it easier for outsiders to single out members as different from others. Frequent social interactions between members of a study population also can create a social equilibrium among members. This equilibrium could be disrupted by genetic research. For example, an American Indian community that makes use of traditional means of disease prevention (e.g., collective preventive rituals) may find those social structures called into question by research on disease susceptibility. In those circumstances, genetic research could undermine the legitimacy of traditional means of disease prevention by suggesting that non-traditional influences play a more important role in the development of disease. Similarly, relationships between communities could be affected by research on population differences. Genetic findings could reveal that a community that views itself as historically or ancestrally related to another community is mistaken and that there are no historic relationships between the two groups.

NOTES AND QUESTIONS

1. What are the advantages and disadvantages of the various forms of community review described above?

2. What makes a particular group of people a "community"? What gives someone the right to act as a "representative" of a community? Recall that similar questions have arisen in connection with the regulations authorizing waivers of consent in emergency research, which require IRBs to consult with the community in which the research will be conducted. *See* Chapter 7, at page 318.

3. Eric Juengst argues that, despite the risks that human groups face from genetics research, "it would be a mistake for scientists and science policymakers to attempt to give groups a gatekeeping role in genomics research." He notes that, apart from "rare geographically isolated exceptions," genetic subgroups — i.e., "groups of individuals more genetically similar to each other than to any other individuals" — bear little relationship to self-defined social or ethnic communities. Using social and ethnic communities as surrogates for genetic subgroups, he argues, would perpetuate the misconception that members of those groups are inherently different from other people in society, "setting the stage for new forms of scientific racism and providing new tools for discrimination." Eric T. Juengst, *Groups as Gatekeepers to Genomic Research:*

Conceptually Confusing, Morally Hazardous, and Practically Useless, 8 KENNEDY INST. ETHICS J. 183 (1998). How might Sharp and Foster respond to these concerns?

4. Organizers of the Human Genome Diversity Project hope to collect DNA from members of approximately five hundred different population groups in the world, in order to permit researchers to study "the diversity and unity of the entire human species." HUMAN GENOME DIVERSITY PROJECT: FREQUENTLY ASKED QUESTIONS, available at http://www.stanford.edu/group/morrinst/hgdp/faq.html. The goal of the project is to develop a database containing information about genetic variations common among different ethnic groups. What are the risks and potential benefits of such an endeavor, and how should the concerns of the affected populations be addressed?

5. In 2004, members of the Havasupai Indian Reservation sued Arizona State University and others based on the alleged misuse of blood samples taken from tribal members during a study of diabetes. The complaint "claims that tribal members were told the samples would be used only for a study of diabetes when, it is alleged, they were used without authorization in unrelated studies of schizophrenia, inbreeding, and theories regarding the migration of humans to North America." William H. Carlile, *Lawsuit Alleges University Mishandled Blood Samples Taken from Arizona Tribe*, 3 MED. RESEARCH L. & POL'Y REP. (BNA) 197 (2004). Recall that the federal regulations would not apply to these secondary uses of the samples if the samples were either stripped of identifying information or coded by the tissue bank before being sent to the researchers. *See supra*, page 704. Do you think the tribe members' concerns had anything to do with whether the samples contained individually identifiable information?

6. The federal regulations direct IRBs not to "consider possible long-range effects of applying knowledge gained in the research (for example, the possible effects of the research on public policy) as among those research risks that fall within the purview of [their] responsibility." 45 C.F.R. § 46.111(a)(2). What are the implications of this provision for IRBs' assessment of the risks of genetics research to nonsubjects? What do you think explains the inclusion of this provision in the regulations?

7. While genetics research targeted to specific populations may expose members of those populations to unique risks, it also holds out the potential for significant benefits. For example, in explaining its decision to create a genetic databank for people of African descent, officials at Howard University emphasized the value of determining whether genetic factors help explain why African Americans suffer higher rates of some diseases than whites, or why African Americans respond differently to particular drugs. *See Howard University Plans Genetic Databank To Study Disease in African-Descent Patients*, 2 MED. RESEARCH L. & POL'Y REP. (BNA) 406 (2003).

[3] Risk Assessment and Eligibility for Expedited Review

If a study involves no more than minimal risks, it may be eligible for expedited IRB review. While the OHRP guidebook states that the "psychosocial risks" of genetics studies "are likely to raise the risk beyond the 'minimal risk' level allowable for expedited review," NBAC concluded that "most research using human biological materials is likely to be considered of minimal risk because much of it focuses on research that is not clinically relevant to the sample source, as compared to research with medical records, for example, which is likely to be filled with clinically relevant findings that could harm the individual if misused or used inappropriately be third parties." NATIONAL BIOETHICS ADVISORY COMMISSION, *supra*, at 67. NBAC recommended that, in assessing whether genetics research involves more than minimal risks, IRBs should consider the following questions:

- How easily identifiable is the source?

- What is the likelihood that the source will be traced?

- If the source is traced, what is the likelihood that persons other than the investigators will obtain information about the source? (Privacy/confidentiality laws may be relevant here, as are the integrity of investigators and their institutional confidentiality protections.)

- If noninvestigators obtain information regarding the source, what is the likelihood that harms will result, including adverse consequences arising from the reporting of uncertain or ambiguous clinical results? (State and federal discrimination laws may be relevant with respect to uses of information by third parties.)

Id. Note that, even if a study involves minimal risks, expedited review is permissible only if the study falls within one of the specific categories of research deemed eligible for expedited consideration. *See* Appendix B. Of particular relevance to genetics research are the following three categories:

(2) Collection of blood samples by finger stick, heel stick, ear stick, or venipuncture [subject to limits on the amount of blood drawn]

(3) Prospective collection of biological specimens for research purposes by noninvasive means.

(5) Research involving materials (data, documents, records, or specimens) that have been collected, or will be collected solely for non-research purposes (such as medical treatment or diagnosis).

63 FED. REG. 60364-60367 (1998).

Would a study examining pre-existing tissue samples that were originally obtained in a prior research project fit within any of these categories?

[E] Informed Consent

[1] Research Involving the Collection of New Tissue Samples ("Prospective Studies")

Statement on Informed Consent for Genetic Research **American Society of Human Genetics**
9 AM. J. HUMAN GENETICS 471 (1996)

Subjects providing consent to prospective studies should be told about the types of information that could result from genetic research. Subjects must be given sufficient information to understand the implications and the limitations of research. Individuals should be told the purpose, limitations, possible outcomes, and means of communicating results and maintaining confidentiality. They should be informed of what information may reasonably be expected to result from the genetic study. Importantly, subjects should also understand that unexpected findings, including identification of medical risk, carrier status, or risk to offspring affected by genetic disease, may arise.

During the course of molecular genetic diagnosis, the results may indicate that the child is not the offspring of one or both the presumed parents. The investigator therefore should consider including in the consent form a statement that misidentified parentage will not be disclosed. Another example of unforeseen outcome is genetic heterogeneity in which disorders which were initially thought to be due to defects in a single allele or locus are associated with new ones.

Additional risks that should be disclosed to subjects of certain genetic research studies include the possibility of adverse psychological sequelae, disruption of family dynamics, and social stigmatization and discrimination. All genetic research studies involving identified or identifiable samples in which disclosure of results is planned should have medical geneticists and/or genetic counselors involved to ensure results are communicated to the subjects accurately and appropriately. The consent form should not promise significant breakthroughs in diagnosis, treatment or outcome to entice participation. Also, careful attention by all parties involved in genetic research should be given to avoiding actions that could be coercive to potential subjects.

Disposition of Samples and Results

Depending on the study, subjects may be given the opportunity to determine if they want to be informed of the results of their testing. Subjects should be informed if the sample will be stored for later study, but they also need to be told that there is always the possibility of storage failure. Decisions related to disposition of results or samples after the subject's death should be specified by the subject. . . .

Subjects involved in studies where the samples are identified or identifiable should indicate if their sample should be used exclusively in the study under consideration. If the sample is to be used more generally, subjects should be given options regarding the scope of the subsequent investigations, such as whether the sample can be used only for a specific disease under investigation, or for other unrelated conditions. It is inappropriate to ask a subject to grant blanket consent for all future unspecified genetic research projects on any disease or in any area if the samples are identifiable in those subsequent studies.

Subjects involved in studies in which the samples are identified or identifiable should indicate if unused portions of the samples may be shared with other researchers. If the subject is willing to have the sample shared with other researchers, it is the responsibility of the principal investigator to distribute the sample, so as to ensure that the agreement embodied in the informed consent is upheld. Finally, subjects should decide if subsequent researchers may receive their samples as anonymous or identifiable specimens.

NOTES AND QUESTIONS

1. Many of the concerns discussed in the preceding excerpt relate to the potential impact on subjects of learning the results of genetic testing. How do the informed consent issues change when subjects will not learn the study results? *See* Laura M. Beskow et al., *Informed Consent for Population-Based Research Involving Genetics*, 286 JAMA 2315 (2001).

2. The preceding excerpt mentions the phenomenon of "genetic heterogeneity," but it does not clearly state how this phenomenon should be addressed in the informed consent process. How do you think researchers should handle this problem?

3. A phenomenon similar to genetic heterogeneity is the "pleiotropic" nature of genes — i.e., the fact that one gene may control several, unrelated phenotypic effects. For example, a particular mutation in the apolipoprotein E (APOE) gene may help determine the appropriate treatment for coronary artery disease, but it also may reveal an individual's likelihood of developing late-onset Alzheimer's disease. *See* NEW YORK STATE TASK FORCE ON LIFE AND THE LAW, *supra*, at 193. It is likely that, as genetic discoveries progress, information originally thought relevant for one condition will turn out to have implications for others. What problems does the pleiotropic nature of genes raise for subjects' ability to provide informed consent to genetics research? How should researchers address these problems?

4. Genetics research can lead to the development of profitable products. Yet, consent forms used by tissue banks "commonly give the impression that banked tissue and blood have no market value and would otherwise be thrown away." David E. Winickoff & Richard N. Winickoff, *The Charitable Trust as a Model for*

Genomic Biobanks, 349 NEW ENG. J. MED. 1180 (2003). What, if anything, should subjects be told about the possible commercial implications of genetics research? We will return to this question below, at page 729.

5. The excerpt from the American Society of Human Genetics recommends that subjects who provide tissue for use in genetics research be asked about their wishes regarding the use of the tissue in future research projects. Assume that a subject expressly states that she does not want her sample used in any future studies — even if the sample is anonymized or coded. If research with anonymized or coded samples does not constitute "human subject" research, do the regulations require the researchers to abide by the subject's wishes? Are there other legal principles that might provide a basis for imposing such an obligation?

6. In addition to obtaining informed consent, researchers conducting prospective studies with identified tissue samples must comply with the HIPAA privacy regulations if the researchers are part of a "covered entity" as defined in HIPAA. *See* Chapter 10, at page 447.

[2] Research Using Existing Tissue Samples ("Retrospective Studies")

When researchers use preexisting samples left over from clinical procedures or prior research projects, contacting all of the individuals who provided the tissue is likely to be extremely difficult, if not impossible. As the next excerpt explains, one option in these situations is to rely on the consent the individuals provided at the time their tissue was originally obtained.

1 RESEARCH INVOLVING HUMAN BIOLOGICAL MATERIALS: ETHICAL ISSUES AND POLICY GUIDANCE NATIONAL BIOETHICS ADVISORY COMMISSION
62-63 (1999)

Research using coded[2] or identified samples requires the consent of the source, unless the criteria for a consent waiver have been satisfied. Unfortunately, the consent signed at the time the specimen was obtained may not always be adequate to satisfy this requirement. Specimens that exist in storage at the time the research is proposed may have been collected under a variety of conditions (e.g., in a clinical setting or as part of an experimental protocol). In some instances, individuals make informed choices about how their sample should be used subsequent to its original research or clinical use. In other cases,

---

[2] As noted above, OHRP has not accepted NBAC's recommendation to treat research with coded samples as a type of human subject research. *See supra*, page 704. However, NBAC's analysis remains relevant to researchers' use of identified samples.

for a variety of reasons, individuals may not understand fully or may not have been given the opportunity to consider carefully how their specimens may be used in the future. When research is contemplated using existing materials, the expressed wishes of the individuals who provided the materials must be respected. Where consent documents exist, they may indicate whether individuals wanted their samples to be used in future research, and in some instances they may specify the type of research.

IRBs should use the following criteria to evaluate the applicability of such documents to the proposed research:

- Does the language or context of the consent form indicate that the source was interested in aiding the type of research being proposed?

- If the source consented to the sample being used in unspecified future studies, is that consent adequate for the type of research being planned, given the circumstances under which the sample was collected (e.g., whether the sample was requested by a treating physician or whether the consent form offered alternatives to allowing the sample to be used in future studies)?

In some cases, an IRB may determine that an existing consent form permitting unspecified future uses is sufficient. For example, Clayton et al. argue that, "[e]ven in the absence of specific language about DNA testing, it may be appropriate to infer consent if the source wished for the sample to be used to determine why his or her family had a particular inherited disorder." In such cases, investigators should consider informing subjects that research is occurring and in certain cases also give subjects the opportunity to "opt out." Rarely, however, does the language that is included in typical surgical and other hospital consent forms provide an adequate basis for inferring consent to future research.

Although an opt-out policy provides significant protection for sources and recognizes that their biological material may have been collected without adequate disclosure, it also provides sources with the opportunity to participate in research. When the IRB determines existing consent documents to be inadequate and when the existing sample is identifiable, the individual should be contacted, offered the option of consenting to the specific proposed protocol, and further offered the option of deciding how the sample may be used in the future.

NOTES AND QUESTIONS

1. As NBAC notes, if it is not possible to rely on the consent provided at the time the tissue was originally obtained, another option is for the researchers to seek a waiver of the requirement to obtain informed consent. Before authorizing a waiver of informed consent, the IRB must determine that "(1) the study involves no more than minimal risks to the subjects; (2) the waiver . . . will not adversely affect the rights and welfare of the subjects; (3) the research could not

practicably be carried out without the waiver . . .; and (4) whenever appropriate, the subjects will be provided with additional pertinent information after participation." 45 C.F.R. § 46.116(d). The first element of this provision ("minimal risk") is discussed *supra*, page 714. Consider the other three elements:

- *Rights and Welfare* — According to NBAC, nonconsensual research with preexisting tissue samples may affect subjects' rights or welfare if it "would violate any state or federal statute or customary practice regarding entitlement to privacy or confidentiality," if it "will examine traits commonly considered to have political, cultural, or economic significance to the study subjects," or if "the study's results might adversely affect the welfare of the subject's community." NATIONAL BIOETHICS ADVISORY COMMISSION, *supra*, at 68. What type of studies might implicate these factors?

- *Impracticability* — How difficult must it be for the researchers to obtain informed consent before it is appropriate to say that "the research could not practicably be carried out" without a waiver of the consent requirement? A workgroup convened by the National Institutes of Health (NIH) and the Centers for Disease Control and Prevention (CDC) concluded that, "given that talking with people always entails some costs, consent cannot be waived on the simple assertion that seeking it would be tedious, burdensome or costly. Rather, there must be proof that requiring consent would be so burdensome or expensive, as might be true were it necessary to contact the entire population, that the research could not go forward." Ellen Wright Clayton et al., *Informed Consent for Genetic Research on Stored Tissue Samples*, 274 JAMA 1786, 1789 (1995). Is this standard appropriate? Is it relevant that delaying the research to contact the sample sources might harm future patients by depriving them of the benefits the study is designed to achieve? In contrast to the NIH/CDC workgroup, NBAC concluded that "IRBs should be permitted to presume that contacting individuals who were the sources of tissues in the past will be impracticable enough to satisfy the regulatory requirements." NATIONAL BIOETHICS ADVISORY COMMISSION, *supra*, at 69. Is this standard preferable?

- *Providing Additional Information as Required* — What sort of additional information, if any, should be given to subjects whose identifiable tissue samples are used in nonconsensual genetics research? Can an argument be made that providing additional information to subjects after the research is concluded would do more harm than good?

Many states have laws that require written informed consent to genetic testing. *See*, e.g., N.Y. CIVIL RIGHTS LAW § 79-l; N.Y. INS. LAW § 2612. What are the implications of such laws for an IRB's ability to waive informed consent under section 46.116(d)?

2. The regulations do not require informed consent for studies that either do not fall within the definition of "human subject" research or are exempt from regulatory scrutiny under 45 C.F.R. § 46.101(b)(4). Thus, if the subjects' prior consent is not sufficient and waiver of the informed consent requirement is not appropriate, the researchers can either strip the samples of identifying information (rendering them "anonymized"), or ask the tissue repository to code the samples and enter into an agreement prohibiting the repository from providing the key to the code to the researchers until the sample sources have died. *See supra*, page 704. While using anonymized samples would make it impossible for the researchers to connect the research findings with the medical records of the sample sources, that problem does not exist with coded samples (although the tissue bank holding the key to the code would have to act as an intermediary). When researchers seek a waiver of the informed consent requirement for studies involving identified samples, does the fact that the research could be conducted with coded samples negate the claim that the research "could not practicably be carried out" without the waiver?

3. As with prospective research using identified tissue samples, the use of existing, identified samples in research may trigger the application of the HIPAA privacy regulations. *See* Chapter 10, at page 459.

[F] Confidentiality Issues

As discussed in Chapter 10, one of the responsibilities of IRBs is to ensure that "there are adequate protections to protect the privacy of subjects and to maintain the confidentiality of data." 45 C.F.R. § 46.111(a)(7). Consider the distinguishing characteristics of genetics information discussed in the excerpt from the New York State Task Force on Life and the Law at the beginning of this chapter. Why might these factors make confidentiality issues particularly important in genetics research?

Although the following excerpt focuses primarily on pedigree studies, it highlights issues that are relevant to genetics research more generally. As you read this excerpt, consider how the issues it raises might apply to the other types of genetics studies outlined at the beginning of this chapter.

INSTITUTIONAL REVIEW BOARD GUIDEBOOK

Chapter 5H

U.S. DEPT. OF HEALTH AND HUMAN SERVICES

OFFICE FOR PROTECTION FROM RESEARCH RISKS

(1993)

Special privacy and confidentiality concerns arise in genetic family studies because of the special relationship between the participants. IRBs should keep in mind that within families, each person is an individual who deserves to have information about him- or herself kept confidential. Family members are not entitled to each other's diagnoses. Before revealing medical or personal information about individuals to other family members, investigators must obtain the consent of the individual.

Another problem that arises in genetic family studies that is also common in other areas of research involving interviews with subjects is the provision by a subject of information about another person. In pedigree studies, for example, the proband or other family member is usually asked to provide information about other members of the family. The ethical question presented by this practice is whether that information can become part of the study without the consent of the person about whom the data pertains. While no consensus on this issue has yet been reached, IRBs may consider collection of data in this manner acceptable, depending on the nature of the risks and sensitivities involved. It may be helpful, for example, to draw a distinction between information about others provided by a subject that is also available to the investigator through public sources (e.g., family names and addresses) and other personal information that is not available through public sources (e.g., information about medical conditions or adoptions).

IRBs should require investigators to establish ahead of time what information will be revealed to whom and under what circumstances, and to communicate these conditions to subjects in clear language. For example, if the pedigree is revealed to the study participants, family members will learn not only about themselves but about each other. The possibility that family members who did not participate might also learn of the pedigree data should not be overlooked. Subjects should know and agree ahead of time to what they might learn (and what they will not learn), both about themselves and others, and what others might learn about them. One approach would be never to reveal the pedigree to participating subjects. Many investigators record their pedigrees using code numbers rather than names. IRBs should note, however, that when a study involves a rare disease or a "known" family, the substitution of numbers for names does not eliminate the problem. . . .

Data must be stored in such a manner that does not directly identify individuals. In general, except where directly authorized by individual subjects, data may not be released to anyone other than the subject. An exception to requiring explicit authorization for the release of data may be secondary research use of the data, where the data are not especially sensitive and where confidentiality can be assured. IRBs should exercise their discretion in reviewing protocols that call for the secondary use of genetic data. Furthermore, when reviewing a consent document, IRBs should note agreements made by investigators not to release information without the express consent of subjects. Subsequent requests for access to the data are subject to agreements made in the consent process. For studies involving socially sensitive traits or conditions, investigators might also consider requesting a certificate of confidentiality. [For a discussion of certificates of confidentiality, see Chapter 10, at page 452.]

NOTES AND QUESTIONS

1. Confidentiality issues are important not only in studies in which individuals are recruited to provide information and/or tissue samples, but also in studies involving pre-existing, identified tissue samples. In studies involving coded samples, the key confidentiality issue is ensuring that the link between the code numbers and any identifying information is secure.

2. In addition to the general legal protections governing the confidentiality of research data, several states have enacted statutes specifically directed at maintaining the confidentiality of genetic information. *See generally* Ellen Wright Clayton, *Ethical, Legal, and Social Implications of Genomic Medicine*, 349 NEW ENG. J. MED. 562 (2003) (identifying 26 such statutes).

3. Should research subjects always have the right to insist that their genetic information not be disclosed to their family members? What if the information would help a relative avert or treat a serious disease, or make a more informed reproductive decision? For example, researchers may discover that a particular subject has a mutation associated with a form of cancer for which early detection and treatment are critical (such as colon cancer). If the subject refuses to disclose this fact to his or her siblings — who are necessarily at risk of having the identical mutation — should the researchers be permitted (or even required) to contact the siblings directly? *See* American Society of Human Genetics, *Professional Disclosure of Familial Genetic Information*, 62 AM. J. HUMAN GENETICS 474 (1998) (arguing, outside the research context, that "disclosure should be permissible where attempts to encourage disclosure on the part of the patient have failed; where the harm is highly likely to occur and is serious and foreseeable; where the at-risk relative is identifiable; . . . where either the disease is preventable/treatable or medically accepted standards indicate that early monitoring will reduce the genetic risk;" and "where the harm that may result from failure to disclose outweighs the harm that may result from the disclosure"); NEW YORK STATE TASK FORCE ON LIFE AND THE LAW, *supra*, at 274 (reaching a similar conclusion but recommending that any nonconsensual disclosures be authorized by a court). In cases arising outside research, two courts have recognized that physicians have a duty to protect the interests of the relatives of patients diagnosed with certain genetic mutations, but one of these courts held that such a duty "will be satisfied by warning the patient." *Pate v. Threlkel*, 661 So. 2d 278 (Fla. 1995). The other court left open the possibility that physicians might have a duty to breach confidentiality to tell the relative directly. *See Safer v. Estate of Pack*, 291 N.J. Super. 619, 677 A.2d 1188 (N.J. Super. Ct. App. Div. 1996); *see also* Kenneth Offit et al., *The "Duty to Warn" a Patient's Family Members about Hereditary Disease Risks*, 292 JAMA 1469 (2004).

[G] Informing Subjects of Study Results

The previous section addressed the importance of protecting genetic information from disclosure to persons other than the research subject. This section considers whether the information may be withheld from the subject him- or herself.

INSTITUTIONAL REVIEW BOARD GUIDEBOOK
Chapter 5H
U.S. DEPT. OF HEALTH AND HUMAN SERVICES
OFFICE FOR PROTECTION FROM RESEARCH RISKS
(1993)

Experts disagree about whether interim or inconclusive findings should be communicated to subjects, although most agree that they should not (that only confirmed, reliable findings constitute "information"). Persons who oppose revealing interim findings argue that the harms that could result from revealing preliminary data whose interpretation changes when more precise or reliable data become available are serious, including anxiety or irrational — and possibly harmful — medical interventions. They argue that such harms are avoidable by controlling the flow of information to subjects and limiting communications to those that constitute reliable information. [One commentator], writing about the development of genetic tests, argues against revealing interim findings, contending that preliminary results do not yet constitute "information" since "until an initial finding is confirmed, there is no reliable information" to communicate to subjects, and that "even . . . confirmed findings may have some unforeseen limitations." He argues that subjects should not be given information about their individual test results until the findings have been confirmed through the "development of a reliable, accurate, safe and valid presymptomatic test." Others have argued that all interim results should be shared with subjects, based on the principle of autonomy — that subjects have a right to know what has been learned about them. . . .

IRBs should consider these arguments, weighing the possible harms and benefits. Investigators should determine, prior to initiation of the study, the point at which the data will be considered solid enough to constitute information that should be provided to subjects. Investigators should further consider coding the data and separating the research records from individuals' medical records, so that neither the investigators nor the subjects may gain access to them.

[One commentator] suggests that IRBs develop general policies governing the disclosure of information to subjects, to help make these determinations. He suggests that at least the following three factors be considered: "(1) the magnitude of the threat posed to the subject, (2) the accuracy with which the data predict that the threat will be realized, and (3) the possibility that action can be taken to avoid or ameliorate the potential injury." IRBs should ask investigators to define three categories of disclosure: (1) "findings that are of such potential importance to the subject that they *must* be disclosed immediately;" (2) "data that are of importance to subjects . . . , but about which [the investigator] should exercise judgment about the decision to disclose. . . . [i]n effect, these are data that trigger a duty to consider the question of disclosure;" and (3) "data that do *not* require special disclosure."

IRBs should consider whether the investigator's approach appropriately balances the risks and benefits involved in providing access to the data. Subjects should be told, as part of the consent process, whether, when, and what information they will receive. Any disclosures of genetic information should be accompanied by appropriate counseling by trained genetic counselors. However the IRB resolves this question, investigators should explain to prospective subjects the basis according to which they will decide which data will be disclosed to whom, and when those disclosures will be made.

Access to Data: The Subjects' "Right Not to Know." Subjects generally retain the right not to receive information about the results of a study that reveals their genetic status. A possible exception involves circumstances where early treatment of genetically-linked disease could improve the subject's prognosis. In such circumstances, investigators may have a duty to inform the subject about the existence of the genetic defect and to advise him or her to seek medical advice. . . .

Access to Data: Incidental Findings. IRBs should also ensure that investigators adequately deal with how they will handle incidental findings; that is, what will be done with genetic information that is learned during the course of the study that does not directly relate to the research. For example, in intergenerational pedigree analyses, questions of paternity or parentage can come up. DNA analysis will reveal information indicating that an individual's biological parents are not who he or she thought they were; blood typing may reveal similar information. DNA analysis may also reveal information about diseases or conditions other than the disease or condition under study. Prospective subjects should be informed during the consent process that the discovery of such information is possible. Appropriate counseling should be provided to educate subjects about the meaning of the genetic information they have received, and to assist them in coping with any psychosocial effects of participation.

NOTES AND QUESTIONS

1. The NIH/CDC workgroup discussed on page 719 noted that "there might be a very small risk that investigators, particularly if they are also the sources' treating physicians, who fail to tell subjects about a mutation that predisposes them to colon cancer, for example, could be found liable if these individuals do not undergo periodic screening and later develop the disease." Clayton et al.,

supra, at 1790. What legal theories might support the imposition of liability in such circumstances? What can researchers do to minimize the risk of liability?

2. The excerpt suggests that investigators "may" have a duty to inform subjects of test results if "early treatment of genetically-linked disease could improve the subject's prognosis," possibly even if the subjects have expressed a desire not to learn the results. Should such a duty be recognized, either as an ethical or legal matter?

3. Even if individual results will not be disclosed to subjects, some commentators suggest that subjects be given "an aggregate report of overall study results, for example, through a newsletter. In the rare event that results unexpectedly have clinical significance, participants could still receive through this mechanism any recommendation to be tested for a particular trait in a clinical laboratory, without revealing individual results." Beskow et al., *supra*, at 2320.

Why might researchers be reluctant to tell subjects that the results of genetic testing will not be disclosed to them? Consider that question as you read the following case.

ANDE v. ROCK
Court of Appeals of Wisconsin, 647 N.W.2d 265 (2002)

C.E.A. was born to Linda and Charles Ande on July 13, 1993. There was then ongoing a cystic fibrosis research project which had begun in 1985. . . . To test for the presence of factors indicative of cystic fibrosis, the study used excess blood that had been drawn from all newborns to conduct statutorily required tests for the presence of other congenital and metabolic disorders. The research protocol required that the parents of half of the newborns in the study were told if their child tested positive for cystic fibrosis. A nutritional plan was made available to them immediately, as it was the researchers' theory that treating the nutritional needs of children with cystic fibrosis before they became symptomatic would result in a less vigorous development of the disease with fewer impairments to overall health. The other half of the children who were tested were placed in the "blinded control" group. Their parents and their treating physicians were not told if they had tested positive for factors indicative of cystic fibrosis. C.E.A. was placed in the blinded group, and therefore, her parents and her primary physician, Dr. Amy Plumb, were not told that she had tested positive.

Prior to testing the blood of newborns for cystic fibrosis, a pamphlet was prepared that told about the different tests that were required to be completed on newborns' blood. It also told of the cystic fibrosis test that would be run as part of a research project. It described the dangers of cystic fibrosis and stated that cystic fibrosis was an inherited disorder. The pamphlet also arguably implied that positive test results would be reported to the infant's physician, and a phone number was listed for parents who wanted additional information about the test. There is no assertion that the Andes were asked for or gave specific, written consent to have the cystic fibrosis test run on C.E.A. or to have the results of that test go unreported to them.

Subsequent to birth, C.E.A. had difficulties thriving. On June 23, 1995, when C.E.A. was almost two years old, she was diagnosed with cystic fibrosis. At the time that the Andes learned that C.E.A. had cystic fibrosis, Linda Ande was pregnant with a second child. The Andes' second child, C.L.A., is also afflicted with cystic fibrosis.

In this lawsuit, the Andes' allegations may be summarized into the assertion that the defendants committed three wrongful acts that give rise to the Andes' various claims: (1) The cystic fibrosis test was run without their informed consent; (2) treatment was withheld from C.E.A. when the investigators had knowledge that nutritional treatment would reduce the severity of her cystic fibrosis; and (3) C.E.A.'s test results were withheld from them. They allege to have been harmed by these acts in two ways: (1) If they had been given the test results, they would have accepted treatment for C.E.A. to lessen the severity of the progression of her illness; and (2) if they had been given the test results, they would not have conceived C.L.A. They do not identify any harm they suffered from the alleged lack of informed consent to run the test in the first instance.

In response, the defendants assert that they did not test C.E.A.'s blood without the Andes' knowledge and consent. They also contend that although all the children in the blinded control group were tested as newborns, no one reviewed the test results for the control group, some of which were negative and some of which were positive for factors indicative of cystic fibrosis. Therefore, the defendants contend they did not withhold information from the Andes. The defendants also raised many affirmative defenses, including failure to state a claim and qualified immunity. . . .

[Most of the plaintiffs' claims were dismissed for failure to satisfy the applicable statute of limitations — in other words, the claims were filed too late. The plaintiffs' malpractice claim, while timely, was dismissed because there was no physician-patient relationship between the plaintiffs and any of the defendants. That left just one claim, which was based on the theory that the defendants had violated the plaintiffs' due process rights under the federal constitution. (The plaintiffs were able to assert their rights under the federal Constitution because the defendants were acting as agents of a state government; constitutional claims would not have been available if the defendants had been purely private actors.) Under the doctrine of "qualified immunity," which applies to claims alleging a violation of constitutional rights, the plaintiffs were required to show not only the existence of a liberty interest in receiving the results of the cystic fibrosis testing, but also that this interest was "clearly established" at the time of the defendants' actions. The remainder of this excerpt addresses that portion of the plaintiffs' claims.]

While neither the Wisconsin Supreme Court nor the United States Supreme Court has yet addressed whether there is a constitutionally protected liberty interest in receiving information from a research project relative to one's genetic predisposition to give birth to a child with a genetically transmitted disorder or in receiving information from a research project that would assist a parent in making informed health care choices for his or her child, we cannot say with certainty that the withholding of the results of C.E.A.'s test did not implicate a liberty interest in either the parents or C.E.A. Therefore, for purposes of our discussion we shall assume, without deciding, that a liberty interest could be established if this case were to go to trial.

Once a liberty interest has been established, it may not be denied without a constitutionally acceptable amount of procedural due process. In regard to the alleged failure to obtain informed consent before the cystic fibrosis test was run in the first instance, the Andes base none of their claimed injuries on an unauthorized disclosure of private information, as they might if the researchers had disclosed C.E.A.'s condition to third parties. And they identify no harm that they suffered by not giving consent to the test in the first instance. For example, they do not allege that they would not have permitted the test if they had known it was being conducted. Instead, all of their alleged injuries flow from not having the *results* of the test at or near the time it was conducted. Therefore, we will not address their claims in regard to an alleged lack of informed consent further.

We now turn to the alleged failure to timely disclose the results of C.E.A.'s cystic fibrosis test. The closest the Andes come in making an argument that the alleged failure to disclose was a clear violation of their rights is to contend that one of the defendants, Richard Aronson, as the Medical Director for the Wisconsin Newborn Screening Program conducted under the direction of the Wisconsin Department of Health and Family Services, had a statutory duty under Wis. Stat. § 253.13(5) to disclose the results of the testing for congenital disorders. Section 253.13(5) stated in relevant part:

> The department shall disseminate information to families whose children suffer from congenital disorders and to women of child-bearing age with a history of congenital disorders concerning the need for and availability of follow-up counseling and special dietary treatment and the necessity for testing infants. The department shall also refer families of children who suffer from congenital disorders to available health and family services programs and shall coordinate the provision of these programs. The department shall periodically consult appropriate experts in reviewing and evaluating the state's infant screening programs.

In 1993, the year C.E.A. was born, Wis. Admin. Code § HSS 115.04 (1993) set out the tests to be done and for which information was required to be provided under § 253.13. Cystic fibrosis was not then a required test under § HSS 115.04. By emergency rule, effective January 31, 1995, cystic fibrosis was added to the list of tests that were required to be performed on newborns, and the Andes were not given C.E.A.'s test results until mid-1995. However, even if we were to conclude that § 253.13 could be construed to implicate a liberty interest in receiving the results of a cystic fibrosis test conducted a year before the testing and reporting of the results became mandatory, the failure to disclose cannot be said to rise to the level of a violation of a "clearly established" right because there is no closely analogous case law which interprets § 253.13 to require the disclosure of tests run before the statute and applicable administrative rules required them.

The Andes also allege a "general" violation of substantive due process, claiming that the actions of the defendants were arbitrary and capricious in the way in which they selected C.E.A for the control group and failed to disseminate the information they had about her. Substantive due process protects individuals from arbitrary, wrongful, governmental actions regardless of the process afforded prior to the deprivation. The Supreme Court has repeatedly explained that the touchstone of substantive due process is the protection of the individual against arbitrary action of government. Substantive due process [protects] against governmental actors who engage in conduct that "shocks the conscience" or conduct that interferes with rights "implicit in the concept of ordered liberty." However, even so generalized a claim of protection still requires the identification of a clearly protected interest that the actor's conduct violates. Due process claims are not a substitute for general tort claims. The Andes have failed to identify any Wisconsin or federal case law clearly establishing such an interest. Therefore, we conclude that qualified immunity bars all their federal claims.

NOTES AND QUESTIONS

1. The investigators in this study explained that they rejected the "traditional approach" to evaluating the efficacy of early intervention for cystic fibrosis — i.e., testing all newborns with the parents' consent and then randomly assigning those who tested positive to treatment or nontreatment groups — because "[i]t was implausible that parents or physicians would be able to resist the temptation to institute early treatment, despite the lack of evidence of its efficacy, or the possibility that it would do more harm than good." Norman Fost & Philip M. Farrell, *A Prospective Randomized Trial of Early Diagnosis and Treatment of Cystic Fibrosis: A Unique Ethical Dilemma*, 37 CLINICAL RESEARCH 495, 496 (1989). After considering and rejecting alternative trial designs, they concluded that the only scientifically valid way of conducting the study was to test all newborns and then disclose the results only to those who would be given the early intervention. They justified this approach on the grounds that (1) no infant was being denied any interventions that had proven value; (2) the interventions involved known risks; and (3) if there were no control group there

would be no study, and with no study the newborns would certainly not have received any testing. *See id.* at 496-97. Do you find those arguments persuasive? *See* Jerry Menikoff, *The Involuntary Research Subject*, 13 CAMBRIDGE Q. HEALTH-CARE ETHICS 338 (2004).

2. Are the issues discussed in the previous note similar to those addressed by the Maryland Supreme Court in *Grimes v. Kennedy Krieger Inst.*, the case about the lead paint study discussed in Chapter 13 at page 567. If the researchers in *Grimes* had a duty to warn parents when their children's test results indicated a possibility of lead paint poisoning, should a similar duty apply to researchers in the type of situation at issue in *Ande*?

[H] Sharing the Profits from Research

While "raw products of nature" are not patentable, the United States Patent and Trademark Office has issued patents to "purified and isolated gene[s], the protein for which the gene codes, cells or biological entities that have been engineered to express the gene, the process by which the gene was purified, and the use of the gene or protein to detect or treat a disease or condition." ANDREWS ET AL., *supra*, at 146. Gene patents raise a number of controversial issues, ranging from whether genetic sequences fall within the statutory definition of patentable subject matter to larger philosophical questions of whether property rights should be granted in forms of human life. This section addresses one aspect of the debate over gene patenting — the rights of the individuals whose tissue is used to isolate genetic sequences and develop patentable inventions. Specifically, when researchers obtain patents on genetic sequences that come from identifiable individuals, are those individuals entitled to share in the proceeds that the patents produce?

MOORE v. REGENTS OF THE UNIVERSITY OF CALIFORNIA
Supreme Court of California, 793 P.2d 479 (1990)

Moore first visited UCLA Medical Center on October 5, 1976, shortly after he learned that he had hairy-cell leukemia. After hospitalizing Moore and "withdr[awing] extensive amounts of blood, bone marrow aspirate, and other bodily substances," Golde confirmed that diagnosis. At this time all defendants, including Golde, were aware that "certain blood products and blood components were of great value in a number of commercial and scientific efforts" and that access to a patient whose blood contained these substances would provide "competitive, commercial, and scientific advantages."

On October 8, 1976, Golde recommended that Moore's spleen be removed. Golde informed Moore "that he had reason to fear for his life, and that the proposed splenectomy operation . . . was necessary to slow down the progress of his disease." Based upon Golde's representations, Moore signed a written consent form authorizing the splenectomy.

Before the operation, Golde and Quan "formed the intent and made arrangements to obtain portions of [Moore's] spleen following its removal" and to take them to a separate research unit. Golde gave written instructions to this effect on October 18 and 19, 1976. These research activities "were not intended to have . . . any relation to [Moore's] medical . . . care." However, neither Golde nor Quan informed Moore of their plans to conduct this research or requested his permission. Surgeons at UCLA Medical Center, whom the complaint does not name as defendants, removed Moore's spleen on October 20, 1976.

Moore returned to the UCLA Medical Center several times between November 1976 and September 1983. He did so at Golde's direction and based upon representations "that such visits were necessary and required for his health and well-being, and based upon the trust inherent in and by virtue of the physician-patient relationship . . . ." On each of these visits Golde withdrew additional samples of "blood, blood serum, skin, bone marrow aspirate, and sperm." On each occasion Moore traveled to the UCLA Medical Center from his home in Seattle because he had been told that the procedures were to be performed only there and only under Golde's direction.

> "In fact, [however,] throughout the period of time that [Moore] was under [Golde's] care and treatment, . . . the defendants were actively involved in a number of activities which they concealed from [Moore] . . . ." Specifically, defendants were conducting research on Moore's cells and planned to "benefit financially and competitively . . . [by exploiting the cells] and [their] exclusive access to [the cells] by virtue of [Golde's] ongoing physician-patient relationship . . . ."

Sometime before August 1979, Golde established a cell line from Moore's T-lymphocytes. On January 30, 1981, the Regents applied for a patent on the cell line, listing Golde and Quan as inventors. "[B]y virtue of an established policy . . . , [the] Regents, Golde, and Quan would share in any royalties or profits . . . arising out of [the] patent." The Regents' patent also covers various methods for using the cell line to produce lymphokines. Moore admits in his complaint that "the true clinical potential of each of the lymphokines . . . [is] difficult to predict, [but] . . . competing commercial firms in these relevant fields have published reports in biotechnology industry periodicals predicting a potential market of approximately $ 3.01 Billion Dollars by the year 1990 for a whole range of [such lymphokines] . . . ." . . .

A. Breach of Fiduciary Duty and Lack of Informed Consent

Moore repeatedly alleges that Golde failed to disclose the extent of his research and economic interests in Moore's cells before obtaining consent to the medical procedures by which the cells were extracted. These allegations, in our view, state a cause of action against Golde for invading a legally protected interest of his patient. This cause of action can properly be characterized either as the breach of a fiduciary duty to disclose facts material to the patient's consent or, alternatively, as the performance of medical procedures without first having obtained the patient's informed consent.

Our analysis begins with three well-established principles. First, "a person of adult years and in sound mind has the right, in the exercise of control over his own body, to determine whether or not to submit to lawful medical treatment." Second, "the patient's consent to treatment, to be effective, must be an informed consent." Third, in soliciting the patient's consent, a physician has a fiduciary duty to disclose all information material to the patient's decision.

These principles lead to the following conclusions: (1) a physician must disclose personal interests unrelated to the patient's health, whether research or economic, that may affect the physician's professional judgment; and (2) a physician's failure to disclose such interests may give rise to a cause of action for performing medical procedures without informed consent or breach of fiduciary duty.

To be sure, questions about the validity of a patient's consent to a procedure typically arise when the patient alleges that the physician failed to disclose medical risks, as in malpractice cases, and not when the patient alleges that the physician had a personal interest, as in this case. The concept of informed consent, however, is broad enough to encompass the latter. "The scope of the physician's communication to the patient . . . must be measured by the patient's need, and that need is whatever information is material to the decision." . . .

It is important to note that no law prohibits a physician from conducting research in the same area in which he practices. Progress in medicine often depends upon physicians, such as those practicing at the university hospital where Moore received treatment, who conduct research while caring for their patients.

Yet a physician who treats a patient in whom he also has a research interest has potentially conflicting loyalties. This is because medical treatment decisions are made on the basis of proportionality — weighing the benefits *to the patient* against the risks *to the patient*. As another court has said, "the determination as to whether the burdens of treatment are worth enduring for any individual patient depends upon the facts unique in each case," and "the patient's interests and desires are the key ingredients of the decision-making process." A physician who adds his own research interests to this balance may be tempted to order a scientifically useful procedure or test that offers marginal, or no, benefits to the patient. The possibility that an interest extraneous to the patient's health has affected the physician's judgment is something that a reasonable patient would want to know in deciding whether to consent to a proposed course of treatment. It is material to the patient's decision and, thus, a prerequisite to informed consent.

Golde argues that the scientific use of cells that have already been removed cannot possibly affect the patient's medical interests. The argument is correct in one instance but not in another. If a physician has no plans to conduct research on a patient's cells at the time he recommends the medical procedure by which they are taken, then the patient's medical interests have not been impaired. In that instance the argument is correct. On the other hand, a physician who does have a preexisting research interest might, consciously or unconsciously, take that into consideration in recommending the procedure. In that instance the argument is incorrect: the physician's extraneous motivation may affect his judgment and is, thus, material to the patient's consent.

We acknowledge that there is a competing consideration. To require disclosure of research and economic interests may corrupt the patient's own judgment by distracting him from the requirements of his health. But California law does not grant physicians unlimited discretion to decide what to disclose. Instead, "it is the prerogative of the patient, not the physician, to determine for himself the direction in which he believes his interests lie." "Unlimited discretion in the physician is irreconcilable with the basic right of the patient to make the ultimate informed decision . . ." . . .

Moore plainly asserts that Golde concealed an economic interest in the postoperative procedures. Therefore, applying the principles already discussed, the allegations state a cause of action for breach of fiduciary duty or lack of informed consent.

B. Conversion

Moore also attempts to characterize the invasion of his rights as a conversion — a tort that protects against interference with possessory and ownership interests in personal property. He theorizes that he continued to own his cells following their removal from his body, at least for the purpose of directing their use, and that he never consented to their use in potentially lucrative medical research. Thus, to complete Moore's argument, defendants' unauthorized use of his cells constitutes a conversion. As a result of the alleged conversion, Moore claims a proprietary interest in each of the products that any of the defendants might ever create from his cells or the patented cell line. . . .

1. Moore's Claim Under Existing Law

. . . Lacking direct authority for importing the law of conversion into this context, Moore relies, as did the Court of Appeal, primarily on decisions addressing privacy rights. One line of cases involves unwanted publicity. These opinions hold that every person has a proprietary interest in his own likeness and that unauthorized, business use of a likeness is redressible as a tort. But in neither opinion did the authoring court expressly base its holding on property law. . . .

Not only are the wrongful-publicity cases irrelevant to the issue of conversion, but the analogy to them seriously misconceives the nature of the genetic materials and research involved in this case. Moore, adopting the analogy originally advanced by the Court of Appeal, argues that "[i]f the courts have found a sufficient proprietary interest in one's persona, how could one not have a right in one's own genetic material, something far more profoundly the essence of one's human uniqueness than a name or a face?" However, as the defendants' patent makes clear — and the complaint, too, if read with an understanding of the scientific terms which it has borrowed from the patent — the goal and result of defendants' efforts has been to manufacture lymphokines. Lymphokines, unlike a name or a face, have the same molecular structure in every human being and the same, important functions in every human being's immune system. Moreover, the particular genetic material which is responsible for the natural production of lymphokines, and which defendants use to manufacture lymphokines in the laboratory, is also the same in every person; it is no more unique to Moore than the number of vertebrae in the spine or the chemical formula of hemoglobin.

Another privacy case offered by analogy to support Moore's claim establishes only that patients have a right to refuse medical treatment. . . . Yet one may earnestly wish to protect privacy and dignity without accepting the extremely problematic conclusion that interference with those interests amounts to a conversion of personal property. Nor is it necessary to force the round pegs of "privacy" and "dignity" into the square hole of "property" in order to protect the patient, since the fiduciary-duty and informed-consent theories protect these interests directly by requiring full disclosure.

The next consideration that makes Moore's claim of ownership problematic is California statutory law, which drastically limits a patient's control over excised cells. . . .

Finally, the subject matter of the Regents' patent — the patented cell line and the products derived from it — cannot be Moore's property. This is because the patented cell line is both factually and legally distinct from the cells taken from Moore's body. Federal law permits the patenting of organisms that represent the product of "human ingenuity," but not naturally occurring organisms. . . . It is this *inventive effort* that patent law rewards, not the discovery of naturally occurring raw materials. Thus, Moore's allegations that he owns the cell line and the products derived from it are inconsistent with the patent, which constitutes an authoritative determination that the cell line is the product of invention. . . .

2. Should Conversion Liability Be Extended?

. . . Of the relevant policy considerations, two are of overriding importance. The first is protection of a competent patient's right to make autonomous medical decisions. That right, as already discussed, is grounded in well-recognized and long-standing principles of fiduciary duty and informed consent. This policy weighs in favor of providing a remedy to patients when physicians act with undisclosed motives that may affect their professional judgment. The second important policy consideration is that we not threaten with disabling civil liability innocent parties who are engaged in socially useful activities, such as researchers who have no reason to believe that their use of a particular cell sample is, or may be, against a donor's wishes. . . .

To be sure, the threat of liability for conversion might help to enforce patients' rights indirectly. This is because physicians might be able to avoid liability by obtaining patients' consent, in the broadest possible terms, to any conceivable subsequent research use of excised cells. Unfortunately, to extend the conversion theory would utterly sacrifice the other goal of protecting innocent parties. Since conversion is a strict liability tort, it would impose liability on all those into whose hands the cells come, whether or not the particular defendant participated in, or knew of, the inadequate disclosures that violated the patient's right to make an informed decision. In contrast to the conversion theory, the fiduciary-duty and informed-consent theories protect the patient directly, without punishing innocent parties or creating disincentives to the conduct of socially beneficial research. . . .

The extension of conversion law into this area will hinder research by restricting access to the necessary raw materials. Thousands of human cell lines already exist in tissue repositories, such as the American Type Culture Collection and those operated by the National Institutes of Health and the American Cancer Society. These repositories respond to tens of thousands of requests for samples annually. Since the patent office requires the holders of patents on cell lines to make samples available to anyone, many patent holders place their cell lines in repositories to avoid the administrative burden of responding to requests. At present, human cell lines are routinely copied and distributed to other researchers for experimental purposes, usually free of charge. This exchange of scientific materials, which still is relatively free and efficient, will surely be compromised if each cell sample becomes the potential subject matter of a lawsuit. . . .

If the scientific users of human cells are to be held liable for failing to investigate the consensual pedigree of their raw materials, we believe the Legislature should make that decision. Complex policy choices affecting all society are involved, and "[l]egislatures, in making such policy decisions, have the ability to gather empirical evidence, solicit the advice of experts, and hold hearings at which all interested parties present evidence and express their views . . ." . . .

Finally, there is no pressing need to impose a judicially created rule of strict liability, since enforcement of physicians' disclosure obligations will protect patients against the very type of harm with which Moore was threatened. So long as a physician discloses research and economic interests that may affect his judgment, the patient is protected from conflicts of interest. Aware of any conflicts, the patient can make an informed decision to consent to treatment, or to withhold consent and look elsewhere for medical assistance. As already discussed, enforcement of physicians' disclosure obligations protects patients directly, without hindering the socially useful activities of innocent researchers.

For these reasons, we hold that the allegations of Moore's third amended complaint state a cause of action for breach of fiduciary duty or lack of informed consent, but not conversion.

NOTES AND QUESTIONS

1. *Moore* involved a patient receiving medical treatment outside a research setting, but the court's discussion of informed consent also is relevant to researchers conducting formal protocols. Recall the discussion in Chapter 5 of whether investigators should inform subjects about conflicts of interest. *See* Chapter 5, at page 239. Under *Moore*, when would such conflicts have to be disclosed? (Note that the *Moore* decision is binding only in California, although courts in other states are free to draw on it for guidance.)

2. Do you agree with the court that California statutes limiting a patient's control over his excised cells made Moore's claim of ownership "problematic"? Is it necessary to have complete control over something in order to claim an ownership interest in it? What about the court's point that the patent was awarded for the researchers' inventive efforts, not simply for the discovery of naturally occurring raw materials? Does the fact that Moore could not have obtained a patent on the cells in their raw form mean that he contributed nothing of value to the ultimate invention?

3. The dissenting opinions in *Moore* disputed the court's assertion that "enforcement of physicians' disclosure obligations will protect patients against the very type of harm with which Moore was threatened." Why might a breach of fiduciary duty claim be insufficient protection for individuals whose tissue is used to develop patentable products without their consent?

4. Do you agree with the court that applying conversion law to the nonconsensual use of human tissue would hinder biotechnology research? *Cf.* Charlotte H. Harrison, *Neither* Moore *Nor the Market: Alternative Models for Compensating Contributors of Human Tissue*, 28 Am. J. L. & Med. 77, 86-88 (2002) (arguing that recognizing property rights in human tissue would be economically inefficient, and that a preferable approach would be to create an administrative mechanism for giving individuals a share of the profits if their tissue proves to have exceptional commercial utility).

5. According to the Nuffield Council on Bioethics, a British organization, "it should be regarded as entailed in consent to medical treatment that tissue removed in the course of treatment will be regarded as having been abandoned by the person from whom it was removed." Nuffield Council on Bioethics, Human Tissue: Ethical and Legal Issues 131 (1995), available at http://www.nuffieldbioethics.org/filelibrary/pdf/human_tissue.pdf. The Council argued that "the altruistic motivation of patients, donors and relatives should be respected and encouraged rather than eroded." *Id.* at 52. Do you agree that it is important to foster the "altruistic motivation" of individuals who provide tissue

for use in biomedical research? If so, is a policy of presuming that patients have "abandoned" their tissue, rather than asking for their consent before using the tissue in research, consistent with the goal of promoting altruism?

6. Some commentators have argued that, rather than treating donated tissue as the property of the tissue bank, it should be held in trust for the benefit of the general public. According to one proposal, the tissue donor would "transfer his or her property interest in the tissue to the trust," and a board of trustees — which would include representatives of the donor group — would govern the use of the tissue. *See* Winickoff & Winickoff, *supra*. What do you think of this proposal? What type of objections is it likely to face?

In contrast to *Moore*, which involved the nonconsensual research use of tissue obtained in a clinical procedure, the following case involves individuals who donated tissue to researchers expressly for the development of a genetic test. As you read the case, consider whether the plaintiffs' claims for a share of the researchers' profits are more or less compelling than the plaintiff's claims in *Moore*.

GREENBERG v. MIAMI CHILDREN'S HOSPITAL RESEARCH INST.

United States District Court for the Southern District of Florida,
264 F. Supp. 2d 1064 (2003)

The Complaint alleges a tale of a successful research collaboration gone sour. In 1987, Canavan disease still remained a mystery — there was no way to identify who was a carrier of the disease, nor was there a way to identify a fetus with Canavan disease. [Canavan disease is a neurological disorder that causes progressive brain atrophy. Most children with the disease die by age 4.] Plaintiff Greenberg [the father of a child with Canavan disease] approached Dr. Matalon, a research physician who was then affiliated with the University of Illinois at Chicago for assistance. Greenberg requested Matalon's involvement in discovering the genes that were ostensibly responsible for this fatal disease, so that tests could be administered to determine carriers and allow for prenatal testing for the disease.

At the outset of the collaboration, Greenberg and the Chicago Chapter of the National Tay-Sachs and Allied Disease Association, Inc. ("NTSAD") located other Canavan families and convinced them to provide tissue (such as blood, urine, and autopsy samples), financial support, and aid in identifying the location of Canavan families internationally. The other individual Plaintiffs began supplying Matalon with the same types of information and samples beginning in the late 1980s. Greenberg and NTSAD also created a confidential database and compilation — the Canavan registry — with epidemiological, medical and other information about the families. . . .

The individual Plaintiffs allege that they provided Matalon with these samples and confidential information "with the understanding and expectations that such samples and information would be used for the specific purpose of researching Canavan disease and identifying mutations in the Canavan disease which could lead to carrier detection within their families and benefit the population at large." Plaintiffs further allege that it was their "understanding that any carrier and prenatal testing developed in connection with the research for which they were providing essential support would be provided on an affordable and accessible basis, and that Matalon's research would remain in the public domain to promote the discovery of more effective prevention techniques and treatments and, eventually, to effectuate a cure for Canavan disease." This understanding stemmed from their "experience in community testing for Tay-Sachs disease, another deadly genetic disease that occurs most frequently in families of Ashkenazi Jewish descent."

There was a breakthrough in the research in 1993. Using Plaintiffs' blood and tissue samples, familial pedigree information, contacts, and financial support, Matalon and his research team successfully isolated the gene responsible for Canavan disease. After this key advancement, Plaintiffs allege that they continued to provide Matalon with more tissue and blood in order to learn more about the disease and its precursor gene.

In September 1994, unbeknownst to Plaintiffs, a patent application was submitted for the genetic sequence that Defendants had identified. This application was granted in October 1997, and Dr. Matalon was listed as an inventor on the gene patent and related applications for the Canavan disease, Patent No. 5,679,635 (the "Patent"). Through patenting, Defendants acquired the ability to restrict any activity related to the Canavan disease gene, including without limitation: carrier and prenatal testing, gene therapy and other treatments for Canavan disease and research involving the gene and its mutations.

Although the Patent was issued in October 1997, Plaintiffs allege that they did not learn of it until November 1998, when MCH [Miami Children's Hospital] revealed their intention to limit Canavan disease testing through a campaign of restrictive licensing of the Patent. Specifically, on November 12, 1998, Plaintiffs allege that Defendants MCH and MCHRI [Miami Children's Hospital Research Institute] began to "threaten" the centers that offered Canavan testing with possible enforcement actions regarding the recently-issued patent. Defendant MCH also began restricting public accessibility through negotiating exclusive licensing agreements and charging royalty fees.

Plaintiffs allege that at no time were they informed that Defendants intended to seek a patent on the research. Nor were they told of Defendants' intentions to commercialize the fruits of the research and to restrict access to Canavan disease testing. . . .

[The plaintiffs asserted a variety of legal theories, including failure to obtain informed consent, breach of fiduciary duty, unjust enrichment, fraudulent concealment, conversion, and misappropriation of trade secrets. The court rejected all of those claims except the one based on unjust enrichment.]

In Count III of the Complaint, Plaintiffs allege that MCH is being unjustly enriched by collecting license fees under the Patent. Under Florida law, the elements of a claim for unjust enrichment are (1) the plaintiff conferred a benefit on the defendant, who had knowledge of the benefit; (2) the defendant voluntarily accepted and retained the benefit; and (3) under the circumstances it would be inequitable for the defendant to retain the benefit without paying for it. The Court finds that Plaintiffs have sufficiently alleged the elements of a claim for unjust enrichment to survive Defendants' motion to dismiss.

While the parties do not contest that Plaintiffs have conferred a benefit to Defendants, including, among other things, blood and tissue samples and soliciting financial contributions, Defendants contend that Plaintiffs have not suffered any detriment, and note that no Plaintiff has been denied access to Canavan testing. Furthermore, the Plaintiffs received what they sought — the successful isolation of the Canavan gene and the development of a screening test. Plaintiffs argue, however, that when Defendants applied the benefits for unauthorized purposes, they suffered a detriment. Had Plaintiffs known that Defendants intended to commercialize their genetic material through patenting and restrictive licensing, Plaintiffs would not have provided these benefits to Defendants under those terms.

Naturally, Plaintiffs allege that the retention of benefits violates the fundamental principles of justice, equity, and good conscience. While Defendants claim that they have invested significant amounts of time and money in research, with no guarantee of success and are thus entitled to seek reimbursement, the same can be said of Plaintiffs. Moreover, Defendants' attempt to seek refuge in the endorsement of the U.S. Patent system, which gives an inventor rights to prosecute patents and negotiate licenses for their intellectual property fails, as obtaining a patent does not preclude the Defendants from being unjustly enriched. The Complaint has alleged more than just a donor-donee relationship for the purposes of an unjust enrichment claim. Rather, the facts paint a picture of a continuing research collaboration that involved Plaintiffs also investing time and significant resources in the race to isolate the Canavan gene. Therefore, given the facts as alleged, the Court finds that Plaintiffs have sufficiently pled the requisite elements of an unjust enrichment claim and the motion to dismiss for failure to state a claim is DENIED as to this count.

NOTES AND QUESTIONS

1. In rejecting the plaintiffs' informed consent claims, the *Greenberg* court distinguished *Moore* as follows:

> *Moore* involved a physician breaching his duty when he asked his patient to return for follow-up tests after the removal of the patient's spleen because he had research and economic interests. The doctors did not inform their patient that they were using his blood and tissue for medical research. The allegations in the Complaint are clearly distinguishable as Defendants here are solely medical researchers and there was no therapeutic relationship as in *Moore*.
>
> In declining to extend the duty of informed consent to cover economic interests, the Court takes note of the practical implications of retroactively imposing a duty of this nature. First, imposing a duty of the character that Plaintiffs seek would be unworkable and would chill medical research as it would mandate that researchers constantly evaluate whether a discloseable event has occurred. Second, this extra duty would give rise to a type of dead-hand control that research subjects could hold because they would be able to dictate how medical research progresses. Finally, these Plaintiffs are more accurately portrayed as donors rather than objects of human experimentation, and thus the voluntary nature of their submissions warrants different treatment.

Greenberg, at 1070-71. Do you find these distinctions persuasive? Do you agree with the court that the donors were not "objects of human experimentation"?

2. In what ways does the unjust enrichment theory accepted in *Greenberg* differ from the conversion theory rejected in *Moore*? Do you think the court that decided *Greenberg* would have allowed the plaintiff in *Moore* to proceed on an unjust enrichment claim?

3. In light of *Greenberg*, how can researchers avoid liability for unjust enrichment when they develop patentable inventions with human tissue? Recall that, under the federal regulations, consent forms may not include "any exculpatory language through which the subject or the representative is made to waive or appear to waive any of the subject's legal rights." 45 C.F.R. § 46.116. In an effort to deal with this problem, a 1996 guidance from the Office for Protection from Research Risks (OPRR, now OHRP) gave examples of both "unacceptable" and "acceptable" language. The "unacceptable" language included:

- "By agreeing to this use, you should understand that you will give up all claim to personal benefit from commercial or other use of these substances."

- "I voluntarily and freely donate any and all blood, urine, and tissue samples to the U.S. Government and hereby relinquish all right, title and interest to said items."

- "By consent to participate in this research, I give up any property rights I may have in bodily fluids or tissue samples obtained in the course of the research."

Acceptable language included:

- "Tissue obtained from you in this research may be used to establish a cell line that could be patented and licensed. There are no plans to provide financial compensation to you should this occur."

- "By consenting to participate, you authorize the use of your bodily fluids and tissue samples for the research described above."

"One possible approach," two commentators recommend,

> might involve language that focuses on a subject's consent to providing his or her material as a gift to the sponsor for future research uses with an express acknowledgment that the subject will not receive financial compensation in return. Although such language likely would not insulate a sponsor from a future claim that the subject has a financial interest in the product derived from his or her material, it hopefully would serve as insulation to a claim of lack of informed consent. Yet even this is uncertain because, as described above, the current regulatory regime is at best utterly confusing and at worst completely self-contradictory. The issue of waivability by subjects of economic and commercial interests in data and tissue awaits resolution by OHRP, the FDA, and the courts. The current confusion benefits no one, and undermines vital public interests in advancing science and medicine.

Mark Barnes & Kate Gallin Heffernan, *The "Future Uses" Dilemma: Secondary Uses of Data and Materials by Researchers and Commercial Research Sponsors*, 3 MED. RESEARCH L. & POL'Y REP. (BNA) 440 (2004).

4. Compare the following scenario to the facts of *Greenberg*:

When Sharon Terry learned that her two young children had inherited PXE (pseudoxanthorma elasticum), a connective tissue disorder that leads to blindness and potential heart attacks, several groups of researchers called to ask for tissue samples from her children to try to find the gene. She inquired as to why they did not get samples from other researchers and was told that scientists would not share the samples. Terry started a bank with tissue samples from her children and began a collaborative project with researchers. When University of Hawaii pathobiologist Charles Boyd isolated the gene, he listed Sharon Terry as a co-inventor on the patent. The PXE patients' group she formed will make the decisions about how to license the rights to the gene. Additionally, the PXE group will give 50% of the resulting royalties to the University. This way the PXE patients' group can keep the price of diagnostic tests down by licensing providers who charge a lower fee.

Lori B. Andrews, *The Gene Patent Dilemma: Balancing Commercial Incentives with Health Needs*, 2002 HOUS. J. HEALTH L. & POL'Y 65, 105 (2002); *see also* Gina Kolata, *Sharing of Profits Is Debated as the Value of Tissue Rises*, N.Y. TIMES, May 15, 2000, at A1 (noting that individuals who provide tissue to researchers are increasingly demanding "money up front" or "writing contracts spelling out what they are entitled to if they help scientists find genes").

§ 17.02　GENE TRANSFER RESEARCH

Unlike the research discussed in the previous section, which is designed to learn about the human genome and particular disease-associated alleles, the research examined in this section seeks to *change* individuals' genetic make-up by correcting defects responsible for the development of disease. In most cases, this is done by inserting a "normal" gene into target cells by means of a carrier molecule known as a "vector." The most commonly used vectors are viruses that have been genetically altered to carry human DNA. It is hoped that the new genes will infect the target cells and produce functional protein products that will restore the cells to a normal state. *See* HUMAN GENOME PROJECT INFORMATION: WHAT IS GENE THERAPY, available at http://www.ornl.gov/TechResources/Human_Genome/medicine/genetherapy.html#work.

The first clinical trial of gene transfer (also known as "gene therapy") research began in 1990, but it was not until 1999 that this research gained widespread public attention. In that year, 18-year-old Jesse Gelsinger, a subject in a gene transfer trial, died from multiple organ failures a few days after his treatment began, apparently as a result of a severe immune response. *See id.*; *see also* Chapter 7, at page 363 (discussing informed consent issues in the Gelsinger study). In January 2003, another setback occurred when it was learned that two children in a French study had developed a leukemia-like condition after having been "successfully" treated with gene transfer techniques for the condition known as "bubble boy syndrome." In response to this news, the FDA temporarily halted all gene transfer studies using retroviral vectors in blood stem cells. The FDA lifted the halt in June 2003. *See FDA Lifts Clinical Hold, Allowing HIV Gene Therapy Trials to Proceed*, 2 MED. RESEARCH L. & POL'Y REP. (BNA) 433 (2003).

Does gene transfer research raise ethical issues not present in other forms of human subject research? If so, does it warrant greater governmental oversight? Consider these questions as you read the following excerpt.

RAC Oversight of Gene Transfer Research:
A Model Worth Extending?
Nancy M.P. King
30 J. L. MED. & ETHICS 381 (2002)

Clinical GTR [gene transfer research] is governed by the same oversight system as most clinical trials, with a significant addition: the RAC [the Recombinant DNA (rDNA) Advisory Committee]. . . . Since the RAC undertook review of clinical GTR, all clinical GTR protocols connected with an institution receiving any federal rDNA funding must be submitted to the Office of Biotechnology Activities (OBA) for RAC review and potentially for public discussion. Since not all GTR takes place at institutions doing federally funded rDNA research, some GTR (especially that taking place outside of the United States) is not required to be reviewed by the RAC. At the urging of the FDA (which reviews any research anywhere that is intended to produce products to be marketed in the United States), however, many such studies are voluntarily submitted to OBA by the sponsor. . . .

Is Gene Transfer Research Unique?

Clinical GTR is generally referred to, in both professional and popular contexts, as "gene therapy." This terminology persists despite extensive — and to some extent successful — efforts to replace it, in scientific and policy documents and consent forms, with "gene transfer research." Clinical gene transfer trials only began in 1990, and the vast majority of trials have been early-phase studies (only 1 percent being Phase III trials), so it is not and should not be surprising that effective treatments have not yet emerged. Nor should it be surprising that, in a complex and technically challenging field that encompasses not only a vast range of diseases and a wide variety of genetic interventions, but also an extraordinary diversity of vectors and routes of administration, definitive promise has only been hinted at in several distinct areas of research. Yet public and professional enthusiasm for the irresistible logic of the concept of gene therapy, and enormously concentrated media attention on this both fascinating and potentially frightening field, have resulted in what might legitimately be termed "irrational exuberance" about the prospects for the field as a whole and the outcome for individual subjects enrolled in gene transfer trials.

Is GTR different enough from other early-phase clinical research to warrant its unique system of oversight? The first step in addressing that question is to consider those characteristics that produce decision-making challenges. One is the field's complexity: gene transfer is a methodology that is used not only for correction of single-gene defects, but also for insertion of genes for other purposes, most notably, to stimulate the immune system (as in anticancer vaccine and immunotherapy studies), to render cancer cells susceptible to antiviral medications, and to stimulate the growth of collateral blood vessels to circumvent blocked arteries in the limbs or in the heart. The technical challenges here are staggeringly multifarious, as is the variety of means of introducing new genetic material. Importantly, the means of achieving dosing consistency across studies is, like the field itself, largely in its beginning stages.

A second characteristic of GTR is the lack of good animal models of disease. This is not, of course, a problem unique to gene transfer, but it may be concentrated here. Certainly there are more mouse models than there are models in larger animals or nonhuman primates, but as a RAC colleague once commented to me, "Everything works in mice." Until Jesse Gelsinger died in September 1999, gene transfer was widely viewed as extremely safe in comparison with other research and treatment modalities, so that moving from preclinical to clinical trials, while necessarily invoking many unknowns, did not appear to pose much danger to human subjects. Yet even before Mr. Gelsinger died, it was recognized that, as is the case for many biologics, dose-dependent safety and efficacy of gene transfer interventions is difficult to predict. Unlike the most common pattern associated with drug research, a reasonably steady rise in both beneficial and harmful effects with increasing doses, many gene transfer interventions show an elbow graph associated with a threshold effect; that is, nothing happens until a threshold dose is reached. In an early trial, then, there may be few clues as to when anything is going to happen, and it can be extremely difficult to anticipate what will happen, good or bad, at the threshold point.

These characteristics produce a great deal of uncertainty in this field — perhaps more uncertainty than in most other clinical research. In addition, some of the unknowns loom especially large, as they include the possibility of permanent changes in subjects, and even inadvertent germ-line transmission of changes to subjects' offspring.[3] Any such changes could be positive, negative, both, or neither. . . .

Several shifts in emphasis and concern in clinical GTR over its short history have compounded these challenges. First, . . . the birth of the field was associated with expectations about potential cures for monogenic diseases. Cystic fibrosis, sickle cell disease, the hemophilias, and a variety of other serious disorders affecting relatively small numbers of persons were the earliest areas of research interest. At present, however, the vast majority of gene transfer studies (about 70 percent) are oncology studies. Oncology research is a very large field, with its own culture, its own model consent forms, its own federal institute complete with clinical trials weblist, and a powerful commitment to clinical research. The shift in emphasis from monogenic disease to cancer has a variety of potential implications. It makes GTR more like other early-phase clinical research, much of which is also cancer research; thus, what happens in GTR may have broader implications for all clinical research. Yet a shift away from seeking cures for rare and largely untreatable disorders could ultimately have broad financial and social justice effects as well.

---

[3] "Germ-line transmission" refers to genetic alterations in an individual's sperm or egg cells, which would be passed on to the individual's offspring.

A second shift relates to perceptions about the most salient risks in GTR. At the outset, insertional mutagenesis and inadvertent germ-line transmission were of great concern. Mr. Gelsinger's death engendered a shift of concern to vector toxicity and helped to spur the ongoing effort to develop safer gene delivery methods, both viral and nonviral. Currently, both vector toxicity and germ-line transmission are areas of heightened concern. The challenge is to determine the magnitude and likelihood of these disparate risks of harm and their appropriate limits. As clinical gene transfer gets closer to demonstrating efficacy, the even greater challenge is to determine whether — and if so, how — to balance the potential for efficacy against the risk of germ-line effects. Germ-line effects pose risks not to subjects but to their offspring. If any germ-line effects materialize at all, they are highly likely to be harmful; however, in theory, they could result in persistent correction of the defect.

Finally, the shift that has garnered the widest attention since September 1999 is the shift in funding sources for clinical GTR, from NIH and the large pharmaceutical companies to small venture biotechnology companies, often investigator-founded in partnership with academia. The problem of financial conflict of interest and the policy question of financial disclosure and what to do with the information (prohibit conflicts, manage conflicts, disclose them to potential subjects and/or to the IRB) long predated Mr. Gelsinger's death, but the revival of interest in conflict of interest management and reporting that directly resulted therefrom extends to all federally funded research and beyond.

The Bench to Bedside Balance

Taken together, the implications of GTR's salient characteristics may be seen as either inherently or only temporarily needing the increased scrutiny that the field has enjoyed. There have been many arguments made over the years by industry, investigators, potential subjects, and at times the FDA, that the RAC is unnecessary, duplicative, burdensome, and an obstacle to research progress. Yet it is undeniable that RAC review provides a public window onto the entirety of an unprecedented and exciting field. From my perspective as a RAC member, this window illuminates, through public meetings and publicly available information, important questions about research design and ethics that are not clearly or systematically showcased in any other forum: when is the right time to move to humans, and who should be the first subjects? Since these are questions that must be answered during the development of any line of research, what marks them as of special interest in GTR? It is simply that, for GTR, these questions are asked by the RAC.

Why does it matter that the RAC asks these questions? There are two reasons. First, the other oversight entities that might also ask have different relationships to the questions and may be inconsistent or incompletely attentive in their approaches. The FDA asks them, but not publicly. Local IRBs may or may not ask them, as local IRBs differ in their capacity and willingness to interrogate the scientific merit of research proposals. The RAC, with its resources and combination of expertises, is the sole entity perfectly positioned to ask these questions about GTR. In addition, because GTR is still highly concentrated on early-phase trials, these questions come up over and over again for the RAC, as they do not in many other fields. Second, by virtue of its public process, the RAC has the opportunity to foster responsible inquiry into these questions, throughout a broadly constituted field in which a range of different answers to the questions may be contemplated.

NOTES AND QUESTIONS

1. Should committees like the RAC be established for other types of research? If so, based on what criteria?

2. While federally funded investigators are required to submit gene transfer protocols to the RAC, the RAC's recommendations are advisory only. *See* FREQUENTLY ASKED QUESTIONS: RECOMBINANT DNA AND GENE TRANSFER, available at http://www4.od.nih.gov/oba/RAC/RAC_FAQs.htm (noting, however, that "[i]nvestigators and sponsors should carefully consider these recommendations as part of optimizing the safe and ethical conduct of the trial"). Does the fact that RAC recommendations are advisory mean that deviating from those recommendations has no legal consequences?

3. In addition to RAC review and IRB approval, gene transfer research also requires the approval of an Institutional Biosafety Committee (IBC), which addresses issues related to biosafety and the containment of recombinant DNA molecules. In addition, because gene transfer techniques fall under the legal definition of a "biologic," researchers may not use them in human subjects without first submitting an investigational new drug application (IND) to the FDA. *See* HUMAN GENE THERAPY AND THE ROLE OF THE FOOD AND DRUG ADMINISTRATION, available at http://www.fda.gov/cber/infosheets/genezn.htm; *see also* Chapter 3, at page 150 (discussing INDs).

4. As noted in the preceding excerpt, one of the risks of gene transfer research is that it will inadvertently alter individuals' germ cells, thereby affecting future generations in potentially damaging ways. Should researchers avoid techniques that pose a substantial risk of germline alteration, even if doing so slows the pace of scientific advances? Alternatively, if inadvertent germline alteration is a real possibility, should researchers design trials that intentionally provoke germline changes, in order to study the safety of germline alteration systematically? Who should decide these questions — researchers, IRBs, the RAC, or some broader societal decision-making process? For further discussion of these issues, see Nancy M.P. King, *Accident and Desire: Inadvertent Germline Effects in Clinical Research*, 33 HASTINGS CENTER REP., Mar.-Apr. 2003, at 23.

5. Rather than viewing germline alterations as a risk of gene transfer research, perhaps we should embrace germline alteration as a valuable scientific goal. After all, germline alteration, at least in theory, "would have the ben-

efit of preventing the inheritance of genetic diseases in families rather than treating it every time it appears, generation after generation." Mark S. Frankel, *Inheritable Genetic Modification and a Brave New World: Did Huxley Have It Wrong*, 33 HASTINGS CENTER REP., Mar.-Apr. 2003, at 31. If you believe that germline alteration is not inherently unethical, would you attempt to distinguish between efforts to prevent disease and efforts to enhance traits beyond the range of what is generally considered "normal"? If so, how would you draw the line between disease prevention and trait enhancement? *See id.* (arguing that, because "the technology developed for therapeutic purposes will be the same as that used for enhancement," the availability of this technology "will likely promote creeping enhancement applications as well"); *see also* Maxwell J. Mehlman, *The Law of Above Averages: Leveling the New Genetic Enhancement Playing Field*, 85 IOWA L. REV. 517 (2000).

APPENDIX A

U.S. Code of Federal Regulations
Title 45—Public Welfare and Human Services
Part 46—Protection of Human Subjects

Subpart A—Basic HHS Policy for Protection of Human Research Subjects

Source: 56 Fed. Reg. 28,003 (1991)

§ 46.101 To what does this policy apply?

(a) Except as provided in paragraph (b) of this section, this policy applies to all research involving human subjects conducted, supported or otherwise subject to regulation by any Federal Department or Agency which takes appropriate administrative action to make the policy applicable to such research. This includes research conducted by Federal civilian employees or military personnel, except that each Department or Agency head may adopt such procedural modifications as may be appropriate from an administrative standpoint. It also includes research conducted, supported, or otherwise subject to regulation by the Federal Government outside the United States.

(1) Research that is conducted or supported by a Federal Department or Agency, whether or not it is regulated as defined in § 46.102(e), must comply with all sections of this policy.

(2) Research that is neither conducted nor supported by a Federal Department or Agency but is subject to regulation as defined in § 46.102(e) must be reviewed and approved, in compliance with § 46.101, § 46.102, and § 46.107 through § 46.117 of this policy, by an Institutional Review Board (IRB) that operates in accordance with the pertinent requirements of this policy.

(b) Unless otherwise required by Department or Agency heads, research activities in which the only involvement of human subjects will be in one or more of the following categories are exempt from this policy:

(1) Research conducted in established or commonly accepted educational settings, involving normal educational practices, such as (i) research on regular and special education instructional strategies, or (ii) research on the effectiveness of or the comparison among instructional techniques, curricula, or classroom management methods.

(2) Research involving the use of educational tests (cognitive, diagnostic, aptitude, achievement), survey procedures, interview procedures or observation of public behavior, unless:

(i) information obtained is recorded in such a manner that human subjects can be identified, directly or through identifiers linked to the subjects; and (ii) any disclosure of the human subjects' responses outside the research could reasonably place the subjects at risk of criminal or civil liability or be damaging to the subjects' financial standing, employability, or reputation.

(3) Research involving the use of educational tests (cognitive, diagnostic, aptitude, achievement), survey procedures, interview procedures, or observation of public behavior that is not exempt under paragraph (b)(2) of this section, if:

(i) the human subjects are elected or appointed public officials or candidates for public office; or (ii) Federal statute(s) require(s) without exception that the confidentiality of the personally identifiable information will be maintained throughout the research and thereafter.

(4) Research involving the collection or study of existing data, documents, records, pathological specimens, or diagnostic specimens, if these sources are publicly available or if the information is recorded by the investigator in such a manner that subjects cannot be identified, directly or through identifiers linked to the subjects.

(5) Research and demonstration projects which are conducted by or subject to the approval of Department or Agency heads, and which are designed to study, evaluate, or otherwise examine:

(i) Public benefit or service programs; (ii) procedures for obtaining benefits or services under those programs; (iii) possible changes in or alternatives to those programs or procedures; or (iv) possible changes in methods or levels of payment for benefits or services under those programs.

(6) Taste and food quality evaluation and consumer acceptance studies, (i) if wholesome foods without additives are consumed or (ii) if a food is consumed that contains a food ingredient at or below the level and for a use found to be safe, or agricultural chemical or environmental contaminant at or below the level found to be safe, by the Food and Drug Administration or approved by the Environmental Protection Agency or the Food Safety and Inspection Service of the U.S. Department of Agriculture.

(c) Department or Agency heads retain final judgment as to whether a particular activity is covered by this policy.

(d) Department or Agency heads may require that specific research activities or classes of research activities conducted, supported, or otherwise subject to regulation by the Department or Agency but not otherwise covered by this policy, comply with some or all of the requirements of this policy.

(e) Compliance with this policy requires compliance with pertinent Federal laws or regulations which provide additional protections for human subjects.

(f) This policy does not affect any State or local laws or regulations which may otherwise be applicable and which provide additional protections for human subjects.

(g) This policy does not affect any foreign laws or regulations which may otherwise be applicable and which provide additional protections to human subjects of research.

(h) When research covered by this policy takes place in foreign countries, procedures normally followed in the foreign countries to protect human subjects may differ from those set forth in this policy. [An example is a foreign institution which complies with guidelines consistent with the World Medical Assembly Declaration (Declaration of Helsinki amended 1989) issued either by sovereign states or by an organization whose function for the protection of human research subjects is internationally recognized.] In these circumstances, if a Department or Agency head determines that the procedures prescribed by the institution afford protections that are at least equivalent to those provided in this policy, the Department or Agency head may approve the substitution of the foreign procedures in lieu of the procedural requirements provided in this policy. Except when otherwise required by statute, Executive Order, or the Department or Agency head, notices of these actions as they occur will be published in the Federal Register or will be otherwise published as provided in Department or Agency procedures.

(i) Unless otherwise required by law, Department or Agency heads may waive the applicability of some or all of the provisions of this policy to specific research activities or classes or research activities otherwise covered by this policy. Except when otherwise required by statute or Executive Order, the Department or Agency head shall forward advance notices of these actions to the Office for Protection from Research Risks, National Institutes of Health, Department of Health and Human Services (DHHS), and shall also publish them in the Federal Register or in such other manner as provided in Department or Agency procedures.[1]

---

[1] Institutions with DHHS-approved assurances on file will abide by provisions of Title 45 CFR Part 46 Subparts A-D. Some of the other departments and agencies have incorporated all provisions of Title 45 CFR Part 46 into their policies and procedures as well. However, the exemptions at 45 CFR 46.101(b) do not apply to research involving prisoners, fetuses, pregnant women, or human in vitro fertilization, Subparts B and C. The exemption at 45 CFR 46.101(b)(2), for research involving survey or interview procedures or observation of public behavior, does not apply to research with children, Subpart D, except for research involving observations of public behavior when the investigator(s) do not participate in the activities being observed.

§ 46.102 Definitions.

(a) *Department or Agency* head means the head of any Federal Department or Agency and any other officer or employee of any Department or Agency to whom authority has been delegated.

(b) *Institution* means any public or private entity or Agency (including Federal, State, and other agencies).

(c) *Legally authorized representative* means an individual or judicial or other body authorized under applicable law to consent on behalf of a prospective subject to the subject's participation in the procedure(s) involved in the research.

(d) *Research* means a systematic investigation, including research development, testing and evaluation, designed to develop or contribute to generalizable knowledge. Activities which meet this definition constitute research for purposes of this policy, whether or not they are conducted or supported under a program which is considered research for other purposes. For example, some demonstration and service programs may include research activities.

(e) *Research subject to regulation*, and similar terms are intended to encompass those research activities for which a Federal Department or Agency has specific responsibility for regulating as a research activity, (for example, Investigational New Drug requirements administered by the Food and Drug Administration). It does not include research activities which are incidentally regulated by a Federal Department or Agency solely as part of the Department's or Agency's broader responsibility to regulate certain types of activities whether research or non-research in nature (for example, Wage and Hour requirements administered by the Department of Labor).

(f) *Human subject* means a living individual about whom an investigator (whether professional or student) conducting research obtains

(1) data through intervention or interaction with the individual, or

(2) identifiable private information.

Intervention includes both physical procedures by which data are gathered (for example, venipuncture) and manipulations of the subject or the subject's environment that are performed for research purposes. *Interaction* includes communication or interpersonal contact between investigator and subject. *Private information* includes information about behavior that occurs in a context in which an individual can reasonably expect that no observation or recording is taking place, and information which has been provided for specific purposes by an individual and which the individual can reasonably expect will not be made public (for example, a medical record). Private information must be individually identifiable (i.e., the identity of the subject is or may readily be ascertained by the investigator or associated with the information) in order for obtaining the information to constitute research involving human subjects.

(g) *IRB* means an Institutional Review Board established in accord with and for the purposes expressed in this policy.

(h) *IRB approval* means the determination of the IRB that the research has been reviewed and may be conducted at an institution within the constraints set forth by the IRB and by other institutional and Federal requirements.

(i) *Minimal risk* means that the probability and magnitude of harm or discomfort anticipated in the research are not greater in and of themselves than those ordinarily encountered in daily life or during the performance of routine physical or psychological examinations or tests.

(j) *Certification* means the official notification by the institution to the supporting Department or Agency, in accordance with the requirements of this policy, that a research project or activity involving human subjects has been reviewed and approved by an IRB in accordance with an approved assurance.

§ 46.103 Assuring compliance with this policy – research conducted or supported by any Federal Department or Agency.

(a) Each institution engaged in research which is covered by this policy and which is conducted or supported by a Federal Department or Agency shall provide written assurance satisfactory to the Department or Agency head that it will comply with the requirements set forth in this policy. In lieu of requiring submission of an assurance, individual Department or Agency heads shall accept the existence of a current assurance, appropriate for the research in question, on file with the Office for Protection from Research Risks, National Institutes Health, DHHS, and approved for Federalwide use by that office. When the existence of an DHHS-approved assurance is accepted in lieu of requiring submission of an assurance, reports (except certification) required by this policy to be made to Department and Agency heads shall also be made to the Office for Protection from Research Risks, National Institutes of Health, DHHS.

(b) Departments and agencies will conduct or support research covered by this policy only if the institution has an assurance approved as provided in this section, and only if the institution has certified to the Department or Agency head that the research has been reviewed and approved by an IRB provided for in the assurance, and will be subject to continuing review by the IRB. Assurances applicable to federally supported or conducted research shall at a minimum include:

(1) A statement of principles governing the institution in the discharge of its responsibilities for protecting the rights and welfare of human subjects of research conducted at or sponsored by the institution, regardless of whether the research is subject to Federal regulation. This may include an appropriate existing code, declaration, or statement of ethical principles, or a statement formulated by the institution itself. This requirement does not preempt provisions of this policy applicable to Department- or Agency-supported or regulated

research and need not be applicable to any research exempted or waived under § 46.101 (b) or (i).

(2) Designation of one or more IRBs established in accordance with the requirements of this policy, and for which provisions are made for meeting space and sufficient staff to support the IRB's review and recordkeeping duties.

(3) A list of IRB members identified by name; earned degrees; representative capacity; indications of experience such as board certifications, licenses, etc., sufficient to describe each member's chief anticipated contributions to IRB deliberations; and any employment or other relationship between each member and the institution; for example: full-time employee, part-time employee, member of governing panel or board, stockholder, paid or unpaid consultant. Changes in IRB membership shall be reported to the Department or Agency head, unless in accord with § 46.103(a) of this policy, the existence of a DHHS-approved assurance is accepted. In this case, change in IRB membership shall be reported to the Office for Protection from Research Risks, National Institutes of Health, DHHS.

(4) Written procedures which the IRB will follow (i) for conducting its initial and continuing review of research and for reporting its findings and actions to the investigator and the institution; (ii) for determining which projects require review more often than annually and which projects need verification from sources other than the investigators that no material changes have occurred since previous IRB review; and (iii) for ensuring prompt reporting to the IRB of proposed changes in a research activity, and for ensuring that such changes in approved research, during the period for which IRB approval has already been given, may not be initiated without IRB review and approval except when necessary to eliminate apparent immediate hazards to the subject.

(5) Written procedures for ensuring prompt reporting to the IRB, appropriate institutional officials, and the Department or Agency head of (i) any unanticipated problems involving risks to subjects or others or any serious or continuing noncompliance with this policy or the requirements or determinations of the IRB; and (ii) any suspension or termination of IRB approval.

(c) The assurance shall be executed by an individual authorized to act for the institution and to assume on behalf of the institution the obligations imposed by this policy and shall be filed in such form and manner as the Department or Agency head prescribes.

(d) The Department or Agency head will evaluate all assurances submitted in accordance with this policy through such officers and employees of the Department or Agency and such experts or consultants engaged for this purpose as the Department or Agency head determines to be appropriate. The Department or Agency head's evaluation will take into consideration the adequacy of the proposed IRB in light of the anticipated scope of the institution's research activities and the types of subject populations likely to be involved, the appropriateness of the proposed initial and continuing review procedures in light of the probable risks, and the size and complexity of the institution.

(e) On the basis of this evaluation, the Department or Agency head may approve or disapprove the assurance, or enter into negotiations to develop an approvable one. The Department or Agency head may limit the period during which any particular approved assurance or class of approved assurances shall remain effective or otherwise condition or restrict approval.

(f) Certification is required when the research is supported by a Federal Department or Agency and not otherwise exempted or waived under § 46.101 (b) or (i). An institution with an approved assurance shall certify that each application or proposal for research covered by the assurance and by § 46.103 of this policy has been reviewed and approved by the IRB. Such certification must be submitted with the application or proposal or by such later date as may be prescribed by the Department or Agency to which the application or proposal is submitted. Under no condition shall research covered by § 46.103 of the policy be supported prior to receipt of the certification that the research has been reviewed and approved by the IRB. Institutions without an approved assurance covering the research shall certify within 30 days after receipt of a request for such a certification from the Department or Agency, that the application or proposal has been approved by the IRB. If the certification is not submitted within these time limits, the application or proposal may be returned to the institution.

(Approved by the Office of Management and Budget under Control Number 9999-0020.)

§§ 46.104 – 46.106 [Reserved]

§ 46.107 IRB membership.

(a) Each IRB shall have at least five members, with varying backgrounds to promote complete and adequate review of research activities commonly conducted by the institution. The IRB shall be sufficiently qualified through the experience and expertise of its members, and the diversity of the members, including consideration of race, gender, and cultural backgrounds and sensitivity to such issues as community attitudes, to promote respect for its advice and counsel in safeguarding the rights and welfare of human subjects. In addition to possessing the professional competence necessary to review specific research activities, the IRB shall be able to ascertain the acceptability of proposed research in terms of institutional commitments and regulations, applicable law, and standards of professional conduct and practice. The IRB shall therefore include persons knowledgeable in these areas. If an IRB regularly reviews research that involves a vulnerable category of subjects, such as children, prisoners, pregnant women, or handicapped or mentally disabled persons, consideration shall be given to the inclusion of one or more individuals who are knowledgeable about and experienced in working with these subjects.

(b) Every nondiscriminatory effort will be made to ensure that no IRB consists entirely of men or entirely of women, including the institution's consideration of qualified persons of both sexes, so long as no selection is made to the IRB on the basis of gender. No IRB may consist entirely of members of one profession.

(c) Each IRB shall include at least one member whose primary concerns are in scientific areas and at least one member whose primary concerns are in non-scientific areas.

(d) Each IRB shall include at least one member who is not otherwise affiliated with the institution and who is not part of the immediate family of a person who is affiliated with the institution.

(e) No IRB may have a member participate in the IRB's initial or continuing review of any project in which the member has a conflicting interest, except to provide information requested by the IRB.

(f) An IRB may, in its discretion, invite individuals with competence in special areas to assist in the review of issues which require expertise beyond or in addition to that available on the IRB. These individuals may not vote with the IRB.

§ 46.108 IRB functions and operations.

In order to fulfill the requirements of this policy each IRB shall:

(a) Follow written procedures in the same detail as described in § 46.103(b)(4) and to the extent required by § 46.103(b)(5).

(b) Except when an expedited review procedure is used (see § 46.110), review proposed research at convened meetings at which a majority of the members of the IRB are present, including at least one member whose primary concerns are in nonscientific areas. In order for the research to be approved, it shall receive the approval of a majority of those members present at the meeting.

§ 46.109 IRB review of research.

(a) An IRB shall review and have authority to approve, require modifications in (to secure approval), or disapprove all research activities covered by this policy.

(b) An IRB shall require that information given to subjects as part of informed consent is in accordance with § 46.116. The IRB may require that information, in addition to that specifically mentioned in § 46.116, be given to the subjects when in the IRB's judgment the information would meaningfully add to the pro-tection of the rights and welfare of subjects.

(c) An IRB shall require documentation of informed consent or may waive doc-umentation in accordance with § 46.117.

(d) An IRB shall notify investigators and the institution in writing of its deci-sion to approve or disapprove the proposed research activity, or of modifications required to secure IRB approval of the research activity. If the IRB decides to disapprove a research activity, it shall include in its written notification a statement of the reasons for its decision and give the investigator an opportunity to respond in person or in writing.

(e) An IRB shall conduct continuing review of research covered by this policy at intervals appropriate to the degree of risk, but not less than once per year, and shall have authority to observe or have a third party observe the consent process and the research.

(Approved by the Office of Management and Budget under Control Number 9999-0020.)

§ 46.110 Expedited review procedures for certain kinds of research involving no more than minimal risk, and for minor changes in approved research.

(a) The Secretary, HHS, has established, and published as a Notice in the Federal Register, a list of categories of research that may be reviewed by the IRB through an expedited review procedure. The list will be amended, as appropriate, after consultation with other departments and agencies, through periodic republication by the Secretary, HHS, in the Federal Register. A copy of the list is available from the Office for Protection from Research Risks, National Institutes of Health, DHHS, Bethesda, Maryland 20892. [This list is reproduced below as Appendix B, and is also available at http://www.hhs.gov/ohrp/human-subjects/guidance/expedited98.htm.]

(b) An IRB may use the expedited review procedure to review either or both of the following:

(1) some or all of the research appearing on the list and found by the reviewer(s) to involve no more than minimal risk,

(2) minor changes in previously approved research during the period (of one year or less) for which approval is authorized.

Under an expedited review procedure, the review may be carried out by the IRB chairperson or by one or more experienced reviewers designated by the chairperson from among members of the IRB. In reviewing the research, the reviewers may exercise all of the authorities of the IRB except that the reviewers may not disapprove the research. A research activity may be disapproved only after review in accordance with the non-expedited procedure set forth in § 46.108(b).

(c) Each IRB which uses an expedited review procedure shall adopt a method for keeping all members advised of research proposals which have been approved under the procedure.

(d) The Department or Agency head may restrict, suspend, terminate, or choose not to authorize an institution's or IRB's use of the expedited review procedure.

§ 46.111 Criteria for IRB approval of research.

(a) In order to approve research covered by this policy the IRB shall determine that all of the following requirements are satisfied:

[handwritten: Belmont, beneficence] (1) Risks to subjects are minimized: (i) by using procedures which are consistent with sound research design and which do not unnecessarily expose subjects to risk, and (ii) whenever appropriate, by using procedures already being performed on the subjects for diagnostic or treatment purposes. *[handwritten: Don't do two tests when one will do]*

[handwritten: Beneficence] (2) Risks to subjects are reasonable in relation to anticipated benefits, if any, to subjects, and the importance of the knowledge that may reasonably be expected to result. In evaluating risks and benefits, the IRB should consider only those risks and benefits that may result from the research (as distinguished from risks and benefits of therapies subjects would receive even if not participating in the research). The IRB should not consider possible long-range effects of applying knowledge gained in the research (for example, the possible effects of the research on public policy) as among those research risks that fall within the purview of its responsibility.

[handwritten: Justice] (3) Selection of subjects is equitable. In making this assessment the IRB should take into account the purposes of the research and the setting in which the research will be conducted and should be particularly cognizant of the special problems of research involving vulnerable populations, such as children, prisoners, pregnant women, mentally disabled persons, or economically or educationally disadvantaged persons.

[handwritten: Resp. for persons] (4) Informed consent will be sought from each prospective subject or the subject's legally authorized representative, in accordance with, and to the extent required by § 46.116.

(5) Informed consent will be appropriately documented, in accordance with, and to the extent required by § 46.117.

[handwritten: Ben.] (6) When appropriate, the research plan makes adequate provision for monitoring the data collected to ensure the safety of subjects.

[handwritten: Resp. for] (7) When appropriate, there are adequate provisions to protect the privacy of subjects and to maintain the confidentiality of data.

(b) When some or all of the subjects are likely to be vulnerable to coercion or undue influence, such as children, prisoners, pregnant women, mentally disabled persons, or economically or educationally disadvantaged persons, additional safeguards have been included in the study to protect the rights and welfare of these subjects.

[handwritten: Resp. for Persons, Justice]

§ 46.112 Review by institution.

Research covered by this policy that has been approved by an IRB may be subject to further appropriate review and approval or disapproval by officials of the institution. However, those officials may not approve the research if it has not been approved by an IRB.

§ 46.113 Suspension or termination of IRB approval of research.

An IRB shall have authority to suspend or terminate approval of research that is not being conducted in accordance with the IRB's requirements or that has been associated with unexpected serious harm to subjects. Any suspension or termination or approval shall include a statement of the reasons for the IRB's action and shall be reported promptly to the investigator, appropriate institutional officials, and the Department or Agency head.

§ 46.114 Cooperative research.

Cooperative research projects are those projects covered by this policy which involve more than one institution. In the conduct of cooperative research projects, each institution is responsible for safeguarding the rights and welfare of human subjects and for complying with this policy. With the approval of the Department or Agency head, an institution participating in a cooperative project may enter into a joint review arrangement, rely upon the review of another qualified IRB, or make similar arrangements for avoiding duplication of effort.

(Approved by the Office of Management and Budget under Control Number 9999-0020.)

§ 46.115 IRB records.

(a) An institution, or when appropriate an IRB, shall prepare and maintain adequate documentation of IRB activities, including the following:

(1) Copies of all research proposals reviewed, scientific evaluations, if any, that accompany the proposals, approved sample consent documents, progress reports submitted by investigators, and reports of injuries to subjects.

(2) Minutes of IRB meetings which shall be in sufficient detail to show attendance at the meetings; actions taken by the IRB; the vote on these actions including the number of members voting for, against, and abstaining; the basis for requiring changes in or disapproving research; and a written summary of the discussion of controverted issues and their resolution.

(3) Records of continuing review activities.

(4) Copies of all correspondence between the IRB and the investigators.

(5) A list of IRB members in the same detail as described in § 46.103(b)(3).

(6) Written procedures for the IRB in the same detail as described in § 46.103(b)(4) and § 46.103(b)(5).

(7) Statements of significant new findings provided to subjects, as required by § 46.116(b)(5).

(b) The records required by this policy shall be retained for at least 3 years, and records relating to research which is conducted shall be retained for at least 3 years after completion of the research. All records shall be accessible for inspection and copying by authorized representatives of the Department or Agency at reasonable times and in a reasonable manner.

(Approved by the Office of Management and Budget under Control Number 9999-0020.)

§ 46.116 General requirements for informed consent.

Except as provided elsewhere in this policy, no investigator may involve a human being as a subject in research covered by this policy unless the investigator has obtained the legally effective informed consent of the subject or the subject's legally authorized representative. An investigator shall seek such consent only under circumstances that provide the prospective subject or the representative sufficient opportunity to consider whether or not to participate and that minimize the possibility of coercion or undue influence. The information that is given to the subject or the representative shall be in language understandable to the subject or the representative. No informed consent, whether oral or written, may include any exculpatory language through which the subject or the representative is made to waive or appear to waive any of the subject's legal rights, or releases or appears to release the investigator, the sponsor, the institution or its agents from liability for negligence.

(a) Basic elements of informed consent. Except as provided in paragraph (c) or (d) of this section, in seeking informed consent the following information shall be provided to each subject:

(1) a statement that the study involves research, an explanation of the purposes of the research and the expected duration of the subject's participation, a description of the procedures to be followed, and identification of any procedures which are experimental;

(2) a description of any reasonably foreseeable risks or discomforts to the subject;

(3) a description of any benefits to the subject or to others which may reasonably be expected from the research;

(4) a disclosure of appropriate alternative procedures or courses of treatment, if any, that might be advantageous to the subject;

(5) a statement describing the extent, if any, to which confidentiality of records identifying the subject will be maintained;

(6) for research involving more than minimal risk, an explanation as to whether any compensation and an explanation as to whether any medical treatments are available if injury occurs and, if so, what they consist of, or where further information may be obtained;

(7) an explanation of whom to contact for answers to pertinent questions about the research and research subjects' rights, and whom to contact in the event of a research-related injury to the subject; and

(8) a statement that participation is voluntary, refusal to participate will involve no penalty or loss of benefits to which the subject is otherwise entitled, and the subject may discontinue participation at any time without penalty or loss of benefits to which the subject is otherwise entitled.

(b) Additional elements of informed consent. When appropriate, one or more of the following elements of information shall also be provided to each subject:

(1) a statement that the particular treatment or procedure may involve risks to the subject (or to the embryo or fetus, if the subject is or may become pregnant) which are currently unforeseeable;

(2) anticipated circumstances under which the subject's participation may be terminated by the investigator without regard to the subject's consent;

(3) any additional costs to the subject that may result from participation in the research;

(4) the consequences of a subject's decision to withdraw from the research and procedures for orderly termination of participation by the subject;

(5) A statement that significant new findings developed during the course of the research which may relate to the subject's willingness to continue participation will be provided to the subject; and

(6) the approximate number of subjects involved in the study.

(c) An IRB may approve a consent procedure which does not include, or which alters, some or all of the elements of informed consent set forth above, or waive the requirement to obtain informed consent provided the IRB finds and documents that:

(1) the research or demonstration project is to be conducted by or subject to the approval of state or local government officials and is designed to study, evaluate, or otherwise examine: (i) public benefit or service programs; (ii) procedures for obtaining benefits or services under those programs; (iii) possible changes in or alternatives to those programs or procedures; or (iv) possible changes in methods or levels of payment for benefits or services under those programs; and

(2) the research could not practicably be carried out without the waiver or alteration.

waiver of informed consent

(d) An IRB may approve a consent procedure which does not include, or which alters, some or all of the elements of informed consent set forth in this section, or waive the requirements to obtain informed consent provided the IRB finds and documents that:

(1) the research involves no more than minimal risk to the subjects;

(2) the waiver or alteration will not adversely affect the rights and welfare of the subjects;

(3) the research could not practicably be carried out without the waiver or alteration; and

(4) whenever appropriate, the subjects will be provided with additional pertinent information after participation.

(e) The informed consent requirements in this policy are not intended to preempt any applicable Federal, State, or local laws which require additional information to be disclosed in order for informed consent to be legally effective.

(f) Nothing in this policy is intended to limit the authority of a physician to provide emergency medical care, to the extent the physician is permitted to do so under applicable Federal, State, or local law.

(Approved by the Office of Management and Budget under Control Number 9999-0020.)

§ 46.117 Documentation of informed consent.

(a) Except as provided in paragraph (c) of this section, informed consent shall be documented by the use of a written consent form approved by the IRB and signed by the subject or the subject's legally authorized representative. A copy shall be given to the person signing the form.

(b) Except as provided in paragraph (c) of this section, the consent form may be either of the following:

(1) A written consent document that embodies the elements of informed consent required by §46.116. This form may be read to the subject or the subject's legally authorized representative, but in any event, the investigator shall give either the subject or the representative adequate opportunity to read it before it is signed; or

(2) A short form written consent document stating that the elements of informed consent required by §46.116 have been presented orally to the subject or the subject's legally authorized representative. When this method is used, there shall be a witness to the oral presentation. Also, the IRB shall approve a written summary of what is to be said to the subject or the representative. Only the short form itself is to be signed by the subject or the representative. However, the witness shall sign both the short form and a copy of the summary, and the person actually obtaining consent shall sign a copy of the summary. A

copy of the summary shall be given to the subject or the representative, in addition to a copy of the short form.

(c) An IRB may waive the requirement for the investigator to obtain a signed consent form for some or all subjects if it finds either:

(1) That the only record linking the subject and the research would be the consent document and the principal risk would be potential harm resulting from a breach of confidentiality. Each subject will be asked whether the subject wants documentation linking the subject with the research, and the subject's wishes will govern; or

(2) That the research presents no more than minimal risk of harm to subjects and involves no procedures for which written consent is normally required outside of the research context.

In cases in which the documentation requirement is waived, the IRB may require the investigator to provide subjects with a written statement regarding the research.

(Approved by the Office of Management and Budget under Control Number 9999-0020.)

§ 46.118 Applications and proposals lacking definite plans for involvement of human subjects.

Certain types of applications for grants, cooperative agreements, or contracts are submitted to departments or agencies with the knowledge that subjects may be involved within the period of support, but definite plans would not normally be set forth in the application or proposal. These include activities such as institutional type grants when selection of specific projects is the institution's responsibility; research training grants in which the activities involving subjects remain to be selected; and projects in which human subjects' involvement will depend upon completion of instruments, prior animal studies, or purification of compounds. These applications need not be reviewed by an IRB before an award may be made. However, except for research exempted or waived under §46.101 (b) or (i), no human subjects may be involved in any project supported by these awards until the project has been reviewed and approved by the IRB, as provided in this policy, and certification submitted, by the institution, to the Department or Agency.

§ 46.119 Research undertaken without the intention of involving human subjects.

In the event research is undertaken without the intention of involving human subjects, but it is later proposed to involve human subjects in the research, the research shall first be reviewed and approved by an IRB, as provided in this policy, a certification submitted, by the institution, to the Department or Agency, and final approval given to the proposed change by the Department or Agency.

§ 46.120 Evaluation and disposition of applications and proposals for research to be conducted or supported by a Federal Department or Agency.

(a) The Department or Agency head will evaluate all applications and proposals involving human subjects submitted to the Department or Agency through such officers and employees of the Department or Agency and such experts and consultants as the Department or Agency head determines to be appropriate. This evaluation will take into consideration the risks to the subjects, the adequacy of protection against these risks, the potential benefits of the research to the subjects and others, and the importance of the knowledge gained or to be gained.

(b) On the basis of this evaluation, the Department or Agency head may approve or disapprove the application or proposal, or enter into negotiations to develop an approvable one.

§ 46.121 [Reserved]

§ 46.122 Use of Federal funds.

Federal funds administered by a Department or Agency may not be expended for research involving human subjects unless the requirements of this policy have been satisfied.

§ 46.123 Early termination of research support: Evaluation of applications and proposals.

(a) The Department or Agency head may require that Department or Agency support for any project be terminated or suspended in the manner prescribed in applicable program requirements, when the Department or Agency head finds an institution has materially failed to comply with the terms of this policy.

(b) In making decisions about supporting or approving applications or proposals covered by this policy the Department or Agency head may take into account, in addition to all other eligibility requirements and program criteria, factors such as whether the applicant has been subject to a termination or suspension under paragraph (a) of this section and whether the applicant or the person or persons who would direct or has/have directed the scientific and technical aspects of an activity has/have, in the judgment of the Department or Agency head, materially failed to discharge responsibility for the protection of the rights and welfare of human subjects (whether or not the research was subject to Federal regulation).

§ 46.124 Conditions.

With respect to any research project or any class of research projects the Department or Agency head may impose additional conditions prior to or at the time of approval when in the judgment of the Department or Agency head additional conditions are necessary for the protection of human subjects.

Subpart B—Additional Protections for Pregnant Women, Human Fetuses and Neonates Involved in Research

Source: 66 Fed. Reg. 56,775 (2001)

§ 46.201 To what do these regulations apply?

(a) Except as provided in paragraph (b) of this section, this subpart applies to all research involving pregnant women, human fetuses, neonates of uncertain viability, or nonviable neonates conducted or supported by the Department of Health and Human Services (DHHS). This includes all research conducted in DHHS facilities by any person and all research conducted in any facility by DHHS employees.

(b) The exemptions at § 46.101(b)(1) through (6) are applicable to this subpart.

(c) The provisions of § 46.101(c) through (i) are applicable to this subpart. Reference to State or local laws in this subpart and in § 46.101(f) is intended to include the laws of federally recognized American Indian and Alaska Native Tribal Governments.

(d) The requirements of this subpart are in addition to those imposed under the other subparts of this part.

§ 46.202 Definitions.

The definitions in § 46.102 shall be applicable to this subpart as well. In addition, as used in this subpart:

(a) Dead fetus means a fetus that exhibits neither heartbeat, spontaneous respiratory activity, spontaneous movement of voluntary muscles, nor pulsation of the umbilical cord.

(b) Delivery means complete separation of the fetus from the woman by expulsion or extraction or any other means.

(c) Fetus means the product of conception from implantation until delivery.

(d) Neonate means a newborn.

(e) Nonviable neonate means a neonate after delivery that, although living, is not viable.

(f) Pregnancy encompasses the period of time from implantation until delivery. A woman shall be assumed to be pregnant if she exhibits any of the pertinent presumptive signs of pregnancy, such as missed menses, until the results of a pregnancy test are negative or until delivery.

(g) Secretary means the Secretary of Health and Human Services and any other officer or employee of the Department of Health and Human Services to whom authority has been delegated.

(h) Viable, as it pertains to the neonate, means being able, after delivery, to survive (given the benefit of available medical therapy) to the point of independently maintaining heartbeat and respiration. The Secretary may from time to time, taking into account medical advances, publish in the Federal Register guidelines to assist in determining whether a neonate is viable for purposes of this subpart. If a neonate is viable then it may be included in research only to the extent permitted and in accordance with the requirements of subparts A and D of this part.

§ 46.203 Duties of IRBs in connection with research involving pregnant women, fetuses, and neonates.

In addition to other responsibilities assigned to IRBs under this part, each IRB shall review research covered by this subpart and approve only research which satisfies the conditions of all applicable sections of this subpart and the other subparts of this part.

§ 46.204 Research involving pregnant women or fetuses.

Pregnant women or fetuses may be involved in research if all of the following conditions are met:

(a) Where scientifically appropriate, preclinical studies, including studies on pregnant animals, and clinical studies, including studies on nonpregnant women, have been conducted and provide data for assessing potential risks to pregnant women and fetuses;

(b) The risk to the fetus is caused solely by interventions or procedures that hold out the prospect of direct benefit for the woman or the fetus; or, if there is no such prospect of benefit, the risk to the fetus is not greater than minimal and the purpose of the research is the development of important biomedical knowledge which cannot be obtained by any other means;

(c) Any risk is the least possible for achieving the objectives of the research;

(d) If the research holds out the prospect of direct benefit to the pregnant woman, the prospect of a direct benefit both to the pregnant woman and the fetus, or no prospect of benefit for the woman nor the fetus when risk to the fetus is not greater than minimal and the purpose of the research is the development of important biomedical knowledge that cannot be obtained by any other means, her consent is obtained in accord with the informed consent provisions of subpart A of this part;

(e) If the research holds out the prospect of direct benefit solely to the fetus then the consent of the pregnant woman and the father is obtained in accord with the informed consent provisions of subpart A of this part, except that the father's consent need not be obtained if he is unable to consent because of unavailability, incompetence, or temporary incapacity or the pregnancy resulted from rape or incest.

(f) Each individual providing consent under paragraph (d) or (e) of this section is fully informed regarding the reasonably foreseeable impact of the research on the fetus or neonate;

(g) For children as defined in § 46.402(a) who are pregnant, assent and permission are obtained in accord with the provisions of subpart D of this part;

(h) No inducements, monetary or otherwise, will be offered to terminate a pregnancy;

(i) Individuals engaged in the research will have no part in any decisions as to the timing, method, or procedures used to terminate a pregnancy; and

(j) Individuals engaged in the research will have no part in determining the viability of a neonate.

§ 46.205 Research involving neonates.

(a) Neonates of uncertain viability and nonviable neonates may be involved in research if all of the following conditions are met:

(1) Where scientifically appropriate, preclinical and clinical studies have been conducted and provide data for assessing potential risks to neonates.

(2) Each individual providing consent under paragraph (b)(2) or (c)(5) of this section is fully informed regarding the reasonably foreseeable impact of the research on the neonate.

(3) Individuals engaged in the research will have no part in determining the viability of a neonate.

(4) The requirements of paragraph (b) or (c) of this section have been met as applicable.

(b) Neonates of uncertain viability. Until it has been ascertained whether or not a neonate is viable, a neonate may not be involved in research covered by this subpart unless the following additional conditions have been met:

(1) The IRB determines that:

(i) The research holds out the prospect of enhancing the probability of survival of the neonate to the point of viability, and any risk is the least possible for achieving that objective, or

(ii) The purpose of the research is the development of important biomedical knowledge which cannot be obtained by other means and there will be no added risk to the neonate resulting from the research; and

(2) The legally effective informed consent of either parent of the neonate or, if neither parent is able to consent because of unavailability, incompetence, or temporary incapacity, the legally effective informed consent of either parent's legally authorized representative is obtained in accord with subpart A of this

part, except that the consent of the father or his legally authorized representative need not be obtained if the pregnancy resulted from rape or incest.

(c) Nonviable neonates. After delivery nonviable neonate may not be involved in research covered by this subpart unless all of the following additional conditions are met:

(1) Vital functions of the neonate will not be artificially maintained;

(2) The research will not terminate the heartbeat or respiration of the neonate;

(3) There will be no added risk to the neonate resulting from the research;

(4) The purpose of the research is the development of important biomedical knowledge that cannot be obtained by other means; and

(5) The legally effective informed consent of both parents of the neonate is obtained in accord with subpart A of this part, except that the waiver and alteration provisions of § 46.116(c) and (d) do not apply. However, if either parent is unable to consent because of unavailability, incompetence, or temporary incapacity, the informed consent of one parent of a nonviable neonate will suffice to meet the requirements of this paragraph (c)(5), except that the consent of the father need not be obtained if the pregnancy resulted from rape or incest. The consent of a legally authorized representative of either or both of the parents of a nonviable neonate will not suffice to meet the requirements of this paragraph (c)(5).

(d) Viable neonates. A neonate, after delivery, that has been determined to be viable may be included in research only to the extent permitted by and in accord with the requirements of subparts A and D of this part.

§ 46.206 Research involving, after delivery, the placenta, the dead fetus or fetal material.

(a) Research involving, after delivery, the placenta; the dead fetus; macerated fetal material; or cells, tissue, or organs excised from a dead fetus, shall be conducted only in accord with any applicable Federal, State, or local laws and regulations regarding such activities.

(b) If information associated with material described in paragraph (a) of this section is recorded for research purposes in a manner that living individuals can be identified, directly or through identifiers linked to those individuals, those individuals are research subjects and all pertinent subparts of this part are applicable.

§ 46.207 Research not otherwise approvable which presents an opportunity to understand, prevent, or alleviate a serious problem affecting the health or welfare of pregnant women, fetuses, or neonates.

The Secretary will conduct or fund research that the IRB does not believe meets the requirements of § 46.204 or § 46.205 only if:

(a) The IRB finds that the research presents a reasonable opportunity to further the understanding, prevention, or alleviation of a serious problem affecting the health or welfare of pregnant women, fetuses or neonates; and

(b) The Secretary, after consultation with a panel of experts in pertinent disciplines (for example: science, medicine, ethics, law) and following opportunity for public review and comment, including a public meeting announced in the Federal Register, has determined either:

(1) That the research in fact satisfies the conditions of § 46.204, as applicable; or

(2) The following:

(i) The research presents a reasonable opportunity to further the understanding, prevention, or alleviation of a serious problem affecting the health or welfare of pregnant women, fetuses or neonates;

(ii) The research will be conducted in accord with sound ethical principles; and

(iii) Informed consent will be obtained in accord with the informed consent provisions of subpart A and other applicable subparts of this part.

Subpart C—Additional Protections Pertaining to Biomedical and Behavioral Research Involving Prisoners as Subjects

Source: 43 Fed. Reg. 53,665 (1978)

§ 46.301 Applicability.

(a) The regulations in this subpart are applicable to all biomedical and behavioral research conducted or supported by the Department of Health and Human Services involving prisoners as subjects.

(b) Nothing in this subpart shall be construed as indicating that compliance with the procedures set forth herein will authorize research involving prisoners as subjects, to the extent such research is limited or barred by applicable State or local law.

(c) The requirements of this subpart are in addition to those imposed under the other subparts of this part.

§ 46.302 Purpose.

Inasmuch as prisoners may be under constraints because of their incarceration which could affect their ability to make a truly voluntary and uncoerced decision whether or not to participate as subjects in research, it is the purpose of this subpart to provide additional safeguards for the protection of prisoners involved in activities to which this subpart is applicable.

§ 46.303 Definitions.

As used in this subpart:

(a) "Secretary" means the Secretary of Health and Human Services and any other officer or employee of the Department of Health and Human Services to whom authority has been delegated.

(b) "DHHS" means the Department of Health and Human Services.

(c) "Prisoner" means any individual involuntarily confined or detained in a penal institution. The term is intended to encompass individuals sentenced to such an institution under a criminal or civil statute, individuals detained in other facilities by virtue of statutes or commitment procedures which provide alternatives to criminal prosecution or incarceration in a penal institution, and individuals detained pending arraignment, trial, or sentencing.

(d) "Minimal risk" is the probability and magnitude of physical or psychological harm that is normally encountered in the daily lives, or in the routine medical, dental, or psychological examination of healthy persons.

§ 46.304 Composition of Institutional Review Boards where prisoners are involved.

In addition to satisfying the requirements in § 46.107 of this part, an Institutional Review Board, carrying out responsibilities under this part with respect to research covered by this subpart, shall also meet the following specific requirements:

(a) A majority of the Board (exclusive of prisoner members) shall have no association with the prison(s) involved, apart from their membership on the Board.

(b) At least one member of the Board shall be a prisoner, or a prisoner representative with appropriate background and experience to serve in that capacity, except that where a particular research project is reviewed by more than one Board only one Board need satisfy this requirement.

§46.305 Additional duties of the Institutional Review Boards where prisoners are involved.

(a) In addition to all other responsibilities prescribed for Institutional Review Boards under this part, the Board shall review research covered by this subpart and approve such research only if it finds that:

(1) the research under review represents one of the categories of research permissible under § 46.306(a)(2);

(2) any possible advantages accruing to the prisoner through his or her participation in the research, when compared to the general living conditions, medical care, quality of food, amenities and opportunity for earnings in the prison, are not of such a magnitude that his or her ability to weigh the risks of the research against the value of such advantages in the limited choice environment of the prison is impaired;

(3) the risks involved in the research are commensurate with risks that would be accepted by nonprisoner volunteers;

(4) procedures for the selection of subjects within the prison are fair to all prisoners and immune from arbitrary intervention by prison authorities or prisoners. Unless the principal investigator provides to the Board justification in writing for following some other procedures, control subjects must be selected randomly from the group of available prisoners who meet the characteristics needed for that particular research project;

(5) the information is presented in language which is understandable to the subject population;

(6) adequate assurance exists that parole boards will not take into account a prisoner's participation in the research in making decisions regarding parole, and each prisoner is clearly informed in advance that participation in the research will have no effect on his or her parole; and

(7) where the Board finds there may be a need for follow-up examination or care of participants after the end of their participation, adequate provision has been made for such examination or care, taking into account the varying lengths of individual prisoners' sentences, and for informing participants of this fact.

(b) The Board shall carry out such other duties as may be assigned by the Secretary.

(c) The institution shall certify to the Secretary, in such form and manner as the Secretary may require, that the duties of the Board under this section have been fulfilled.

§46.306 Permitted research involving prisoners.

(a) Biomedical or behavioral research conducted or supported by DHHS may involve prisoners as subjects only if:

(1) the institution responsible for the conduct of the research has certified to the Secretary that the Institutional Review Board has approved the research under § 46.305 of this subpart; and

(2) in the judgment of the Secretary the proposed research involves solely the following:

(i) study of the possible causes, effects, and processes of incarceration, and of criminal behavior, provided that the study presents no more than minimal risk and no more than inconvenience to the subjects;

(ii) study of prisons as institutional structures or of prisoners as incarcerated persons, provided that the study presents no more than minimal risk and no more than inconvenience to the subjects;

(iii) research on conditions particularly affecting prisoners as a class (for example, vaccine trials and other research on hepatitis which is much more prevalent in prisons than elsewhere; and research on social and psychological problems such as alcoholism, drug addiction, and sexual assaults) provided that the study may proceed only after the Secretary has consulted with appropriate experts including experts in penology, medicine, and ethics, and published notice, in the Federal Register, of his intent to approve such research; or

(iv) research on practices, both innovative and accepted, which have the intent and reasonable probability of improving the health or well-being of the subject. In cases in which those studies require the assignment of prisoners in a manner consistent with protocols approved by the IRB to control groups which may not benefit from the research, the study may proceed only after the Secretary has consulted with appropriate experts, including experts in penology, medicine, and ethics, and published notice, in the Federal Register, of the intent to approve such research.

(b) Except as provided in paragraph (a) of this section, biomedical or behavioral research conducted or supported by DHHS shall not involve prisoners as subjects.

Subpart D—Additional Protections for Children Involved as Subjects in Research

Source: 48 Fed. Reg. 9818 (1991)

§ 46.401 To what do these regulations apply?

(a) This subpart applies to all research involving children as subjects, conducted or supported by the Department of Health and Human Services.

(1) This includes research conducted by Department employees, except that each head of an Operating Division of the Department may adopt such non-substantive, procedural modifications as may be appropriate from an administrative standpoint.

(2) It also includes research conducted or supported by the Department of Health and Human Services outside the United States, but in appropriate circumstances, the Secretary may, under paragraph (i) of § 46.101 of Subpart A, waive the applicability of some or all of the requirements of these regulations for research of this type.

(b) Exemptions at § 46.101(b)(1) and (b)(3) through (b)(6) are applicable to this subpart. The exemption at § 46.101(b)(2) regarding educational tests is also applicable to this subpart. However, the exemption at § 46.101(b)(2) for research involving survey or interview procedures or observations of public behavior does not apply to research covered by this subpart, except for research involving observation of public behavior when the investigator(s) do not participate in the activities being observed.

(c) The exceptions, additions, and provisions for waiver as they appear in paragraphs (c) through (i) of § 46.101 of Subpart A are applicable to this subpart.

§ 46.402 Definitions.

The definitions in § 46.102 of Subpart A shall be applicable to this subpart as well. In addition, as used in this subpart:

(a) "Children" are persons who have not attained the legal age for consent to treatments or procedures involved in the research, under the applicable law of the jurisdiction in which the research will be conducted.

(b) "Assent" means a child's affirmative agreement to participate in research. Mere failure to object should not, absent affirmative agreement, be construed as assent.

(c) "Permission" means the agreement of parent(s) or guardian to the participation of their child or ward in research.

(d) "Parent" means a child's biological or adoptive parent.

(e) "Guardian" means an individual who is authorized under applicable State or local law to consent on behalf of a child to general medical care.

§ 46.403 IRB duties.

In addition to other responsibilities assigned to IRBs under this part, each IRB shall review research covered by this subpart and approve only research which satisfies the conditions of all applicable sections of this subpart.

§ 46.404 Research not involving greater than minimal risk.

DHHS will conduct or fund research in which the IRB finds that no greater than minimal risk to children is presented, only if the IRB finds that adequate provisions are made for soliciting the assent of the children and the permission of their parents or guardians, as set forth in § 46.408.

Defined at 46.102 i

§ 46.405 Research involving greater than minimal risk but presenting the prospect of direct benefit to the individual subjects.

DHHS will conduct or fund research in which the IRB finds that more than minimal risk to children is presented by an intervention or procedure that holds out the prospect of direct benefit for the individual subject, or by a monitoring procedure that is likely to contribute to the subject's well-being, only if the IRB finds that:

(a) the risk is justified by the anticipated benefit to the subjects;

(b) the relation of the anticipated benefit to the risk is at least as favorable to the subjects as that presented by available alternative approaches; and

(c) adequate provisions are made for soliciting the assent of the children and permission of their parents or guardians, as set forth in § 46.408.

§ 46.406 Research involving greater than minimal risk and no prospect of direct benefit to individual subjects, but likely to yield generalizable knowledge about the subject's disorder or condition.

DHHS will conduct or fund research in which the IRB finds that more than minimal risk to children is presented by an intervention or procedure that does not hold out the prospect of direct benefit for the individual subject, or by a monitoring procedure which is not likely to contribute to the well-being of the subject, only if the IRB finds that:

(a) the risk represents a minor increase over minimal risk;

(b) the intervention or procedure presents experiences to subjects that are reasonably commensurate with those inherent in their actual or expected medical, dental, psychological, social, or educational situations;

(c) the intervention or procedure is likely to yield generalizable knowledge about the subjects' disorder or condition which is of vital importance for the understanding or amelioration of the subjects' disorder or condition; and

(d) adequate provisions are made for soliciting assent of the children and permission of their parents or guardians, as set forth in § 46.408.

§ 46.407 Research not otherwise approvable which presents an opportunity to understand, prevent, or alleviate a serious problem affecting the health or welfare of children.

DHHS will conduct or fund research that the IRB does not believe meets the requirements of § 46.404, § 46.405, or § 46.406 only if:

(a) the IRB finds that the research presents a reasonable opportunity to further the understanding, prevention, or alleviation of a serious problem affecting the health or welfare of children; and

(b) the Secretary, after consultation with a panel of experts in pertinent disciplines (for example: science, medicine, education, ethics, law) and following opportunity for public review and comment, has determined either:

(1) that the research in fact satisfies the conditions of § 46.404, § 46.405, or § 46.406, as applicable, or

(2) the following:

(i) the research presents a reasonable opportunity to further the understanding, prevention, or alleviation of a serious problem affecting the health or welfare of children;

(ii) the research will be conducted in accordance with sound ethical principles;

(iii) adequate provisions are made for soliciting the assent of children and the permission of their parents or guardians, as set forth in § 46.408.

§ 46.408 Requirements for permission by parents or guardians and for assent by children.

(a) In addition to the determinations required under other applicable sections of this subpart, the IRB shall determine that adequate provisions are made for soliciting the assent of the children, when in the judgment of the IRB the children are capable of providing assent. In determining whether children are capable of assenting, the IRB shall take into account the ages, maturity, and psychological state of the children involved. This judgment may be made for all children to be involved in research under a particular protocol, or for each child, as the IRB deems appropriate. If the IRB determines that the capability of some or all of the children is so limited that they cannot reasonably be consulted or that the intervention or procedure involved in the research holds out a prospect of direct benefit that is important to the health or well-being of the children and is available only in the context of the research, the assent of the children is not a necessary condition for proceeding with the research. Even where the IRB determines that the subjects are capable of assenting, the IRB may still waive the assent requirement under circumstances in which consent may be waived in accord with § 46.116 of Subpart A.

(b) In addition to the determinations required under other applicable sections of this subpart, the IRB shall determine, in accordance with and to the extent that consent is required by § 46.116 of Subpart A, that adequate provisions are made for soliciting the permission of each child's parents or guardian. Where parental permission is to be obtained, the IRB may find that the permission of one parent is sufficient for research to be conducted under § 46.404 or § 46.405. Where research is covered by § 46.406 and § 46.407 and permission is to be obtained from parents, both parents must give their permission unless one parent is deceased, unknown, incompetent, or not reasonably available, or when only one parent has legal responsibility for the care and custody of the child.

(c) In addition to the provisions for waiver contained in § 46.116 of Subpart A, if the IRB determines that a research protocol is designed for conditions or for a subject population for which parental or guardian permission is not a reasonable requirement to protect the subjects (for example, neglected or abused children), it may waive the consent requirements in Subpart A of this part and paragraph (b) of this section, provided an appropriate mechanism for protecting the children who will participate as subjects in the research is substituted, and provided further that the waiver is not inconsistent with Federal, State, or local law. The choice of an appropriate mechanism would depend upon the nature and purpose of the activities described in the protocol, the risk and anticipated benefit to the research subjects, and their age, maturity, status, and condition.

(d) Permission by parents or guardians shall be documented in accordance with and to the extent required by § 46.117 of Subpart A.

(e) When the IRB determines that assent is required, it shall also determine whether and how assent must be documented.

§ 46.409 Wards.

(a) Children who are wards of the State or any other agency, institution, or entity can be included in research approved under § 46.406 or § 46.407 only if such research is:

(1) related to their status as wards; or

(2) conducted in schools, camps, hospitals, institutions, or similar settings in which the majority of children involved as subjects are not wards.

(b) If the research is approved under paragraph (a) of this section, the IRB shall require appointment of an advocate for each child who is a ward, in addition to any other individual acting on behalf of the child as guardian or in loco parentis. One individual may serve as advocate for more than one child. The advocate shall be an individual who has the background and experience to act in, and agrees to act in, the best interests of the child for the duration of the child's participation in the research and who is not associated in any way (except in the role as advocate or member of the IRB) with the research, the investigator(s), or the guardian organization.

APPENDIX B

Department of Health and Human Services

Categories of Research That May Be Reviewed by the Institutional Review Board (IRB) through an Expedited Review Procedure[1]

Applicability

(A) Research activities that (1) present no more than minimal risk to human subjects, and (2) involve only procedures listed in one or more of the following categories, may be reviewed by the IRB through the expedited review procedure authorized by 45 CFR 46.110 and 21 CFR 56.110. The activities listed should not be deemed to be of minimal risk simply because they are included on this list. Inclusion on this list merely means that the activity is eligible for review through the expedited review procedure when the specific circumstances of the proposed research involve no more than minimal risk to human subjects.

(B) The categories in this list apply regardless of the age of subjects, except as noted.

(C) The expedited review procedure may not be used where identification of the subjects and/or their responses would reasonably place them at risk of criminal or civil liability or be damaging to the subjects' financial standing, employability, insurability, reputation, or be stigmatizing, unless reasonable and appropriate protections will be implemented so that risks related to invasion of privacy and breach of confidentiality are no greater than minimal.

(D) The expedited review procedure may not be used for classified research involving human subjects.

(E) IRBs are reminded that the standard requirements for informed consent (or its waiver, alteration, or exception) apply regardless of the type of review — expedited or convened — utilized by the IRB.

(F) Categories one (1) through seven (7) pertain to both initial and continuing IRB review.

---

[1] An expedited review procedure consists of a review of research involving human subjects by the IRB chairperson or by one or more experienced reviewers designated by the chairperson from among members of the IRB in accordance with the requirements set forth in 45 CFR 46.110.

Research Categories

(1) Clinical studies of drugs and medical devices only when condition (a) or (b) is met.

(a) Research on drugs for which an investigational new drug application (21 CFR Part 312) is not required. (Note: Research on marketed drugs that significantly increases the risks or decreases the acceptability of the risks associated with the use of the product is not eligible for expedited review.)

(b) Research on medical devices for which (i) an investigational device exemption application (21 CFR Part 812) is not required; or (ii) the medical device is cleared/approved for marketing and the medical device is being used in accordance with its cleared/approved labeling.

(2) Collection of blood samples by finger stick, heel stick, ear stick, or venipuncture as follows:

(a) from healthy, nonpregnant adults who weigh at least 110 pounds. For these subjects, the amounts drawn may not exceed 550 ml in an 8 week period and collection may not occur more frequently than 2 times per week; or

(b) from other adults and children,[2] considering the age, weight, and health of the subjects, the collection procedure, the amount of blood to be collected, and the frequency with which it will be collected. For these subjects, the amount drawn may not exceed the lesser of 50 ml or 3 ml per kg in an 8 week period and collection may not occur more frequently than 2 times per week.

(3) Prospective collection of biological specimens for research purposes by non-invasive means.

Examples: (a) hair and nail clippings in a nondisfiguring manner; (b) deciduous teeth at time of exfoliation or if routine patient care indicates a need for extraction; (c) permanent teeth if routine patient care indicates a need for extraction; (d) excreta and external secretions (including sweat); (e) uncannulated saliva collected either in an unstimulated fashion or stimulated by chewing gumbase or wax or by applying a dilute citric solution to the tongue; (f) placenta removed at delivery; (g) amniotic fluid obtained at the time of rupture of the membrane prior to or during labor; (h) supra- and subgingival dental plaque and calculus, provided the collection procedure is not more invasive than routine prophylactic scaling of the teeth and the process is accomplished in accordance with accepted prophylactic techniques; (i) mucosal and skin cells collected by buccal scraping or swab, skin swab, or mouth washings; (j) sputum collected after saline mist nebulization.

---

[2] Children are defined in the HHS regulations as "persons who have not attained the legal age for consent to treatments or procedures involved in the research, under the applicable law of the jurisdiction in which the research will be conducted." 45 CFR 46.402(a).

(4) Collection of data through noninvasive procedures (not involving general anesthesia or sedation) routinely employed in clinical practice, excluding procedures involving x-rays or microwaves. Where medical devices are employed, they must be cleared/approved for marketing. (Studies intended to evaluate the safety and effectiveness of the medical device are not generally eligible for expedited review, including studies of cleared medical devices for new indications.)

Examples: (a) physical sensors that are applied either to the surface of the body or at a distance and do not involve input of significant amounts of energy into the subject or an invasion of the subject's privacy; (b) weighing or testing sensory acuity; (c) magnetic resonance imaging; (d) electrocardiography, electroencephalography, thermography, detection of naturally occurring radioactivity, electroretinography, ultrasound, diagnostic infrared imaging, Doppler blood flow, and echocardiography; (e) moderate exercise, muscular strength testing, body composition assessment, and flexibility testing where appropriate given the age, weight, and health of the individual.

(5) Research involving materials (data, documents, records, or specimens) that have been collected, or will be collected solely for nonresearch purposes (such as medical treatment or diagnosis). (NOTE: Some research in this category may be exempt from the HHS regulations for the protection of human subjects. 45 CFR 46.101(b)(4). This listing refers only to research that is not exempt.)

(6) Collection of data from voice, video, digital, or image recordings made for research purposes.

(7) Research on individual or group characteristics or behavior (including, but not limited to, research on perception, cognition, motivation, identity, language, communication, cultural beliefs or practices, and social behavior) or research employing survey, interview, oral history, focus group, program evaluation, human factors evaluation, or quality assurance methodologies. (NOTE: Some research in this category may be exempt from the HHS regulations for the protection of human subjects. 45 CFR 46.101(b)(2) and (b)(3). This listing refers only to research that is not exempt.)

(8) Continuing review of research previously approved by the convened IRB as follows:

(a) where (i) the research is permanently closed to the enrollment of new subjects; (ii) all subjects have completed all research-related interventions; and (iii) the research remains active only for long-term follow-up of subjects; or

(b) where no subjects have been enrolled and no additional risks have been identified; or

(c) where the remaining research activities are limited to data analysis.

(9) Continuing review of research, not conducted under an investigational new drug application or investigational device exemption where categories two (2)

through eight (8) do not apply but the IRB has determined and documented at a convened meeting that the research involves no greater than minimal risk and no additional risks have been identified.

Source: 63 Fed. Reg. 60,364 (1998)

APPENDIX C

Food and Drug Administration

Significant Differences in FDA and HHS Regulations for Protection of Human Subjects

The Department of Health and Human Services (HHS) regulations [45 CFR part 46] apply to research involving human subjects conducted by the HHS or funded in whole or in part by the HHS. The Food and Drug Administration (FDA) regulations [21 CFR parts 50 and 56] apply to research involving products regulated by the FDA. Federal support is not necessary for the FDA regulations to be applicable. When research involving products regulated by the FDA is funded, supported or conducted by FDA and/or HHS, both the HHS and FDA regulations apply.

IRB Regulations

Section Numbers	Description
§ 56.102 (FDA) § 46.102 (HHS)	FDA definitions are included for terms specific to the type of research covered by the FDA regulations (test article, application for research or marketing permit, clinical investigation). A definition for emergency use is provided in the FDA regulations.
§ 56.104 (FDA) § 46.116 (HHS)	FDA provides exemption from the prospective IRB review requirement for "emergency use" of test article in specific situations. HHS regulations state that they are not intended to limit the provision of emergency medical care.
§ 56.105 (FDA) § 46.101 (HHS)	FDA provides for sponsors and sponsor-investigators to request a waiver of IRB review requirements (but not informed consent requirements). HHS exempts certain categories of research and provides for a Secretarial waiver.
§ 56.109 (FDA) § 46.109 (HHS) § 46.117(c) (HHS)	Unlike HHS, FDA does not provide that an IRB may waive the requirement for signed consent when the principal risk is a breach of confidentiality because FDA does not regulate studies which would fall into that category of research. (Both regulations allow for IRB waiver of documentation of informed consent in instances of minimal risk.)

§ 56.110 (FDA) § 46.110 (HHS)	The FDA list of investigations eligible for expedited review (published in the Federal Register) does not include the studies described in category 9 of the HHS list because these types of studies are not regulated by FDA
§ 56.114 (FDA) § 46.114 (HHS)	FDA does not discuss administrative matters dealing with grants and contracts because they are irrelevant to the scope of the Agency's regulation. (Both regulations make allowances for review of multi-institutional studies.)
§ 56.115 (FDA) § 46.115 (HHS)	FDA has neither an assurance mechanism nor files of IRB membership. Therefore, FDA does not require the IRB or institution to report changes in membership whereas HHS does require such notification.
§ 56.115(c) (FDA)	FDA may refuse to consider a study in support of a research or marketing permit if the IRB or the institution refuses to allow FDA to inspect IRB records. HHS has no such provision because it does not issue research or marketing permits.
§§ 56.120-124 (FDA)	FDA regulations provide sanctions for non-compliance with regulations.

Informed Consent Regulations

Section Numbers	**Description**
§ 50.23 (FDA)	FDA, but not HHS, provides for an exception from the informed consent requirements in emergency situations. The provision is based on the Medical Device Amendments of 1976, but may be used in investigations involving drugs, devices, and other FDA regulated products in situations described in § 50.23.
§ 46.116(c)&(d) (HHS)	HHS provides for waiving or altering elements of informed consent under certain conditions. FDA has no such provision because the types of studies which would qualify for such waivers are either not regulated by FDA or are covered by the emergency treatment provisions (§ 50.23).
§ 50.25(a)(5) (FDA) § 46.116(a)(5) (HHS)	FDA explicitly requires that subjects be informed that FDA may inspect the records of the study because FDA may occasionally examine a subject's medical records when they pertain to the study. While HHS has the right to inspect records of studies it funds, it does not impose that same informed consent requirement.

§ 50.27(a) (FDA)   FDA explicitly requires that consent forms be dated as well as signed by the subject or the subject's legally authorized representative. The HHS regulations do not explicitly require consent forms to be dated.

Source: Food and Drug Administration, INFORMATION SHEETS: GUIDANCE FOR INSTITUTIONAL REVIEW BOARDS AND CLINICAL INVESTIGATORS, *Appendix E*, 97-98 (1998), *available at* http://www.fda.gov/oc/ohrt/irbs/default.htm

APPENDIX D

Nuremberg Code

1. The voluntary consent of the human subject is absolutely essential.

   This means that the person involved should have legal capacity to give consent; should be so situated as to be able to exercise free power of choice, without the intervention of any element of force, fraud, deceit, duress, over-reaching, or other ulterior form of constraint or coercion; and should have sufficient knowledge and comprehension of the elements of the subject matter involved as to enable him to make an understanding and enlightened decision. This latter element requires that before the acceptance of an affirmative decision by the experimental subject there should be made known to him the nature, duration, and purpose of the experiment; the method and means by which it is to be conducted; all inconveniences and hazards reasonably to be expected; and the effects upon his health or person which may possibly come from his participation in the experiment.

   The duty and responsibility for ascertaining the quality of the consent rests upon each individual who initiates, directs or engages in the experiment. It is a personal duty and responsibility which may not be delegated to another with impunity.

2. The experiment should be such as to yield fruitful results for the good of society, unprocurable by other methods or means of study, and not random and unnecessary in nature.

3. The experiment should be so designed and based on the results of animal experimentation and a knowledge of the natural history of the disease or other problem under study that the anticipated results will justify the performance of the experiment.

4. The experiment should be so conducted as to avoid all unnecessary physical and mental suffering and injury.

5. No experiment should be conducted where there is an a priori reason to believe that death or disabling injury will occur; except, perhaps, in those experiments where the experimental physicians also serve as subjects.

6. The degree of risk to be taken should never exceed that determined by the humanitarian importance of the problem to be solved by the experiment.

7. Proper preparations should be made and adequate facilities provided to protect the experimental subject against even remote possibilities of injury, disability, or death.

8. The experiment should be conducted only by scientifically qualified persons. The highest degree of skill and care should be required through all stages of the experiment of those who conduct or engage in the experiment.

9. During the course of the experiment the human subject should be at liberty to bring the experiment to an end if he has reached the physical or mental state where continuation of the experiment seems to him to be impossible.

10. During the course of the experiment the scientist in charge must be prepared to terminate the experiment at any stage, if he has probably cause to believe, in the exercise of the good faith, superior skill and careful judgment required of him that a continuation of the experiment is likely to result in injury, disability, or death to the experimental subject.

Source: II TRIALS OF WAR CRIMINALS BEFORE THE NUERNBERG MILITARY TRIBUNALS UNDER CONTROL COUNCIL LAW NO. 10, 181-83 (U.S. Gov't Printing Office 1946-1949)

APPENDIX E

Declaration of Helsinki

A. Introduction

1. The World Medical Association has developed the Declaration of Helsinki as a statement of ethical principles to provide guidance to physicians and other participants in medical research involving human subjects. Medical research involving human subjects includes research on identifiable human material or identifiable data.

2. It is the duty of the physician to promote and safeguard the health of the people. The physician's knowledge and conscience are dedicated to the fulfillment of this duty.

3. The Declaration of Geneva of the World Medical Association binds the physician with the words, "The health of my patient will be my first consideration," and the International Code of Medical Ethics declares that, "A physician shall act only in the patient's interest when providing medical care which might have the effect of weakening the physical and mental condition of the patient."

4. Medical progress is based on research which ultimately must rest in part on experimentation involving human subjects.

5. In medical research on human subjects, considerations related to the well-being of the human subject should take precedence over the interests of science and society.

6. The primary purpose of medical research involving human subjects is to improve prophylactic, diagnostic and therapeutic procedures and the understanding of the aetiology and pathogenesis of disease. Even the best proven prophylactic, diagnostic, and therapeutic methods must continuously be challenged through research for their effectiveness, efficiency, accessibility and quality.

7. In current medical practice and in medical research, most prophylactic, diagnostic and therapeutic procedures involve risks and burdens.

8. Medical research is subject to ethical standards that promote respect for all human beings and protect their health and rights. Some research populations are vulnerable and need special protection. The particular needs of the economically and medically disadvantaged must be recognized. Special attention is also required for those who cannot give or refuse consent for

themselves, for those who may be subject to giving consent under duress, for those who will not benefit personally from the research and for those for whom the research is combined with care.

9. Research Investigators should be aware of the ethical, legal and regulatory requirements for research on human subjects in their own countries as well as applicable international requirements. No national ethical, legal or regulatory requirement should be allowed to reduce or eliminate any of the protections for human subjects set forth in this Declaration.

B. Basic Principles for All Medical Research

10. It is the duty of the physician in medical research to protect the life, health, privacy, and dignity of the human subject.

11. Medical research involving human subjects must conform to generally accepted scientific principles, be based on a thorough knowledge of the scientific literature, other relevant sources of information, and on adequate laboratory and, where appropriate, animal experimentation.

12. Appropriate caution must be exercised in the conduct of research which may affect the environment, and the welfare of animals used for research must be respected.

13. The design and performance of each experimental procedure involving human subjects should be clearly formulated in an experimental protocol. This protocol should be submitted for consideration, comment, guidance, and where appropriate, approval to a specially appointed ethical review committee, which must be independent of the investigator, the sponsor or any other kind of undue influence. This independent committee should be in conformity with the laws and regulations of the country in which the research experiment is performed. The committee has the right to monitor ongoing trials. The researcher has the obligation to provide monitoring information to the committee, especially any serious adverse events. The researcher should also submit to the committee, for review, information regarding funding, sponsors, institutional affiliations, other potential conflicts of interest and incentives for subjects.

14. The research protocol should always contain a statement of the ethical considerations involved and should indicate that there is compliance with the principles enunciated in this Declaration.

15. Medical research involving human subjects should be conducted only by scientifically qualified persons and under the supervision of a clinically competent medical person. The responsibility for the human subject must always rest with a medically qualified person and never rest on the subject of the research, even though the subject has given consent.

16. Every medical research project involving human subjects should be preceded by careful assessment of predictable risks and burdens in comparison

with foreseeable benefits to the subject or to others. This does not preclude the participation of healthy volunteers in medical research. The design of all studies should be publicly available.

17. Physicians should abstain from engaging in research projects involving human subjects unless they are confident that the risks involved have been adequately assessed and can be satisfactorily managed. Physicians should cease any investigation if the risks are found to outweigh the potential benefits or if there is conclusive proof of positive and beneficial results.

18. Medical research involving human subjects should only be conducted if the importance of the objective outweighs the inherent risks and burdens to the subject. This is especially important when the human subjects are healthy volunteers.

19. Medical research is only justified if there is a reasonable likelihood that the populations in which the research is carried out stand to benefit from the results of the research.

20. The subjects must be volunteers and informed participants in the research project.

21. The right of research subjects to safeguard their integrity must always be respected. Every precaution should be taken to respect the privacy of the subject, the confidentiality of the patient's information and to minimize the impact of the study on the subject's physical and mental integrity and on the personality of the subject.

22. In any research on human beings, each potential subject must be adequately informed of the aims, methods, sources of funding, any possible conflicts of interest, institutional affiliations of the researcher, the anticipated benefits and potential risks of the study and the discomfort it may entail. The subject should be informed of the right to abstain from participation in the study or to withdraw consent to participate at any time without reprisal. After ensuring that the subject has understood the information, the physician should then obtain the subject's freely-given informed consent, preferably in writing. If the consent cannot be obtained in writing, the non-written consent must be formally documented and witnessed.

23. When obtaining informed consent for the research project the physician should be particularly cautious if the subject is in a dependent relationship with the physician or may consent under duress. In that case the informed consent should be obtained by a well-informed physician who is not engaged in the investigation and who is completely independent of this relationship.

24. For a research subject who is legally incompetent, physically or mentally incapable of giving consent or is a legally incompetent minor, the investigator must obtain informed consent from the legally authorized representative in accordance with applicable law. These groups should not be

included in research unless the research is necessary to promote the health of the population represented and this research cannot instead be performed on legally competent persons.

25. When a subject deemed legally incompetent, such as a minor child, is able to give assent to decisions about participation in research, the investigator must obtain that assent in addition to the consent of the legally authorized representative.

26. Research on individuals from whom it is not possible to obtain consent, including proxy or advance consent, should be done only if the physical/mental condition that prevents obtaining informed consent is a necessary characteristic of the research population. The specific reasons for involving research subjects with a condition that renders them unable to give informed consent should be stated in the experimental protocol for consideration and approval of the review committee. The protocol should state that consent to remain in the research should be obtained as soon as possible from the individual or a legally authorized surrogate.

27. Both authors and publishers have ethical obligations. In publication of the results of research, the investigators are obliged to preserve the accuracy of the results. Negative as well as positive results should be published or otherwise publicly available. Sources of funding, institutional affiliations and any possible conflicts of interest should be declared in the publication. Reports of experimentation not in accordance with the principles laid down in this Declaration should not be accepted for publication.

C. Additional Principles for Medical Research Combined with Medical Care

28. The physician may combine medical research with medical care, only to the extent that the research is justified by its potential prophylactic, diagnostic or therapeutic value. When medical research is combined with medical care, additional standards apply to protect the patients who are research subjects.

29. The benefits, risks, burdens and effectiveness of a new method should be tested against those of the best current prophylactic, diagnostic, and therapeutic methods. This does not exclude the use of placebo, or no treatment, in studies where no proven prophylactic, diagnostic or therapeutic method exists. (*See note.*)

30. At the conclusion of the study, every patient entered into the study should be assured of access to the best proven prophylactic, diagnostic and therapeutic methods identified by the study. (*See note.*)

31. The physician should fully inform the patient which aspects of the care are related to the research. The refusal of a patient to participate in a study must never interfere with the patient-physician relationship.

32. In the treatment of a patient, where proven prophylactic, diagnostic and therapeutic methods do not exist or have been ineffective, the physician, with informed consent from the patient, must be free to use unproven or new prophylactic, diagnostic and therapeutic measures, if in the physician's judgment it offers hope of saving life, re-establishing health or alleviating suffering. Where possible, these measures should be made the object of research, designed to evaluate their safety and efficacy. In all cases, new information should be recorded and, where appropriate, published. The other relevant guidelines of this Declaration should be followed.

Note: Note of clarification on paragraph 29 of the WMA Declaration of Helsinki

The WMA hereby reaffirms its position that extreme care must be taken in making use of a placebo-controlled trial and that in general this methodology should only be used in the absence of existing proven therapy. However, a placebo-controlled trial may be ethically acceptable, even if proven therapy is available, under the following circumstances:

• Where for compelling and scientifically sound methodological reasons its use is necessary to determine the efficacy or safety of a prophylactic, diagnostic or therapeutic method; or

• Where a prophylactic, diagnostic or therapeutic method is being investigated for a minor condition and the patients who receive placebo will not be subject to any additional risk of serious or irreversible harm.

All other provisions of the Declaration of Helsinki must be adhered to, especially the need for appropriate ethical and scientific review.

Note: Note of clarification on paragraph 30 of the WMA Declaration of Helsinki

The WMA hereby reaffirms its position that it is necessary during the study planning process to identify post-trial access by study participants to prophylactic, diagnostic and therapeutic procedures identified as beneficial in the study or access to other appropriate care. Post-trial access arrangements or other care must be described in the study protocol so the ethical review committee may consider such arrangements during its review.

Source: The Declaration of Helsinki (Document 17.C) is an official policy document of the World Medical Association, the global representative body for physicians. It was first adopted in 1964 (Helsinki, Finland) and revised in 1975 (Tokyo, Japan), 1983 (Venice, Italy), 1989 (Hong Kong), 1996 (Somerset-West, South Africa) and 2000 (Edinburgh, Scotland). Note of clarification on Paragraph 29 added by the WMA General Assembly, Washington 2002. Note of clarification on Paragraph 30 added by the WMA General Assembly, Tokyo 2004.

The Belmont Report
Ethical Principles & Guidelines for Research Involving Human Subjects

Scientific research has produced substantial social benefits. It has also posed some troubling ethical questions. Public attention was drawn to these questions by reported abuses of human subjects in biomedical experiments, especially during the Second World War. During the Nuremberg War Crime Trials, the Nuremberg code was drafted as a set of standards for judging physicians and scientists who had conducted biomedical experiments on concentration camp prisoners. This code became the prototype of many later codes[1] intended to assure that research involving human subjects would be carried out in an ethical manner.

The codes consist of rules, some general, others specific, that guide the investigators or the reviewers of research in their work. Such rules often are inadequate to cover complex situations; at times they come into conflict, and they are frequently difficult to interpret or apply. Broader ethical principles will provide a basis on which specific rules may be formulated, criticized and interpreted.

Three principles, or general prescriptive judgments, that are relevant to research involving human subjects are identified in this statement. Other principles may also be relevant. These three are comprehensive, however, and are stated at a level of generalization that should assist scientists, subjects, reviewers and interested citizens to understand the ethical issues inherent in research involving human subjects. These principles cannot always be applied so as to resolve beyond dispute particular ethical problems. The objective is to provide an analytical framework that will guide the resolution of ethical problems arising from research involving human subjects.

This statement consists of a distinction between research and practice, a discussion of the three basic ethical principles, and remarks about the application of these principles.

---

[1] Since 1945, various codes for the proper and responsible conduct of human experimentation in medical research have been adopted by different organizations. The best known of these codes are the Nuremberg Code of 1947, the Helsinki Declaration of 1964 (revised in 1975), and the 1971 Guidelines (codified into Federal Regulations in 1974) issued by the U.S. Department of Health, Education, and Welfare Codes for the conduct of social and behavioral research have also been adopted, the best known being that of the American Psychological Association, published in 1973.

Part A: Boundaries Between Practice & Research

It is important to distinguish between biomedical and behavioral research, on the one hand, and the practice of accepted therapy on the other, in order to know what activities ought to undergo review for the protection of human subjects of research. The distinction between research and practice is blurred partly because both often occur together (as in research designed to evaluate a therapy) and partly because notable departures from standard practice are often called "experimental" when the terms "experimental" and "research" are not carefully defined.

For the most part, the term "practice" refers to interventions that are designed solely to enhance the well-being of an individual patient or client and that have a reasonable expectation of success. The purpose of medical or behavioral practice is to provide diagnosis, preventive treatment or therapy to particular individuals.[2] By contrast, the term "research' designates an activity designed to test an hypothesis, permit conclusions to be drawn, and thereby to develop or contribute to generalizable knowledge (expressed, for example, in theories, principles, and statements of relationships). Research is usually described in a formal protocol that sets forth an objective and a set of procedures designed to reach that objective.

When a clinician departs in a significant way from standard or accepted practice, the innovation does not, in and of itself, constitute research. The fact that a procedure is "experimental," in the sense of new, untested or different, does not automatically place it in the category of research. Radically new procedures of this description should, however, be made the object of formal research at an early stage in order to determine whether they are safe and effective. Thus, it is the responsibility of medical practice committees, for example, to insist that a major innovation be incorporated into a formal research project.[3]

Research and practice may be carried on together when research is designed to evaluate the safety and efficacy of a therapy. This need not cause any confusion

---

[2] Although practice usually involves interventions designed solely to enhance the well-being of a particular individual, interventions are sometimes applied to one individual for the enhancement of the well-being of another (e.g., blood donation, skin grafts, organ transplants) or an intervention may have the dual purpose of enhancing the well-being of a particular individual, and, at the same time, providing some benefit to others (e.g., vaccination, which protects both the person who is vaccinated and society generally). The fact that some forms of practice have elements other than immediate benefit to the individual receiving an intervention, however, should not confuse the general distinction between research and practice. Even when a procedure applied in practice may benefit some other person, it remains an intervention designed to enhance the well-being of a particular individual or groups of individuals; thus, it is practice and need not be reviewed as research.

[3] Because the problems related to social experimentation may differ substantially from those of biomedical and behavioral research, the Commission specifically declines to make any policy determination regarding such research at this time. Rather, the Commission believes that the problem ought to be addressed by one of its successor bodies.

regarding whether or not the activity requires review; the general rule is that if there is any element of research in an activity, that activity should undergo review for the protection of human subjects.

Part B: Basic Ethical Principles

The expression "basic ethical principles" refers to those general judgments that serve as a basic justification for the many particular ethical prescriptions and evaluations of human actions. Three basic principles, among those generally accepted in our cultural tradition, are particularly relevant to the ethics of research involving human subjects: the principles of respect of persons, beneficence and justice.

1. Respect for Persons. — Respect for persons incorporates at least two ethical convictions: first, that individuals should be treated as autonomous agents, and second, that persons with diminished autonomy are entitled to protection. The principle of respect for persons thus divides into two separate moral requirements: the requirement to acknowledge autonomy and the requirement to protect those with diminished autonomy.

An autonomous person is an individual capable of deliberation about personal goals and of acting under the direction of such deliberation. To respect autonomy is to give weight to autonomous persons' considered opinions and choices while refraining from obstructing their actions unless they are clearly detrimental to others. To show lack of respect for an autonomous agent is to repudiate that person's considered judgments, to deny an individual the freedom to act on those considered judgments, or to withhold information necessary to make a considered judgment, when there are no compelling reasons to do so.

However, not every human being is capable of self-determination. The capacity for self-determination matures during an individual's life, and some individuals lose this capacity wholly or in part because of illness, mental disability, or circumstances that severely restrict liberty. Respect for the immature and the incapacitated may require protecting them as they mature or while they are incapacitated.

Some persons are in need of extensive protection, even to the point of excluding them from activities which may harm them; other persons require little protection beyond making sure they undertake activities freely and with awareness of possible adverse consequence. The extent of protection afforded should depend upon the risk of harm and the likelihood of benefit. The judgment that any individual lacks autonomy should be periodically reevaluated and will vary in different situations.

In most cases of research involving human subjects, respect for persons demands that subjects enter into the research voluntarily and with adequate information. In some situations, however, application of the principle is not obvious. The involvement of prisoners as subjects of research provides an instructive example. On the one hand, it would seem that the principle of respect for persons requires that prisoners not be deprived of the opportunity to volunteer for research. On the other hand, under prison conditions they may be subtly coerced or unduly influenced to engage in research activities for which they would not otherwise volunteer. Respect for persons would then dictate that prisoners be protected. Whether to allow prisoners to "volunteer" or to "protect" them presents a dilemma. Respecting persons, in most hard cases, is often a matter of balancing competing claims urged by the principle of respect itself.

2. Beneficence. — Persons are treated in an ethical manner not only by respecting their decisions and protecting them from harm, but also by making efforts to secure their well-being. Such treatment falls under the principle of beneficence. The term "beneficence" is often understood to cover acts of kindness or charity that go beyond strict obligation. In this document, beneficence is understood in a stronger sense, as an obligation. Two general rules have been formulated as complementary expressions of beneficent actions in this sense: (1) do not harm and (2) maximize possible benefits and minimize possible harms.

The Hippocratic maxim "do no harm" has long been a fundamental principle of medical ethics. Claude Bernard extended it to the realm of research, saying that one should not injure one person regardless of the benefits that might come to others. However, even avoiding harm requires learning what is harmful; and, in the process of obtaining this information, persons may be exposed to risk of harm. Further, the Hippocratic Oath requires physicians to benefit their patients "according to their best judgment." Learning what will in fact benefit may require exposing persons to risk. The problem posed by these imperatives is to decide when it is justifiable to seek certain benefits despite the risks involved, and when the benefits should be foregone because of the risks.

The obligations of beneficence affect both individual investigators and society at large, because they extend both to particular research projects and to the entire enterprise of research. In the case of particular projects, investigators and members of their institutions are obliged to give forethought to the maximization of benefits and the reduction of risk that might occur from the research investigation. In the case of scientific research in general, members of the larger society are obliged to recognize the longer term benefits and risks that may result from the improvement of knowledge and from the development of novel medical, psychotherapeutic, and social procedures.

The principle of beneficence often occupies a well-defined justifying role in many areas of research involving human subjects. An example is found in research involving children. Effective ways of treating childhood diseases and fostering healthy development are benefits that serve to justify research involving children — even when individual research subjects are not direct beneficiaries. Research also makes it possible to avoid the harm that may result from the application of previously accepted routine practices that on closer investigation turn out to be dangerous. But the role of the principle of beneficence is not always so unambiguous. A difficult ethical problem remains, for example, about research that presents more than minimal risk without immediate prospect of direct benefit to the children involved. Some have argued that such research is inadmissible, while others have pointed out that this limit would rule out much research promising great benefit to children in the future. Here again, as with all hard cases, the different claims covered by the principle of beneficence may come into conflict and force difficult choices.

3. Justice. — Who ought to receive the benefits of research and bear its burdens? This is a question of justice, in the sense of "fairness in distribution" or "what is deserved." An injustice occurs when some benefit to which a person is entitled is denied without good reason or when some burden is imposed unduly. Another way of conceiving the principle of justice is that equals ought to be treated equally. However, this statement requires explication. Who is equal and who is unequal? What considerations justify departure from equal distribution? Almost all commentators allow that distinctions based on experience, age, deprivation, competence, merit and position do sometimes constitute criteria justifying differential treatment for certain purposes. It is necessary, then, to explain in what respects people should be treated equally. There are several widely accepted formulations of just ways to distribute burdens and benefits. Each formulation mentions some relevant property on the basis of which burdens and benefits should be distributed. These formulations are (1) to each person an equal share, (2) to each person according to individual need, (3) to each person according to individual effort, (4) to each person according to societal contribution, and (5) to each person according to merit.

Questions of justice have long been associated with social practices such as punishment, taxation and political representation. Until recently these questions have not generally been associated with scientific research. However, they are foreshadowed even in the earliest reflections on the ethics of research involving human subjects. For example, during the 19th and early 20th centuries the burdens of serving as research subjects fell largely upon poor ward patients, while the benefits of improved medical care flowed primarily to private patients. Subsequently, the exploitation of unwilling prisoners as research subjects in Nazi concentration camps was condemned as a particularly flagrant injustice. In this country, in the 1940's, the Tuskegee syphilis study used disadvantaged, rural black men to study the untreated course of a disease that is by no means confined to that population. These subjects were deprived of demonstrably effective treatment in order not to interrupt the project, long after such treatment became generally available.

Against this historical background, it can be seen how conceptions of justice are relevant to research involving human subjects. For example, the selection of research subjects needs to be scrutinized in order to determine whether some classes (e.g., welfare patients, particular racial and ethnic minorities, or persons confined to institutions) are being systematically selected simply because of their easy availability, their compromised position, or their manipulability, rather than for reasons directly related to the problem being studied. Finally, whenever research supported by public funds leads to the development of therapeutic devices and procedures, justice demands both that these not provide advantages only to those who can afford them and that such research should not unduly involve persons from groups unlikely to be among the beneficiaries of subsequent applications of the research.

Part C: Applications

Applications of the general principles to the conduct of research leads to consideration of the following requirements: informed consent, risk/benefit assessment, and the selection of subjects of research.

1. Informed Consent. — Respect for persons requires that subjects, to the degree that they are capable, be given the opportunity to choose what shall or shall not happen to them. This opportunity is provided when adequate standards for informed consent are satisfied.

While the importance of informed consent is unquestioned, controversy prevails over the nature and possibility of an informed consent. Nonetheless, there is widespread agreement that the consent process can be analyzed as containing three elements: information, comprehension and voluntariness.

Information. Most codes of research establish specific items for disclosure intended to assure that subjects are given sufficient information. These items generally include: the research procedure, their purposes, risks and anticipated benefits, alternative procedures (where therapy is involved), and a statement offering the subject the opportunity to ask questions and to withdraw at any time from the research. Additional items have been proposed, including how subjects are selected, the person responsible for the research, etc.

However, a simple listing of items does not answer the question of what the standard should be for judging how much and what sort of information should be provided. One standard frequently invoked in medical practice, namely the information commonly provided by practitioners in the field or in the locale, is inadequate since research takes place precisely when a common understanding does not exist. Another standard, currently popular in malpractice law, requires the practitioner to reveal the information that reasonable persons would wish to know in order to make a decision regarding their care. This, too, seems insufficient since the research subject, being in essence a volunteer, may wish to know considerably more about risks gratuitously undertaken than do patients who deliver themselves into the hand of a clinician for needed care. It may be that a standard of "the reasonable volunteer" should be proposed: the extent and nature of information should be such that persons, knowing that the procedure is neither necessary for their care nor perhaps fully understood, can decide whether they wish to participate in the furthering of knowledge. Even when some direct benefit to them is anticipated, the subjects should understand clearly the range of risk and the voluntary nature of participation.

A special problem of consent arises where informing subjects of some pertinent aspect of the research is likely to impair the validity of the research. In many cases, it is sufficient to indicate to subjects that they are being invited to participate in research of which some features will not be revealed until the research is concluded. In all cases of research involving incomplete disclosure, such research is justified only if it is clear that (1) incomplete disclosure is truly necessary to accomplish the goals of the research, (2) there are no undisclosed risks to subjects that are more than minimal, and (3) there is an adequate plan for debriefing subjects, when appropriate, and for dissemination of research results to them. Information about risks should never be withheld for the purpose of eliciting the cooperation of subjects, and truthful answers should always be given to direct questions about the research. Care should be taken to distinguish cases in which disclosure would destroy or invalidate the research from cases in which disclosure would simply inconvenience the investigator.

Comprehension. The manner and context in which information is conveyed is as important as the information itself. For example, presenting information in a disorganized and rapid fashion, allowing too little time for consideration or curtailing opportunities for questioning, all may adversely affect a subject's ability to make an informed choice.

Because the subject's ability to understand is a function of intelligence, rationality, maturity and language, it is necessary to adapt the presentation of the information to the subject's capacities. Investigators are responsible for ascertaining that the subject has comprehended the information. While there is always an obligation to ascertain that the information about risk to subjects is complete and adequately comprehended, when the risks are more serious, that obligation increases. On occasion, it may be suitable to give some oral or written tests of comprehension.

Special provision may need to be made when comprehension is severely limited — for example, by conditions of immaturity or mental disability. Each class of subjects that one might consider as incompetent (e.g., infants and young children, mentally disable patients, the terminally ill and the comatose) should be considered on its own terms. Even for these persons, however, respect requires giving them the opportunity to choose to the extent they are able, whether or not to participate in research. The objections of these subjects to involvement should be honored, unless the research entails providing them a therapy unavailable elsewhere. Respect for persons also requires seeking the permission of other parties in order to protect the subjects from harm. Such persons are thus respected both by acknowledging their own wishes and by the use of third parties to protect them from harm.

The third parties chosen should be those who are most likely to understand the incompetent subject's situation and to act in that person's best interest. The person authorized to act on behalf of the subject should be given an opportunity to observe the research as it proceeds in order to be able to withdraw the subject from the research, if such action appears in the subject's best interest.

Voluntariness. An agreement to participate in research constitutes a valid consent only if voluntarily given. This element of informed consent requires conditions free of coercion and undue influence. Coercion occurs when an overt threat of harm is intentionally presented by one person to another in order to obtain compliance. Undue influence, by contrast, occurs through an offer of an excessive, unwarranted, inappropriate or improper reward or other overture in order to obtain compliance. Also, inducements that would ordinarily be acceptable may become undue influences if the subject is especially vulnerable.

Unjustifiable pressures usually occur when persons in positions of authority or commanding influence — especially where possible sanctions are involved — urge a course of action for a subject. A continuum of such influencing factors exists, however, and it is impossible to state precisely where justifiable persuasion ends and undue influence begins. But undue influence would include actions such as manipulating a person's choice through the controlling influence of a close relative and threatening to withdraw health services to which an individual would otherwise be entitle.

2. Assessment of Risks and Benefits. — The assessment of risks and benefits requires a careful arrayal of relevant data, including, in some cases, alternative ways of obtaining the benefits sought in the research. Thus, the assessment presents both an opportunity and a responsibility to gather systematic and comprehensive information about proposed research. For the investigator, it is a means to examine whether the proposed research is properly designed. For a review committee, it is a method for determining whether the risks that will be presented to subjects are justified. For prospective subjects, the assessment will assist the determination whether or not to participate.

The Nature and Scope of Risks and Benefits. The requirement that research be justified on the basis of a favorable risk/benefit assessment bears a close relation to the principle of beneficence, just as the moral requirement that informed consent be obtained is derived primarily from the principle of respect for persons. The term "risk" refers to a possibility that harm may occur. However, when expressions such as "small risk" or "high risk" are used, they usually refer (often ambiguously) both to the chance (probability) of experiencing a harm and the severity (magnitude) of the envisioned harm.

The term "benefit" is used in the research context to refer to something of positive value related to health or welfare. Unlike, "risk," "benefit" is not a term that expresses probabilities. Risk is properly contrasted to probability of benefits, and benefits are properly contrasted with harms rather than risks of harm. Accordingly, so-called risk/benefit assessments are concerned with the probabilities and magnitudes of possible harm and anticipated benefits. Many kinds of possible harms and benefits need to be taken into account. There are, for example, risks of psychological harm, physical harm, legal harm, social harm and economic harm and the corresponding benefits. While the most likely types of harms to research subjects are those of psychological or physical pain or injury, other possible kinds should not be overlooked.

Risks and benefits of research may affect the individual subjects, the families of the individual subjects, and society at large (or special groups of subjects in society). Previous codes and Federal regulations have required that risks to subjects be outweighed by the sum of both the anticipated benefit to the subject, if any, and the anticipated benefit to society in the form of knowledge to be gained from the research. In balancing these different elements, the risks and benefits affecting the immediate research subject will normally carry special weight. On the other hand, interests other than those of the subject may on some occasions be sufficient by themselves to justify the risks involved in the research, so long as the subjects' rights have been protected. Beneficence thus requires that we protect against risk of harm to subjects and also that we be concerned about the loss of the substantial benefits that might be gained from research.

The Systematic Assessment of Risks and Benefits. It is commonly said that benefits and risks must be "balanced" and shown to be "in a favorable ratio." The metaphorical character of these terms draws attention to the difficulty of making precise judgments. Only on rare occasions will quantitative techniques be available for the scrutiny of research protocols. However, the idea of systematic, nonarbitrary analysis of risks and benefits should be emulated insofar as possible. This ideal requires those making decisions about the justifiability of research to be thorough in the accumulation and assessment of information about all aspects of the research, and to consider alternatives systematically. This procedure renders the assessment of research more rigorous and precise, while making communication between review board members and investigators less subject to misinterpretation, misinformation and conflicting judgments. Thus, there should first be a determination of the validity of the presuppositions of the research; then the nature, probability and magnitude of risk should be distinguished with as much clarity as possible. The method of ascertaining risks should be explicit, especially where there is no alternative to the use of such vague categories as small or slight risk. It should also be determined whether an investigator's estimates of the probability of harm or benefits are reasonable, as judged by known facts or other available studies.

Finally, assessment of the justifiability of research should reflect at least the following considerations: (i) Brutal or inhumane treatment of human subjects is never morally justified. (ii) Risks should be reduced to those necessary to achieve the research objective. It should be determined whether it is in fact necessary to use human subjects at all. Risk can perhaps never be entirely eliminated, but it can often be reduced by careful attention to alternative procedures. (iii) When research involves significant risk of serious impairment, review committees should be extraordinarily insistent on the justification of the risk (looking usually to the likelihood of benefit to the subject — or, in some rare cases, to the manifest voluntariness of the participation). (iv) When vulnerable populations are involved in research, the appropriateness of involving them should itself be demonstrated. A number of variables go into such judgments, including the nature and degree of risk, the condition of the particular population involved, and the nature and level of the anticipated benefits. (v) Relevant risks and benefits must be thoroughly arrayed in documents and procedures used in the informed consent process.

3. Selection of Subjects. — Just as the principle of respect for persons finds expression in the requirements for consent, and the principle of beneficence in risk/benefit assessment, the principle of justice gives rise to moral require- ments that there be fair procedures and outcomes in the selection of research subjects.

Justice is relevant to the selection of subjects of research at two levels: the social and the individual. Individual justice in the selection of subjects would require that researchers exhibit fairness: thus, they should not offer poten- tially beneficial research only to some patients who are in their favor or select only "undesirable" persons for risky research. Social justice requires that dis- tinction be drawn between classes of subjects that ought, and ought not, to participate in any particular kind of research, based on the ability of members of that class to bear burdens and on the appropriateness of placing further burdens on already burdened persons. Thus, it can be considered a matter of social justice that there is an order of preference in the selection of classes of subjects (e.g., adults before children) and that some classes of potential subjects (e.g., the institutionalized mentally infirm or prisoners) may be involved as research subjects, if at all, only on certain conditions.

Injustice may appear in the selection of subjects, even if individual subjects are selected fairly by investigators and treated fairly in the course of research. Thus injustice arises from social, racial, sexual and cultural biases institution- alized in society. Thus, even if individual researchers are treating their research subjects fairly, and even if IRBs are taking care to assure that subjects are selected fairly within a particular institution, unjust social patterns may nev- ertheless appear in the overall distribution of the burdens and benefits of research. Although individual institutions or investigators may not be able to resolve a problem that is pervasive in their social setting, they can consider dis- tributive justice in selecting research subjects.

Some populations, especially institutionalized ones, are already burdened in many ways by their infirmities and environments. When research is proposed that involves risks and does not include a therapeutic component, other less bur- dened classes of persons should be called upon first to accept these risks of research, except where the research is directly related to the specific condi- tions of the class involved. Also, even though public funds for research may often flow in the same directions as public funds for health care, it seems unfair that populations dependent on public health care constitute a pool of preferred research subjects if more advantaged populations are likely to be the recipients of the benefits.

One special instance of injustice results from the involvement of vulnerable sub- jects. Certain groups, such as racial minorities, the economically disadvantaged, the very sick, and the institutionalized may continually be sought as research subjects, owing to their ready availability in settings where research is conducted. Given their dependent status and their frequently compromised capacity for free consent, they should be protected against the danger of being involved in research solely for administrative convenience, or because they are easy to manipulate as a result of their illness or socioeconomic condition.

Source: Department of Health, Education and Welfare, *Report of the National Commission for the Protection of Human Subjects of Biomedical and Behavioral Research*, 44 Fed. Reg. 23,192 (1979)

Author Index

References are to pages.

A

Addicott, Christian, 127–129
Advisory Committee on Human
  Radiation Experiments, 358–359
Albert Einstein College of Medicine,
  384–386, 405–406
Alvino, Lori A., 137
American Association of Pediatrics,
  536–537, 539
American Medical Association Council on
  Ethical and Judicial Affairs, 303
American Society for Human Genetics,
  715–716
American Society for Reproductive
  Medicine, 683–685
Angell, Marcia, 220–224
Appelbaum, Paul S., 355–357
Association of American Medical
  Colleges, Task Force on Financial
  Conflicts of Interest in Clinical
  Research, 235–236, 238

B

Barnes, Mark, 232–234
Beauchamp, Tom L., 443–445
Beh, Hazel Glenn, 189–193
Bellin, Eran, 115–118
Blackhall, Leslie J., 366
Brennan, Troyen A., 496–499
Brody, Howard, 262–266
Bush, George W., 676–680

C

Campbell, Paulette Walker, 57–58
Centers for Disease Control and
  Prevention, 119–120
Childress, James F., 443–445
Clark, Randall Baldwin, 529–530,
  533–536
Coleman, Carl H., 187–188, 502–508
Committee on Bioethics of the American
  Association of Pediatrics, 536–537,
  539

Comprehensive Working Group on
  Informed Consent in Cancer Clinical
  Trials for the National Cancer
  Institute, 328–334
Congregation for the Doctrine of the
  Faith, 663–664
Crigger, Bette-Jane, 182–185

D

Department of Health and Human
  Services, 196, 227–231, 237–238,
  254–255, 371–375, 381–383, 388–389,
  391–393, 397–399, 412–415, 415–416,
  426–429, 433–435, 449–450, 456–458,
  707–708, 720–721, 723–724
DeRenzo, Evan G., 617–618
Dresser, Rebecca, 90–94, 95–96, 99,
  100–102, 359–361, 417–424, 609–610
Dubler, Nancy, 84–85, 115–118, 348–349,
  351–354, 591–592, 629–630, 648–649

E

Elliott, Carl, 597, 598
Ethics Committee of the American
  Society for Reproductive Medicine,
  683–685

F

FDA Consumer, 161
Finke, Dr., 24
Fisher, Celia B., 346–347
Fleischman, Alan R., 81–83
Florencio, Patrik S., 232–234
Food and Drug Administration, 143,
  154–155, 159–160, 378–380, 395–396,
  415–416, 426–429
Fost, Norman, 304–305
Foster, Morris W., 710–712
Freedman, Benjamin, 257–260

G

Gartside, Peter S., 479–480

George Washington University
    Committee on Human Research
    Institutional Review Board, 314–315
Glantz, Leonard H., 527–529, 551–553
Goldner, Jesse A., 14–15, 51–54, 67–68,
    207–215
Gordon, Bruce G., 250–252, 286–287,
    472–473

H

Hoffman, Sharona, 635–637
Hoffmann, Diane E., 617–618
Holzloehner, Dr., 24
Hoopengardner, Joan L., 559
Horowitz, Joy, 271–275
Human Rights Watch, 632–633

I

Institute of Medicine, National Academy
    of Sciences, 344–346, 349–350,
    522–523

J

Jones, James H., 42–43

K

Katz, Jay, 307–309
King, Nancy M.P., 284–285, 340–342,
    742–745
Klein, Jason E., 81–83
Koski, Greg, 645–646
Kuszler, Patricia C., 69–72, 215–220

L

Lavery, James V., 475–476
Lemmens, Trudo, 266–268
Levine, Robert J., 282–284
Lo, Bernard, 591, 597, 598

M

Martin, Douglas K., 290–292
McHenry, Christine, 479–480
Mello, Michelle M., 496–499
Menikoff, Jerry, 336–339
Merrill, Richard A., 148–149
Meyer, Michael J., 668–671
Miechalowski, Leo, 22–24
Miller, Franklin G., 262–266

Miller, Paul B., 266–268
Moore, Mary Tyler, 662–663
Morreim, E. Haavi, 511–517

N

National Academy of Sciences, 344–346,
    349–350, 524–525
National Bioethics Advisory Commission,
    129–136, 163–167, 279, 280–281,
    292–294, 589, 592–595, 598–600,
    602–605, 610, 614–617, 701–702,
    717–718
National Breast Cancer Coalition,
    481–483
National Cancer Institute, 327–328,
    328–334
National Commission for the Protection
    of Human Subjects of Biomedical and
    Behavioral Research, 54, 109–110,
    289–290, 409–411, 586–588, 612
National Commission on Correctional
    Health Care, 630–631
National Human Research Protections
    Advisory Committee, 239–241
National Institute of Child Health and
    Human Development, 351–354
National Institutes of Health, 87–90,
    430–431, 436–437, 453–454, 665–667
Nelson, Deborah, 363–365
Nelson, Lawrence J., 668–671
New York State Department of Health
    Workgroup on IRB Guidelines, 296,
    387
New York State Task Force on Life and
    the Law, 672–674, 698–700

O

Office for Human Research Protections,
    138–141, 179–180, 465–468, 704
Office for Protection from Research
    Risks, 254–255, 321–323, 381–383,
    388–389, 391–393, 397–399, 412–415,
    433–435, 449–450, 456–458, 707–708,
    720–721, 723–724
Office of Extramural Research, National
    Institutes of Health, 453–454
Office of Inspector General, Department
    of Health and Human Services,
    169–170, 197–201, 371–375

Office of Public Health and Science, Department of Health and Human Services, 227–231, 237–238

P

Peckman, Steven, 171–174, 176–178
Pharmaceutical Research and Manufacturers of America, 61–62
Prentice, Ernest D., 250–252, 286–287, 472–473
President's Commission for the Study of Ethical Problems in Medicine and Biomedical and Behavioral Research, 487–494
President's Council on Bioethics, 686–687, 688–690
Public Health Service, 415–416, 426–429

R

Rascher, Dr., 24
Rettig, Richard A., 79–81
Rockwell, Don A., 275–278
Rose, Gerhard, 25–26
Rotenberg, Marc, 446–447
Rothenberg, Karen H., 368–369
Rothman, David J., 12–13
Rubenstein, Ronald C., 558–559

S

Saint Louis University Institutional Review Board, 476–478
Santelli, John S., 541–542
Saver, Richard S., 318–321
Schonfeld, David J., 545–546, 548–550
Schwartz, Jack, 163–167, 617–618
Scott, Larry D., 203–204
Sharp, Richard R., 710–712
Sidel, Victor, 629–630, 648–649
Silver, Lee M., 690–692
Slovic, Paul, 247–249
Slutsky, Arthur S., 475–476
Solove, Daniel J., 446–447
Stephenson, Joan, 595–596
Stolberg, Sheryl Gay, 97–99
Stone, T. Howard, 125–127
Studdert, David M., 496–499

T

Taylor, Telford, 19–22
Tuskegee Syphilis Study Legacy Committee, 41–42

U

University of Washington, 520–521

V

Veressayev, Vikenty, 9–11
Veterans Administration, Office of Research Oversight, 313–314

W

Weinbaum, Cindy, 631–632, 650
Weiss, Rick, 363–365
Wells, Robert J., 479–480
World Medical Association, 245–246
Wyman, Brian, 651–652

Index

References are to pages.

A

ABORTED FETAL TISSUE
Generally . . . 657
Federal law . . . 657–658; App. A–21
State law . . . 658–661

ACADEMIC HEALTH CENTERS (AHCs)
Bayh-Dole Act . . . 67–69
Biotech companies . . . 76–77
Changing role of . . . 65–73
Conflicts of interest . . . 232-237
Current funding streams . . . 69–73
Federal funding
    Generally . . . 69–70
    Agency for Healthcare Research and Quality (AHRQ) . . . 75
    Centers for Disease Control and Prevention (CDC) . . . 74
    Congressionally Directed Medical Research Programs (CDMRP) . . . 75
    National Institutes of Health . . . 73–74
    NIOSH research . . . 74–75
    Veterans Affairs, Department of . . . 75
Movement of research to private physicians' offices . . . 77–86
Patient "out-of-pocket" payment . . . 72
Pharmaceutical companies . . . 76
Private sponsors . . . 70
Third-party payers . . . 70–72

ADOLESCENTS
Decision-making authority . . . 541–544
Informed consent script . . . 351–354

ADVERSE EVENTS
Reporting . . . 470–475; App. A–6

ADVERTISING AND PROMOTION
(See RECRUITING STUDY SUBJECTS)

AGENCY FOR HEALTHCARE RESEARCH AND QUALITY (AHRQ)
Federal funding . . . 75

AIDS/HIV RESEARCH
Prisoners . . . 629–631; 648–650

AMERICAN MEDICAL EDUCATION
"Revolutionary" developments . . . 8–9

ANCIENT TIMES
Human experimentation . . . 4–6

B

BAYH-DOLE ACT
Generally . . . 67–69

BEECHER ARTICLE
Generally . . . 37–39

BEHAVIORAL RESEARCH
Juvenile inmates . . . 651–653
Milgram experiments . . . 48–50

BELMONT REPORT
Accepted therapy, practice of . . . 109–110
Generally . . . 52-56
Justice in research . . . 409–411
Text of . . . App. F–1 to F–11

BIOMEDICAL ADVANCES
1980s to 1990s . . . 61–63
Academic health centers
    (See ACADEMIC HEALTH CENTERS (AHCs))
Funding research . . . 63–64
    (See also FUNDING RESEARCH)

BIOTECH COMPANIES
Academic health centers . . . 76–77

**BRAINWASHING AND
  INTERROGATION**
U.S. servicemen . . . 48

C

CANCER RESEARCH
Jewish Chronic Disease Hospital
  study . . . 39
Radiation experiments . . . 44-48

**CENTERS FOR DISEASE CONTROL
  AND PREVENTION (CDC)**
Federal funding . . . 74

**CERTIFICATES OF
  CONFIDENTIALITY**
Generally . . . 452–456

CHALLENGE STUDIES
Generally . . . 271

CHILD SUBJECTS
Generally . . . 527–533
Cystic fibrosis in neonates . . . 555–562
Decision-making authority
  Minor's assent
    adolescents . . . 541–544
    soliciting . . . 538–540; App.
      A–29 to A–30
  Parental authority
    generally . . . 533–538
    adolescents . . . 541–544
DHHS review of research not otherwise
  approvable
  Generally . . . 554
  Cystic fibrosis in neonates . . . 555–562
  Regulation, text of . . . App. A–29
  Smallpox vaccination in young
    children . . . 562–567
FDA Modernization Act . . . 531–532
Fenfluramine Study . . . 551–554
Incarcerated children . . . 650–653
Judicial opinion . . . 567–583
Pediatric Rule . . . 531–532
Permissible risk(s)
  Categories . . . 544–545
  Fenfluramine Study . . . 551–554
  Greater than minimal risk and
    no prospect of direct benefit
    . . . 548–551

Greater than minimal risk with
  prospect of direct benefit . . . 547–548
Minimal risk . . . 545–547
Smallpox vaccination in young children
  . . . 562–567

CLINICAL EQUIPOISE
Concept of . . . 256–262
Placebo controls and . . . 262–270

CLINICAL INNOVATION
Research *versus* . . . 109–115

CLONING
Generally . . . 686
Federal law . . . 693–695
State law . . . 695–696
Views on . . . 688–693
What is . . . 686–687

COMMON RULE
Generally . . . 106–107
Clinical innovation, research *versus*
  . . . 109–115
Coverage . . . 107; App. A–1
Enforcement authority (See OFFICE
  FOR HUMAN RESEARCH
  PROTECTIONS (OHRP))
Exempt research . . . 123–125; App. A–1
  to A–2
"Human subject," defined . . . 121–123
Public health initiatives, research *versus*
  . . . 119–121
Quality improvement, research *versus*
  . . . 115–118
"Research," defined . . . 107–121
Research protocol . . . 108–109

CONFIDENTIALITY
AMA Canon 5.05 . . . 443
Autonomy arguments . . . 445
Certificates of confidentiality . . . 452–456
Consequentialist arguments . . . 444–445
Ethical principle, as . . . 443–445
Fidelity-based arguments . . . 445
Freedom of Information Act . . . 451–452
Genetics research . . . 720–722
HIPPA privacy regulations
  Generally . . . 447–448
  Medical records . . . 459–464

Hippocratic oath . . . 443
IRB Guidebook . . . 449–450
Medical records
    HIPPA privacy regulations
      . . . 459–464
    IRB guidelines . . . 456–459
Privacy rights arguments . . . 445
Research data
    Generally . . . 448–452
    Certificates of confidentiality
      . . . 452–456
    Federal regulation . . . 444
    IRB Guidebook . . . 449–450
State laws . . . 446–447

CONFLICTS OF INTEREST
Academic institutions . . . 232–237
Disclosure to subjects . . . 239–242
Institutional review boards . . . 237–239
Investigators (See INVESTIGATORS)

**CONGRESSIONALLY DIRECTED
    MEDICAL RESEARCH
    PROGRAMS (CDMRP)**
Federal funding . . . 75

CONSENT (See INFORMED
    CONSENT)

**CONTRACT RESEARCH
    ORGANIZATIONS**
Rise of . . . 79–86

CRITICAL CARE RESEARCH
Informed consent . . . 318–321

CYSTIC FIBROSIS
Neonates research . . . 555–562

D

DATA-SAFETY MONITORING
Boards . . . 475–485
Guidelines . . . 476–478
Letrozole clinical trial . . . 481–485
When interim data restricted to
    independent DMCs . . . 479–481

**DECISIONALLY IMPAIRED
    PERSONS**
Beneficence, principle of . . . 586–587

Constitutional considerations
    . . . 621–628
Decision making
    Capacity (See subhead: Decision-
      making capacity)
    Surrogates, by . . . 601–609
Decision-making capacity
    Assessing . . . 591; 598–601
    Defining . . . 591–598
    Persistent decisional impairments
      . . . 593–595
Guardianship . . . 601
Health care proxy statutes . . . 601–605
Informed consent
    Capacity to consent . . . 591–592
    Research living wills . . . 609–611
    Schizophrenia research . . . 595–596
    Subject's "assent" . . . 612
    Subject's refusal . . . 612–613
    Surrogate decision making
      . . . 601–609
Justice in research . . . 587–588
Living wills . . . 609–611
Permissible risks . . . 613–620
Prisoners . . . 632–635
Schizophrenia research . . . 595–596
Surrogate decision making . . . 601–609

**DEPARTMENT OF HEALTH AND
    HUMAN SERVICES (DHHS)**
Generally . . . 105
Accreditation . . . 202–205
Child subjects (See CHILD SUBJECTS)
Common Rule (See COMMON RULE)
Expedited reviews . . . 195–197; App. A–9
    to A–10
"Full" reviews . . . 179–195; App. A–8
    to A–9
IRB oversight . . . 170
"Local" character of review . . . 173–175
Membership
    Generally . . . 175–177
    Regulation covering . . . App. A–7
    to A–8
OHRP (See OFFICE FOR HUMAN
    RESEARCH PROTECTIONS (OHRP))
Origins and purpose . . . 171–173
Proprietary and independent boards
    . . . 197–202
Reforms needed . . . 189–195

Regulations
    Common Rule (See COMMON RULE)
    Vulnerable populations (See
        VULNERABLE POPULATIONS)
Review process
    Generally . . . 179
    Expedited reviews . . . 195–197;
        App. A–9 to A–10
    "Full" reviews . . . 179–195; App. A–8
        to A–9
Risk assessment process . . . 187–189
Vulnerable populations (See
    VULNERABLE POPULATIONS)

DEVICE APPROVAL
FDA process . . . 157–160

DHHS (See DEPARTMENT OF
    HEALTH AND HUMAN SERVICES
    (DHHS))

**DIETHYLSTILBESTROL (DES)
    RESEARCH**
Generally . . . 36

DISCLOSURE
Confidentiality (See
    CONFIDENTIALITY)
Conflicts of interest . . . 239–242
Freedom of Information Act . . . 451–452
HIPPA privacy regulations
    Generally . . . 447–448
    Medical records . . . 459–464
Informed consent (See INFORMED
    CONSENT)
Medical records
    HIPPA privacy regulations
        . . . 459–464
    IRB guidelines . . . 456–459

DNA RESEARCH (See GENETICS
    RESEARCH)

DRUG APPROVAL
FDA process . . . 144–157

DUKE MEDICAL CENTER
Suspension of research . . . 57–59

E

**EDUCATIONALLY
    DISADVANTAGED**
Vulnerable populations . . . 125–127

**EMBRYO AND EMBRYONIC STEM
    CELL RESEARCH**
Generally . . . 661–662
Consent to research . . . 683–686
Federal law and policy
    Embryonic stem cell research
        . . . 676–681
    Embryo research . . . 672–675
Juvenile diabetes . . . 662–663
Pluralistic approach . . . 666–667
Single criterion views . . . 665–666
State law and policy . . . 681–682
Vatican II . . . 663–665
Views on . . . 662–672

EMPLOYEES
Soliciting for studies . . . 391–394

ETHNIC MINORITIES
Justice in research . . . 433–442

EUROPEAN MEDICINE
Historical antecedents . . . 6–7

EXEMPT RESEARCH
Common Rule . . . 123–125; App. A–1
    to A–2
Genetics research . . . 706–707

EXPEDITED REVIEW
Generally . . . 195–197

F

FEDERAL OVERSIGHT
1960s to 1990s . . . 51–56
1996 to 2003 . . . 57–61
Aborted fetal tissue . . . 657–658
CFR, Title 45, Part 46 . . . App. A–1
    to A–31
Cloning . . . 693–695
DHHS (See DEPARTMENT OF HEALTH
    AND HUMAN SERVICES (DHHS))
Embryonic stem cell research
    . . . 676–681

Embryo research . . . 672–675
FDA (See FOOD AND DRUG
     ADMINISTRATION (FDA))
Informed consent (See INFORMED
     CONSENT, subhead: Research, to)
IRB jurisdiction and . . . 53–54
Legal structure . . . 105–106
"Minimal risk" research . . . 280–281
OHRP (See OFFICE FOR HUMAN
     RESEARCH PROTECTIONS (OHRP))
Prison research . . . 642–647
Research *not* subject to . . . 161–163

FENFLURAMINE STUDIES
Child subjects . . . 551–554

FETAL RESEARCH
Generally . . . 655
Aborted fetal tissue
     Generally . . . 657
     Federal law . . . 657–658; App. A–21
     State law . . . 658–661
Fetuses *in utero* . . . 655–657; App. A–19
     to A–20

**FOOD AND DRUG
     ADMINISTRATION (FDA)**
Generally . . . 142
Device approval process . . . 157–160
Drug approval process . . . 144–157
Human subject protections . . . 143–144;
     Appx. C
Office for Good Clinical Practice
     . . . 160–161
Paying subjects, guidance for . . . 395–396
Recruiting subjects, guidance for
     . . . 378–381
Regulations
     Generally . . . 142
     Device approval process . . . 157–160
     Drug approval process . . . 144–157
     Human subject protections . . .
     143–144; App. C–1 to C–3

**FREEDOM OF INFORMATION ACT
     (FOIA)**
Research data . . . 451–452

FUNDING RESEARCH
1900 to 1940, in the U.S. . . . 32–34

Biomedical advances . . . 63–64
NIH priorities . . . 87–99

G
GELSINGER, JESSE
Death in study at University of
     Pennsylvania . . . 363–365, 496–497,
     500, 741, 743–744

GENDER-BASED BARRIERS (See
     WOMEN)

GENETICS RESEARCH
Generally . . . 697–698
Biological materials, sources of
     . . . 701–702
Confidentiality . . . 720–722
DNA diagnostic studies . . . 697
DNA stability . . . 698–699
Exempt research . . . 706–707
Familial nature of genetic information
     . . . 699–700
Gene expression studies . . . 697
Genetic sequencing studies . . . 697
Gene transfer research . . . 741–746
Informed consent
     Existing tissue samples . . . 717–720
     New tissue samples . . . 715–717
Informing subjects of study results
     . . . 723–729
IRB review
     Eligibility for expedited review . . . 714
     Exempt research . . . 706–707
     "Human subject," defined . . . 703–706
Limited sample requirement . . . 699
Misuse and misunderstanding of genetics
     . . . 700
Pedigree studies . . . 697
Personal nature of genetic information
     . . . 699
Precision of genetic information . . . 699
Predictive power of genetic information
     . . . 698
Profits from research, sharing of
     . . . 729–741
Proteomics research . . . 697
Risks to others . . . 709–713
Risks to subjects . . . 707–709

GENTAMICIN
Innovative treatment . . . 110–115

GUARDIANSHIP
Decisionally impaired persons . . . 601

H

HEALTH CARE PROXY STATUTES
Decisionally impaired persons
. . . 601–605

HELSINKI, DECLARATION OF
Risk-benefit assessment . . . 245–246
Text of . . . App. E–1 to E–6

HEPATITIS RESEARCH
Incarcerated children . . . 650–653
Prisoners . . . 631–632
Willowbrook study . . . 39–41

HIPAA PRIVACY REGULATIONS
Generally . . . 447–448
Medical records . . . 459–464

HIPPOCRATIC OATH
Confidentiality . . . 443

HIPPOCRATICS
Human experimentation . . . 4–5

HISTORICAL ANTECEDENTS
Generally . . . 3
Ancient activity . . . 4–6
Beecher article . . . 37–39
Diethylstilbestrol (DES) research . . . 36
European medicine . . . 6–7
Jewish Chronic Disease Hospital study
. . . 39
Mid-twentieth century, through . . . 6–13
Milgram experiments . . . 48–50
Nazi Germany (See NUREMBERG
TRIAL(S))
Prison research . . . 635–642
Rabies . . . 12–13
Radiation experiments . . . 44–47
Sexually transmitted disease
experiments . . . 9-12
Statistics in research . . . 7–8
Thalidomide research . . . 35–36
Tuskegee syphilis study . . . 41–44

United States
Judicial reaction to experimentation
. . . 14–16
1900 to early 1970s
Beecher article . . . 37–39
Diethylstilbestrol (DES) research
. . . 36
funding research, through World
War II . . . 32–34
Jewish Chronic Disease Hospital
study . . . 39
Milgram experiments . . . 48–50
post-World War I activities
. . . 31–32
public's developing role . . . 34–35
radiation experiments . . . 44–48
Thalidomide research . . . 35–36
Tuskegee syphilis study . . . 41–44
Willowbrook study . . . 39–41
"Revolutionary" developments . . . 8–9
Willowbrook study . . . 39–41
Yellow fever . . . 12–13

HUMAN GENOME PROJECT
Generally . . . 697–698
Genetics research (See GENETICS
RESEARCH)

"HUMAN SUBJECT," DEFINED
Common Rule . . . 121–123
Genetic testing research . . . 703–706
Regulation, text of . . . App. A–4 to A–5

**HUTCHINSON (FRED) CANCER
RESEARCH CENTER**
Lawsuit against . . . 225, 497

I

INCARCERATED SUBJECTS
Children . . . 650–653
Prisoners (See PRISONERS)

INCOMPETENTS
Children (See CHILD SUBJECTS)
Mental (See DECISIONALLY IMPAIRED
PERSONS)

INFORMED CONSENT
Generally . . . 297
Adolescent trials, script for . . . 351–354

Boilerplate "benefit" statements
... 340–343
Children (See CHILD SUBJECTS,
    subhead: Decision-making authority)
Concept ... 345–346
Cultural barriers ... 366–367
Decisionally impaired persons (See
    DECISIONALLY IMPAIRED
    PERSONS)
Embryo and embryonic stem cell
    research ... 683–686
Emergency research waivers
    ... 304–306; 318–327
Failure to convey information
    ... 363–365
Form(s)
    Generally ... 327–343
    Role of ... 349–350
Gender-based barriers ... 368–369
Genetics research
    Existing tissue samples ... 717–720
    New tissue samples ... 715–717
Goodness-of-fit ethic ... 346–347
Injury compensation (See INJURY
    COMPENSATION, subhead: Consent)
Innovative treatment, to ... 304–306
Investigational treatments off-study
    ... 336–339
Medical care, to
    AMA guidelines ... 303–304
    Case law ... 298–303
Nuremberg Code ... 311–312
Process, as ... 344–351
Process deficiencies
    Failure to convey information
        ... 363–365
    Therapeutic misconception
        ... 355–363
"Prospective" genetics studies
    ... 715–717
Research, to ... 307–312
    Boilerplate "benefit" statements
        ... 340–343
    Consent as a process ... 344–351
    Consent form(s)
        generally ... 327–343
        role of ... 349–350
    Consent script ... 351–354
    Federal regulations
        generally ... 312–313
    emergency research waivers
        ... 318–327
    general waivers ... 313–318
    implementing ... 327–354
    text of ... App. A–12 to A–15
    Role of ... 349–350
"Retrospective" genetics studies
    ... 717–720
Schizophrenia research ... 595–596
Script for ... 351–354
Therapeutic misconception ... 355–363

INJURY COMPENSATION
Generally ... 487
Consent
    Fairness versus ... 491–494
    Requirements ... 495
    (See also INFORMED CONSENT)
    Tort issues ... 510–518
Ethical considerations ... 487–494
Fairness argument ... 488–489
Gift-of-security argument ... 489–491
No-fault compensation
    Generally ... 519–520
    Comprehensive compensation system
        proposals ... 522–524
    Voluntary compensation schemes
        ... 520–522
Researchers' duties to subjects
    ... 502–510
Tort litigation
    Generally ... 495
    Duties to subjects ... 502–510
    Emerging role of ... 496-502
    Informed consent cases ... 510–518

INNOVATIVE TREATMENT
Gentamicin ... 110–115
Informed consent ... 304–306

INSTITUTIONAL CONFLICTS
Financial interests ... 232–237

**INSTITUTIONAL REVIEW BOARDS
    (IRBs)**
Approval of research ... 412–415
Confidentiality guidelines
    Medical records ... 456–459
    Research data ... 449–450
Conflicts of interest ... 237–239

DHHS oversight . . . 170
Federal oversight
    DHHS oversight . . . 170
    Jurisdiction and . . . 53–54
Genetics research review (See
    GENETICS RESEARCH)
Location . . . 170
OHRP oversight . . . 170
Ongoing research, review . . . 465–470
Organization . . . 170
Responsibilities . . . 169–170

INVESTIGATIONAL DEVICES
IDE regulations . . . 159–160

INVESTIGATIONAL TREATMENTS
OFF-STUDY
Informed consent . . . 336–339

INVESTIGATIONAL USE OF
MARKETED DRUGS
Biologics and medical devices . . . 155

INVESTIGATORS
Clinical research in the office setting
    . . . 77–86
Conflicts of interest
    Generally . . . 207–208
    Academic research environment
        . . . 213–215
    Curing conflicts . . . 215–220
    Finder's fees . . . 211
    Gifts from industry sponsors
        . . . 211–212
    Institutional policies . . . 218–220
    Laws and regulations . . . 216–218
    NIH conference testimony . . . 220–227
    OPHS guidelines . . . 227–231
    Per capita payments . . . 210–211
    Primary, secondary, and non-financial
        . . . 208–210
    Redressing conflicts . . . 220
    Stock ownership and similar interests
        . . . 212–213

IRBs (See INSTITUTIONAL REVIEW
    BOARDS (IRBS))

J
JEWISH CHRONIC DISEASE
HOSPITAL STUDY
Cancer research . . . 39

JOHNS HOPKINS MEDICAL
SCHOOL
Suspension of research . . . 59, 182-186

JUSTICE IN RESEARCH
Decisionally impaired persons
    . . . 587-588
Generally . . . 409–415
Belmont Report . . . 409–411
IRB approval of research . . . 412–415
Racial and ethnic minorities . . . 433–442
Women
    Pre-1993 federal policy . . . 415–425
    FDA policy revisions . . . 426–429;
        432–433
    NIH policy revisions . . . 430–432

JUVENILE DIABETES
Embryo and embryonic stem cell
    research . . . 662–663

K
KANT, IMMANUEL
"Categorical imperative" . . . 6

L
LEGISLATIVE ADVOCACY
Priorities in research . . . 96–99

LETROZOLE CLINICAL TRIAL
Halting of . . . 481–485

LIVING WILLS
Decisionally impaired persons . . .
    609–611

LSD EXPERIMENTS
U.S. servicemen . . . 46–48

M
MIDDLE AGES
Medical care . . . 5–6

MILGRAM EXPERIMENTS
Generally . . . 48–50

"MINIMAL RISK" RESEARCH
Child subjects . . . 545–547
Federal regulations, under . . . 280–281

MINORITIES
Justice in research . . . 433–442

N

NATIONAL INSTITUTES OF HEALTH
Biomedical advances . . . 62–63
Federal funding
    Generally . . . 73–74
    Priorities, setting . . . 87–94
Gender-based barriers, policy revisions
    . . . 430–432
Investigator—conflicts of interest
    . . . 220–227
Research priorities, setting . . . 87–99

NATIONAL RESEARCH ACT OF 1974
Generally . . . 52–53

NAZI GERMANY (See NUREMBERG TRIAL(S))

"NEW DRUG" APPROVAL
FDA process . . . 144–157

NO-FAULT INJURY COMPENSATION
Generally . . . 519–521
Comprehensive compensation system
    proposals . . . 522–524
Voluntary compensation schemes
    . . . 522–524

NUREMBERG CODE
Informed consent . . . 311–312
Risk-benefit assessment . . . 245
Text of . . . App. D–1 to D–2

NUREMBERG TRIAL(S)
Generally . . . 16–17
Defendants' final statements . . . 25–26
Documentary evidence . . . 24
Indictment . . . 17–19

Judgment excerpts . . . 26–31
Opening statement . . . 19–22
Testimonial evidence . . . 22–24

O

OFFICE FOR HUMAN RESEARCH PROTECTIONS (OHRP)
Generally . . . 105
Compliance oversight procedures
    Memorandum . . . 138–141
    Regulation, text of . . . App. A–5 to A–7
Enforcement authority
    Generally . . . 136–138
    Compliance oversight procedures,
        memorandum . . . 138–141
    Regulation covering . . . App. A–5
        to A–7
IRB oversight . . . 170
Paying subjects, guidance for . . . 397–402
Recruiting subjects, guidance for
    . . . 381–384

"OFF-LABEL" USE OF MARKETED DRUGS
Biologics and medical devices
    . . . 154–157

OHRP (See OFFICE FOR HUMAN RESEARCH PROTECTIONS (OHRP))

ONGOING RESEARCH
Generally . . . 465
Adverse event reporting . . . 470–475;
    App. A–6
Data-safety monitoring
    Boards . . . 475–485
    Guidelines . . . 476–478
    Letrozole clinical trial . . . 481–485
    When interim data restricted to
        independent DMCs . . . 479–481
IRB continuing review . . . 465–470

P

PAYING STUDY SUBJECTS
Generally . . . 395
Agency guidance . . . 395–402
Amount of payment . . . 402–405
FDA guidance . . . 395–396
OHRP guidance . . . 397–402
Structuring payments . . . 405–407

PEDIATRIC RULE
Generally . . . 531–532

PEDIGREE STUDIES
Genetics research . . . 697

PHARMACEUTICAL COMPANIES
Academic health centers, as . . . 76

PHYSICAL RISKS
Study subjects . . . 250–251

PLACEBO CONTROLS
Clinical equipoise . . . 262–270

POOR PERSONS
Vulnerable populations . . . 125–127

PRIORITIES IN RESEARCH
Generally . . . 86–87
Advocacy, role of
    Generally . . . 95–96
    Conduct of research, manner of
        . . . 100–103
    Legislative advocacy . . . 96–99
Legislative advocacy . . . 96–99
NIH priorities, setting . . . 87–99

PRISONERS
Access *versus* protection . . . 647–650
AIDS/HIV research . . . 629–631; 648–650
Child subjects . . . 650–653
Federal regulation
    Generally . . . 642–645
    Interpretation questions . . . 645–647
    Text of . . . App. A–23 to A–26
Health care/status in prisons . . . 629–635
Hepatitis research . . . 631–632
History of medical research . . . 635–642

PRIVACY
Confidentiality (See
    CONFIDENTIALITY)
HIPAA privacy regulations
    Generally . . . 447–448
    Medical records . . . 459–464

PRIVATE PRACTICING PHYSICIAN-
    INVESTIGATORS (See
    INVESTIGATORS)

PROTEOMICS RESEARCH
Generally . . . 697

PSYCHOLOGICAL RISKS
Study subjects . . . 251

PUBLIC HEALTH INITIATIVES
Research *versus* . . . 119–121

Q

QUALITY IMPROVEMENT
Research *versus* . . . 115–118

R

RABIES
Early experiments . . . 12–13

RACIAL MINORITIES
Inclusion in research . . . 430–442

RADIATION EXPERIMENTS
Cancer research . . . 48
United States, 1944-1974 . . . 44–48

RECRUITING STUDY SUBJECTS
Generally . . . 371–377
Additional patient bases, seeking
    . . . 373–374
Advertising and promotion
    Generally . . . 374–375, 378–380
    AECOM policy . . . 384–386
Agency guidance . . . 378–384
Employees of researchers, soliciting
    . . . 393
FDA guidance . . . 378–381
Incentives, offering . . . 371–372
Institutional policies . . . 384–386
Normal, healthy subjects . . . 386–391
OHRP guidance . . . 381–384
Patients, targeting own . . . 372–373
Students, soliciting . . . 391–394

REGULATION
Federal (See FEDERAL OVERSIGHT)
State (See STATE LAWS)

RESEARCH DATA (See
    CONFIDENTIALITY)

"RESEARCH," DEFINED
Common Rule . . . 107–121

RESEARCH FUNDING (See
FUNDING RESEARCH)

RESEARCH PRIORITIES (See
PRIORITIES IN RESEARCH)

RESEARCH PROTOCOL
Common Rule . . . 108–109

RISK-BENEFIT ASSESSMENT
Balancing risks and benefits . . . 289–295
Helsinki, Declaration of . . . 245–246
IRB expedited review, eligibility for
. . . 715
Knowledge as a benefit . . . 286–289
Nuremberg Code . . . 245
Potential benefits . . . 282–286
Role of . . . 245–247

RISK(S)
Generally . . . 245
Assessment (See RISK-BENEFIT
ASSESSMENT)
Child subjects (See CHILD SUBJECTS,
subhead: Permissible risk(s))
Concept of . . . 247–249
Decisionally impaired subjects
. . . 613-620
Interventions . . . 254–256
"Minimal risk" research
Generally . . . 280–281
Child subjects . . . 545–547
Minimizing . . . 295–296
Others, to . . . 279
Genetics research . . . 709–713
Subjects, to (See RISKS TO RESEARCH
SUBJECTS)

RISKS TO RESEARCH SUBJECTS
Challenge studies . . . 271
Clinical equipoise
Concept of . . . 256–262
Placebo controls and . . . 262–270
Economic risks . . . 252
Genetics research . . . 707–709
Legal risks . . . 252
Physical risks . . . 250–251

Psychological risks . . . 251
Risks of interventions, distinguishing
. . . 254–256
Social risks . . . 251–252
Types of . . . 250–254
Washouts . . . 271–278

ROCHE, ELLEN
Death in study at John Hopkins
. . . 182–186

S

SCHIZOPHRENIA RESEARCH
Informed consent . . . 595–596

**SEXUALLY TRANSMITTED
DISEASES**
Early experiments . . . 9–12
Tuskegee Syphilis Study . . . 41–44

SMALLPOX
Human experimentation . . . 6

SMALLPOX VACCINATION
Young children . . . 562–567

SOCIAL RISKS
Study subjects . . . 251–252

SOCIAL SCIENCE RESEARCH
Milgram experiments . . . 48–50

**SR/NSR
(SIGNIFICANT/NONSIGNIFICANT
RISK) DEVICES**
IDE regulations . . . 160

STATE LAWS
Generally . . . 163–168
Aborted fetal tissue . . . 658–661
Cloning . . . 695–696
Confidentiality . . . 446–447
Embryo and embryonic stem cell
research . . . 681–682

STATISTICS IN RESEARCH
Historical antecedents . . . 7

STEM CELL RESEARCH (See
EMBRYO AND EMBRYONIC STEM
CELL RESEARCH)

STUDENTS
Soliciting for studies . . . 391–394

SURROGATE DECISION MAKING
Decisionally impaired persons
. . . 601–609

SYPHILIS (See SEXUALLY
TRANSMITTED DISEASES)

T

TERMINALLY ILL PATIENTS
Vulnerable populations . . . 127–129

THALIDOMIDE RESEARCH
Generally . . . 35–36

THERAPEUTIC MISCONCEPTION
Informed consent . . . 355–363

TORT LITIGATION (See INJURY
COMPENSATION)

TUSKEGEE STUDY
Syphilis research . . . 41–44

U

UNIVERSITIES
Conflicts of interest . . . 232–237

V

**VETERANS AFFAIRS,
DEPARTMENT OF**
Federal funding . . . 75

VULNERABLE POPULATIONS
Generally . . . 125–127
Aligning protections with vulnerabilities
. . . 134–136
Cognitive or communicative vulnerability
. . . 131
Deferential vulnerability . . . 132–133
DHHS regulations
Generally . . . 125–127; 129–131
Text of . . . App. A–10

Economic vulnerability . . . 134
Institutional vulnerability . . . 131–132
Medical vulnerability . . . 133
Social vulnerability . . . 134
Terminally ill patients . . . 127–129

W

WASHOUTS
Generally . . . 271–278

WILLOWBROOK STUDY
Hepatitis treatment . . . 39–41

WOMEN
Informed consent barriers . . . 368–369
Justice in research
Exclusion of women . . . 415–425
Inclusion of women . . . 426–429;
430–433

Y

YELLOW FEVER
Early experiments . . . 12–13

Table of Cases

A

Abigail Alliance v. McClellan,
No. 03-1601 (RMU) (D.D.C. Aug. 30,
2004), 147

Ancheff v. Hartford Hosp., 799 A.2d 1067
(Conn. 2002), 110–112

Ande v. Rock, 647 N.W.2d 265
(2002), 725–728

Association of Am. Physicians &
Surgeons v. FDA, 226 F. Supp. 2d 204
(D.D.C. 2002), 532

A.Z. v. B.Z., 725 N.E.2d 1051 (Mass.
2000), 686

B

Bailey v. Lally, 481 F. Supp. 203 (D. Md.
1979), 637–641, 643

C

Canterbury v. Spence, 464 F.2d 772 (D.C.
Cir. 1972), 299–301, 507

Carey v. Population Serv. Int'l, 431 U.S.
678 (1977), 543

Carpenter v. Blake, 14

Central Intelligence Agency v. Sims, 471
U.S. 159 (1985), 48

Cincinnati Radiation Litig., In re, 874 F.
Supp. 796 (S.D. Ohio 1995), 48

D

Dahl v. HEM Pharm. Corp., 485

Diaz v. Hillsborough County Hosp. Auth.,
2000 U.S. Dist. LEXIS 14061 (M.D.
Fla. 2000), 367

Diaz v. Tampa Gen. Hosp., 514

Doe v. Illinois Masonic Med. Ctr., 696
N.E.2d 707 (Ill. Ct. App. 1st Dist.
1998), 452

Doe v. Mills (Mich. App. 1995), 446

Doe v. Rumsfeld, 2004 U.S. Dist. LEXIS
21668 (2004), 30

E

Eli Lilly & Co. v. Commissioner, 84 T.C.
996 91985), aff'd in part and rev'd
in part, 856 F.2d 855 (7th Cir.
1988), 150–153

Estelle v. Gamble, 429 U.S. 97 (1976),
633, 640

Estrada v. Jacques, 321 S.E.2d 240 (N.C.
Ct. App. 1984), 113, 306

F

Forbes v. Napolitano, 236 F.3d 1009 (9th
Cir. 2000), 658–660, 682

Fortner v. Koch, 14

G

Gaston v. Hunter, 588 P.2d 326 (Ariz. Ct.
App. 1978), 508

Gault, In re, 387 U.S. 1 (1967), 542

Gelsinger v. University of Pa. Hosp., 496

Greenberg v. Miami Children's Hosp.
Research Inst., 265 F. Supp. 2d 1064
(2003), 736–738

Grimes v. Kennedy-Krieger Inst., 782
A.2d 807 (Md. 2001), 498, 509, 513,
567–578, 730

H

Hartke v. McKelway, 707 F.2d 1544
(D.D.C. 1983), 302

Heinrich v. Sweet, 512

I

In re, see party name

International Union, United Auto.,
Aerospace & Agric. Implement
Workers of Am. v. Johnson Controls,
499 U.S. 187 (1991), 425

J

Jane L. v. Bangerter, 61 F.3d 1493 (10th
Cir. 1995), 661

J.B. v. M.B., 783 A.2d 707 (N.J.
2001), 686

K

Ketchup v. Howard, 543 S.E.2d 371 (Ga. Ct. App. 2000), 302

Kirk v. Michael Reese Hosp., 513 N.E.2d 387 (Ill. 1987), 510

Kus v. Sherman Hosp., 268 Ill. App. 3d 771 (2d Dist. 1995), 518

L

Lifchez v. Hartigan, 735 F. Supp. 1361 (N.D. Ill.), aff'd, 914 F.2d 260 (7th Cir. 1990), 661, 682

M

Mapp v. Ohio, 38

Margaret S. v. Edwards, 794 F.2d 994 (5th Cir. 1986), 661

Marriage of Arthur Lee Witten, III & Tamera Jean Witten, In re the, 672 N.W.2d 768 (Iowa 2003), 686

Medtronic, Inc. v. Lohr, 518 U.S. 470 (1996), 157–159

Mele v. Sherman Hosp., 838 F.2d 923 (7th Cir. 1988), 518

Mink v. University of Chicago, 460 F. Supp. 713 (N.D. Ill. 1978), 518

Moore v. Regents of the Univ. of Cal., 793 P.2d 479 (Cal. 1990), 241, 729–735

P

Parham v. J.R., 442 U.S. 584 (1979), 585

Pate v. Threlkel, 661 So. 2d 278 (Fla. 1995), 723

Payette v. Rockefeller Univ., 643 N.Y.S.2d 79 (N.Y. App. Div. 1996), 391

Planned Parenthood v. Casey, 505 U.S. 833 (1992), 656, 661, 667

R

Rivers v. Katz, 623

Robertson v. Oklahoma, 497

Roe v. Wade, 410 U.S. 113 (1973), 655, 660, 661, 667

Rutherford, United States v., 442 U.S. 544 (1979), 144–147

S

Safer v. Estate of Pack, 291 N.J. Super 619, 677 A.2d 1188 (N.J. Super. Ct. App. Div. 1996), 447, 723

Salgo v. Leland Stanford Jr. Univ. Bd. of Trs., 317 P.2d 170 (Cal. Ct. App. 1957), 299

Schiff v. Prados, 112 Cal. Rptr. 2d 171 (Cal. Ct. App. 2001), 339

Schloendorff v. Society of N.Y. Hosp. (1914), 298

Schneider v. Rivici, 817 F.2d 987 (2d Cir. 1987), 261

Skillings v. Allen, 173 N.W. 663 (Minn. 1919), 447

Stanley, United States v., 483 U.S. 669 (1987), 46–48

Stewart v. Cleveland Clinic Found., 736 N.E.2d 491 (Ohio Ct. App. 1999), 340

Susan S. v. Israels (Cal. Ct. App. 1997), 446

Synergen, Inc., In re, 863 F. Supp. 1409 (D. Colo. 1994), 153

T

Tarasoff v. Regents of the Univ. of Cal., 551 P.2d 334 (Cal. 1976), 447

T.D. v. New York State Office of Mental Health, 650 N.Y.S.2d 173 (1996), 582, 621–627, 628

U

United States v., see party name

Urbaniak v. Newton (Cal. App. 1991), 446

V

Vodopest v. MacGregor, 913 P.2d 779 (Wash. 1996), 391

W

Washington v. Glucksberg, 521 U.S. 702 (1997), 147

Washington Legal Found. v. Friedman, 13 F. Supp. 2d 51 :(D.D.C. 1998), 156

Washington Legal Found. v. Henney, 202 F.3d 331 (D.C. Cir. 2000), 156

Welke v. Kuzilla, 375 N.W.2d 403 (Mich. Ct. App. 1985), 510

Wright v. Fred Hutchinson Cancer
    Ctr., 497

Y

Y.G. & L.G. v. Jewish Hosp. of St. Louis
    (Mo. App. 1990), 446

Z

Zalazar v. Vercimak, 515